Mosby's

Ocular Drug Consult

GANNAM

Mosby's Ocular Drug Consult

MILTON M. HOM, OD, FAAO

Private Practice

Azusa, California

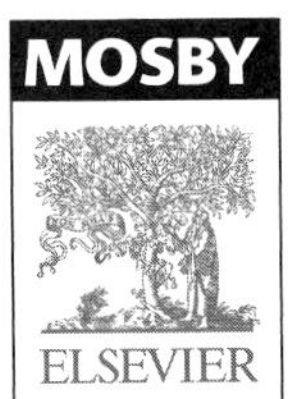

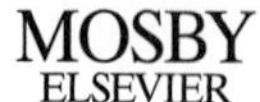

11830 Westline Industrial Drive
St. Louis, Missouri 63146

MOSBY'S OCULAR DRUG CONSULT

ISBN 13 978-0-323-02447-1
ISBN 10 0-323-02447-5

Notice

Knowledge and best practice in this field are constantly changing. As new research and experience broaden our knowledge, changes in practice, treatment, and drug therapy may become necessary or appropriate. Readers are advised to check the most current information provided (i) on procedures featured or (ii) by the manufacturer of each product to be administered, to verify the recommended dose or formula, the method and duration of administration, and contraindications. It is the responsibility of the practitioner, relying on his or her own experience and knowledge of the patient, to make diagnoses, to determine dosages and the best treatment for each individual patient, and to take all appropriate safety precautions. To the fullest extent of the law, neither the Publisher nor the Author assumes any liability for any injury and/or damage to persons or property arising out or related to any use of the material contained in this book.

ISBN 13 978-0-323-02447-1
ISBN 10 0-323-02447-5

Publishing Director: Linda Duncan
Acquisitions Editor: Kathy Falk
Senior Developmental Editor: Christie M. Hart
Publishing Services Manager: Patricia Tannian
Senior Project Manager: Anne Altepeter
Design Direction: Teresa McBryan

Printed in the United States of America

Last digit is the print number: 9 8 7 6 5 4 3 2 1

Reviewers

Diane T. Adamczyk, OD, FAAO
Associate Professor
Director of Residency Education and Externships
State University of New York State
College of Optometry
New York, New York

Steven Bratman, MD
AltmedConsult.com

Arthur B. Epstein, OD, FAAO
Senior partner, North Shore Contact Lens and Vision Consultants, PC
Roslyn Heights, New York
Director of the Contact Lens Service
North Shore University Hospital
New York University School of Medicine
New York, New York
Clinical Adjunct Assistant Professor
Northeastern State University College of Optometry
Tahlequah, Oklahoma

Nicky R. Holdeman, OD, MD
Associate Dean for Clinical Education
Executive Director, University Eye Institute
University of Houston College of Optometry
Houston, Texas

Alan G. Kabat, OD, FAAO
Associate Professor/Director of Residency Programs
Nova Southeastern University College of Optometry
Fort Lauderdale, Florida

Jennifer A. Palombi, OD
Dayton Veterans Administration Medical Center
Dayton, Ohio

SP Srinivas, PhD
Associate Professor
School of Optometry
Indiana University

To Jill, Jennifer, and Zachary Milton;
Norma Hom; and Katherine Chan

Preface

With the proliferation of new drugs in recent years, *Mosby's Ocular Drug Consult* is designed to be a portable chairside reference to aid the eye care practitioner. *Mosby's Ocular Drug Consult* was conceived in response to eye care professionals' need for an up-to-date, comprehensive drug reference for use at point of care.

Mosby's Ocular Drug Consult covers not only prescription ophthalmic drugs but also the 100 most commonly prescribed drugs. Herbal supplements that may have ocular implications and over-the-counter (OTC) artificial tears are included. The source on which most of the material is based is the renowned and authoritative *Mosby's Drug Consult.* For information not included in this book, further study of *Mosby's Drug Consult* is highly recommended.

I thank Christie M. Hart of Elsevier for asking me to write *Mosby's Ocular Drug Consult.* Every book has a period during which the author just needs to "grind it out." This book would not have been possible without Christie's constant encouragement and unwavering support during those times.

I also thank Anne Altepeter for her wonderful efforts in managing this project.

Milton M. Hom

How to Use This Book

Detailed entries provide all the information you need about the generic drugs in an A to Z format. In every drug entry, you will find:

- ***Generic name, pronunciation, and trade names.*** Each generic drug name is listed alphabetically—and spelled phonetically—for quick identification.
- ***Do not confuse with.*** This unique feature identifies generic and trade names that resemble the featured drug to help you avoid drug errors.
- ***Category and schedule.*** This section lists the drug's pregnancy risk category and, when appropriate, its controlled substance schedule or over-the-counter (OTC) status.
- ***Mechanism of action.*** Expanding on the chapter overview information, this section clearly and concisely details the drug's mechanism of action and therapeutic effects.
- ***Pharmacokinetics.*** Under this heading, a quick-reference chart outlines the drug's route, onset, peak, and duration, when known. This information is followed by a discussion of the drug's absorption, distribution, metabolism, excretion, and half-life.
- ***Availability.*** This section identifies the forms in which the drug is available (e.g., tablets, sustained-release capsules, or injectable solution). In addition, this section lists the available doses and concentrations.
- ***Indications and dosages.*** Here you will find approved indications and routes, as well as dosage information for all age groups, including adults, seniors, children, neonates, and patients with preexisting conditions such as liver or kidney disease.
- ***Unlabeled uses.*** This section brings you up to date on the unlabeled uses commonly seen in practice.
- ***Contraindications.*** In this section, conditions that prohibit use of the drug are listed.
- ***Interactions.*** This section supplies vital information about interactions between the topic drug and other drugs, herbal supplements, and food.
- ***Diagnostic test effects.*** Under this heading, you will find a brief description of the drug's effects on laboratory and diagnostic test results, such as liver enzyme levels and electrocardiogram tracings.
- ***Intravenous (IV) compatibilities and incompatibilities.*** These twin sections provide information about which IV drugs can or cannot be

given with the featured drug, whether by IV push, Y-site, or IV piggyback administration.

- ***Side effects.*** Unlike other handbooks that mix common, deadly effects with rare, minor ones in a long, undifferentiated list, this book ranks side effects by frequency of occurrence as expected, frequent, occasional, or rare. This section also includes the percentage of occurrence, when known.
- ***Serious reactions.*** Because serious reactions are life-threatening responses that require prompt intervention, this section highlights them, apart from other side effects, for easy identification.
- ***Special considerations.*** This section presents special considerations in the following categories:

  Precautions—alerts you to specific conditions or circumstances that call for caution when administering the drug.

  Patient Teaching—explains exactly what to teach your patients to help them achieve the maximum therapeutic response to drugs while minimizing possible adverse effects.

  Pregnancy and Lactation—provides the pertinent information you need to determine what is safe to prescribe for your pregnant or lactating patients.

  Ocular Considerations—provides information specific to ocular-related topics.

Most of the ophthalmic medications are topical. Reports exist of multidose droppers or containers and bacterial keratitis. Instruct patients to avoid allowing the tip of the dispensing container to contact the eye or surrounding structures. Also instruct patients that ocular solutions, if handled improperly, can become contaminated by common bacteria known to cause ocular infections. Serious damage to the eye and subsequent loss of vision may result from using contaminated solutions. Advise patients that if they develop an intercurrent ocular condition (e.g., trauma, ocular surgery, or infection), they should immediately seek their eye care practitioner's advice concerning the continued use of the multidose container in its present form.

We think you will agree that *Mosby's Ocular Drug Consult* is an indispensable tool for delivering the best possible patient care. We know you will love the way this unique, comprehensive reference book is organized to help you focus on the drugs used in your daily practice. Whether you keep this book in your laboratory coat pocket, on the drug cart, or at the nurse's station, you will surely turn to it again and again for drug information you can trust.

The following references were used in the preparation of this manuscript:

Bartlett JD, et al: *Ophthalmic drug facts 2005,* St Louis, 2005, Facts and Comparisons.

Bartlett JD, Janus SD: *Clinical ocular pharmacology,* ed 4, St Louis, 2001, Butterworth-Heinemann.

Cullom RD, Chang B: *The Wills eye manual,* ed 4, Philadelphia, 2004, JB Lippincott.

Ellsworth AJ, Witt DM, Dugdale DC, et al: *Mosby's 2005 medical drug reference,* St Louis, 2005, Mosby.

Gage TW, Pickett FA: *Mosby's dental drug reference,* ed 7, St Louis, 2005, Mosby.

Mosby's drug consult, ed 15, St Louis, 2005, Mosby.

Weisbecker CA, Fraunfelder FT, Tippermann R: *Physician's desk reference for ophthalmic medicines,* Montvale, NJ, 2002, Medical Economics.

Contents

acarbose

(a-car'bose)

Rx: Precose

Drug Class: Alpha glucosidase inhibitors; Antidiabetic agents

Pregnancy Category: B

Do not confuse Precose with PreCare.

CLINICAL PHARMACOLOGY

Mechanism of Action: An alpha glucosidase inhibitor that delays glucose absorption and digestion of carbohydrates, resulting in a smaller rise in blood glucose concentration after meals. *Therapeutic Effect:* Lowers postprandial hyperglycemia.

AVAILABLE FORMS

• *Tablets:* 25 mg, 50 mg, 100 mg.

INDICATIONS AND DOSAGES

Diabetes mellitus

PO

Adults, Elderly. Initially, 25 mg 3 times a day with first bite of each main meal. Increase at 4- to 8-wk intervals. Maximum: For patients weighing more than 60 kg, 100 mg 3 times a day; for patients weighing 60 kg or less, 50 mg 3 times a day.

CONTRAINDICATIONS: Chronic intestinal diseases associated with marked disorders of digestion or absorption, cirrhosis, colonic ulceration, conditions that may deteriorate as a result of increased gas formation in the intestine, diabetic ketoacidosis, hypersensitivity to acarbose, inflammatory bowel disease, partial intestinal obstruction or predisposition to intestinal obstruction, significant renal dysfunction (serum creatinine level greater than 2 mg/dl)

INTERACTIONS

Drug

Digestive enzymes, intestinal absorbents (such as charcoal): Reduces effects of acarbose.

Herbal

None known.

Food

None known.

DIAGNOSTIC TEST EFFECTS: May increase AST (SGOT) levels.

SIDE EFFECTS

Side effects diminish in frequency and intensity over time.

Frequent

Transient GI disturbances: flatulence (77%), diarrhea (33%), abdominal pain (21%)

SERIOUS REACTIONS

• None known.

SPECIAL CONSIDERATIONS

PRECAUTIONS

• Because acarbose given in combination with a sulfonylurea or insulin will cause a further lowering of blood glucose, it may increase the potential for hypoglycemia. When diabetic patients are exposed to stress such as fever, trauma, infection, or surgery, a temporary loss of control of blood glucose may occur. At such times, temporary insulin therapy may be necessary.

PATIENT INFORMATION

• Tell patients to take acarbose orally 3 times a day at the start (with the first bite) of each main meal. It is important that patients continue to adhere to dietary instructions, a regular exercise program, and regular testing of urine and/or blood glucose.

PREGNANCY AND LACTATION

• Pregnancy Category B. The safety of acarbose in pregnant women has not been established. A small amount of radioactivity has been found in the milk of lactating rats after administration of radiolabeled acarbose. Excretion into human milk is not known.

acetaminophen; codeine phosphate

(a-seat-a-min'-oh-fen; koe'-deen foss'-fate)

Rx: Capital with Codeine Suspension, EZ III, Tylenol with Codeine, Tylenol with Codeine #2, Tylenol with Codeine #3, Tylenol with Codeine #4

Drug Class: Analgesics, narcotic

Pregnancy Category: C

DEA Class: Schedule III; Schedule V

CLINICAL PHARMACOLOGY

Mechanism of Action: Codeine is an opioid agonist that binds at opiate receptor sites in central nervous system (CNS). Has direct action in the medulla. Acetaminophen is a peripherally acting analgesic that appears to inhibit prostaglandin synthetase centrally. *Therapeutic Effect:* Inhibits ascending pain pathways, altering perception of and response to pain, causes cough suppression.

Pharmacokinetics

Well absorbed from gastrointestinal (GI) tract. Protein binding: 20%-50%. Widely distributed to most body tissues. Metabolized in liver. Excreted in urine. **Half-life:** 1-4 hrs (half-life is increased in those with liver disease, elderly, neonates; decreased in children).

AVAILABLE FORMS

- *Capsules:* 325 mg acetaminophen and 30 mg codeine (Phenaphen with Codeine).
- *Liquid:* 120 mg acetaminophen and 12 mg codeine/5 ml (Tylenol with Codeine).
- *Suspension:* 120 mg acetaminophen and 12 mg codeine/5 ml (Capital with Codeine Suspension).
- *Tablets:* 300 mg acetaminophen and 15 mg codeine (Tylenol with Codeine #2), 300 mg acetaminophen and 30 mg codeine (Tylenol with Codeine #3), 300 mg acetaminophen and 60 mg codeine (Tylenol with Codeine #4), 650 mg acetaminophen and 30 mg codeine (EZ III).

INDICATIONS AND DOSAGES

Analgesic

PO

Adults, Elderly, Children 12 yr and older. 30 mg q4-6h based on codeine. Range: 15-60 mg.

Children less than 12 yr. 0.5-1 mg codeine/kg/dose q4-6h; 10-15 mg/kg/dose q4-6h up to a maximum of 2.6 g/24h.

Antitussive

PO

Adults, Elderly, Children 12 yr and older. 15-30 mg q4-6h based on codeine, up to a maximum of 360 mg/24h.

Dosage in renal impairment

Creatinine Clearance	*Dosage*
10-50 ml/min	75% dose
less than 10 ml/min	50% dose

CONTRAINDICATIONS: Active alcoholism, liver disease, or viral hepatitis, all of which increase the risk of hepatotoxicity, hypersensitivity to acetaminophen, codeine or any other component of the formulation.

INTERACTIONS

Drug

Alcohol, central nervous system (CNS) depressants: May increase CNS or respiratory depression, and hypotension.

MAOIs: May produce severe, fatal reaction unless dosage reduced by one quarter.

Warfarin: May increase the risk of bleeding with regular use.

Herbal

None known.

Food

None known.

DIAGNOSTIC TEST EFFECTS: May increase serum amylase and lipase levels.

SIDE EFFECTS

Frequent

Constipation, drowsiness, nausea, vomiting.

Occasional

Paradoxical excitement, confusion, pounding heartbeat, facial flushing, decreased urination, blurred vision, dizziness, dry mouth, headache, hypotension, decreased appetite, redness, burning, pain at injection site.

Rare

Hallucinations, depression, stomach pain, insomnia, hypersensitivity reaction.

SERIOUS REACTIONS

- Too frequent use may result in paralytic ileus.
- Acetaminophen toxicity is the primary serious reaction.
- Early signs and symptoms of acetaminophen toxicity include anorexia, nausea, diaphoresis, and generalized weakness within the first 12 to 24 hrs.
- Later signs of acetaminophen toxicity include vomiting, right upper quadrant tenderness, and elevated liver function tests within 48 to 72 hrs after ingestion.
- Overdosage of codeine results in cold or clammy skin, confusion, convulsions, decreased blood pressure (BP), restlessness, pinpoint pupils, bradycardia, respiratory depression, decreased level of consciousness (LOC), and severe weakness.
- Tolerance to analgesic effect and physical dependence may occur with repeated use.

SPECIAL CONSIDERATIONS

PRECAUTIONS

- Acetaminophen and codeine phosphate may elevate cerebrospinal fluid pressure with head injury. This combination may obscure the diagnosis or clinical course of patients with acute abdominal conditions. This combination is given with caution to certain patients such as the elderly or debilitated and those with severe impairment of hepatic or renal function, hypothyroidism, Addison's disease, and prostatic hypertrophy or urethral stricture.
- Codeine can produce drug dependence of the morphine type and therefore has the potential for being abused. Psychic dependence, physical dependence, and tolerance may develop upon repeated administration of this drug, and it should be prescribed and administered with the same degree of caution appropriate to the use of other oral narcotic-containing medications.

PATIENT INFORMATION

- This drug combination may impair the mental and/or physical abilities required for the performance of potentially hazardous tasks such as driving a car or operating machinery. Caution the patient who is using this drug accordingly. The patient should understand the single-dose and 24-hour dose limits and the time interval between doses.

PREGNANCY AND LACTATION

- Pregnancy Category C. Codeine: A study in rats and rabbits reported no teratogenic effect of codeine administered during the period of organogenesis. Dependence has been reported in newborns whose mothers took opiates regularly during pregnancy. Narcotic analgesics cross the placental barrier. Some studies, but not others, have reported detectable amounts of codeine in breast milk. The levels are probably not clinically significant after usual therapeutic dosage. Consider the possibility of clinically important amounts being excreted in breast milk in individuals abusing codeine.

OCULAR CONSIDERATIONS

• Acetaminophen and codeine phosphate are indicated for the relief of mild to moderately severe pain. The combination can be used for pain-related photorefractive keratectomy, radial keratotomy, and corneal abrasions. Acetaminophen and codeine phosphate tablets and capsules are a Schedule III controlled substance. Acetaminophen with codeine phosphate oral solution USP is a Schedule V controlled substance.

acetaminophen; hydrocodone bitartrate

(a-seat-a-min'-oh-fen; hye-droe-koe'-done bye-tar'-trate)

Rx: Anexsia, Anolor DH5, Bancap HC, Ceta Plus, Co-Gesic, Dolacet, Hy-Phen, Lorcet 10/650, Lorcet HD, Lorcet Plus, Lortab 10, Lortab 2.5/500, Lortab 5/500, Lortab 7.5/500, Lortab Elixir, Maxidone, Norco, Panacet, Stagesic, Stagesic-10, T-Gesic, Vanacet, Vicodin, Vicodin ES, Vicodin HP, Zydone

Drug Class: Analgesics, narcotic

Pregnancy Category: C

DEA Class: Schedule III

CLINICAL PHARMACOLOGY

Mechanism of Action: Hydrocodone blocks pain perception in the cerebral cortex by binding to specific opiate receptors (mu and kappa) neuronal membranes of synapses. This binding results in a decreased synaptic chemical transmission throughout the CNS thus inhibiting the flow of pain sensations into the higher centers and cause analgesia. Acetaminophen is a central analgesic whose exact mechanism is unknown, but appears to inhibit prostaglandin synthesis in the central nervous system (CNS) and, to a lesser extent, block pain impulses through peripheral action. Acetaminophen acts centrally on hypothalamic heat-regulating center, producing peripheral vasodilation (heat loss, skin erythema, sweating).

Therapeutic Effect: Alters perception of pain and produces analgesic effect.

Pharmacokinetics

Well absorbed from gastrointestinal (GI) tract. Protein binding: 20%-50%. Widely distributed to most body tissues. Metabolized in liver; excreted in urine. Removed by hemodialysis. **Half-life:** 3-4 hrs (half-life is increased in those with liver disease, elderly, neonates; decreased in children).

AVAILABLE FORMS

- *Capsules:* Hydrocodone bitartrate 5 mg and acetaminophen 500 mg (Anolor DH5, Bancap HC, Ceta-Plus, Dolacet, Lorcet-HD, T-Gesic, Zydone).
- *Elixir:* Hydrocodone bitartrate 7.5 mg and acetaminophen 500 mg/15 ml (Lortab Elixir).
- *Tablets:* Hydrocodone bitartrate 2.5 mg and acetaminophen 500 mg (Lortab 2.5/500), hydrocodone bitartrate 5 mg and acetaminophen 325 mg (Norco), hydrocodone bitartrate 5 mg and acetaminophen 400 mg (Zydone), hydrocodone bitartrate 5 mg and acetaminophen 500 mg (Anexsia, Co-Gesic, Hy-Phen, Lortab 5/500, Panacet, Vanacet, Vicodin), hydrocodone bitartrate 7.5 mg and acetaminophen 325 mg (Norco), hydrocodone bitartrate 7.5 mg and acetaminophen 400 mg (Zydone), hydrocodone bitartrate 7.5 mg and acetaminophen 500 mg (Lortab 7.5/500), hydrocodone bitartrate 7.5 mg and acetaminophen 650 mg (Anexsia, Lorcet Plus), hydrocodone bitartrate 7.5 mg and acetaminophen 750 mg (Vicodin ES), hydrocodone bitartrate 10 mg and acetaminophen 325 mg (Norco), hydrocodone bitartrate 10 mg and acetaminophen 400 mg (Zydone), hydrocodone bitartrate 10 mg and acetaminophen 500 mg (Lortab 10), hydrocodone bitartrate 10 mg and acetaminophen 650 mg (Lorcet 10/650), hydrocodone bitartrate 10 mg and acetaminophen 660 mg (Anexsia), hydrocodone bitartrate 10 mg and acetaminophen 750 mg (Maxidone).

INDICATIONS AND DOSAGES

Analgesia

PO

Adults, Children older than 13 yr or more than 50 kg. 2.5-10 mg q4-6h. Maximum: 60 mg/day hydrocodone. Maximum dose of acetaminophen: 4 g/day.

Elderly. 2.5-5 mg hydrocodone q4-6h. Titrate dose to appropriate analgesic effect. Maximum: 4 g/day acetaminophen.

Children 2-13 yr or less than 50 kg. 0.135 mg/kg/dose hydrocodone q4-6h. Maximum: 6 doses/day of hydrocodone or maximum recommended dose of acetaminophen.

CONTRAINDICATIONS: CNS depression, severe respiratory depression, hypersensitivity to hydrocodone, acetaminophen, or any component of the formulation.

INTERACTIONS

Drug

Alcohol, central nervous system (CNS) depressants: May increase CNS or respiratory depression, and hypotension.

CYP2D6 inhibitors (e.g., chlorpromazine): May decrease the effects of hydrocodone.

Hepatotoxic medications (e.g., phenytoin), liver enzyme inducers (e.g., cimetidine): May increase risk of hepatotoxicity associated with acetaminophen with prolonged high dose or single toxic dose.

MAOIs, tricyclic antidepressants: May increase effects of MAOIs and TCAs and hydrocodone.

Warfarin: May increase the risk of bleeding with regular use.

Herbal

Valerian, St John's wort, SAMe, kava kava: May increase risk of excessive sedation.

Food

None known.

DIAGNOSTIC TEST EFFECTS: Acetaminophen may increase serum bilirubin, prothrombin time (may indicate hepatotoxicity), SGOT (AST), and SGPT (ALT). Therapeutic serum level: 10-30 mcg/ml; toxic serum level: greater than 200 mcg/ml.

SIDE EFFECTS

Frequent

Dizziness, sedation, drowsiness, bradycardia.

Occasional

Anxiety, dysphoria, euphoria, fear, lethargy, lightheadedness, malaise, mental clouding, mental impairment, mood changes, physiological dependence, sedation, somnolence, constipation, bradycardia, heartburn, nausea, vomiting.

Rare

Hypersensitivity reaction, rash.

SERIOUS REACTIONS

- Cardiac arrest, circulatory collapse, coma, hypotension, hypoglycemic coma, ureteral spasm, urinary retention, vesical sphincter spasm, agranulocytosis, bleeding time prolonged, hemolytic anemia, iron deficiency anemia, occult blood loss, thrombocytopenia, hepatic necrosis, hepatits, skeletal muscle rigidity, renal toxicity, renal tubular necrosis have been reported.
- Hearing impairment or loss have been reported with chronic overdose.
- Acute airway obstruction, apnea, dyspnea, and respiratory depression occur rarely and are usually dose related.
- Acetaminophen toxicity is the primary serious reaction.
- Early signs and symptoms of acetaminophen toxicity include anorexia, nausea, diaphoresis, and generalized weakness within the first 12 to 24 hrs.
- Later signs of acetaminophen toxicity include vomiting, right upper quadrant tenderness, and elevated liver function tests within 48 to 72 hrs after ingestion.
- The antidote to acetaminophen toxicity is acetylcysteine.
- Tolerance to analgesic effect and physical dependence may occur with repeated use.

SPECIAL CONSIDERATIONS

PRECAUTIONS

- Use acetaminophen and hydrocodone bitartrate with caution in elderly or debilitated patients and in those with severe impairment of hepatic or renal function, hypothyroidism, Addison's disease, prostatic hypertrophy, or urethral stricture. Exercise caution when acetaminophen and hydrocodone bitartrate tablets are used postoperatively and in patients with pulmonary disease because they suppress the cough reflex.

PATIENT INFORMATION

- This drug combination may impair the mental and/or physical abilities required for the performance of potentially hazardous tasks such as driving a car or operating machinery. Caution patients accordingly. Alcohol and other central nervous system depressants may produce an additive central nervous system depression when taken with this combination product and should be avoided. Hydrocodone may be habit forming. Patients should take the drug only for as long as it is prescribed, in the amounts prescribed, and no more frequently than prescribed.

PREGNANCY AND LACTATION

- Pregnancy Category C. Hydrocodone has been shown to be teratogenic in hamsters.
- Babies born to mothers who have been taking opioids regularly before delivery will be physically dependent. Acetaminophen is excreted in breast milk in small amounts, but the significance of its effects on nursing infants is not known. Whether hydrocodone is excreted in human milk is not known.

OCULAR CONSIDERATIONS

- This drug combination is indicated for the relief of moderate to moderately severe pain and pain from photorefractive keratectomy radial keratotomy, and corneal abrasions.

OCULAR DOSAGE

- Photorefractive keratectomy, radial keratotomy, and corneal abrasions: Use 400 mg/5 mg or 400 mg/7.5 mg, 1 to 2 tablets q4-6 hrs.

acetaminophen; propoxyphene napsylate

(a-seat-a-min'-oh-fen; proe-pox'-i-feen nap'-si-late)

Rx: Darvocet A500, Darvocet N 100, Darvocet N 50, Propacet 100

Drug Class: Analgesics, narcotic

Pregnancy Category: C

DEA Class: Schedule IV

CLINICAL PHARMACOLOGY

Mechanism of Action: Propoxyphene is an opioid agonist that binds with opioid receptors within the central nervous system (CNS). Acetaminophen is a central analgesic whose exact mechanism is unknown, but appears to inhibit prostaglandin synthesis in the central nervous system (CNS) and, to a lesser extent, block pain impulses through peripheral action. It acts centrally on hypothalamic heat-regulating center, producing peripheral vasodilation (heat loss, skin erythema, sweating). *Therapeutic Effect:* Alters processes affecting pain perception, emotional response to pain. Produces analgesic effect.

Pharmacokinetics

Well absorbed from the gastrointestinal (GI) tract. Widely distributed. Metabolized in liver. Primarily excreted in urine. Not removed by hemodialysis. **Half-life:** 6-12 hrs; metabolite: 30-36 hrs.

AVAILABLE FORMS

- *Tablets:* 50 mg propoxyphene napsylate and 325 mg acetaminophen (Darvocet N 50), 100 mg propoxyphene napsylate and 500 mg acetaminophen (Darvocet A500), 100 mg propoxyphene napsylate and 650 mg acetaminophen (Darvocet N 100, Propacet 100).

INDICATIONS AND DOSAGES

Relief of mild to moderate pain

PO

Adults, Elderly. 1-2 tablets q4h as needed. Maximum: 600 mg propoxyphene napsylate/day. Dosage of acetaminophen should not exceed 4 g/day (6 tablets of Darvocet-N 100).

CONTRAINDICATIONS: Active alcoholism, liver disease, or viral hepatitis, all of which increase the risk of hepatotoxicity, hypersensitivity to propoxyphene napsylate, acetaminophen, or any other component of the formulation.

INTERACTIONS

Drug

Alcohol, CNS depressants: May increase CNS or respiratory depression and risk of hypotension.

Buprenorphine: Effects may be decreased with buprenorphine.

Carbamazepine: May increase the blood concentration and risk of toxicity of carbamazepine.

Hepatotoxic medications (e.g., phenytoin), liver enzyme inducers (e.g., cimetidine): May increase risk of hepatotoxicity with prolonged high dose or single toxic dose.

MAOIs: May produce severe, fatal reaction; plan to reduce to one quarter usual dose.

Warfarin: May increase the risk of bleeding with regular use.

Herbal

None known.

Food

None known.

DIAGNOSTIC TEST EFFECTS: Propoxyphene napsylate

May increase serum alkaline phosphatase, amylase, bilirubin, LDH, lipase, SGOT (AST), and SGPT (ALT) levels. Therapeutic blood serum level is 100-400 ng/ml; toxic blood serum level is greater than 500 ng/ml.

Acetaminophen

May increase serum bilirubin, prothrombin time (may indicate hepatotoxicity), SGOT (AST), and SGPT (ALT). Therapeutic serum level: 10-30 mcg/ml; toxic serum level: greater than 200 mcg/ml.

SIDE EFFECTS

Frequent

Dizziness, drowsiness, dry mouth, euphoria, hypotension, nausea, vomiting, unusual tiredness.

Occasional

Histamine reaction, including decreased blood pressure (BP), increased sweating, flushing, and wheezing, trembling, decreased urination, altered vision, constipation, headache.

Rare

Confusion, increased BP, depression, stomach cramps, anorexia, hypersensitivity reaction.

SERIOUS REACTIONS

- Overdosage results in respiratory depression, skeletal muscle flaccidity, cold or clammy skin, cyanosis, extreme somnolence progressing to convulsions, stupor, and coma.
- Liver toxicity may occur with overdosage of acetaminophen component of fixed-combination.
- Acetaminophen toxicity is the primary serious reaction.
- Early signs and symptoms of acetaminophen toxicity include anorexia, nausea, diaphoresis, and generalized weakness within the first 12 to 24 hrs.
- Later signs of acetaminophen toxicity include vomiting, right upper quadrant tenderness, and elevated liver function tests within 48 to 72 hrs after ingestion.
- Tolerance to propoxyphene's analgesic effect and physical dependence may occur with repeated use.

SPECIAL CONSIDERATIONS

PRECAUTIONS

- Do not prescribe propoxyphene for patients who are suicidal or addiction-prone. Prescribe propoxyphene with caution for patients taking tranquilizers or antidepressant drugs and patients who use alcohol in excess. Tell patients not to exceed the recommended dose and to limit their intake of alcohol. Propoxyphene products in excessive doses, alone or combined with other central nervous system depressants, including alcohol, are a major cause of drug-related deaths. Administer propoxyphene with caution to patients with hepatic or renal impairment because higher serum concentrations or delayed elimination may occur.

PREGNANCY AND LACTATION

• Pregnancy Category C. Safe use in pregnancy has not been established relative to possible adverse effects on fetal development. Low levels of propoxyphene have been detected in human milk.

---

acetazolamide

(a-seat-a-zole'a-mide)

Rx: Diamox, Diamox Sequels

Drug Class: Carbonic anhydrase inhibitors

Pregnancy Category: C

Do not confuse with acetohexamide.

CLINICAL PHARMACOLOGY

Mechanism of Action: A carbonic anhydrase inhibitor that reduces formation of hydrogen and bicarbonate ions from carbon dioxide and water by inhibiting, in proximal renal tubule, the enzyme carbonic anhydrase, thereby promoting renal excretion of sodium, potassium, bicarbonate, water. Ocular: Reduces rate of aqueous humor formation, lowers intraocular pressure. *Therapeutic Effect:* Produces anticonvulsant activity.

Pharmacokinetics

Rapidly absorbed. Protein binding: 95%. Widely distributed throughout body tisses including erythrocytes, kidneys, and blood brain barrier. Not metabolized. Excreted unchanged in urine. Removed by hemodialysis. **Half-life:** 2.4-5.8 hrs.

AVAILABLE FORMS

• *Capsules, sustained release:* 500 mg (Diamox Sequels).

• *Powder for reconstitution:* 500 mg.

• *Tablets:* 125 mg, 250 mg (Diamox).

INDICATIONS AND DOSAGES

Glaucoma

PO

Adults. 250 mg 1-4 times/day. Extended-Release: 500 mg 1-2 times/day usually given in morning and evening.

Secondary glaucoma, preop treatment of acute congestive glaucoma

PO/IV

Adults. 250 mg q4h, 250 mg q12h; or 500 mg, then 125-250 mg q4h.

PO

Children. 10-15 mg/kg/day in divided doses.

IV

Children. 5-10 mg/kg q6h.

Edema

IV

Adults. 25-375 mg once daily.

Children. 5 mg/kg or 150 mg/m^2 once daily.

Epilepsy

Oral

Adults, Children. 375-1000 mg/day in 1-4 divided doses.

Acute mountain sickness

PO

Adults. 500-1000 mg/day in divided doses. If possible, begin 24-48 hrs before ascent; continue at least 48 hrs at high altitude.

Usual elderly dosage

PO

Initially, 250 mg 2 times/day; use lowest effective dose.

Dosage in renal impairment

Creatinine Clearance	*Dosage Interval*
10- 50 ml/min	q12h
less than 10 ml/min	avoid use

UNLABELED USES: Urine alkalinization, respiratory stimulant in COPD

CONTRAINDICATIONS: Severe renal disease, adrenal insufficiency, hypochloremic acidosis, hypersensitivity to acetazolamide, to any component of the formulation, or to sulfonamides.

INTERACTIONS

Drug

Amphetamines: May increase effects and toxicity of amphetamines

Cyclosporine: May increase cyclosporine trough concentrations and possible neprotoxicity and neurotoxicity.

Digoxin: May increase the risk of digoxin toxicity caused by hypokalemia.

Lithium: May increase lithium excretion and decrease serum levels.

Methenamine: May decrease effects of methenamine.

Phenytoin: May increase serum concentrations of phenytoin.

Primidone: May decrease serum concentrations of primidone.

Quinidine: May decrease urinary excretion of quinidine and increase effects.

Salicylates: May increase risk of acetazolamide accumulation and toxicity including CNS depression and metabolic acidosis.

Herbal

None known.

Food

None known.

DIAGNOSTIC TEST EFFECTS: May increase ammonia, bilirubin, glucose, chloride, uric acid, calcium. May decrease bicarbonate, potassium.

IV INCOMPATIBILITIES: No drug incompatibilities reported.

IV COMPATIBILITIES: Cimetidine (Tagament), procaine, ranitidine (Zantac)

SIDE EFFECTS

Frequent

Unusually tired/weak, diarrhea, increased urination/frequency, decreased appetite/weight, altered taste (metallic), nausea, vomiting, numbness in extremities, lips, mouth

Occasional

Depression, drowsiness

Rare

Headache, photosensitivity, confusion, tinnitus, severe muscle weakness, loss of taste

SERIOUS REACTIONS

- Long-term therapy may result in acidotic state.
- Nephrotoxicity / hepatotoxicity occurs occasionally, manifested as dark urine/stools, pain in lower back, jaundice, dysuria, crystalluria, renal colic/calculi.
- Bone marrow depression may be manifested as aplastic anemia, thrombocytopenia, thrombocytopenic purpura, leukopenia, agranulocytosis, hemolytic anemia.

SPECIAL CONSIDERATIONS

PRECAUTIONS

- Increasing the dose does not increase the diuresis and may increase the incidence of drowsiness and/or paresthesia. Increasing the dose often results in a decrease in diuresis. Under certain circumstances, however, very large doses have been given with other diuretics to secure diuresis in complete refractory failure.

PATIENT INFORMATION

- Adverse reactions common to all sulfonamide derivatives may occur: anaphylaxis, fever, rash (including erythema multiforme, Stevens-Johnson syndrome, and toxic epidermal necrolysis), crystalluria, renal calculus, bone marrow depression, thrombocytopenic purpura, hemolytic anemia, leukopenia, pancytopenia, and agranulocytosis. Precaution is advised for early detection of such reactions, and the drug should be discontinued and appropriate therapy instituted.

- In patients with pulmonary obstruction or emphysema in whom alveolar ventilation may be impaired, use acetazolamide (which may precipitate or aggravate acidosis) with caution.
- Gradual ascent is desirable to try to avoid acute mountain sickness. If rapid ascent is undertaken and acetazolamide is used, such use does not obviate the need for prompt descent if severe forms of high-altitude sickness occur, that is, high-altitude pulmonary edema or high-altitude cerebral edema.
- Advise receiving concomitant high-dose aspirin and acetazolamide to be cautious because anorexia, tachypnea, lethargy, coma, and death have been reported.

PREGNANCY AND LACTATION

- Pregnancy Category C. Acetazolamide, administered orally or parenterally, has been shown to be teratogenic (defects of the limbs) in mice, rats, hamsters, and rabbits. No adequate and well-controlled studies have been performed in pregnant women. Excretion into human milk is not known.

OCULAR DOSAGE AND ADMINISTRATION

- Glaucoma: Acetazolamide should be used as an adjunct to the usual therapy. The dosage used in the treatment of chronic simple (open-angle) glaucoma ranges from 250 mg to 1 g of acetazolamide per 24 hours, usually in divided doses for amounts over 250 mg. A dosage in excess of 1 g per 24 hours usually has been found not to produce an increased effect.
- In all cases, adjust the dosage with careful individual attention to symptomatology and ocular tension. Continuous supervision by a physician is advisable.
- In treatment of secondary glaucoma and in the preoperative treatment of some cases of acute congestive (closed-angle) glaucoma, the preferred dosage is 250 mg every 4 hours, although some patients have responded to 250 mg twice daily on short-term therapy. In some acute cases, it may be more satisfactory to administer an initial dose of 500 mg followed by 125 mg every 4 hours depending on the individual case.
- Intravenous therapy may be used for rapid relief to ocular tension in acute cases. A complementary effect has been noted when acetazolamide has been used with miotics or mydriatics as the case demanded.

acetohexamide

(a-seat-oh-hex′-a-mide)

Drug Class: Antidiabetic agents; Sulfonylureas, first generation

Pregnancy Category: C

Do not confuse with acetazolamide.

CLINICAL PHARMACOLOGY

Mechanism of Action: An intermediate acting sulfonylurea that promotes the release of insulin from beta cells of pancreas, increases insulin sensitivity at peripheral sites. *Therapeutic Effect:* Lowers blood glucose concentration.

Pharmacokinetics

Well absorbed from the gastrointestinal (GI) tract. Protein binding: 65%-90%. Metabolized in liver. Excreted in urine. Not removed by hemodialysis. **Half-life:** 1.3 hrs.

AVAILABLE FORMS

- *Tablets:* 250 mg, 500 mg (Dymelor).

INDICATIONS AND DOSAGES

Diabetes mellitus

PO

Adults, Elderly. Initially, 250 mg/day. Adjust dosage in 250- to 500-mg increments at intervals of 5-7 days. Maximum daily dose: 1.5 g. Elderly patients may be more sensitive and should be started at a lower dosage initially.

CONTRAINDICATIONS: Diabetic ketoacidosis with or without coma, Type 1 diabetes mellitus, hypersensitivity to acetohexamide or any component of the formulation

INTERACTIONS

Drug

Acarbose, clofibrate, fluoroquinolones, NSAIDs, thioctic acid: May increase risk of hypoglycemia.

Beta-blockers: May increase the hypoglycemic effect and mask signs of hypoglycemia.

Cotrimoxazole, MAOIs, sulfadiazine, sulfamethoxazole, sulfisoxazole: May increase the effects of acetohexamide.

Herbal

Bitter melon, eucalyptus, fenugreek, ginseng, guar gum, gymnema extracts, psyllium, St. John's wort: May increase risk of hypoglycemia.

Glucosamine, licorice: May decrease acetohexamide effectiveness.

Food

None known.

DIAGNOSTIC TEST EFFECTS: *None known.*

SIDE EFFECTS

Frequent

Altered taste sensation, dizziness, drowsiness, weight gain, constipation, diarrhea, heartburn, nausea, vomiting, stomach fullness, headache.

Occasional

Increased sensitivity of skin to sunlight, peeling of skin, itching, rash.

SERIOUS REACTIONS

- Hypoglycemia may occur because of overdosage or insufficient food intake, especially with increased glucose demands.
- GI hemorrhage, cholestatic hepatic jaundice, leukopenia, thrombocytopenia, pancytopenia, agranulocytosis, aplastic or hemolytic anemia occurs rarely.

SPECIAL CONSIDERATIONS

PRECAUTIONS

- Acetohexamide administration is associated with increased cardiovascular mortality compared with treatment with diet alone or diet plus insulin. All sulfonylurea drugs are capable of producing severe hypoglycemia. Renal or hepatic insufficiency may cause elevated blood levels of acetohexamide, and the latter also may diminish gluconeogenic capacity, both of which increase the risk of serious hypoglycemic reactions. Elderly, debilitated, or malnourished patients and those with adrenal or pituitary insufficiency are particularly susceptible to the hypoglycemic action of glucose-lowering drugs. When a patient stabilized on any diabetic regimen is exposed to stress, such as fever, trauma, infection, or surgery, a loss of control may occur. At such times, it may be necessary to discontinue acetohexamide and administer insulin.

PREGNANCY AND LACTATION

• Pregnancy Category C. Acetohexamide has been shown to be teratogenic in animals. Excretion into human milk is not known.

acetylcholine chloride

(a-se-teel-koe'-leen)

Rx: Miochol-E, Miochol-E/Steri-Tags, Miochol-E System Pak

Drug Class: Cholinergics; Miotics; Ophthalmics

Pregnancy Category: C

CLINICAL PHARMACOLOGY

Mechanism of Action: A cholinergic agonist that causes contraction of the sphincter muscles of the iris. *Therapeutic Effect:* Results in miosis and contraction of ciliary muscle, leading to accommodation spasm.

Pharmacokinetics

Rapid miosis of short duration.

AVAILABLE FORMS

• *Powder for reconstitution (intraocular):* 1% (Miochol-E, Miochol-E/Steri-Tags, Miochol-E System Pak).

INDICATIONS AND DOSAGES

Production of miosis

Intraocular

Adults, Elderly. 0.5-2 ml instilled into anterior chamber before or after securing one or more sutures.

CONTRAINDICATIONS: Acute iritis and acute inflammatory disease of the anterior chamber, hypersensitivity to acetylcholine chloride or any component of the formulation

INTERACTIONS

Drug

Flurbiprofen, suprofen (ophthalmic): May decrease the effects of acetylcholine.

Tacrine: May increase or prolong the effects of acetylcholine.

Thioridazine: May increase risk of cardiotoxicity.

Herbal

None known.

Food

None known.

DIAGNOSTIC TEST EFFECTS: *None known.*

SIDE EFFECTS

Rare

Corneal clouding, corneal decompensation

SERIOUS REACTIONS

• Systemic effects rarely occur. These effects include bradycardia, hypotension, flushing, breathing difficulties, and sweating.

SPECIAL CONSIDERATIONS

PRECAUTIONS

• Anterior or posterior synechiae may occur. In cataract surgery, use acetylcholine only after delivery of the lens. NOTE: Do not use solution that is not clear and colorless.

PREGNANCY AND LACTATION

• Pregnancy Category C. Fetal harm is not known with topical administration. Excretion into human milk is not known.

OCULAR CONSIDERATIONS

• Indications: Complete miosis of the iris in seconds after delivery of the lens in cataract surgery, in penetrating keratoplasty, iridectomy, and other anterior segment surgery.

• Reactions: Ocular—infrequent cases of corneal edema, corneal clouding, and corneal decompensation.

• Administration: Instill with a needle into the anterior chamber before or after securing sutures.

acetylcysteine

(a-see-til-sis'tay-een)

Rx: Acetadote, Acys-5, Mucomyst-10, Mucomyst-20

Drug Class: Antidotes; Mucolytics

Pregnancy Category: B

Do not confuse acetylcysteine with acetylcholine.

CLINICAL PHARMACOLOGY

Mechanism of Action: An intratracheal respiratory inhalant that splits the linkage of mucoproteins, reducing the viscosity of pulmonary secretions. *Therapeutic Effect:* Facilitates the removal of pulmonary secretions by coughing, postural drainage, mechanical means. Protects against acetaminophen overdose–induced hepatotoxicity.

AVAILABLE FORMS

• *Injection (Acedote):* 20% (200 mg/ml).

• *Inhalation Solution (Mucomyst):* 10% (100 mg/ml), 20% (200 mg/ml).

INDICATIONS AND DOSAGES

Adjunctive treatment of viscid mucus secretions from chronic bronchopulmonary disease and for pulmonary complications of cystic fibrosis

Nebulization

Adults, Elderly, Children. 3-5 ml (20% solution) 3-4 times a day or 6-10 ml (10% solution) 3-4 times a day. Range: 1-10 ml (20% solution) q2-6h or 2-20 ml (10% solution) q2-6h.

Infants. 1-2 ml (20%) or 2-4 ml (10%) 3-4 times a day.

Treatment of viscid mucus secretions in patients with a tracheostomy

Intratracheal

Adults, Children. 1-2 ml of 10% or 20% solution instilled into tracheostomy q1-4h.

Acetaminophen overdose

PO (Oral solution 5%)

Adults, Elderly, Children. Loading dose of 140 mg/kg, followed in 4 hr by maintenance dose of 70 mg/kg q4h for 17 additional doses (unless acetaminophen assay reveals nontoxic level).

IV

Adults, Elderly, Children. 150 mg/kg infused over 15 minutes, then 50 mg/kg infused over 4 hr, then 100 mg/kg infused over 16 hr. See administration and handling. Repeat dose if emesis occurs within 1 hr of administration. Continue until all doses are given, even if acetaminophen plasma level drops below toxic range.

Prevention of renal damage from dyes used during certain diagnostic tests

PO (Oral solution 5%)

Adults, Elderly. 600 mg twice a day for 4 doses starting the day before the procedure.

UNLABELED USES: Prevention of renal damage from dyes given during certain diagnostic tests (such as CT scans)

CONTRAINDICATIONS: None known.

INTERACTIONS

Drug

None known.

Herbal

None known.

Food

None known.

DIAGNOSTIC TEST EFFECTS: *None known.*

SIDE EFFECTS

Frequent

Inhalation: Stickiness on face, transient unpleasant odor

Occasional

Inhalation: Increased bronchial secretions, throat irritation, nausea, vomiting, rhinorrhea

Rare

Inhalation: Rash

Oral: Facial edema, bronchospasm, wheezing

SERIOUS REACTIONS

• Large doses may produce severe nausea and vomiting.

SPECIAL CONSIDERATIONS

PRECAUTIONS

• With the administration of acetylcysteine the patient initially may notice a slight disagreeable odor that soon is not noticeable. With a face mask there may be a stickiness on the face after nebulization, which is removed easily by washing with water.

• Under certain conditions, a color change may take place in the solution of acetylcysteine in the opened bottle. The light purple color is the result of a chemical reaction that does not significantly impair the safety or mucolytic effectiveness of acetylcysteine.

PREGNANCY AND LACTATION

• Pregnancy Category B. Reproduction studies of acetylcysteine with isoproterenol have been performed in rats and of acetylcysteine alone in rabbits at doses up to 2.6 times the human dose. These studies have revealed no evidence of impaired fertility or harm to the fetus from acetylcysteine. Excretion into human milk is not known.

OCULAR CONSIDERATIONS

• Off-label uses include the dissolving of mucus filaments and decrease in tear viscosity for vernal, giant papillary conjunctivitis, and filamentary keratitis. Mucomyst needs to be diluted to 2% to 5% for ocular use.

• For moderate to severe chemical burns with corneal melting: 10% to 20% Mucomyst q4h may be used.

acitretin

(a-si-tre′tin)

Rx: Soriatane

Drug Class: Antipsoriatics; Dermatologics; Retinoids

Pregnancy Category: X

CLINICAL PHARMACOLOGY

Mechanism of Action: A second-generation retinoid that adjusts factors influencing epidermal proliferation, RNA/DNA synthesis, controls glycoprotein, and governs immune response. *Therapeutic Effect:* Regulates keratinocyte growth and differentiation.

Pharmacokinetics

Well absorbed from the gastrointestinal (GI) tract. Food increases rate of absorption. Protein binding: greater than 99%. Metabolized in liver. Excreted in bile and urine. Not removed by hemodialysis. **Half-life:** 49 hrs.

AVAILABLE FORMS

• *Capsules:* 10 mg, 25 mg (Soriatane).

INDICATIONS AND DOSAGES

Psoriasis

PO

Adults, Elderly. 25-50 mg/day as a single dose with main meal. May increase to 75 mg/day if necessary and dose tolerated. Maintenance: 25-50 mg/day after the initial response is noted. Continue until lesions have resolved.

UNLABELED USES: Treatment of Darier's disease, palmoplantar pustulosis, lichen planus; children with lameliar ichthyosis, nonbullous and bullous ichthyosiform erythroderma, Sjögren-Larsson syndrome

CONTRAINDICATIONS: Pregnancy or those who intend to become pregnant within 3 years following discontinuation of therapy, severely impaired liver or kidney function, chronic abnormal elevated lipid levels, concomitant use of methotrexate or tetracyclines, ingestion of alcohol (in females of reproductive potential), hypersensitivity to acitretin, etretinate or other retinoids, sensitivity to parabenz (used as preservative in gelatin capsule)

INTERACTIONS

Drug

Alcohol: May prevent elimination of acitretin.

"Minipill" oral contraceptive: May interfere with contraceptive effect.

Methotrexate: May increase risk of hepatotoxicity.

Tetracyclines: May increase risk of increased intracranial pressure.

Herbal

St. John's wort: May increase risk of unplanned pregnancy and birth defects.

Vitamin A: May increase risk of vitamin A toxicity.

Food

None known.

DIAGNOSTIC TEST EFFECTS: May increase triglucerides, SGOT (AST), SGPT (ALT). May decrease LDH (high density lipoprotein).

SIDE EFFECTS

Frequent

Lip inflammation, alopecia, skin peeling, shakiness, dry eyes, rash, hyperesthesia, paresthesia, sticky skin, dry mouth, epistaxis, dryness/thickening of conjunctiva

Occasional

Eye irritation, brow and lash loss, sweating, chills, sensation of cold, flushing, edema, blurred vision, diarrhea, nausea, thirst

SERIOUS REACTIONS

- Benign intracranial hypertension (pseudotumor cerebri) occurs rarely.

SPECIAL CONSIDERATIONS

PRECAUTIONS

- The eyes and vision of 329 patients treated with acitretin were examined. The findings included dry eyes (23%), irritation of eyes (9%), and brow and lash loss (5%). The following were reported in less than 5% of patients: Bell's palsy, blepharitis and/or crusting of lids, blurred vision, conjunctivitis, corneal epithelial abnormality, cortical cataract, decreased night vision, diplopia, itchy eyes or eyelids, nuclear cataract, pannus, papilledema, photophobia, posterior subcapsular cataract, recurrent sties, and subepithelial corneal lesions.
- Adverse reactions reported are as follows: 10% to 25%, xerophthalmia; 1% to 10%, abnormal/blurred vision, blepharitis, conjunctivitis/irritation, corneal epithelial abnormality, decreased night vision/night blindness, eye abnormality, eye pain, and photophobia; less than 1%, abnormal lacrimation, chalazion, conjunctival hemorrhage, corneal ulceration, diplopia, ectropion, itchy eyes and lids, papilledema, recurrent sties, subepithelial corneal lesions.

PATIENT INFORMATION

- Any patient treated with acitretin who is experiencing visual difficulties should discontinue the drug and undergo an eye examination.

• Decreased night vision has been reported with acitretin therapy. Advise patients of this potential problem and warn them to be cautious when driving or operating any vehicle at night. Monitor visual problems carefully. Advise patients that they may experience decreased tolerance to contact lenses during the treatment period and sometimes after treatment has stopped.

PREGNANCY AND LACTATION

• Pregnancy Category X. Acitretin can cause severe birth defects. Female patients must not be pregnant when acitretin therapy is initiated, and they must not become pregnant while taking acitretin and for at least 3 years after stopping acitretin so that the drug can be eliminated to below a blood concentration that would be associated with an increased incidence of birth defects. Because this threshold has not been established for acitretin in human beings and because elimination rates vary among patients, the duration of posttherapy contraception to achieve adequate elimination cannot be calculated precisely.

• Also advise females of reproductive potential that they must not ingest beverages or products containing ethanol while taking acitretin and for 2 months after acitretin treatment has been discontinued. This allows for elimination of the acitretin that can be converted to etretinate in the presence of alcohol.

• Advise female patients that any method of birth control can fail, including tubal ligation, and that microdosed progestin "minipill" preparations are not recommended for use with acitretin. Data from one patient who received a very low-dosed progestin contraceptive (levonorgestrel 0.03 mg) indicate that she had a significant increase of the progesterone level after three menstrual cycles during acitretin treatment.

• Female patients should sign a consent form before beginning acitretin therapy.

• Studies on lactating rats have shown that etretinate is excreted in the milk. One prospective case report indicates that acitretin is excreted in human milk. Therefore nursing mothers should not receive acitretin before or during nursing because of the potential for serious adverse reactions in nursing infants.

---

acyclovir

(ay-sye'kloe-ver)

Rx: Zovirax, Zovirax Topical

Drug Class: Antivirals

Pregnancy Category: C; B

Do not confuse with Zostrix, Zyvox.

CLINICAL PHARMACOLOGY

Mechanism of Action: A synthetic nucleoside that converts to acyclovir triphosphate, becoming part of the DNA chain. *Therapeutic Effect:* Interferes with DNA synthesis and viral replication. Virustatic.

Pharmacokinetics

Poorly absorbed from the GI tract; minimal absorption following topical application. Protein binding: 9%-36%. Widely distributed. Partially metabolized in liver. Excreted primarily in urine. Removed by hemodialysis. **Half-life:** 2.5 hr (increased in impaired renal function).

AVAILABLE FORMS

- *Capsules:* 200 mg.
- *Tablets:* 400 mg, 800 mg.
- *Injection, solution:* 50 mg/ml.
- *Oral Suspension:* 200 mg/5 ml.

• *Powder for Injection:* 500 mg, 1000 mg.
• *Ointment:* 5%/50 mg.

INDICATIONS AND DOSAGES

Genital herpes (initial episode)

IV

Adults, Elderly, Children 12 yr and older. 5 mg/kg q8h for 5 days.

PO

Adults, Elderly, Children 12 yr and older. 200 mg q4h 5 times a day.

Genital herpes (recurrent)

Less than 6 episodes per year:

PO

Adults, Elderly, Children 12 yr and older. 200 mg q4h 5 times a day for 5 days.

6 episodes or more per year:

PO

Adults, Elderly, Children 12 yr and older. 400 mg 2 times a day or 200 mg 3-5 times a day for up to 12 months.

Herpes simplex mucocutaneous

IV

Adults, Elderly, Children 12 yr and older. 5 mg/kg/dose q8h for 7 days.

Children younger than 12 yr. 10 mg/kg q8h for 7 days.

Herpes simplex neonatal

IV

Children younger than 4 mo. 10 mg/kg q8h for 10 days.

Herpes simplex encephalitis

IV

Adults, Elderly, Children 12 yr and older. 10 mg/kg q8h for 10 days.

Children 3 mos to younger than 12 yr. 20 mg/kg q8h for 10 days.

Herpes zoster (caused by varicella)

IV

Adults, Elderly, Children 12 yr and older. 10 mg/kg q8h for 7 days.

Children younger than 12 yr. 20 mg/kg q8h for 7 days.

Herpes zoster (shingles)

PO

Adults, Elderly, Children 12 yr and older. 800 mg q4h 5 times a day for 7-10 days.

Topical

Adults, Elderly. Apply to affected area 3-6 times a day for 7 days.

Varicella (chickenpox)

PO

Adults, Elderly, Children older than 12 yr or children 2-12 yr, weighing 40 kg or more. 800 mg 4 times a day for 5 days.

Children 2-12 yr, weighing less than 40 kg. 20 mg/kg 4 times a day for 5 days. Maximum: 800 mg/dose.

Children younger than 2 yr. 80 mg/kg/day.

Dosage in renal impairment

Dosage and frequency are modified based on severity of infection and degree of renal impairment.

PO

For creatinine clearance of 10 ml/min or less, dosage is 200 mg q12h.

IV

Creatinine Clearance	*Dosage Percent*	*Dosage Interval*
greater than 50 ml/min	100	8 hr
25-50 ml/min	100	12 hr
10-25 ml/min	100	24 hr
less than 10 ml/min	50	24 hr

UNLABELED USES: Treatment of herpes simplex ocular infections, infectious mononucleosis

CONTRAINDICATIONS: Use in neonates when acyclovir is reconstituted with bacteriostatic water containing benzyl alcohol.

INTERACTIONS

Drug

Nephrotoxic medications (such as aminoglycosides): May increase the nephrotoxicity of acyclovir.

Probenecid: May increase acyclovir half-life.

Herbal

None known.

Food

None known.

DIAGNOSTIC TEST EFFECTS: May increase BUN and serum creatinine concentrations.

IV INCOMPATIBILITIES: Aztreonam (Azactam), cefepime (Maxipime), diltiazem (Cardizem), dobutamine (Dobutrex), dopamine (Intropin), levofloxacin (Levaquin), meropenem (Merrem IV), ondansetron (Zofran), piperacillin and tazobactam (Zosyn)

IV COMPATIBILITIES: Allopurinol (Alloprim), amikacin (Amikin), ampicillin, cefazolin (Ancef), cefotaxime (Claforan), ceftazidime (Fortaz), ceftriaxone (Rocephin), cimetidine (Tagamet), clindamycin (Cleocin), famotidine (Pepcid), fluconazole (Diflucan), gentamicin, heparin, hydromorphone (Dilaudid), imipenem (Primaxin), lorazepam (Ativan), magnesium sulfate, methylprednisolone (SoluMedrol), metoclopramide (Reglan), metronidazole (Flagyl), morphine, multivitamins, potassium chloride, propofol (Diprivan), ranitidine (Zantac), vancomycin

SIDE EFFECTS

Frequent

Parenteral (9%-7%): Phlebitis or inflammation at IV site, nausea, vomiting

Topical (28%): Burning, stinging

Occasional

Parenteral (3%): Pruritus, rash, urticaria

Oral (12%-6%): Malaise, nausea

Topical (4%): Pruritus

Rare

Oral (3%-1%): Vomiting, rash, diarrhea, headache

Parenteral (2%-1%): Confusion, hallucinations, seizures, tremors

Topical (less than 1%): Rash

SERIOUS REACTIONS

- Rapid parenteral administration, excessively high doses, or fluid and electrolyte imbalance may produce renal failure exhibited by such signs and symptoms as abdominal pain, decreased urination, decreased appetite, increased thirst, nausea, and vomiting.
- Toxicity has not been reported with oral or topical use.

SPECIAL CONSIDERATIONS

PRECAUTIONS

- Dosage adjustment is recommended when administering acyclovir to patients with renal impairment. Also exercise caution when administering acyclovir to patients receiving potentially nephrotoxic agents because this may increase the risk of renal dysfunction and the risk of reversible central nervous system symptoms such as those that have been reported in patients treated with acyclovir intravenously.

PATIENT INFORMATION

- Instruct patients to consult with their physician if they experience severe or troublesome adverse reactions, they become pregnant or intend to become pregnant, they intend to breast-feed while taking orally administered acyclovir, or they have any other questions.
- Herpes Zoster: No data exist on treatment initiated more than 72 hours after onset of the zoster rash. Advise patients to initiate treatment as soon as possible after a diagnosis of herpes zoster.

• Genital Herpes Infections: Inform patients that acyclovir is not a cure for genital herpes. No data exist evaluating whether acyclovir will prevent transmission of infection to others. Because genital herpes is a sexually transmitted disease, patients should avoid contact with lesions or intercourse when lesions and/or symptoms are present to avoid infecting partners. Genital herpes also can be transmitted in the absence of symptoms through asymptomatic viral shedding. If medical management of a genital herpes recurrence is indicated, advise patients to initiate therapy at the first sign or symptom of an episode.
• Chickenpox: Chickenpox in otherwise healthy children is usually a self-limited disease of mild to moderate severity. Adolescents and adults tend to have more severe disease. Treatment was initiated within 24 hours of the typical chickenpox rash in the controlled studies, and there is no information regarding the effects of treatment begun later in the disease course.

PREGNANCY AND LACTATION

• Pregnancy Category B. No adequate and well-controlled studies have been performed in pregnant women. A prospective epidemiologic registry of acyclovir use during pregnancy was established in 1984 and completed in April 1999. The study followed 756 pregnancies in women exposed to systemically effective acyclovir during the first trimester of pregnancy. The occurrence rate of birth defects approximates that found in the general population.
• However, the small size of the registry is insufficient to evaluate the risk for less common defects or to permit reliable and definitive conclusions regarding the safety of acyclovir in pregnant women and their developing fetuses. Acyclovir concentrations have been documented in breast milk in two women following oral administration of acyclovir.

OCULAR CONSIDERATIONS

• Herpes simplex virus epithelial keratitis: Use 2g/day for 10 days.
• Herpex simplex virus keratouveitis: Use 200-400 mg 5 times/day.

albuterol

(al-byoo'ter-ole)

Rx: Accuneb, Proventil, Proventil HFA, Proventil Repetabs, Ventolin, Ventolin HFA, Ventolin Rotacaps, Volmax, Vospire

Drug Class: Adrenergic agonists; Bronchodilators

Pregnancy Category: C

Do not confuse albuterol with Albutein or atenolol, or Proventil with Prinivil.

CLINICAL PHARMACOLOGY

Mechanism of Action: A sympathomimetic that stimulates beta$_2$-adrenergic receptors in the lungs, resulting in relaxation of bronchial smooth muscle. *Therapeutic Effect:* Relieves bronchospasm and reduces airway resistance.

Pharmacokinetics

Route	Onset	Peak	Duration
PO	15-30 min	2-3 hr	4-6 hr
PO (extended-release)	30 min	2-4 hr	12 hr
Inhalation	5-15 min	0.5-2 hr	2-5 hr

Rapidly, well absorbed from the GI tract; gradually absorbed from the bronchi after inhalation. Metabolized in the liver. Primarily excreted in urine. **Half-life:** 2.7-5 hr (PO); 3.8 hr (inhalation).

AVAILABLE FORMS

- *Syrup:* 2 mg/5ml.
- *Tablet:* 2 mg, 4 mg.
- *Tablet (Extended-Release [Proventil Repetabs]):* 4 mg.
- *Tablets (Extended-Release [Volmax, VoSpire ER]):* 4 mg, 8 mg.
- *Inhalation (Aerosol [Proventil, Ventolin]):* 90 mcg/spray.
- *Inhalation (Solution [AccuNeb]):* 0.75 mg/3 ml, 1.5 mg/3 ml.
- *Inhalation (Solution [Proventil]):* 0.083%, 0.5%.

INDICATIONS AND DOSAGES

Bronchospasm

PO

Adults, Children older than 12 yr. 2-4 mg 3-4 times a day. Maximum: 8 mg 4 times/day.

Elderly. 2 mg 3-4 times a day. Maximum: 8 mg 4 times a day.

Children 6-12 yr. 2 mg 3-4 times a day. Maximum: 24 mg/day.

PO (Extended-Release)

Adults, Children older than 12 yr. 4-8 mg q12h.

Inhalation

Adults, Elderly, Children older than 12 yr. 1-2 puffs by metered dose inhaler q4-6h as needed.

Children 4-12 yr. 1-2 puffs 4 times a day.

Nebulization

Adults, Elderly, Children older than 12 yr. 2.5 mg 3-4 times a day.

Children 2-12 yr. 0.63-1.25 mg 3-4 times a day.

Exercise-induced bronchospasm

Inhalation

Adults, Elderly, Children 4 yr and older. 2 puffs 15-30 min before exercise.

CONTRAINDICATIONS: History of hypersensitivity to sympathomimetics

INTERACTIONS

Drug

Beta-blockers: Antagonize effects of albuterol.

Digoxin: May increase the risk of arrhythmias.

MAOIs, tricyclic antidepressants: May potentiate cardiovascular effects.

Herbal

None known.

Food

None known.

DIAGNOSTIC TEST EFFECTS: May increase blood glucose level. May decrease serum potassium level.

SIDE EFFECTS

Frequent

Headache (27%); nausea (15%); restlessness, nervousness, tremors (20%); dizziness (less than 7%); throat dryness and irritation, pharyngitis (less than 6%); BP changes, including hypertension (5%-3%); heartburn, transient wheezing (less than 5%)

Occasional (3%-2%)

Insomnia, asthenia, altered taste

Inhalation: Dry, irritated mouth or throat; cough; bronchial irritation

Rare

Somnolence, diarrhea, dry mouth, flushing, diaphoresis, anorexia

SERIOUS REACTIONS

- Excessive sympathomimetic stimulation may produce palpitations, extrasystole, tachycardia, chest pain, a slight increase in BP followed by a substantial decrease, chills, diaphoresis, and blanching of skin.
- Too-frequent or excessive use may lead to decreased bronchodilating effectiveness and severe, paradoxical bronchoconstriction.

SPECIAL CONSIDERATIONS

PRECAUTIONS

- Use albuterol with caution in patients with cardiovascular disorders, especially coronary insufficiency, cardiac arrhythmias, hypertension, convulsive disorders, hyperthyroidism, or diabetes mellitus and in patients who are unusually responsive to sympathomimetic amines. Clinically significant changes in systolic and diastolic blood pressure have been seen. Albuterol may produce significant hypokalemia.

PATIENT INFORMATION

- The action of Ventolin inhalation aerosol may last up to 6 hours or longer. Ventolin inhalation aerosol should not be used more frequently than recommended. Instruct patients not to increase the dose or frequency of Ventolin inhalation aerosol without consulting their physician. Instruct patients that if they find that treatment with Ventolin inhalation aerosol becomes less effective for symptomatic relief, their symptoms become worse, and/or they need to use the product more frequently than usual, they should seek medical attention immediately. While using Ventolin inhalation aerosol, patients should take other inhaled drugs and asthma medications only as directed by their physician. Common adverse effects include palpitations, chest pain, rapid heart rate, and tremor or nervousness. Pregnant or nursing patients should contact their physician about use of Ventolin inhalation aerosol. Effective and safe use of Ventolin inhalation aerosol includes an understanding of the way that it should be administered.
- In general, the technique for administering Ventolin inhalation aerosol to children is similar to that for adults because children's smaller ventilatory exchange capacity automatically provides proportionally smaller aerosol intake. Children should use Ventolin inhalation aerosol under adult supervision, as instructed by the patient's physician.

PREGNANCY AND LACTATION

- Pregnancy Category C. Albuterol sulfate has been shown to be teratogenic in mice. Fetal harm is not known. Excretion into human milk is not known.

alendronate sodium

(a-len'dro-nate)

Rx: Fosamax

Drug Class: Bisphosphonates

Pregnancy Category: C

Do not confuse Fosamax with Flomax.

CLINICAL PHARMACOLOGY

Mechanism of Action: A bisphosphonate that inhibits normal and abnormal bone resorption, without retarding mineralization. *Therapeutic Effect:* Leads to significantly increased bone mineral density; reverses the progression of osteoporosis.

Pharmacokinetics

Poorly absorbed after oral administration. Protein binding: 78%. After oral administration, rapidly taken into bone, with uptake greatest at sites of active bone turnover. Excreted in urine. **Terminal half-life:** Greater than 10 yr (reflects release from skeleton as bone is resorbed).

AVAILABLE FORMS

- *Tablets:* 5 mg, 10 mg, 35 mg, 40 mg, 70 mg.
- *Oral Solution:* 70 mg/75 ml.

INDICATIONS AND DOSAGES

Osteoporosis (in men)

PO

Adults, Elderly. 10 mg once a day in the morning.

Glucocorticoid-induced osteoporosis
PO
Adults, Elderly. 5 mg once a day in the morning.
Postmenopausal women not receiving estrogen. 10 mg once a day in the morning.

Postmenopausal osteoporosis
PO (treatment)
Adults, Elderly. 10 mg once a day in the morning or 70 mg weekly.
PO (prevention)
Adults, Elderly. 5 mg once a day in the morning or 35 mg weekly.

Paget's disease
PO
Adults, Elderly. 40 mg once a day in the morning.

UNLABELED USES: Treatment of breast cancer

CONTRAINDICATIONS: GI disease, including dysphagia, frequent heartburn, gastrointestinal reflux disease, hiatal hernia, and ulcers, inability to stand or sit upright for at least 30 minutes; renal impairment; sensitivity to alendronate

INTERACTIONS

Drug
Aspirin: May increase GI disturbances.
IV ranitidine: May double the bioavailability of alendronate.

Herbal
None known.

Food
Beverages other than plain water, dietary supplements, food: May interfere with absorption of alendronate.

DIAGNOSTIC TEST EFFECTS: Reduces serum calcium and serum phosphate concentrations. Significantly decreases serum alkaline phosphatase level in patients with Paget's disease.

SIDE EFFECTS
Frequent (8%-7%)
Back pain, abdominal pain
Occasional (3%-2%)
Nausea, abdominal distention, constipation, diarrhea, flatulence
Rare (less than 2%)
Rash

SERIOUS REACTIONS
- Overdose causes hypocalcemia, hypophosphatemia, and significant GI disturbances.
- Esophageal irritation occurs if alendronate is not given with 6-8 ounces of plain water or if the patient lies down within 30 minutes of drug administration.

SPECIAL CONSIDERATIONS

PRECAUTIONS
- Alendronate sodium may cause local irritation of the upper gastrointestinal mucosa. Esophageal adverse experiences such as esophagitis, esophageal ulcers, and esophageal erosions have been reported. There have been postmarketing reports of gastric and duodenal ulcers, some severe and with complications. Consider causes of osteoporosis other than estrogen deficiency, aging, and glucocorticoid use. Hypocalcemia must be corrected before initiation of therapy with alendronate sodium. Ensuring adequate calcium and vitamin D intake is especially important in patients with Paget's disease of bone and in patients receiving glucocorticoids. Alendronate sodium is not recommended for patients with renal insufficiency. Treatment of glucocorticoid-induced osteoporosis has been shown in patients with a median bone mineral density that was 1.2 SD below the mean for healthy young adults.

PATIENT INFORMATION

• Physicians should instruct their patients to read the patient package insert before starting therapy with alendronate sodium and to reread it each time the prescription is renewed.

• Instruct patients to take supplemental calcium and vitamin D if daily dietary intake is inadequate. Weight-bearing exercise should be considered along with the modification of certain behavioral factors, such as cigarette smoking and excessive alcohol consumption, if these factors exist.

• Dosing Instructions: Instruct patients that the expected benefits of alendronate sodium may be obtained only when each tablet is swallowed with plain water the first thing upon arising for the day and at least 30 minutes before the first food, beverage, or medication of the day. Even dosing with orange juice or coffee has been shown to reduce the absorption of alendronate sodium greatly. To facilitate delivery to the stomach and thus reduce the potential for esophageal irritation, instruct patients to swallow alendronate sodium with a full glass of water (6 to 8 oz) and not to lie down for at least 30 minutes and until after their first food of the day. Patients should not chew or suck on the tablet because of a potential for oropharyngeal ulceration. Specifically instruct patients not to take alendronate sodium at bedtime or before arising for the day. Patients should be informed that failure to follow these instructions may increase their risk of esophageal problems. Instruct patients that if they develop symptoms of esophageal disease (such as difficulty or pain on swallowing, retrosternal pain, or new or worsening heartburn), they should stop taking alendronate sodium and consult their physician. Instruct patients that if they miss a dose of once weekly alendronate sodium, they should take 1 tablet on the morning after they remember. They should not take 2 tablets on the same day but should return to taking 1 tablet once a week, as originally scheduled on their chosen day.

PREGNANCY AND LACTATION

• Pregnancy Category C. Reproduction studies in rats showed decreased postimplantation survival and decreased body weight gain in normal pups. Fetal harm is not known. Excretion into human milk is not known.

---

alprazolam

(al-pray'zoe-lam)

Rx: Xanax, Xanax XR

Drug Class: Anxiolytics; Benzodiazepines; Sedatives/hypnotics

Pregnancy Category: D

DEA Class: Schedule IV

Do not confuse alprazolam with lorazepam, or Xanax with Tenex or Zantac.

CLINICAL PHARMACOLOGY

Mechanism of Action: A benzodiazepine that enhances the action of the inhibitory neurotransmitter gamma-aminobutyric acid in the brain. *Therapeutic Effect*: Produces anxiolytic effect from its CNS depressant action.

Pharmacokinetics

Well absorbed from GI tract. Protein binding: 80%. Metabolized in the liver. Primarily excreted in urine. Minimal removal by hemodialysis. **Half-life:** 11-16 hr.

AVAILABLE FORMS

- *Oral Solution:* 1 mg/ml.
- *Tablets:* 0.25 mg (Xanax), 0.5 mg (Xanax), 1 mg (Xanax), 2 mg (Xanax).
- *Tablets (Extended-Release):* 0.5 mg (Xanax XR), 1 mg (Xanax XR), 2 mg (Xanax XR), 3 mg (Xanax XR).

INDICATIONS AND DOSAGES

Anxiety disorders

PO

Adults (immediate release). Initially, 0.25-0.5 mg 3 times a day. May titrate q3-4 days. Maximum: 4 mg/day in divided doses.

Elderly, Debilitated patients, Patients with hepatic disease or low serum albumin. Initially, 0.25 mg 2-3 times a day. Gradually increase to optimum therapeutic response.

Panic disorder

PO, immediate release

Adults. Initially, 0.5 mg 3 times a day. May increase at 3- to 4-day intervals. Range: 5-6 mg/day. Maximum: 10 mg/day.

PO, extended release

Adults. Initially, 0.5-1 mg once a day. May titrate at 3- to 4-day intervals. Range: 3-6 mg/day. Maximum: 10 mg/day.

Elderly. Initially, 0.125-0.25 mg 2 times a day; may increase in 0.125-mg increments until desired effect attained.

Premenstrual syndrome

PO

Adults. 0.25 mg 3 times a day.

UNLABELED USES: Management of premenstrual syndrome symptoms (mood disturbances, insomnia, and cramps), irritable bowel syndrome

CONTRAINDICATIONS: Acute alcohol intoxication with depressed vital signs, acute angle-closure glaucoma, concurrent use of itraconazole or ketoconazole, myasthenia gravis, severe COPD

INTERACTIONS

Drug

Alcohol, other CNS depressants: Potentiate effects of alprazolam and may increase sedation.

Fluvoxamine, itraconazole, ketoconazole, nefazodone: May inhibit metabolism and increase serum concentrations of alprazolam.

Herbal

Kava kava, valerian: May increase CNS depressant effect of alprazolam.

Food

Grapefruit, grapefruit juice: May inhibit alprazolam's metabolism.

DIAGNOSTIC TEST EFFECTS: *None known.*

SIDE EFFECTS

Frequent

Ataxia); lightheadedness; transient, mild somnolence; slurred speech (particularly in elderly or debilitated patients)

Occasional

Confusion, depression, blurred vision, constipation, diarrhea, dry mouth, headache, nausea

Rare

Behavioral problems such as anger, impaired memory, paradoxical reactions such as insomnia, nervousness, or irritability

SERIOUS REACTIONS

- Abrupt or too-rapid withdrawal may result in pronounced restlessness, irritability, insomnia, hand tremors, abdominal and muscle cramps, diaphoresis, vomiting, and seizures.
- Overdose results in somnolence, confusion, diminished reflexes, and coma.
- Blood dyscrasias have been reported rarely.

SPECIAL CONSIDERATIONS

PRECAUTIONS

• Caution patients against engaging in hazardous occupations or activities that require complete mental alertness, such as operating machinery or driving a motor vehicle. For the same reason, caution patients about the simultaneous ingestion of alcohol and other central nervous system depressants during treatment with alprazolam. Episodes of hypomania and mania and suicidal tendencies have been reported.

PATIENT INFORMATION

• To ensure safe and effective use of benzodiazepines, provide all patients prescribed alprazolam with the following guidance. In addition, advise panic disorder patients, for whom doses greater than 4 mg/day typically are prescribed, about the risks associated with the use of higher doses.

• Patients should inform their physician about any alcohol consumption and medicine they are taking now, including medication they may buy without a prescription. Generally, the patient should not use alcohol during treatment with benzodiazepines.

• Alprazolam is not recommended for use in pregnancy. Therefore patients should inform their physician if they are pregnant, if they are planning to have a child, or if they become pregnant while taking this medication.

• Patients should inform their physician if they are nursing.

• Until patients experience how this medication affects them, they should not drive a car or operate potentially dangerous machinery.

• Patients should not increase the dose even if they think the medication "does not work anymore" without consulting their physician. Benzodiazepines, even when used as recommended, may produce emotional and/or physical dependence.

• Patients should not stop taking this medication abruptly or decrease the dose without consulting their physician because withdrawal symptoms can occur.

PREGNANCY AND LACTATION

• Pregnancy Category D. Consider that the child born of a mother who is receiving benzodiazepines may be at some risk for withdrawal symptoms from the drug during the postnatal period. Neonatal flaccidity and respiratory problems have been reported in children born of mothers who have been receiving benzodiazepines. Benzodiazepines are known to be excreted in human milk.

OCULAR CONSIDERATIONS

• Alprazolam may be used in patients with open-angle glaucoma who are receiving appropriate therapy, but it is contraindicated in patients with acute narrow-angle glaucoma.

• When rats were treated with alprazolam at 3, 10, and 30 mg/kg per day (15 to 150 times the maximum recommended human dose) orally for 2 years, a tendency for a dose-related increase in the number of cataracts was observed in females, and a tendency for a dose-related increase in corneal vascularization was observed in males. These lesions did not appear until after 11 months of treatment.

aminocaproic acid

(a-mee-noe-ka-proe'ik)

Rx: Amicar

Drug Class: Hemostatics

Pregnancy Category: C

Do not confuse Amicar with amikacin or Amikin.

CLINICAL PHARMACOLOGY

Mechanism of Action: A systemic hemostatic that acts as an antifibrinolytic and antihemorrhagic by inhibiting the activation of plasminogen activator substances. *Therapeutic Effect:* Prevents formation of fibrin clots.

AVAILABLE FORMS

- *Syrup:* 250 mg/ml.
- *Tablets*: 500 mg.
- *Injection:* 250 mg/ml.

INDICATIONS AND DOSAGES

Acute bleeding

PO, IV Infusion

Adults, Elderly. 4-5 g over first hr; then 1-1.25 g/hr. Continue for 8 hr or until bleeding is controlled. Maximum: 30 g/24 hr.

Children. 3 g/m^2 over first hr; then 1 g/m^2/hr. Maximum: 18 g/m^2/24 hr.

Dosage in renal impairment

Decrease dose to 25% of normal.

UNLABELED USES: Prevention of recurrence of subarachnoid hemorrhage, prevention of hemorrhage in hemophiliacs following dental surgery

CONTRAINDICATIONS: Evidence of active intravascular clotting process, disseminated intravascular coagulation without concurrent heparin therapy, hematuria of upper urinary tract origin (unless benefit outweighs risk); newborns (parenteral form).

INTERACTIONS

Drug

None known.

Herbal

None known.

Food

None known.

DIAGNOSTIC TEST EFFECTS: May elevate serum potassium level.

IV INCOMPATIBILITIES: Sodium lactate

SIDE EFFECTS

Occasional

Nausea, diarrhea, cramps, decreased urination, decreased BP, dizziness, headache, muscle fatigue and weakness, myopathy, bloodshot eyes

SERIOUS REACTIONS

- Too rapid IV administration produces tinnitus, rash, arrhythmias, unusual fatigue, and weakness.
- Rarely, a grand mal seizure occurs, generally preceded by weakness, dizziness, and headache.

SPECIAL CONSIDERATIONS

PRECAUTIONS

- Aminocaproic acid contains benzyl alcohol as a preservative and is not recommended for use in newborns. The drug inhibits the action of plasminogen activators and, to a lesser degree, plasmin activity. Avoid rapid intravenous administration of the drug because this may induce hypotension, bradycardia, and arrhythmia. Inhibition of fibrinolysis by aminocaproic acid theoretically may result in clotting or thrombosis. Reports have appeared in the literature of an increased incidence of certain neurologic deficits such as hydrocephalus, cerebral ischemia, or cerebral vasospasm associated with the use of antifibrinolytic agents in the treatment of subarachnoid hemorrhage. Guard against thrombophlebitis, a possibility with all intravenous therapy, by strict attention to the proper insertion of the needle and the fixing of its position.

Epsilon-amniocaproic acid should not be administered with factor IX complex concentrates or antiinhibitor coagulant concentrates because the risk of thrombosis may be increased.

PREGNANCY AND LACTATION

• Pregnancy Category C. Whether aminocaproic acid can cause fetal harm when administered to a pregnant woman or can affect reproduction capacity is not known. Excretion into human milk is not known.

amiodarone hydrochloride

(a-mee'oh-da-rone)

Rx: Cordarone, Cordarone I.V., Pacerone

Drug Class: Antiarrhythmics, class III

Pregnancy Category: D

Do not confuse amiodarone with amiloride or Cordarone with Cardura.

CLINICAL PHARMACOLOGY

Mechanism of Action: A cardiac agent that prolongs duration of myocardial cell action potential and refractory period by acting directly on all cardiac tissue. Decreases AV and sinus node function. *Therapeutic Effect:* Suppresses arrhythmias.

Pharmacokinetics

Route	*Onset*	*Peak*	*Duration*
PO	3 days - 3 wk	1 wk - 5 mo	7-50 days after discontinuation

Slowly, variably absorbed from GI tract. Protein binding: 96%. Extensively metabolized in the liver to active metabolite. Excreted via bile; not removed by hemodialysis. **Half-life:** 26-107 days; metabolite, 61 days.

AVAILABLE FORMS

• *Tablets (Cordarone):* 200 mg.

• *Tablets (Pacerone):* 100 mg, 200 mg, 400 mg.

• *Injection (Cordarone):* 50 mg/ml.

INDICATIONS AND DOSAGES

Life-threatening recurrent ventricular fibrillation or hemodynamically unstable ventricular tachycardia

PO

Adults, Elderly. Initially, 800-1,600 mg/day in 2-4 divided doses for 1-3 wk. After arrhythmia is controlled or side effects occur, reduce to 600-800 mg/day for about 4 wk. Maintenance: 200-600 mg/day.

Children. Initially, 10-15 mg/kg/day for 4-14 days, then 5 mg/kg/day for several wk. Maintenance: 2.5 mg/kg or lowest effective maintenance dose for 5 of 7 days/wk.

IV Infusion

Adults. Initially, 1050 mg over 24 hr; 150 mg over 10 min, then 360 mg over 6 hr; then 540 mg over 18 hr. May continue at 0.5 mg/min for up to 2-3 wk regardless of age or renal or left ventricular function.

UNLABELED USES: Treatment and prevention of supraventricular arrhythmias and symptomatic atrial flutter refractory to conventional treatment

CONTRAINDICATIONS: Bradycardia-induced syncope (except in the presence of a pacemaker), second- and third-degree AV block, severe hepatic disease, severe sinus-node dysfunction

INTERACTIONS

Drug

Antiarrhythmics: May increase cardiac effects.

Beta-blockers, oral anticoagulants: May increase effect of beta-blockers and oral anticoagulants.

Digoxin, phenytoin: May increase drug concentration and risk of toxicity of digoxin and phenytoin.

Herbal

None known.

Food

None known.

DIAGNOSTIC TEST EFFECTS: May increase antinuclear antibody titers and AST (SGOT), ALT (SGPT), and serum alkaline phosphatase levels. May cause changes in EKG and thyroid function test results. Therapeutic serum level is 0.5-2.5 mcg/ml; toxic serum level has not been established.

IV INCOMPATIBILITIES: Aminophylline (theophylline), cefazolin (Ancef), heparin, sodium bicarbonate

IV COMPATIBILITIES: Dobutamine (Dobutrex), dopamine (Intropin), furosemide (Lasix), insulin (regular), labetalol (Normodyne), lidocaine, midazolam (Versed), morphine, nitroglycerin, norepinephrine (Levophed), phenylephrine (Neo-Synephrine), potassium chloride, vancomycin

SIDE EFFECTS

Expected

Corneal microdeposits are noted in almost all patients treated for more than 6 months (can lead to blurry vision).

Frequent (greater than 3%)

Parenteral: Hypotension, nausea, fever, bradycardia.

Oral: Constipation, headache, decreased appetite, nausea, vomiting, paresthesias, photosensitivity, muscular incoordination.

Occasional (less than 3%)

Oral: Bitter or metallic taste; decreased libido; dizziness; facial flushing; blue-gray coloring of skin (face, arms, and neck); blurred vision; bradycardia; asymptomatic corneal deposits.

Rare (less than 1%)

Oral: Rash, vision loss, blindness.

SERIOUS REACTIONS

- Serious, potentially fatal pulmonary toxicity (alveolitis, pulmonary fibrosis, pneumonitis, acute respiratory distress syndrome) may begin with progressive dyspnea and cough with crackles, decreased breath sounds, pleurisy, CHF or hepatotoxicity.
- Amiodarone may worsen existing arrhythmias or produce new arrhythmias (called proarrhythmias).

SPECIAL CONSIDERATIONS

PRECAUTIONS

- Cases of optic neuropathy and optic neuritis and corneal microdeposits have been reported.
- Photosensitivity, peripheral neuropathy, hypothyroidism, hyperthyroidism, adult respiratory distress syndrome, and elevations in liver enzymes (serum glutamic-oxaloacetic transaminase and serum glutamic-pyruvic transaminase) can occur. Correct potassium or magnesium deficiency before instituting amiodarone hydrochloride therapy.

PREGNANCY AND LACTATION

- Pregnancy Category D. In addition to causing infrequent congenital goiter/hypothyroidism and hyperthyroidism, amiodarone has caused a variety of adverse effects in animals. Whether the use of amiodarone hydrochloride during labor or delivery has any immediate or delayed adverse effects is not known. Amiodarone hydrochloride is excreted in human milk, suggesting that breast-feeding could expose the nursing infant to a significant dose of the drug.

OCULAR CONSIDERATIONS

- Cases of optic neuropathy and optic neuritis, usually resulting in visual impairment, have been reported in patients treated with amiodarone. In some cases, visual impairment has progressed to permanent blindness. Optic neuropathy and optic neuritis may occur at any time following initiation of therapy. A causal relationship to the drug has not been clearly established. If symptoms of visual impairment appear, such as changes in visual acuity and decreases in peripheral vision, prompt eye examination is recommended. Appearance of optic neuropathy and/or neuritis calls for reevaluation of amiodarone hydrochloride therapy. The risks and complications of antiarrhythmic therapy with amiodarone hydrochloride must be weighed against its benefits in patients whose lives are threatened by cardiac arrhythmias. Regular eye examination, including fundoscopy and slit-lamp examination, is recommended during administration of amiodarone hydrochloride.

• Corneal microdeposits appear in the majority of adults treated with amiodarone hydrochloride. The microdeposits are usually discernible only by slit-lamp examination but give rise to symptoms such as visual halos or blurred vision in as many as 10% of patients. Corneal microdeposits are reversible upon reduction of dose or termination of treatment. Asymptomatic microdeposits are not a reason to reduce dose or discontinue treatment.

amitriptyline hydrochloride

(a-mee-trip'ti-leen)

Rx: Elavil, Vanatrip

Drug Class: Antidepressants, tricyclic

Pregnancy Category: C

Do not confuse amitriptyline with aminophylline or nortriptyline, or Elavil with Equanil or Mellaril.

CLINICAL PHARMACOLOGY

Mechanism of Action: A tricyclic antidepressant that blocks the reuptake of neurotransmitters, including norepinephrine and serotonin, at presynaptic membranes, thus increasing their availability at postsynaptic receptor sites. Also has strong anticholinergic activity. *Therapeutic Effect:* Relieves depression.

Pharmacokinetics

Rapidly and well absorbed from the GI tract. Protein binding: 90%. Undergoes first-pass metabolism in the liver. Primarily excreted in urine. Minimal removal by hemodialysis. **Half-life:** 10-26 hr.

AVAILABLE FORMS

- *Tablets:* 10 mg, 25 mg, 50 mg, 75 mg, 100 mg, 150 mg.
- *Injection:* 10 mg/ml.

INDICATIONS AND DOSAGES

Depression

PO

Adults. 30-100 mg/day as a single dose at bedtime or in divided doses. May gradually increase up to 300 mg/day. Titrate to lowest effective dosage.

Elderly. Initially, 10-25 mg at bedtime. May increase by 10-25 mg at weekly intervals. Range: 25-150 mg/day.

Children 6-12 yr. 1-5 mg/kg/day in 2 divided doses.

IM

Adults. 20-30 mg 4 times a day.

Pain management

PO

Adults, Elderly. 25-100 mg at bedtime.

UNLABELED USES: Relief of neuropathic pain, such as that experienced by patients with diabetic neuropathy or postherpetic neuralgia; treatment of bulimia nervosa

CONTRAINDICATIONS: Acute recovery period after MI, use within 14 days of MAOIs

INTERACTIONS

Drug

Antithyroid agents: May increase the risk of agranulocytosis.

Cimetidine, valproic acid: May increase amitriptyline blood concentration and risk of toxicity.

Clonidine, guanadrel: May decrease the effects of these drugs.

CNS depressants (including alcohol, anticonvulsants, barbiturates, phenothiazines, and sedative-hypnotics): May increase CNS and respiratory depression and the hypotensive effects of amitriptyline.

MAOIs: May increase the risk of neuroleptic malignant syndrome, seizures, hypertensive crisis, and hyperpyresis.

Phenothiazines: May increase the sedative and anticholinergic effects of amitriptyline.

Sympathomimetics: May increase the risk of cardiac effects.

Herbal

None known.

Food

None known.

DIAGNOSTIC TEST EFFECTS: May alter blood glucose levels and EKG readings. Therapeutic serum drug level is 120-250 ng/ml; toxic serum drug level is greater than 500 ng/ml.

SIDE EFFECTS

Frequent

Dizziness, somnolence, dry mouth, orthostatic hypotension, headache, increased appetite, weight gain, nausea, unusual fatigue, unpleasant taste

Occasional

Blurred vision, confusion, constipation, hallucinations, delayed micturition, eye pain, arrhythmias, fine muscle tremors, parkinsonian syndrome, anxiety, diarrhea, diaphoresis, heartburn, insomnia

Rare

Hypersensitivity, alopecia, tinnitus, breast enlargement, photosensitivity

SERIOUS REACTIONS

• Overdose may produce confusion, seizures, severe somnolence, arrhythmias, fever, hallucinations, agitation, dyspnea, vomiting, and unusual fatigue or weakness.

• Abrupt discontinuation after prolonged therapy may produce headache, malaise, nausea, vomiting, and vivid dreams.

• Blood dyscrasias and cholestatic jaundice occur rarely.

SPECIAL CONSIDERATIONS

PRECAUTIONS

• Schizophrenic patients may develop increased symptoms of psychosis; patients with paranoid symptomatology may have an exaggeration of such symptoms. Depressed patients, particularly those with known manic-depressive illness, may experience a shift to mania or hypomania. The possibility of suicide in depressed patients remains until significant remission occurs. Potentially suicidal patients should not have access to large quantities of this drug. Concurrent administration of amitriptyline hydrochloride and electroshock therapy may increase the hazards associated with such therapy. When possible, the drug should be discontinued several days before elective surgery. Elevation and lowering of blood sugar levels have been reported. Use amitriptyline hydrochloride with caution in patients with impaired liver function.

PATIENT INFORMATION

• For patients receiving amitriptyline hydrochloride therapy, advise them of the possible impairment of mental and/or physical abilities required for performance of hazardous tasks such as operating machinery or driving a motor vehicle.

PREGNANCY AND LACTATION

• Pregnancy Category C. Studies in literature have shown amitriptyline to be teratogenic in mice and hamsters. Amitriptyline has been shown to cross the placenta. Amitriptyline is excreted into breast milk.

OCULAR CONSIDERATIONS

• Cycloplegia can occur.

amlodipine

(am-low'di-peen)

Rx: Norvasc

Drug Class: Calcium channel blockers

Pregnancy Category: C

Do not confuse amlodipine with amiloride, or Norvasc with Navane or Vascor.

CLINICAL PHARMACOLOGY

Mechanism of Action: A calcium channel blocker that inhibits calcium movement across cardiac and vascular smooth-muscle cell membranes. *Therapeutic Effect:* Relieves angina by dilating coronary arteries, peripheral arteries, and arterioles. Decreases total peripheral vascular resistance and BP by vasodilation.

Pharmacokinetics

Route	*Onset*	*Peak*	*Duration*
PO	0.5-1 hr	6-12 hr	24 hr

Slowly absorbed from the GI tract. Protein binding: 93%. Undergoes first-pass metabolism in the liver. Excreted primarily in urine. Not removed by hemodialysis. **Half-life:** 30-50 hr (increased in the elderly and those with liver cirrhosis).

AVAILABLE FORMS

• *Tablets:* 2.5 mg, 5 mg, 10 mg.

INDICATIONS AND DOSAGES

Hypertension

PO

Adults. Initially, 5 mg/day as a single dose. Maximum: 10 mg/day.

Small-Frame, Fragile, Elderly. Initially, 2.5 mg/day as a single dose.

Angina (chronic stable or vasospastic)

PO

Adults. 5-10 mg/day as a single dose.

Elderly, Patients with hepatic insufficiency: 5 mg/day as a single dose.

Dosage in renal impairment

For adults and elderly patients, give 2.5 mg/day.

CONTRAINDICATIONS: Severe hypotension

INTERACTIONS

Drug

None known.

Herbal

None known.

Food

Grapefruit, grapefruit juice: May increase amlodipine blood concentration and hypotensive effects.

DIAGNOSTIC TEST EFFECTS: *None known.*

SIDE EFFECTS

Frequent (greater than 5%)

Peripheral edema, headache, flushing

Occasional (less than 5%)

Dizziness, palpitations, nausea, unusual fatigue or weakness (asthenia)

Rare (less than 1%)

Chest pain, bradycardia, orthostatic hypotension

SERIOUS REACTIONS

• Overdose may produce excessive peripheral vasodilation and marked hypotension with reflex tachycardia.

SPECIAL CONSIDERATIONS

PRECAUTIONS

• Exercise caution when administering amlodipine besylate as with any other peripheral vasodilator, particularly in patients with severe aortic stenosis. Use the drug with caution in patients with heart failure. Amlodipine besylate is not a beta-blocker and therefore gives no protection against the dangers of abrupt beta-blocker withdrawal.

• Exercise caution when administering amlodipine besylate to patients with severe hepatic impairment.

PREGNANCY AND LACTATION

• Pregnancy Category C. Fetal harm is not known. Excretion into human milk is not known.

amoxicillin

(a-mox'i-sill-in)

Rx: Amoxicot, Amoxil, Amoxil Pediatric Drops, Biomox, Dispermox, Moxilin, Trimox, Wymox

Drug Class: Antibiotics, penicillins

Pregnancy Category: B

Do not confuse amoxicillin with amoxapine or DisperMox with Diamox or Trimox with Tylox.

CLINICAL PHARMACOLOGY

Mechanism of Action: A penicillin that inhibits bacterial cell wall synthesis. *Therapeutic Effect:* Bactericidal in susceptible microorganisms.

Pharmacokinetics

Well absorbed from the GI tract. Protein binding: 20%. Partially metabolized in the liver. Primarily excreted in urine. Removed by hemodialysis. **Half-life:** 1-1.3 hr (increased in impaired renal function).

AVAILABLE FORMS

• *Capsules (Amoxil, Moxillin, Trimox):* 250 mg, 500 mg.

• *Oral drops (Amoxil):* 125 mg/5 ml, 200 mg/5 ml, 250 mg/5 ml, 400 mg/5 ml.

• *Tablets (Amoxil):* 500 mg, 875 mg.

• *Tablets (Chewable [Amoxil]):* 200 mg, 250 mg, 400 mg.

• *Tablets for Oral Suspension (DisperMox):* 200 mg, 400 mg.

INDICATIONS AND DOSAGES

Ear, nose, throat, GU, skin, and skin-structure infections

PO

Adults, Elderly, Children weighing more than 20 kg. 250-500 mg q8h or 500-875 mg (tablets) twice a day

Children weighing less than 20 kg. 20-40 mg/kg/day in divided doses q8-12h.

Lower respiratory tract infections

PO

Adults, Elderly, Children weighing more than 20 kg. 500 mg q8h or 875 mg (tablets) twice a day.

Children weighing less than 20 kg. 40 mg/kg/day in divided doses q8-12h.

Acute, uncomplicated gonorrhea

PO

Adults. 3 g one time with 1 g probenecid. Follow with tetracycline or erythromycin therapy.

Children 2 yr and older. 50 mg/kg plus probenecid 25 mg/kg as a single dose.

Acute otitis media

PO

Children. 80-90 mg/kg/day in divided doses q12h.

Helicobacter pylori infection

PO

Adults, Elderly. 1 g twice a day for 10 days (in combination with other antibiotics).

Prevention of endocarditis

PO

Adults, Elderly. 2 g 1 hr before procedure.

Children. 50 mg/kg 1 hr before procedure.

Usual pediatric dosage

Children younger than 3 mo, Neonates. 20-30 mg/kg/day in divided doses q12h.

Dosage in renal impairment

Dosage interval is modified based on creatinine clearance.

Creatinine clearance 10-30 ml/min. Usual dose q12h.

Creatinine clearance less than 10 ml/min. Usual dose q24h.

UNLABELED USES: Treatment of Lyme disease and typhoid fever

CONTRAINDICATIONS: Hypersensitivity to any penicillin, infectious mononucleosis

INTERACTIONS

Drug

Allopurinol: May increase incidence of rash.

Oral contraceptives: May decrease effectiveness of oral contraceptives.

Probenecid: May increase amoxicillin blood concentration and risk of toxicity.

Herbal

None known.

Food

None known.

DIAGNOSTIC TEST EFFECTS: May increase BUN and serum LDH, bilirubin, creatinine, AST (SGOT), and ALT (SGPT) levels. May cause a positive Coombs' test.

SIDE EFFECTS

Frequent

GI disturbances (mild diarrhea, nausea, or vomiting), headache, oral or vaginal candidiasis

Occasional

Generalized rash, urticaria

SERIOUS REACTIONS

• Antibiotic-associated colitis and other superinfections may result from altered bacterial balance.

• Severe hypersensitivity reactions, including anaphylaxis and acute interstitial nephritis occur rarely.

SPECIAL CONSIDERATIONS

PRECAUTIONS

• Serious and occasionally fatal hypersensitivity (anaphylactic) reactions have been reported in patients receiving penicillin therapy. Pseudomembranous colitis has been reported with nearly all antibacterial agents, including amoxicillin, and may range in severity from mild to life threatening. Keep in mind the possibility of superinfections with mycotic or bacterial pathogens during therapy.

PREGNANCY AND LACTATION

• Pregnancy Category B. Reproduction studies performed in mice and rats have revealed no evidence of impaired fertility or harm to the fetus from amoxicillin. Fetal harm is not known. Penicillins have been shown to be excreted in human milk.

---

amoxicillin; clarithromycin; lansoprazole

(a-mox-i-sill'in; clare-i-thro-mye'sin; lance-ah-pra'zol)

Rx: Prevpac

Drug Class: Antibiotics, macrolides; Antibiotics, penicillins; Gastrointestinals; Proton pump inhibitors

Pregnancy Category: C

CLINICAL PHARMACOLOGY

Mechanism of Action: A combination of a penicillin, a macrolide and a proton pump inhibitor. Amoxicillin acts as a bactericidal in susceptible microorganisms. Clarithromycin is a macrolide that is bacteriostatic and binds to ribosomal receptor sites; may be bactericidal with high dosage or very susceptible microorganisms. Lansoprazole is a proton pump inhibitor that selectively inhibits parietal cell membrane enzyme system H^+, K^+, ATPase or proton pump. *Therapeutic Effect:* Inhibits bacterial cell wall synthesis. Inhibits protein synthesis of bacterial cell wall.

Pharmacokinetics

Amoxicillin

Well absorbed from gastrointestinal (GI) tract. Protein binding: 20%. Partially metabolized in liver. Primarily excreted in urine. Removed by hemodialysis. **Half-life:** 1-1.3 hrs (half-life increased in reduced renal function).

Clarithromycin

Well absorbed from the gastrointestinal (GI) tract. Protein binding: 65%-75%. Widely distributed. Metabolized in liver to active metabolite. Primarily excreted in urine. Not removed by hemodialysis. **Half-life:** 3-7 hrs; metabolite: 5-7 hrs (half-life is increased in those with impaired renal function).

Lansoprazole

Once leaving stomach, rapid and complete absorption (food may decrease absorption). Protein binding: 97%. Distributed primarily to gastric parietal cells, converted to two active metabolites. Extensively metabolized in liver. Eliminated from body in bile and urine. Not removed by hemodialysis. **Half-life:** 1.5 hrs (half-life is increased in elderly, those with liver impairment).

AVAILABLE FORMS

• *Combination kit, oral:* 500 mg amoxicillin capsules [4 capsules/day], 50 mg clarithromycin [2 tablets/day], 30 mg lansoprazole capsules [2 capsules/day] (Prevpac).

INDICATIONS AND DOSAGES

H. pylori to reduce risk of recurrent duodenal ulcer

PO

Adults, Elderly. 30 mg lansoprazole, 1 g amoxicillin, and 500 mg clarithromycin taken together or twice daily for 10 to 14 days.

CONTRAINDICATIONS: Concomitant administration with cisapride, pimozide, astemizole, or terfenadine, infectious mononucleosis, hypersensitivity to any penicillin, clarithromycin, erythromycins, any macrolide antibiotic, lansoprazole or any component of the formulation

INTERACTIONS

Drug

Allopurinol: May increase incidence of rash.

Ampicillin, digoxin, iron salts, ketoconazole: May interfere with the absorption of ampicillin, digoxin, iron salts, and ketoconazole.

Carbamazepine, digoxin, theophylline: May increase blood concentration and toxicity of these drugs.

Cisapride, pimozide, astemizole, terfenadine: May result in cardiac arrhythmias (QT prolongation, ventricular tachycardia, ventricular fibrillation, and torsades de pointes) and even death.

Oral contraceptives: May decrease effects of oral contraceptives.

Probenecid: May increase amoxicillin blood concentration and risk for amoxicillin toxicity.

Rifampin: May decrease clarithromycin blood concentration.

Sucralfate: May delay the absorption of lansoprazole; give lansoprazole 30 min before sucralfate.

Warfarin: May increase warfarin effects.

Zidovudine: May decrease blood concentration of zidovudine.

Herbal

None known.

Food

None known.

DIAGNOSTIC TEST EFFECTS: Amoxicillin may increase BUN, LDH, serum bilirubin, serum creatinine, SGOT (AST), and SGPT (ALT) levels. May cause positive Coombs' test.

Clarithromycin may rarely increase BUN, SGOT (AST), and SGPT (ALT) levels.

Lansoprazole may increase LDH concentrations, serum alkaline phosphatase, bilirubin, cholesterol, creatinine, SGOT (AST), SGPT (ALT), triglycerides, and uric acid levels. May produce abnormal albumin/globulin ratio, electrolyte balance, and platelet, red blood cell (RBC), and white blood cell (WBC) counts. May increase blood Hgb and Hct.

SIDE EFFECTS

Frequent

Amoxicillin: Gastrointestinal (GI) disturbances (mild diarrhea, nausea, or vomiting), headache, oral or vaginal candidiasis

Occasional

Amoxicillin: Generalized rash, urticaria

Clarithromycin: Headache, dyspepsia

Lansoprazole: Diarrhea, abdominal pain, rash, pruritus, altered appetite

Rare

Lansoprazole: Nausea, headache

SERIOUS REACTIONS

- Severe hypersensitivity reactions, including anaphylaxis and acute interstitial nephritis occur rarely.
- Antibiotic-associated colitis as evidenced by severe abdominal pain and tenderness, fever, and watery and severe diarrhea, and other superinfections may result from altered bacterial balance.
- Hepatotoxicity and thrombocytopenia occur rarely.
- Bilirubinemia, eosinophilia, and hyperlipemia occur rarely.

SPECIAL CONSIDERATIONS

PRECAUTIONS

- Serious and occasionally fatal hypersensitivity (anaphylactoid) reactions have been reported in patients receiving penicillin therapy. Pseudomembranous colitis has been reported with nearly all antibacterial agents, including clarithromycin, and may range in severity from mild to life threatening. Keep in mind the possibility of superinfections with mycotic organisms or bacterial pathogens.

PATIENT INFORMATION

• Each dose of Prevpac contains four pills: 1 pink and black capsule (lansoprazole), 2 maroon and light-pink capsules (amoxicillin), and 1 yellow tablet (clarithromycin). Each dose should be taken twice per day before eating. Instruct patients to swallow each pill whole.

PREGNANCY AND LACTATION

• Pregnancy Category C. Category C is based on the pregnancy category for clarithromycin. Fetal harm is not known. Clarithromycin has demonstrated adverse effects of pregnancy outcome and embryo-fetal development in monkeys, rats, mice, and rabbits. Amoxicillin is excreted in human milk in very small amounts. Because of the potential for serious adverse reactions in nursing infants from Prevpac, decide whether to discontinue nursing or to discontinue the drug therapy, taking into account the importance of the therapy to the mother.

amoxicillin/ clavulanate potassium

(a-mox'i-sill-in clav-u-lan'ate)

Rx: Augmentin, Augmentin ES-600, Augmentin XR

Drug Class: Antibiotics, penicillins

Pregnancy Category: B

Do not confuse amoxicillin with amoxapine.

CLINICAL PHARMACOLOGY

Mechanism of Action: Amoxicillin inhibits bacterial cell wall synthesis, while clavulanate inhibits bacterial beta-lactamase. *Therapeutic Effect:* Amoxicillin is bactericidal in susceptible microorganisms. Clavulanate protects amoxicillin from enzymatic degradation.

Pharmacokinetics

Well absorbed from the GI tract. Protein binding: 20%. Partially metabolized in the liver. Primarily excreted in urine. Removed by hemodialysis. **Half-life:** 1-1.3 hr (increased in impaired renal function).

AVAILABLE FORMS

• *Powder for Oral Suspension:* 125 mg/5 ml, 200 mg/5 ml, 250 mg/5 ml, 400 mg/5 ml, 600 mg/5 ml.

• *Tablets:* 250 mg, 500 mg, 875 mg.

• *Tablets (Extended-Release):* 1000 mg.

• *Tablets (Chewable):* 125 mg, 200 mg, 250 mg, 400 mg.

INDICATIONS AND DOSAGES

Mild to moderate infections

PO

Adults, Elderly, Children weighing more than 40 kg. 250 mg q8h or 500 mg q12h.

Children weighing less than 40 kg. 20 mg/kg/day in divided doses q8h.

Respiratory tract and other severe infections

PO

Adults, Elderly, Children weighing more than 40 kg. 500 mg q8h or 875 mg q12h.

Children weighing less than 40 kg. 40 mg/kg/day in divided doses q8h.

Otitis media

PO

Children. 90 mg/kg/day in divided doses q12h for 10 days.

Sinusitis, lower respiratory tract infections

PO

Children. 40 mg/kg/day in divided doses q8h or 45 mg/kg/day in divided doses q12h.

Usual neonate dosage

PO

Neonates, Children younger than 3 mos. 30 mg/kg/day in divided doses q12h.

Dosage in renal impairment

Dosage and frequency are modified based on creatinine clearance.

Creatinine clearance 10-30 ml/min. 250-500 mg q12h.

Creatinine clearance less than 10 ml/min. 250-500 mg q24h.

UNLABELED USES: Treatment of bronchitis and chancroid

CONTRAINDICATIONS: Hypersensitivity to any penicillins, infectious mononucleosis

INTERACTIONS

Drug

Allopurinol: May increase incidence of rash.

Oral contraceptives: May decrease effects of oral contraceptives.

Probenecid: May increase amoxicillin and clavulanate blood concentration and risk of toxicity.

Herbal

None known.

Food

None known.

DIAGNOSTIC TEST EFFECTS: May increase serum AST (SGOT) and ALT (SGPT) levels. May cause a positive Coombs' test.

SIDE EFFECTS

Frequent

GI disturbances (mild diarrhea, nausea, vomiting), headache, oral or vaginal candidiasis

Occasional

Generalized rash, urticaria

SERIOUS REACTIONS

• Antibiotic-associated colitis and other superinfections may result from altered bacterial balance.

• Severe hypersensitivity reactions, including anaphylaxis and acute interstitial nephritis occur rarely.

SPECIAL CONSIDERATIONS

PRECAUTIONS

• Although amoxicillin and clavulanate potassium together possess the characteristic low toxicity of the penicillin group of antibiotics, periodic assessment of organ system functions, including renal, hepatic, and hematopoietic function, is advisable during prolonged therapy. A high percentage of patients with mononucleosis who receive ampicillin develop an erythematous skin rash. Thus ampicillin-class antibiotics should not be administered to patients with mononucleosis. Keep in mind the possibility of superinfections with mycotic or bacterial pathogens during therapy. If superinfections occur (usually involving *Pseudomonas* or *Candida*), discontinue the drug and/or institute appropriate therapy.

PATIENT INFORMATION

• Oral Suspension and Chewable Tablets Only: Amoxicillin and clavulanate potassium may be taken every 8 hours or every 12 hours, depending on the strength of the product prescribed. Each dose should be taken with a meal or snack to reduce the possibility of gastrointestinal upset. Many antibiotics can cause diarrhea. Instruct patients to call their physician if diarrhea is severe or lasts more than 2 or 3 days.

• Parents should ensure their child completes the entire prescribed course of treatment, even if the child begins to feel better after a few days. Keep suspension refrigerated. Shake well before using. When dosing a child with amoxicillin and clavulanate potassium suspension (liquid), use a dosing spoon or medicine dropper. Be sure to rinse the spoon or dropper after each use. Bottles of amoxicillin and clavulanate potassium suspension may contain more liquid than required. Instruct patients to follow their doctor's instructions about the amount to use and the days of treatment their child requires. Discard any unused medicine.

PREGNANCY AND LACTATION

• Pregnancy Category B. Reproduction studies performed in pregnant rats and mice given amoxicillin revealed no evidence of harm to the fetus from amoxicillin and clavulanate potassium. Ampicillin-class antibiotics are excreted in the milk.

---

amphetamine; dextroamphetamine

(am-fet'-a-meen; dex-troe-am-fet'-a-meen)

Rx: Adderall, Adderall XR

Drug Class: Adrenergic agonists; Amphetamines; Anorexiants; Stimulants, central nervous system

Pregnancy Category: C

DEA Class: Schedule II

CLINICAL PHARMACOLOGY

Mechanism of Action: A combination of amphetamines that enhances release, action of catecholamine (dopamine, norepinephrine) by blocking reuptake, inhibiting monoamine oxidase. *Therapeutic Effect:* Increases motor activity, mental alertness; decreases drowsiness, fatigue.

Pharmacokinetics

Well absorbed in the gastrointestinal (GI) tract. Widely distributed including the cerebrospinal fluid (CSF). Extensively metabolized in liver. Primarily excreted in the urine. **Half-life** depends on formulation.

AVAILABLE FORMS

• *Tablets:* 5 mg (Adderall), 10 mg (Adderall), 20 mg (Adderall), 30 mg (Adderall).

• *Capsules:* 10 mg (Adderall XR), 20 mg (Adderall XR), 30 mg (Adderall XR).

INDICATIONS AND DOSAGES

Attention deficit hyperactive disorder (ADHD)

PO, extended-release

Adults. Initially, 10 mg/day. 20 mg daily.

Children 6 yr and older. Initially, 10 mg every morning. May increase daily dose in 10 mg increments at weekly intervals until optimal response. Maximum: 30 mg/day

PO, immediate release

Children 6 yr and older. Initially 5 mg once or twice daily. May increase daily dose in 5 mg increments at weekly intervals until optimal response. Maximum: 40 mg/day.

Children 3-5 yr. Initially, 2.5 mg every morning. May increase daily dose in 2.5 mg increments at weekly intervals until optimal response.

Narcolepsy

PO, immediate release

Adults. 5-60 mg/day in divided doses.

Children 12 yr and older. 10 mg once daily. May increase daily dose in 10 mg increments at weekly intervals until optimal response.

Children 6-12 yr. 5 mg once daily. May increase daily dose in 5 mg increments at weekly intervals until optimal response.

CONTRAINDICATIONS: Advanced arteriosclerosis, agitated states, glaucoma, history of drug abuse, history of hypersensitivity to sympathomimetic amines, hyperthyroidism, moderate to severe hypertension, symptomatic cardiovascular disease, within 14 days following discontinuation of an MAOI, hypersensitivity to any component of the formulation.

INTERACTIONS

Drug

Beta-blockers: May increase risk of bradycardia, heart block, and hypertension.

Central nervous system (CNS) stimulants: May increase the effects of dextroamphetamine.

Digoxin: May increase the risk of arrhythmias with this drug.

Haloperidol: May decrease stimulant effects of amphetamines.

Lithium: May decrease stimulatory effects of amphetamines.

MAOIs: May prolong and intensify the effects of dextroamphetamine.

Meperidine: May increase the risk of hypotension, respiratory depression, seizures, and vascular collapse.

Phenobarbital, phenytoin: May decrease absorption of these drugs.

Thyroid hormones: May increase the effects of thyroid this drug and of dextroamphetamine.

Tricyclic antidepressants: May increase cardiovascular effects.

Veratrum alkaloids: May decrease the hypotensive effect of veratrum alkaloids.

Herbal

None known.

Food

Acidic food: May alter serum concentrations.

DIAGNOSTIC TEST EFFECTS: May interfere with urinary steroid determinations. May increase plasma corticosteroid levels.

SIDE EFFECTS

Frequent

Irregular pulse, increased motor activity, talkativeness, nervousness, mild euphoria, insomnia

Occasional

Headache, chills, dry mouth, gastrointestinal (GI) distress, worsening depression in patients who are clinically depressed, tachycardia, palpitations, chest pain

SERIOUS REACTIONS

- Overdose may produce skin pallor or flushing, arrhythmias, and psychosis.
- Abrupt withdrawal following prolonged administration of high dosage may produce lethargy (may last for weeks).
- Prolonged administration to children with ADD may produce a temporary suppression of normal weight and height patterns.

SPECIAL CONSIDERATIONS

PRECAUTIONS

- Clinical experience suggests that in psychotic children, administration of amphetamine may exacerbate symptoms of behavior disturbance and thought disorder. Exercise caution in prescribing amphetamine for patients with even mild hypertension.

PATIENT INFORMATION

- Amphetamine may impair the ability of the patient to engage in potentially hazardous activities such as operating machinery or vehicles; therefore caution the patient accordingly.

PREGNANCY AND LACTATION

- Pregnancy Category C. Infants born to mothers dependent on amphetamine have an increased risk of premature delivery and low birth weight. These infants also may experience symptoms of withdrawal as demonstrated by dysphoria, including agitation, and significant lassitude. Amphetamine is excreted in human milk. Advise mothers who are taking amphetamine to refrain from nursing.

amphotericin B liposome

(am-foe-ter'i-sin bee lye-po'soem)

Rx: AmBisome

Drug Class: Antifungals

Pregnancy Category: B

CLINICAL PHARMACOLOGY

Mechanism of Action: A lipophilic polyene antibiotic that binds to sterols in the fungal cell membrane. *Therapeutic Effect:* Increases fungal cell-membrane permeability, allowing loss of potassium, and other cellular components.

Pharmacokinetics

Widely distributed. Metabolic pathways are unknown. Excretion has not been established. **Half-life:** Terminal: 174 hrs.

AVAILABLE FORMS

- *Injection, powder for reconstitution:* 50 mg (AmBisone).

INDICATIONS AND DOSAGES

Empiric treatment for fungal infection in patients with febrile neutropenia; for aspergillus, candida, or cryptococcus infections unresponsive to Fungizone; or for patients with renal impairment or toxicity from Fungizone

IV Infusion

Adults, Children. 3-5 mg/kg over 1 hr.

CONTRAINDICATIONS: Hypersensitivity to amphotericin B deoxycholate or any amphotericin B–containing formulation

INTERACTIONS

Drug

Bone marrow depressants: May increase risk for anemia.

Digoxin: May increase risk of digoxin toxicity from hypokalemia.

Nephrotoxic medications: May increase risk of nephrotoxicity.

Steroids: May cause severe hypokalemia.

Herbal

None known.

Food

None known.

DIAGNOSTIC TEST EFFECTS: May increase BUN, serum alkaline phosphatase, serum creatinine, SGOT (AST), and SGPT (ALT) levels. May decrease serum calcium, magnesium, and potassium levels.

IV INCOMPATIBILITIES: Do not mix with any other drug, diluent, or solution.

IV COMPATIBILITIES: None known; do not mix with other medications or electrolytes.

SIDE EFFECTS

Frequent (greater than 10%)

Hypokalemia, hypomagnesemia, hyperglycemia, hypocalcemia, edema, abdominal pain, back pain, chills, chest pain, hypotension, diarrhea, nausea, vomiting, headache, fever, rigors, insomnia, dyspnea, epistaxis, increased liver/renal function test results

SERIOUS REACTIONS

- Cardiovascular toxicity as evidenced by hypotension and ventricular fibrillation and anaphylaxis occur rarely.
- Vision and hearing alterations, seizures, liver failure, coagulation defects, multiple organ failure, and sepsis may be noted.

SPECIAL CONSIDERATIONS

PRECAUTIONS

- As with any amphotericin B–containing product, the drug should be administered by medically trained personnel. During the initial dosing period, patients should be under close clinical observation. AmBisome has been shown to be significantly less toxic than amphotericin B deoxycholate; however, adverse events still may occur.

PREGNANCY AND LACTATION

• Pregnancy Category B. Studies in rats and rabbits have concluded that AmBisome had no teratogenic potential in these species. Excretion into human milk is not known.

apraclonidine hydrochloride

(ap-raa-kloe'-ni-deen)

Rx: Iopidine

Drug Class: Adrenergic agonists; Ophthalmics

Pregnancy Category: C

Do not confuse with Cetapred, clomiphene, Klonopin, or quinidine.

CLINICAL PHARMACOLOGY

Mechanism of Action: An ocular alpha-adrenergic agent that is a relatively selective for $alpha_2$ receptor agonist. *Therapeutic Effect:* Reduces intraocular pressure.

Pharmacokinetics

Onset of action occurs within 1 hour. The duration of a single dose is about 12 hours. **Half-life:** 8 hrs.

AVAILABLE FORMS

• *Ophthalmic solution:* 0.5%, 1% (Iodipine).

INDICATIONS AND DOSAGES

Glaucoma

Ophthalmic

Adults, Elderly. Instill 1 drop of 0.5% solution to affected eye(s) 3 times daily.

Intraocular hypertension, post–laser surgery

Ophthalmic

Adults, Elderly. Instill 1 drop of 1% solution in operative eye(s) 1 hour before surgery and 1 drop postoperatively.

UNLABELED USES: Postcycloplegic intraocular pressure spikes, intraocular pressure from post–cataract surgery.

CONTRAINDICATIONS: Hypersensitivity to apraclonidine or clonidine or any component of the formulation.

INTERACTIONS

Drug

MAOIs: May potentiate effects of MAOIs.

Herbal

None known.

Food

None known.

DIAGNOSTIC TEST EFFECTS: *None known.*

SIDE EFFECTS

Frequent

Eye discomfort, dry mouth.

Occasional

Headache, constipation, redness around eye, conjunctivitis, changes in visual acuity, mydriasis, ocular inflammation.

Rare

Nasal decongestion.

SERIOUS REACTIONS

• Allergic reaction occurs rarely.

• Peripheral edema and arrhythmias have been reported.

SPECIAL CONSIDERATIONS

PRECAUTIONS

• Severe cardiovascular disease, hypertension, impaired liver function, coronary insufficiency, recent myocardial infarction, cerebrovascular disease, chronic renal failure, Raynaud's disease, or thromboangiitis obliterans infrequently are associated with depression. Apraclonidine hydrochloride can cause dizziness, somnolence, and decreased mental alertness. The possibility exists of a vasovagal attack occurring during laser surgery.

PREGNANCY AND LACTATION
• Pregnancy Category C. Fetal harm is not known with topical administration. Excretion into human milk is not known.

ascorbic acid (vitamin C)

(a-skor'bic)
Rx: Ascor L 500, Cee-500, Cenolate, Mega-C/A Plus, Vitamin C
Drug Class: Vitamins/minerals

CLINICAL PHARMACOLOGY
Mechanism of Action: Assists in collagen formation and tissue repair and is involved in oxidation reduction reactions and other metabolic reactions. *Therapeutic Effect:* Involved in carbohydrate use and metabolism, as eell as synthesis of carnitine, lipids, and proteins. Preserves blood vessel integrity.
Pharmacokinetics
Readily absorbed from the GI tract. Protein binding: 25%. Metabolized in the liver. Excreted in urine. Removed by hemodialysis.
AVAILABLE FORMS
• *Capsules (Controlled-Release):* 500 mg.
• *Liquid:* 500 mg/5 ml.
• *Oral Solution:* 500 mg/5 ml.
• *Tablets:* 100 mg, 250 mg, 500 mg, 1 g.
• *Tablets (Chewable):* 100 mg, 250 mg, 500 mg.
• *Tablets (Controlled-Release):* 500 mg, 1 g, 1500 mg.
• *Injection:* 250 mg/ml, 500 mg/ml.
INDICATIONS AND DOSAGES
Dietary supplement
PO
Adults, Elderly. 50-200 mg/day.
Children. 35-100 mg/day.
Acidification of urine
PO
Adults, Elderly. 4-12 g/day in 3-4 divided doses.
Children. 500 mg q6-8h.
Scurvy
PO
Adults, Elderly. 100-250 mg 1-2 times a day.
Children. 100-300 mg/day in divided doses.
Prevention and reduction of severity of colds
PO
Adults, Elderly. 1-3 g/day in divided doses.
UNLABELED USES: Prevention of common cold, control of idiopathic methemoglobinemia, urine acidifier
CONTRAINDICATIONS: None known.
INTERACTIONS
Drug
Deferoxamine: May increase iron toxicity.
Herbal
None known.
Food
None known.
DIAGNOSTIC TEST EFFECTS: May decrease serum bilirubin level and urinary pH. May increase urine uric acid and urine oxalate levels.
IV INCOMPATIBILITIES: No information available for Y-site administration.
IV COMPATIBILITIES: Calcium gluconate, heparin
SIDE EFFECTS
Rare
Abdominal cramps, nausea, vomiting, diarrhea, increased urination with doses exceeding 1 g
Parenteral: Flushing, headache, dizziness, sleepiness or insomnia, soreness at injection site.
SERIOUS REACTIONS
• Ascorbic acid may acidify urine, leading to crystalluria.

• Large doses of IV ascorbic acid may lead to deep vein thrombosis.

• Abrupt discontinuation after prolonged use of large doses may produce rebound ascorbic acid deficiency.

SPECIAL CONSIDERATIONS

PRECAUTIONS

• Excessive doses for prolonged periods should not be taken by diabetic patients, patients with renal calculi, patients undergoing anticoagulant therapy, or patients with a history of gout.

PREGNANCY AND LACTATION

• Pregnancy Category A if doses do not exceed the recommended daily allowance; Pregnancy Category C if doses exceed the recommended daily allowance. Ascorbic acid is excreted in breast milk. The recommended daily allowance in lactating mothers is 90 to 100 mg.

OCULAR CONSIDERATIONS

• Some studies show that patients with a higher intake of vitamin C have a lower incidence of cataracts and macular degeneration. The findings do not indicate that vitamin C supplements will help prevent or treat these conditions. (Alleghany Regional Hospital. Retrieved May 16, 2004, from http://www.alleghanyregional.com/healthcontent.asp?page=/choice/demonstration/TheNaturalPharmacist-Consumer.)

aspirin/acetylsalicylic acid/ASA

(as′pir-in)

Rx: Entaprin, YSP Aspirin, Zero-Order Release, Zorprin

Drug Class: Analgesics, nonnarcotic; Antipyretics; Salicylates

Pregnancy Category: D

Do not confuse aspirin or Ascriptin with Aricept, Afrin, or Asendin, or Ecotrin with Edecrin.

CLINICAL PHARMACOLOGY

Mechanism of Action: A nonsteroidal salicylate that inhibits prostaglandin synthesis, acts on the hypothalamus heat-regulating center, and interferes with the production of thromboxane A, a substance that stimulates platelet aggregation. *Therapeutic Effect:* Reduces inflammatory response and intensity of pain; decreases fever; inhibits platelet aggregation.

Pharmacokinetics

Route	Onset	Peak	Duration
PO	1 hr	2-4 hr	24 hr

Rapidly and completely absorbed from GI tract; enteric-coated absorption delayed; rectal absorption delayed and incomplete. Protein binding: High. Widely distributed. Rapidly hydrolyzed to salicylate. **Half-life:** 15-20 min (aspirin); 2-3 hr (salicylate at low dose); more than 20 hr (salicylate at high dose).

AVAILABLE FORMS

• *Tablets (Bayer):* 325 mg, 500 mg.

• *Tablets (Chewable [Bayer and St. Joseph]):* 81 mg.

• *Tablets (Enteric-Coated [Bayer, Ecotrin, St. Joseph]):* 81 mg, 325 mg, 500 mg, 650 mg.

- *Tablets (Hafprin):* 162 mg.
- *Caplets (Bayer):* 81 mg, 325 mg, 500 mg.
- *Gelcaps (Bayer):* 325 mg, 500 mg.
- *Suppositories:* 60 mg, 120 mg, 125 mg, 200 mg, 325 mg, 600 mg, 650 mg.

INDICATIONS AND DOSAGES

Analgesia, fever

PO, Rectal

Adults, Elderly. 325-1000 mg q4-6h

Children. 10-15 mg/kg/dose q4-6h. Maximum: 4 g/day.

Antiinflammatory

PO

Adults, Elderly. Initially, 2.4-3.6 g/day in divided doses; then 3.6-5.4 g/day.

Children. Initially, 60-90 mg/kg/day in divided doses; then 80-100 mg/kg/day.

Suspected MI

PO

Adults, Elderly. 162 mg as soon as the MI is suspected, then daily for 30 days after the MI.

Prevention of MI

PO

Adults, Elderly. 75-325 mg/day.

Prevention of stroke after transient ischemic attack

PO

Adults, Elderly. 50-325 mg/day.

Kawasaki disease

PO

Children. 80-100 mg/kg/day in divided doses.

UNLABELED USES: Prevention of thromboembolism, treatment of Kawasaki disease

CONTRAINDICATIONS: Allergy to tartrazine dye, bleeding disorders, chickenpox or flu in children and teenagers, GI bleeding or ulceration, hepatic impairment, history of hypersensitivity to aspirin or NSAIDs

INTERACTIONS

Drug

Alcohol, NSAIDs: May increase the risk of adverse GI effects, including ulceration.

Antacids, urinary alkalinizers: Increase the excretion of aspirin.

Anticoagulants, heparin, thrombolytics: Increase the risk of bleeding.

Insulin, oral antidiabetics: May increase the effects of these drugs (with large doses of aspirin).

Methotrexate, zidovudine: May increase the risk of toxicity of these drugs.

Ototoxic medications, vancomycin: May increase the risk of ototoxicity.

Platelet aggregation inhibitors, valproic acid: May increase the risk of bleeding.

Probenecid, sulfinpyrazone: May decrease the effects of these drugs.

Herbal

None known.

Food

None known.

DIAGNOSTIC TEST EFFECTS: May alter serum alkaline phosphatase, uric acid, AST (SGOT), and ALT (SGPT) levels. May prolong PT and bleeding time. May decrease serum cholesterol, serum potassium, and T_3 and T_4 levels.

SIDE EFFECTS

Occasional

GI distress (including abdominal distention, cramping, heartburn, and mild nausea); allergic reaction (including bronchospasm, pruritus, and urticaria)

SERIOUS REACTIONS

- High doses of aspirin may produce GI bleeding and gastric mucosal lesions.

• Dehydrated, febrile children may experience aspirin toxicity quickly. Reye's syndrome may occur in children with the chickenpox or the flu.
• Low-grade toxicity characterized is by tinnitus, generalized pruritus (possibly severe), headache, dizziness, flushing, tachycardia, hyperventilation, diaphoresis, and thirst.
• Market toxicity is characterized by hyperthermia, restlessness, seizures, abnormal breathing patterns, respiratory failure, and coma.

SPECIAL CONSIDERATIONS

PRECAUTIONS

• Administer aspirin tablets with caution to patients with asthma, nasal polyps, or nasal allergies. Instruct patients to consult a physician before giving this medicine to children, including teenagers, with chicken pox or flu. In patients receiving large doses of aspirin and/or prolonged therapy, mild salicylate intoxication (salicylism) may develop that may be reversed by reduction in dosage. Although the fecal blood loss with enteric-coated aspirin is less than that with uncoated aspirin tablets, administer enteric-coated aspirin tablets with caution to patients with a history of gastric distress, ulcer, or bleeding problems. Sodium excretion produced by spironolactone may be decreased in the presence of salicylates. Salicylates can produce changes in thyroid function tests. Use salicylates with caution in patients with severe hepatic damage, preexisting hypoprothrombinemia, or vitamin K deficiency and in those undergoing surgery.

PREGNANCY AND LACTATION

• Pregnancy Category D. An increase in adverse effects has been reported in the mother and fetus following chronic ingestion of aspirin. Prolonged pregnancy and labor with increased bleeding before and after delivery, as well as decreased birth weight and increased rate of stillbirth, were correlated with high blood levels of salicylate. Excretion into human milk is not known.

OCULAR CONSIDERATIONS

• Aspirin can affect extraocular muscles. Off-label uses include oral treatment of vernal conjunctivitis. Aspirin can be added to the treatment regimen of cromolyn sodium and steroids.

atenolol

(a-ten'oh-lol)

Rx: Tenormin

Drug Class: Antiadrenergics, beta blocking

Pregnancy Category: C

Do not confuse atenolol with albuterol or timolol.

CLINICAL PHARMACOLOGY

Mechanism of Action: A beta$_1$-adrenergic blocker that acts as an antianginal, antiarrhythmic, and antihypertensive agent by blocking beta$_1$-adrenergic receptors in cardiac tissue. *Therapeutic Effect:* Slows sinus node heart rate, decreasing cardiac output and BP. Decreases myocardial oxygen demand.

Pharmacokinetics

Route	*Onset*	*Peak*	*Duration*
PO	1 hr	2-4 hr	24 hr

Incompletely absorbed from the GI tract. Protein binding: 6%-16%. Minimal liver metabolism. Primarily excreted unchanged in urine. Removed by hemodialysis. **Half-life:** 6-7 hr (increased in impaired renal function).

AVAILABLE FORMS

- *Tablets:* 25 mg, 50 mg, 100 mg.
- *Injection:* 5 mg/10 ml.

INDICATIONS AND DOSAGES

Hypertension

PO

Adults. Initially, 25-50 mg once a day. May increase dose up to 100 mg once a day.

Elderly. Usual initial dose, 25 mg a day.

Children. Initially, 0.8-1 mg/kg/dose given once a day. Range: 0.8-1.5 mg/kg/day. **Maximum:** 2 mg/kg/day or 100 mg/day.

Angina pectoris

PO

Adults. Initially, 50 mg once a day. May increase dose up to 200 mg once a day.

Elderly. Usual initial dose, 25 mg a day.

Acute MI

IV

Adults. Give 5 mg over 5 min; may repeat in 10 min. In those who tolerate full 10-mg IV dose, begin 50-mg tablets 10 min after last IV dose followed by another 50-mg oral dose 12 hr later. Thereafter, give 100 mg once a day or 50 mg twice a day for 6-9 days. Or, for those who do not tolerate full IV dose, give 50 mg orally twice a day or 100 mg once a day for at least 7 days.

Dosage in renal impairment

Dosage interval is modified based on creatinine clearance.

Creatinine Clearance	*Dosage interval*
15-35 ml/min	50 mg a day
less than 15 ml/min	50 mg every other day

UNLABELED USES: Improved survival in diabetics with heart disease; treatment of hypertrophic cardiomyopathy, pheochromocytoma, and syndrome of mitral valve prolapse; prevention of migraine, thyrotoxicosis, tremors

CONTRAINDICATIONS: Cardiogenic shock, overt heart failure, second- or third-degree heart block, severe bradycardia

INTERACTIONS

Drug

Cimetidine: May increase atenolol blood concentration.

Diuretics, other antihypertensives: May increase hypotensive effect of atenolol.

Insulin, oral hypoglycemics: May mask symptoms of hypoglycemia and prolong hypoglycemic effect of insulin and oral hypoglycemics.

NSAIDs: May decrease antihypertensive effect of atenolol.

Sympathomimetics, xanthines: May mutually inhibit effects.

Herbal

None known.

Food

None known.

DIAGNOSTIC TEST EFFECTS: May increase serum antinuclear antibody titer and BUN, serum creatinine, potassium, lipoprotein, triglyceride, and uric acid levels.

IV INCOMPATIBILITIES: Amphotericin complex (Abelcet, AmBisome, Amphotec)

SIDE EFFECTS

Atenolol is generally well tolerated, with mild and transient side effects.

Frequent

Hypotension manifested as cold extremities, constipation or diarrhea, diaphoresis, dizziness, fatigue, headache, and nausea

Occasional

Insomnia, flatulence, urinary frequency, impotence or decreased libido, depression

Rare
Rash, arthralgia, myalgia, confusion (especially in the elderly), altered taste

SERIOUS REACTIONS

- Overdose may produce profound bradycardia and hypotension.
- Abrupt atenolol withdrawal may result in diaphoresis, palpitations, headache, and tremors.
- Atenolol administration may precipitate CHF or MI in patients with cardiac disease; thyroid storm in those with thyrotoxicosis; and peripheral ischemia in those with existing peripheral vascular disease.
- Hypoglycemia may occur in patients with previously controlled diabetes.
- Thrombocytopenia, manifested as unusual bruising or bleeding, occurs rarely.

SPECIAL CONSIDERATIONS

PRECAUTIONS

- Carefully evaluate patients already taking a beta-blocker before administering atenolol. Initial and subsequent atenolol dosages can be adjusted downward depending on clinical observations including pulse and blood pressure. Atenolol may aggravate peripheral arterial circulatory disorders. Use atenolol with caution in patients with impaired renal function

PREGNANCY AND LACTATION

- Pregnancy Category D. Atenolol can cause fetal harm when administered to a pregnant woman. Atenolol crosses the placental barrier and appears in cord blood. Atenolol is excreted in human breast milk at a ratio of 1.5 to 6.8 compared with the concentration in plasma.

OCULAR CONSIDERATIONS

- Reports have been made of skin rashes and dry eyes associated with the use of beta-adrenergic blocking drugs. The reported incidence is small, and in most cases, the symptoms have cleared when treatment was withdrawn. Consider discontinuance of the drug if any such reaction is not otherwise explicable. Closely monitor patients following cessation of therapy.

---

atorvastatin

(ah-tore-vah'-stah-tin)
Rx: Lipitor
Drug Class: Antihyperlipidemics; HMG CoA reductase inhibitors
Pregnancy Category: X
Do not confuse Lipitor with Levatol.

CLINICAL PHARMACOLOGY

Mechanism of Action: An antihyperlipidemic that inhibits HMG-CoA reductase, the enzyme that catalyzes the early step in cholesterol synthesis. *Therapeutic Effect:* Decreases LDL and VLDL cholesterol, and plasma triglyceride levels; increases HDL cholesterol concentration.

Pharmacokinetics

Poorly absorbed from the GI tract. Protein binding: greater than 98%. Metabolized in the liver. Minimally eliminated in urine. Plasma levels are markedly increased in chronic alcoholic hepatic disease, but are unaffected by renal disease. **Half-life:** 14 hr.

AVAILABLE FORMS

- *Tablets:* 10 mg, 20 mg, 40 mg, 80 mg.

INDICATIONS AND DOSAGES

Hyperlipidemia, Reduction of risk of MI, angina revascularization procedures

PO

Adults, Elderly. Initially, 10-40 mg a day given as a single dose. Dose range: Increase at 2- to 4-wk intervals to maximum of 80 mg/day.

Children 10-17 yr. Initially, 10 mg/day, may increase to 20 mg/day.

Familial hypercholesterolemia

PO

Children 10-17 yr. Initially, 10 mg/day. May increase to 20 mg/day.

CONTRAINDICATIONS: Active hepatic disease, lactation, pregnancy, unexplained elevated hepatic function test results

INTERACTIONS

Drug

Antacids, colestipol, propranolol: Decreases atorvastatin activity.

Cyclosporine, erythromycin, gemfibrozil, nicotinic acid: Increases the risk of acute renal failure and rhabdomyolysis with these drugs.

Digoxin, itraconazole, oral contraceptives, warfarin: May increase atorvastatin blood concentration, producing severe muscle inflammation, pain, and weakness.

Herbal

None known.

Food

None known.

DIAGNOSTIC TEST EFFECTS: May increase serum CK and transaminase concentrations.

SIDE EFFECTS

Atorvastatin is generally well tolerated. Side effects are usually mild and transient.

Frequent (16%)

Headache

Occasional (5%-2%)

Myalgia, rash or pruritus, allergy

Rare (2%-1%)

Flatulence, dyspepsia

SERIOUS REACTIONS

• Cataracts may develop, and photosensitivity may occur.

SPECIAL CONSIDERATIONS

PRECAUTIONS

• 3-Hydroxy-3-methylglutaryl-coenzyme A (HMG-CoA) reductase inhibitors interfere with cholesterol synthesis and theoretically might blunt adrenal and/or gonadal steroid production. Exercise caution if an HMG-CoA reductase inhibitor is administered concomitantly with drugs that may decrease the levels or activity of endogenous steroid hormones such as ketoconazole, spironolactone, and cimetidine. Brain hemorrhage was seen in a treated female dog.

PATIENT INFORMATION

• Advise patients to report unexplained muscle pain, tenderness, or weakness promptly, particularly if accompanied by malaise or fever.

PREGNANCY AND LACTATION

• Pregnancy Category X. Atorvastatin crosses the rat placenta and reaches a level in fetal liver equivalent to that of the maternal plasma. Nursing rat pups had plasma and liver drug levels of 50% and 40%, respectively, of that in their mother's milk. Because of the potential for adverse reactions in nursing infants, women taking atorvastatin should not breast-feed.

atropine sulfate

(a'troe-peen)

Rx: Atropine-Care, Atropisol, Atrosulf-1, Isopto Atropine, Ocu-Tropine, Sal-Tropine

Drug Class: Antiarrhythmics; Anticholinergics; Antidotes; Cycloplegics; Mydriatics; Ophthalmics; Preanesthetics

Pregnancy Category: B

Do not confuse atropine sulfate with Akarpine or Aplisol.

CLINICAL PHARMACOLOGY

Mechanism of Action: Anticholinergics act directly on the smooth muscles and secretory glands innervated by postganglionic cholinergic nerves. Blocks the parasympathomimetic (muscarinic) effects of acetylcholine and parasympathomimetic drugs at these sites. *Therapeutic Effect:* Decreases GI motility and secretory activity, and GU muscle tone (ureter, bladder); produces ophthalmic cycloplegia, and mydriasis.

AVAILABLE FORMS

- *Ophthalmic:* ointment 1%; solution 1%.
- *Injection:* 0.05 mg/ml, 0.1 mg/ml, 0.4 mg/0.5 ml, 0.4 mg/ml, 0.5 mg/ml, 1 mg/ml.

INDICATIONS AND DOSAGES

Mydriasis and cycloplegia for refraction; dilation and relaxation of the ciliary muscle in anterior uveitis

1 or 2 drops in the eyes 3 times/day.

Asystole, slow pulseless electrical activity

IV

Adults, Elderly. 1 mg; may repeat q3-5min up to total dose of 0.04 mg/kg.

Preanesthetic

IV/IM/Subcutaneous

Adults, Elderly. 0.4-0.6 mg 30-60 min pre-op.

Children weighing 5 kg and more. 0.01-0.02 mg/kg/dose to maximum of 0.4 mg/dose.

Children weighing less than 5 kg. 0.02 mg/kg/dose 30-60 min pre-op.

Bradycardia

IV

Adults, Elderly. 0.5-1 mg q5min not to exceed 2 mg or 0.04 mg/kg.

Children. 0.02 mg/kg with a minimum of 0.1 mg to a maximum of 0.5 mg in children and 1 mg in adolescents. May repeat in 5 min. Maximum total dose: 1 mg in children, 2 mg in adolescents.

CONTRAINDICATIONS: Bladder neck obstruction due to prostatic hypertrophy, cardiospasm, intestinal atony, myasthenia gravis in those not treated with neostigmine, narrow-angle glaucoma, obstructive disease of the GI tract, paralytic ileus, severe ulcerative colitis, tachycardia secondary to cardiac insufficiency or thyrotoxicosis, toxic megacolon, unstable cardiovascular status in acute hemorrhage

INTERACTIONS

Drug

Antacids, antidiarrheals: May decrease absorption of atropine.

Anticholinergics: May increase effects of atropine.

Ketoconazole: May decrease absorption of ketoconazole.

Potassium chloride: May increase severity of GI lesions (wax matrix).

Herbal

None known.

Food

None known.

DIAGNOSTIC TEST EFFECTS: *None known.*

IV INCOMPATIBILITIES: Pentothal (Thiopental)

IV COMPATIBILITIES: Diphenhydramine (Benadryl), droperidol (Inapsine), fentanyl (Sublimaze), glycopyrrolate (Robinul), heparin, hydromorphone (Dilaudid), midazolam (Versed), morphine, potassium chloride, propofol (Diprivan)

SIDE EFFECTS

Frequent

Dry mouth, nose, and throat that may be severe; decreased sweating, constipation, irritation at subcutaneous or IM injection site

Occasional

Swallowing difficulty, blurred vision, bloated feeling, impotence, urinary hesitancy

Rare

Allergic reaction, including rash and urticaria; mental confusion or excitement, particularly in children, fatigue

SERIOUS REACTIONS

- Overdosage may produce tachycardia, palpitations, hot, dry or flushed skin, absence of bowel sounds, increased respiratory rate, nausea, vomiting, confusion, somnolence, slurred speech, dizziness and CNS stimulation.
- Overdosage may also produce psychosis as evidenced by agitation, restlessness, rambling speech, visual hallucinations, paranoid behavior, and delusions, followed by depression.

SPECIAL CONSIDERATIONS

PRECAUTIONS

- Keep out of reach of children.

PREGNANCY AND LACTATION

- Pregnancy Category B. Fetal harm is not known. Atropine may be excreted in milk, causing infant toxicity, and may reduce breast milk production.

OCULAR CONSIDERATIONS

- Prolonged use may cause general systemic reactions, allergic lid reactions, local irritation, hyperemia, edema, follicular conjunctivitis, or dermatitis.

auranofin/ aurothioglucose

(ah-ran'-oh-fin/ah-row-thigh-oh-glue'-cose)

Rx: Ridaura

Drug Class: Disease modifying antirheumatic drugs; Gold compounds

Pregnancy Category: C

Do not confuse Ridaura with Cardura.

CLINICAL PHARMACOLOGY

Mechanism of Action: Gold compounds that alter cellular mechanisms, collagen biosynthesis, enzyme systems, and immune responses. *Therapeutic Effect:* Suppress synovitis in the active stage of rheumatoid arthritis.

Pharmacokinetics

Auranofin (29% gold): Moderately absorbed from the GI tract. Protein binding: 60%. Rapidly metabolized. Primarily excreted in urine. **Half-life:** 21-31 days. Aurothioglucose (50% gold): Slowly and erraticly absorbed after IM administration. Protein binding: 95%-99%. Primarily excreted in urine. **Half-life:** 3-27 days (increased with increased number of doses).

AVAILABLE FORMS

- *Capsules (Ridaura):* 3 mg.
- *Injection (Solganal):* 50-mg/ml suspension.

INDICATIONS AND DOSAGES

Rheumatoid arthritis

PO

Adults, Elderly. 6 mg/day as a single or 2 divided doses. If there is no response in 6 mo, may increase to 9 mg/day in 3 divided doses. If response is still inadequate, discontinue.

Children. 0.1 mg/kg/day as a single or 2 divided doses. Maintenance: 0.15 mg/kg/day. Maximum: 0.2 mg/kg/day.

IM

Adults, Elderly. Initially, 10 mg, followed by 25 mg for 2 doses, then 50 mg weekly until total dose of 0.8-1 g has been given. If patient has improved and shows no signs of toxicity, may give 50 mg q3-4wk for many months.

Children. 0.25 mg/kg; may increase by 0.25 mg/kg each week. Maintenance: 0.75-1 mg/kg/dose. Maximum: 25 mg/dose for 20 doses, then repeated q2-4wk.

UNLABELED USES: Treatment of pemphigus, psoriatic arthritis

CONTRAINDICATIONS: Bone marrow aplasia, history of gold-induced pathologies (including blood dyscrasias, exfoliative dermatitis, necrotizing enterocolitis, and pulmonary fibrosis), severe blood dyscrasias

INTERACTIONS

Drug

Bone marrow depressants; hepatotoxic and nephrotoxic medications: May increase the risk of aurothioglucose toxicity.

Penicillamine: May increase the risk of hematologic or renal adverse effects.

Herbal

None known.

Food

None known.

DIAGNOSTIC TEST EFFECTS: May decrease Hgb level, Hct, and WBC and platelet counts. May increase urine protein level. May alter hepatic function test results.

SIDE EFFECTS

Frequent

Auranofin: Diarrhea (50%), pruritic rash (26%), abdominal pain (14%), stomatitis (13%), nausea (10%)

Aurothioglucose: Rash (39%), stomatitis (19%), diarrhea (13%).

Occasional

Aurothioglucose: Nausea, vomiting, anorexia, abdominal cramps

SERIOUS REACTIONS

- Signs and symptoms of gold toxicity, the primary serious reaction, include decreased Hgb level, decreased granulocyte count (less than 150,000/mm^3), proteinuria, hematuria, stomatitis, blood dyscrasias (anemia, leukopenia [WBC count less than 4000/mm^3], thrombocytopenia, and eosinophilia), glomerulonephritis, nephrotic syndrome, and cholestatic jaundice.

SPECIAL CONSIDERATIONS

PRECAUTIONS

- The safety of concomitant use of auranofin with injectable gold, hydroxychloroquine, penicillamine, immunosuppressive agents (e.g., cyclophosphamide, azathioprine, or methotrexate), or high doses of corticosteroids has not been established. Medical problems that might affect the signs or symptoms used to detect auranofin toxicity should be under control before starting auranofin. Weigh the potential benefits of using auranofin in patients with progressive renal disease, significant hepatocellular disease, inflammatory bowel disease, skin rash, or history of bone marrow depression against (1) the potential risks of gold toxicity on organ systems previously compromised or with decreased reserve and (2) the difficulty in quickly detecting and correctly attributing the toxic effect.

PATIENT INFORMATION

- Advise patients of the possibility of toxicity from auranofin and of the signs and symptoms that they should report promptly. Warn women of childbearing potential of the potential risks of auranofin therapy during pregnancy.

PREGNANCY AND LACTATION

- Pregnancy Category C. Use of auranofin by pregnant women is not recommended. Nursing during auranofin therapy is not recommended. Following auranofin administration to rats and mice, gold is excreted in milk.

OCULAR CONSIDERATIONS

- Gold deposits in the lens or cornea unassociated clinically with eye disorders or visual impairment occur in less than 1% of patients.

azatadine maleate

(a-za'-ta-deen mal'-ee-ate)

Rx: Optimine

Drug Class: Antihistamines, H1

Pregnancy Category: B

Do not confuse with azelastine or azacitidine.

CLINICAL PHARMACOLOGY

Mechanism of Action: A piperazine-derivative antihistamine that has both anticholinergic an antiserotonin activity. Inhibits mediator release from mast cells and prevents calcium entry into mast cells through voltage-dependent calcium channels. *Therapeutic Effect:* Relieves allergic conditions, including urticaria and pruritus. Anticholinergic effects cause drying of nasal mucosa.

Pharmacokinetics

Rapidly and extensively absorbed from the gastrointestinal (GI) tract. Protein binding: minimal. Metabolized in liver. Excreted in urine. **Half-life:** 8.7 hrs

AVAILABLE FORMS

- *Tablets:* 1 mg (Optimine).

INDICATIONS AND DOSAGES

Allergic rhinitis

PO

Adults, Elderly, Children 12 yr or older. 1-2 mg 2 times a day.

CONTRAINDICATIONS: History of hypersensitivity to azatadine, antihistamines, or any other component of the formulation or to other related antihistamines including cyproheptadine, concomitant use MAO inhibitors

INTERACTIONS

Drug

Alcohol, central nervous system (CNS) depressants, tricylic antidepressants, procarbazine: May increase CNS depression.

Herbal

None known.

Food

None known.

DIAGNOSTIC TEST EFFECTS: *None known.*

SIDE EFFECTS

Frequent

Slight to moderate drowsiness, thickening of bronchial secretions.

Rare

Headache, fatigue, nervousness, dizziness, appetite increase, weight gain, nausea, diarrhea, abdominal pain, dry mouth, arthralgia, pharyngitis.

SERIOUS REACTIONS

- Hepatitis, bronchospasm, and epistaxis have been reported.

SPECIAL CONSIDERATIONS

PRECAUTIONS

- Azatadine maleate has an atropine-like action and therefore should be used with caution in patients with a history of bronchial asthma, increased intraocular pressure, hyperthyroidism, cardiovascular disease, or hypertension. Use the drug with caution in patients with urinary bladder obstruction caused by symptomatic prostatic hypertrophy and narrowing of the bladder neck. Azatadine maleate has additive effects with alcohol and other central nervous system depressants (e.g., hypnotics, sedatives, and tranquilizers). Warn patients about engaging in activities requiring mental alertness, such as driving a car or operating certain appliances and machinery until their response to this medication has been determined. Azatadine maleate is more likely to cause dizziness, sedation, and hypotension in patients over 60 years of age.

PATIENT INFORMATION

• Antihistamines may cause drowsiness.

• Patients taking antihistamines should not engage in activities requiring mental alertness, such as driving a car or operating machinery and certain appliances until their response to this medication has been determined.

• Alcohol or other sedative drugs may enhance the drowsiness caused by antihistamines.

• Patients should not take this medication if they are receiving a monoamine oxidase inhibitor or if they are receiving oral anticoagulants.

• This medication should not be given to children less than 12 years of age.

PREGNANCY AND LACTATION

• Pregnancy Category B. Reproduction studies in rats and rabbits revealed no evidence of impaired fertility or harm to the fetus. Antihistamines should not be used in the third trimester of pregnancy because newborn and premature infants may have severe reactions to them, such as convulsions. Whether this drug is excreted in human milk is not known. However, certain antihistamines are known to be excreted in human milk in low concentration.

azathioprine

(ay-za-thye'oh-preen)

Rx: Azasan, Azathioprine Sodium, Imuran

Drug Class: Disease modifying antirheumatic drugs; Immunosuppressives

Pregnancy Category: D

Do not confuse azathioprine with Azulfidine or azatadine, or Imuran with Elmiron or Imferon.

CLINICAL PHARMACOLOGY

Mechanism of Action: An immunologic agent that antagonizes purine metabolism and inhibits DNA, protein, and RNA synthesis. *Therapeutic Effect:* Suppresses cell-mediated hypersensitivities; alters antibody production and immune response in transplant recipients; reduces the severity of arthritis symptoms.

AVAILABLE FORMS

• *Tablets (Azasan):* 25 mg, 50 mg, 75 mg, 100 mg.

• *Tablets (Imuran):* 50 mg.

• *Injection:* 100-mg vial.

INDICATIONS AND DOSAGES

Adjunct in prevention of renal allograft rejection

PO, IV

Adults, Elderly, Children. 2-5 mg/kg/day on day of transplant, then 1-3 mg/kg/day as maintenance dose.

Rheumatoid arthritis

PO

Adults. Initially, 1 mg/kg/day as a single dose or in 2 divided doses. May increase by 0.5 mg/kg/day after 6-8 wk at 4-wk intervals up to maximum of 2.5 mg/kg/day. Maintenance: Lowest effective dosage. May decrease dose by 0.5 mg/kg or 25 mg/day q4wk (while other therapies, such as rest, physiotherapy, and salicylates, are maintained).

Elderly. Initially, 1 mg/kg/day (50-100 mg); may increase by 25 mg/day until response or toxicity.

Dosage in renal impairment

Dosage is modified based on creatinine clearance.

Creatinine Clearance	*Dose*
10-50 ml/min	75% of usual dose
less than 10 ml/min	50% of usual dose

UNLABELED USES: Treatment of biliary cirrhosis, chronic active hepatitis, glomerulonephritis, inflammatory bowel disease, inflammatory myopathy, multiple sclerosis, myasthenia gravis, nephrotic syndrome, pemphigoid, pemphigus, polymyositis, systemic lupus erythematosus

CONTRAINDICATIONS: Pregnant patients with rheumatoid arthritis

INTERACTIONS

Drug

Allopurinol: May increase activity and risk of toxicity of azathioprine.

Bone marrow depressants: May increase myelosuppression.

Live-virus vaccines: May potentiate virus replication, increase the vaccine's side effects, and decrease the patient's antibody response to the vaccine.

Other immunosuppressants: May increase the risk of infection or neoplasms.

Herbal

None known.

Food

None known.

DIAGNOSTIC TEST EFFECTS: May decrease serum albumin, Hgb, and serum uric acid levels. May increase serum alkaline phosphatase, amylase, bilirubin, AST (SGOT), and ALT (SGPT) levels.

IV INCOMPATIBILITIES: Methyl and propyl parabens, phenol

SIDE EFFECTS

Frequent

Nausea, vomiting, anorexia (particularly during early treatment and with large doses)

Occasional

Rash

Rare

Severe nausea and vomiting with diarrhea, abdominal pain, hypersensitivity reaction

SERIOUS REACTIONS

- Azathioprine use increases the risk of developing neoplasia (new abnormal-growth tumors).
- Significant leukopenia and thrombocytopenia may occur, particularly in those undergoing kidney transplant rejection.
- Hepatotoxicity occurs rarely.

SPECIAL CONSIDERATIONS

PRECAUTIONS

- A gastrointestinal hypersensitivity reaction characterized by severe nausea and vomiting has been reported. These symptoms also may be accompanied by diarrhea, rash, fever, malaise, myalgias, elevations in liver enzymes, and occasionally, hypotension.
- Symptoms of gastrointestinal toxicity most often develop within the first several weeks of azathioprine therapy and are reversible upon discontinuation of the drug. The reaction can recur within hours after rechallenge with a single dose of azathioprine.

PATIENT INFORMATION

• Inform patients being started on azathioprine of the necessity of periodic blood counts while they are receiving the drug, and encourage them to report any unusual bleeding or bruising to their physician. Inform patients of the danger of infection while receiving azathioprine, and ask them to report signs and symptoms of infection to their physician. Give careful dosage instructions to patients, especially when azathioprine is being administered in the presence of impaired renal function or concomitantly with allopurinol. Advise patients of the potential risks of the use of azathioprine during pregnancy and during the nursing period. Explain to the patient the increased risk of neoplasia following azathioprine therapy.

PREGNANCY AND LACTATION

• Pregnancy Category D. Azathioprine can cause fetal harm when administered to a pregnant woman. Do not use azathioprine to treat rheumatoid arthritis in pregnant women. Use in nursing mothers is not recommended. Azathioprine or its metabolites are transferred at low levels transplacentally and in breast milk.

azelastine

(a'zel-ah-steen)

Rx: Astelin, Optivar

Drug Class: Antihistamines, H1; Antihistamines, inhalation; Antihistamines, ophthalmic; Ophthalmics

Pregnancy Category: C

Do not confuse Optivar with Optiray.

CLINICAL PHARMACOLOGY

Mechanism of Action: An antihistamine that competes with histamine for histamine receptor sites on cells in the blood vessels, GI tract, and respiratory tract. *Therapeutic Effect:* Relieves symptoms associated with seasonal allergic rhinitis such as increased mucus production and sneezing and symptoms associated with allergic conjunctivitis, such as redness, itching, and excessive tearing.

Pharmacokinetics

Route	*Onset*	*Peak*	*Duration*
Nasal spray	0.5-1 hr	2-3 hr	12 hr
Ophthalmic	N/A	3 min	8 hr

Well absorbed through nasal mucosa. Primarily excreted in feces. **Half-life:** 22 hr.

AVAILABLE FORMS

• *Nasal Spray (Astelin):* 137 mcg.

• *Ophthalmic Solution (Optivar):* 0.05%.

INDICATIONS AND DOSAGES

Allergic rhinitis

Nasal

Adults, Elderly, Children 12 yr and older. 2 sprays in each nostril twice a day.

Children 5-11 yr. 1 spray in each nostril twice a day.

Allergic conjunctivitis
Ophthalmic
Adults, Elderly, Children 3 yr or older. 1 drop into affected eye twice a day.

CONTRAINDICATIONS: Breast-feeding women, history of hypersensitivity to antihistamines, neonates or premature infants, third trimester of pregnancy

INTERACTIONS

Drug
Alcohol, other CNS depressants: May increase CNS depression.
Cimetidine: May increase azelastine blood concentration.

Herbal
None known.

Food
None known.

DIAGNOSTIC TEST EFFECTS: May increase ALT (SGPT) levels. May suppress flare and wheal reactions to antigen skin testing unless drug is discontinued 4 days before testing.

SIDE EFFECTS

Frequent (20%-15%)
Headache, bitter taste

Rare
Nasal burning, paroxysmal sneezing
Ophthalmic: Transient eye burning or stinging, bitter taste, headache

SERIOUS REACTIONS

• Epistaxis occurs rarely.

SPECIAL CONSIDERATIONS

PATIENT INFORMATION

• Azelastine should not be used to treat contact lens-related irritation. Instruct patients to wait at least 10 minutes before they insert their contact lenses because of benzalkonium chloride.

PREGNANCY AND LACTATION

• Pregnancy Category C. Azelastine hydrochloride has been shown to be embryotoxic, fetotoxic, and teratogenic (external and skeletal abnormalities) in mice with oral doses. Fetal harm is not known with topical administration. Excretion into human milk is not known.

---

azithromycin

(ay-zi-thro-mye′sin)

Rx: Zithromax, Zithromax IV, Zithromax TRI-PAK, Zithromax Z-Pak

Drug Class: Antibiotics, macrolides

Pregnancy Category: B

Do not confuse azithromycin with erythromycin.

CLINICAL PHARMACOLOGY

Mechanism of Action: A macrolide antibiotic that binds to ribosomal receptor sites of susceptible organisms, inhibiting RNA-dependent protein synthesis. *Therapeutic Effect:* Bacteriostatic or bactericidal, depending on the drug dosage.

Pharmacokinetics
Rapidly absorbed from the GI tract. Protein binding: 7%-50%. Widely distributed. Eliminated primarily unchanged by biliary excretion. **Half-life:** 68 hr.

AVAILABLE FORMS

• *Oral Suspension:* 100 mg/5 ml, 200 mg/5 ml.

• *Tablets:* 250 mg, 500 mg, 600 mg. Tri-Pak: 3x500 mg. Z-Pak: 6x250 mg.

• *Injection:* 500 mg.

INDICATIONS AND DOSAGES

Respiratory tract, skin, and skin-structure infections
PO
Adults, Elderly. 500 mg once, then 250 mg/day for 4 days.

Children 6 mo and older. 10 mg/kg once (maximum 500 mg) then 5 mg/kg/day for 4 days (maximum 250 mg).

Acute bacterial exacerbations of COPD

PO

Adults. 500 mg/day for 3 days.

Otitis media

PO

Children 6 mo and older. 10 mg/kg once (maximum 500 mg) then 5 mg/kg/day for 4 days (maximum 250 mg). Single dose: 30 mg/kg. Maximum: 1500 mg. Three day regimen: 10 mg/kg/day as single daily dose. Maximum: 500 mg/day.

Pharyngitis, tonsillitis

PO

Children older than 2 yr. 12 mg/kg/day (maximum 500 mg) for 5 days.

Chancroid

PO

Adults, Elderly: 1 g as single dose.

Children: 20 mg/kg as single dose. Maximum: 1 g.

Treatment of* Mycobacterium avium *complex (MAC)

PO

Adults, Elderly. 500 mg/day in combination.

Children. 5 mg/kg/day (maximum 250 mg) in combination.

Prevention of MAC

PO

Adults, Elderly. 1200 mg/wk alone or with rifabutin.

Children. 5 mg/kg/day (maximum 250 mg) or 20 mg/kg/wk (maximum 1200 mg) alone or with rifabutin.

***Nongonococcal urethritis and cervicitis caused by* Chlamydia trachomatis**

PO

Adults. 1 g as a single dose.

Usual pediatric dosage

PO

Children older than 6 mo. 10 mg/kg once (maximum: 500 mg) then 5 mg/kg/day for 4 days (maximum 250 mg).

Usual parenteral dosage (Community Acquired Pneumonia, PID)

IV

Adults. 500 mg/day, followed by oral therapy.

UNLABELED USES: Chlamydial infections, gonococcal pharyngitis, uncomplicated gonococcal infections of the cervix, urethra, and rectum

CONTRAINDICATIONS: Hypersensitivity to azithromycin or other macrolide antibiotics

INTERACTIONS

Drug

Aluminum- or magnesium-containing antacids: May decrease azithromycin blood concentration.

Carbamazepine, cyclosporine, theophylline, warfarin: May increase the serum concentrations of these drugs.

Herbal

None known.

Food

None known.

DIAGNOSTIC TEST EFFECTS: May increase serum CK, AST (SGOT), and ALT (SGPT) levels.

IV INCOMPATIBILITIES: Information is not available.

IV COMPATIBILITIES: None known; do not mix with other medications.

SIDE EFFECTS

Occasional

Nausea, vomiting, diarrhea, abdominal pain

Rare

Headache, dizziness, allergic reaction

SERIOUS REACTIONS

- Antibiotic-associated colitis and other superinfections may result from altered bacterial balance.
- Acute interstitial nephritis and hepatotoxicity occur rarely.

SPECIAL CONSIDERATIONS

PRECAUTIONS

- Exercise caution when administering azithromycin to patients with impaired hepatic function. The following adverse events have been reported with macrolide products: ventricular arrhythmias, including ventricular tachycardia, and torsades de pointes, in individuals with prolonged Q-T intervals.

PATIENT INFORMATION

- Caution patients to take azithromycin capsules and azithromycin suspension at least 1 hour before a meal or at least 2 hours after a meal. These medications should not be taken with food. Azithromycin tablets may be taken with or without food. However, increased tolerability has been observed when tablets are taken with food. Direct patients to discontinue azithromycin and contact a physician if any signs of an allergic reaction occur.

PREGNANCY AND LACTATION

- Pregnancy Category B. In the animal studies, no evidence of harm to the fetus from azithromycin was found. Excretion into human milk is not known.

OCULAR CONSIDERATIONS

- Azithromycin (AzaSite) in a topical form is in clinical trials for the treatment of corneal infections. Another potential indication for topical azithromycin is the treatment of trachoma. (Bonner H: Ocular drug preview: spotlight on emerging pharmaceuticals, Review of Optometry Online vol 141, issue 12, 2004. http://www.revoptom.com/index.asp?page=2_1309.htm.)
- Dosage and Administration: Adult inclusion (chlamydial) conjunctivitis—1 gram orally once daily. Patient may require only a single dose.

---

bacitracin

(bass-i-tray' sin)

Rx: AK-Tracin, Baci-IM, Baci-Rx, Ocu-Tracin, Ziba-Rx

Drug Class: Anti-infectives, ophthalmic; Anti-infectives, topical; Antibiotics, miscellaneous; Dermatologics; Ophthalmics

Pregnancy Category: C

Do not confuse bacitracin with Bactrim or Bactroban.

CLINICAL PHARMACOLOGY

Mechanism of Action: An antibiotic that interferes with plasma membrane permeability and inhibits bacterial cell wall synthesis in susceptible bacteria. *Therapeutic Effect:* Bacteriostatic.

AVAILABLE FORMS

- *Powder for Irrigation:* 50,000 units.
- *Ophthalmic Ointment.* 500 units/g.
- *Topical Ointment.* 500 units/g.

INDICATIONS AND DOSAGES

Superficial ocular infections

Ophthalmic

Adults. ½-inch ribbon in conjunctival sac q3-4h.

Skin abrasions, superficial skin infections

Topical

Adults, Children. Apply to affected area 1-5 times a day.

Surgical treatment and prophylaxis

Irrigation

Adults, Elderly. 50,000-150,000 units, as needed.

CONTRAINDICATIONS: None known.

INTERACTIONS

Drug

None known.

Herbal

None known.

Food

None known.

DIAGNOSTIC TEST EFFECTS: *None known.*

SIDE EFFECTS

Rare

Ophthalmic: Burning, itching, redness, swelling, pain

Topical: Hypersensitivity reaction (allergic contact dermatitis, burning, inflammation, pruritus)

SERIOUS REACTIONS

• Severe hypersensitivity reactions, including apnea and hypotension, occur rarely.

SPECIAL CONSIDERATIONS

PRECAUTIONS

• Overgrowth of nonsusceptible organisms may result. If new infections caused by bacteria or fungi appear during therapy, take appropriate measures.

• For severe eye pain, headache, rapid change in vision (side or straight ahead), sudden appearance of floating spots, acute redness of the eyes, pain on exposure to light, or double vision, instruct patients to consult an eye care practitioner immediately.

PATIENT INFORMATION

• Advise patients to discontinue use of this product and consult an eye care practitioner if symptoms persist or become worse.

OCULAR CONSIDERATIONS

• Ocular Indications and Usage: Conjunctivitis and keratitis

---

bacitracin zinc; neomycin sulfate; polymyxin B sulfate

(bass-i-tray'-sin zink; nee-oh-mye'-sin sul'-fate; pol-ee-mix'-in bee sul'-fate)

Rx: AK-Spore Ointment, Neocin, Neosporin Ophthalmic Ointment, Ocu-Spore-B, Ocutricin

Drug Class: Anti-infectives, ophthalmic; Anti-infectives, topical; Dermatologics; Ophthalmics

Pregnancy Category: C

CLINICAL PHARMACOLOGY

Mechanism of Action: Bacitracin is an antibiotic that interferes with plasma membrane permeability in susceptible bacteria. Polymyxin B damages bacterial cytoplasmic membrane which causes leakage of intracellular components. Neomycin is an aminoglycoside antibiotic that binds to the 30s subunit of the ribosome. *Therapeutic Effect:* Inhibits bacterial cell wall synthesis.

Pharmacokinetics

Not absorbed through topical administration. Neomycin may be absorbed following topical administration to the eye if tissue damage is present.

AVAILABLE FORMS

• *Ointment, ophthalmic:* 400 units bacitracin, 3.5 mg neomycin, 10,000 units polymyxin B/g (AK-Spore, Neocin, Ocu-Spore-B, Ocutricin).

INDICATIONS AND DOSAGES

Superficial ocular infections

Ophthalmic

Adults. Instill ½ inch into conjunctival sac every 3-4 hrs for 7-10 days for acute infections. Apply ½ inch 2-3 times/day for mild to moderate infections for 7-10 days.

CONTRAINDICATIONS: Hypersensitivity to bacitracin, polymyxin B, neomycin, or any component of the formulation

INTERACTIONS

Drug

None known.

Herbal

None known.

Food

None known.

DIAGNOSTIC TEST EFFECTS: *None known.*

SIDE EFFECTS

Rare

Burning, itching, redness, swelling, pain

SERIOUS REACTIONS

• Severe hypersensitivity reaction, including apnea and hypotension, occurs rarely.

SPECIAL CONSIDERATIONS

PRECAUTIONS

• Bacterial resistance to this product may develop. If purulent discharge, inflammation, or pain becomes aggravated, the patient should discontinue use of the medication and consult an eye care practitioner. Allergic cross-reactions may occur with kanamycin, paromomycin, streptomycin, and possibly gentamicin.

PATIENT INFORMATION

• If the condition persists or gets worse or if a rash or allergic reaction develops, advise patients to stop use and consult an eye care practitioner. Instruct patients not to use this product if they are allergic to any of the listed ingredients.

PREGNANCY AND LACTATION

• Pregnancy Category C. Fetal harm is not known with topical administration. Excretion into human milk is not known.

bacitracin zinc; polymyxin B sulfate

(bah-cih-tray'-sin zink; pol-i-miks'-in bee sul'-fate)

Rx: AK-Poly-Bac, Polysporin Ophthalmic, Polytracin Ophthalmic

Drug Class: Anti-infectives, ophthalmic; Anti-infectives, topical; Dermatologics; Ophthalmics

Pregnancy Category: C

CLINICAL PHARMACOLOGY

Mechanism of Action: Bacitracin is an antibiotic that interferes with plasma membrane permeability in susceptible bacteria. Polymyxin B damages bacterial cytoplasmic membrane which causes leakage of intracellular components. *Therapeutic Effect:* Inhibits bacterial cell wall synthesis.

Pharmacokinetics

Not absorbed through topical administration.

AVAILABLE FORMS

• *Ointment, ophthalmic:* 500 units bacitracin, 10,000 units polymyxin B/g (AK-Poly-Bac, Polysporin Ophthalmic, Polytracin Ophthalmic).

INDICATIONS AND DOSAGES

Superficial ocular infections

Ophthalmic ointment

Adults. Instill ½-inch ribbon in the affected eyes every 3-4 hours for acute infections or 2-3 times/day for mild to moderate infections for 7-10 days.

CONTRAINDICATIONS: Hypersensitivity to bacitracin, polymyxin B, or any component of the formulation

INTERACTIONS

Drug

None known.

Herbal

None known.

Food

None known.

DIAGNOSTIC TEST EFFECTS: *None known.*

SIDE EFFECTS

Rare

Burning, itching, redness, swelling, pain.

SERIOUS REACTIONS

• Severe hypersensitivity reaction, including apnea and hypotension, occurs rarely.

SPECIAL CONSIDERATIONS

PRECAUTIONS

• Overgrowth of nonsusceptible organisms including fungi may occur. Bacterial resistance to bacitracin zinc and polymyxin B sulfate eye ointment also may develop. Allergic cross-reactions may occur with kanamycin, paromomycin, streptomycin, and possibly gentamicin.

PATIENT INFORMATION

• If the condition persists or worsens or if a rash or other allergic reaction develops, advise patients to stop use and consult an eye care practitioner. Instruct patients not to use this product if they are allergic to any of the listed ingredients.

PREGNANCY AND LACTATION

• Pregnancy Category C. Fetal harm is not known with topical administration. Excretion into human milk is not known.

bacitracin; hydrocortisone acetate; neomycin sulfate; polymyxin B sulfate

(bah-cih-tray'-sin; high-droe-core'-tah-sewn; nee-oh-mye'-sin; pol-i-miks'-in bee sul'-fate)

Rx: Cortisporin, Cortisporin Ophthalmic, Neotricin HC, Ocu-Cort

Drug Class: Anti-infectives, ophthalmic; Anti-infectives, topical; Dermatologics; Ophthalmics

Pregnancy Category: C

Do not confuse with Bactrim or Bactroban.

CLINICAL PHARMACOLOGY

Mechanism of Action: Bacitracin is an antibiotic that interferes with plasma membrane permeability in susceptible bacteria. Hydrocortisone is an adrenal corticosteroid that inhibits accumulation of inflammatory cells at inflammation sites, phagocytosis, lysosomal enzyme release and synthesis or release of mediators of inflammation. Polymyxin B damages bacterial cytoplasmic membrane which causes leakage of intracellular components. Neomycin is an aminoglycoside antibiotic that binds to the 30s subunit of the ribosome. *Therapeutic Effect:* Inhibits bacterial cell wall synthesis. Decreases or prevents tissue response to inflammatory process.

Pharmacokinetics

Not absorbed through topical administration. Neomycin and hydrocortisone may be absorbed following topical administration to the eye if tissue damage is present. Neomyin, polymyxin B, and hydrocortisone may be absorbed following topical application to the ear if eardrum perforation in present.

AVAILABLE FORMS

- *Ointment, ophthalmic:* 400 units bacitracin, 10 mg hydrocortisone, 3.5 mg neomycin, 10,000 units polymyxin B/g (Cortisporin Ophthalmic, Neotricin HC, Ocu-Cort).
- *Ointment, topical:* 400 units bacitracin, 10 mg hydrocortisone, 3.5 mg neomycin, 10,000 units polymyxin B/g (Cortisporin).

INDICATIONS AND DOSAGES

Superficial ocular infections

Ophthalmic

Adults. Apply ½-inch ribbon to inside of lower lid every 3-4 hrs until improvement occurs.

Skin abrasions, superficial skin infections

Topical

Adults. Apply 2-4 times/day to infected area and cover with sterile bandage as needed.

CONTRAINDICATIONS: Hypersensitivity to bacitracin, hydrocortisone, polymyxin B, neomycin, or any component of the formulation

INTERACTIONS

Drug

None known.

Herbal

None known.

Food

None known.

DIAGNOSTIC TEST EFFECTS: *None known.*

SIDE EFFECTS

Rare

Topical: Hypersensitivity reaction as evidenced by allergic contact dermatitis, burning, inflammation, and itching

Ophthalmic: Burning, itching, redness, swelling, pain

SERIOUS REACTIONS

- Severe hypersensitivity reaction, including apnea and hypotension, occurs rarely.

SPECIAL CONSIDERATIONS

PRECAUTIONS

- Fungal infections of the cornea may occur after prolonged corticosteroid dosing. If this drug combination is used for 10 days or longer, monitor intraocular pressure. Bacterial keratitis is associated with the use of topical drugs in multiple-dose containers. Allergic cross-reactions may occur with kanamycin, paromomycin, streptomycin, and possibly gentamicin.

PATIENT INFORMATION

- Instruct the patient to avoid allowing the tip of the dispensing container to contact the eye, eyelid, fingers, or any other surface. If the condition persists or gets worse or if a rash or allergic reaction develops, advise the patient to stop use and consult an eye care practitioner.

PREGNANCY AND LACTATION

- Pregnancy Category C. This drug combination is teratogenic in rabbits. Systemically administered corticosteroids appear in human milk.

balanced salt solution

Rx: B.S.S., BSS Plus, Endosol Extra
Drug Class: Ophthalmics

CLINICAL PHARMACOLOGY
Mechanism of Action: An irrigating solution that provides corneal detumescne and maintains corneal endothelial integrity during ocular perfusion. *Therapeutic Effect:* Inhibits symptoms associated with seasonal allergic rhinitis such as increased mucus production and sneezing.
Pharmacokinetics
None reported.

AVAILABLE FORMS
• *Ophthalmic Solution:* Balanced Salt Solution (B.S.S.), Balanced Salt Solution Plus (BSS Plus, Endosol Extra).

INDICATIONS AND DOSAGES
Intraocular irrigating solution during intraocular surgical procedures involving perfusion of the eye
Ophthalmic
Adults, Elderly. Based on standard for each surgical procedure.
Surgical procedures of the eyes, ears, nose, and/or throat
Irrigation
Adults, Elderly. Based on standard for each surgical procedure

CONTRAINDICATIONS: History of hypersensitivity to balanced salt solution or any component of the formulation

INTERACTIONS
Drug
None known.
Herbal
None known.
Food
None known.

DIAGNOSTIC TEST EFFECTS: *None known.*

SIDE EFFECTS
Rare
Bullous keratopathy, corneal clouding, corneal decompensation, corneal edema, corneal swelling, inflammatory reactions, lens changes

SERIOUS REACTIONS
• Epistaxis or nosebleed occurs rarely.

SPECIAL CONSIDERATIONS

PRECAUTIONS
• Discard unused contents. Do not use for more than one patient. Do not mix with additives. Corneal clouding or edema can occur following ocular surgery.

benazepril

(be-naze'a-pril)
Rx: Lotensin
Drug Class: Angiotensin converting enzyme inhibitors
Pregnancy Category: D
Do not confuse benazepril with Benadryl, or Lotensin with Loniten or lovastatin.

CLINICAL PHARMACOLOGY
Mechanism of Action: An ACE inhibitor that decreases the rate of conversion of angiotensin I to angiotensin II, a potent vasoconstrictor. Reduces peripheral arterial resistance. *Therapeutic Effect:* Lowers BP.
Pharmacokinetics

Route	*Onset*	*Peak*	*Duration*
PO	1 hr	2-4 hr	24 hr

Partially absorbed from the GI tract. Protein binding: 97%. Metabolized in the liver to active metabolite. Primarily excreted in urine. Minimal removal by hemodialysis. **Half-life:** 35 min; metabolite 10-11 hr.

AVAILABLE FORMS

• *Tablets:* 5 mg, 10 mg, 20 mg, 40 mg.

INDICATIONS AND DOSAGES

Hypertension (monotherapy)

PO

Adults. Initially, 10 mg/day. Maintenance: 20-40 mg/day as single or in 2 divided doses. Maximum: 80 mg/day.

Elderly. Initially, 5-10 mg/day. Range: 20-40 mg/day.

Hypertension (combination therapy)

PO

Adults. Discontinue diuretic 2-3 days prior to initiating benazepril, then dose as noted above. If unable to discontinue diuretic, begin benazepril at 5 mg/day.

Dosage in renal impairment

For adult patients with creatinine clearance less than 30 ml/min, initially, 5 mg/day titrated up to maximum of 40 mg/day.

UNLABELED USES: Treatment of CHF

CONTRAINDICATIONS: History of angioedema from previous treatment with ACE inhibitors

INTERACTIONS

Drug

Alcohol, antihypertensives, diuretics: May increase the effects of benazepril.

Lithium: May increase the lithium blood concentration and risk of lithium toxicity.

NSAIDs: May decrease the effects of benazepril.

Potassium-sparing diuretics, potassium supplements: May cause hyperkalemia.

Herbal

None known.

Food

None known.

DIAGNOSTIC TEST EFFECTS: May increase BUN, serum alkaline phosphatase, serum bilirubin, serum potassium, AST (SGOT), and ALT (SGPT) levels. May decrease serum sodium levels. May cause positive antinuclear antibody titer.

SIDE EFFECTS

Frequent (6%-3%)

Cough, headache, dizziness

Occasional (2%)

Fatigue, somnolence or drowsiness, nausea

Rare (less than 1%)

Rash, fever, myalgia, diarrhea, loss of taste

SERIOUS REACTIONS

• Excessive hypotension ("first-dose syncope") may occur in patients with CHF and in those who are severely salt or volume depleted.

• Angioedema (swelling of the face and lips) and hyperkalemia occur rarely.

• Agranulocytosis and neutropenia may be noted in those with collagen vascular disease, including scleroderma and systemic lupus erythematosus, and impaired renal function.

• Nephrotic syndrome may be noted in patients with history of renal disease.

SPECIAL CONSIDERATIONS

PRECAUTIONS

• As a consequence of inhibiting the renin-angiotensin-aldosterone system, changes in renal function may occur in susceptible individuals. Anaphylactoid reactions have been reported in patients dialyzed with high-flux membranes and treated concomitantly with a angiotensin-converting enzyme inhibitor. Hyperkalemia occurred in hypertensive patients receiving benazepril hydrochloride. Cough has been reported with the use of angiotensin-converting enzyme inhibitors.

PREGNANCY AND LACTATION

- Pregnancy Category C (first trimester) and D (second and third trimesters). Angiotensin-converting enzyme inhibitors can cause fetal and neonatal morbidity and death when administered to pregnant women. Minimal amounts of unchanged benazepril and of benazeprilat are excreted into the breast milk of lactating women.

benoxinate hydrochloride; fluorescein sodium

(be-nox'-in-ate hye-droe-klor'-ide; flure'-e-seen soe'-dee-um)

Rx: Flurate, Fluress, Flurox

Drug Class: Anesthetics, ophthalmic; Diagnostics, nonradioactive; Ophthalmics

CLINICAL PHARMACOLOGY

Mechanism of Action: A combination of a disclosing agent with an anesthetic agent. *Therapeutic Effect:* Local anesthetic effect and an indicator dye.

Pharmacokinetics

None reported.

AVAILABLE FORMS

- *Ophthalmic Solution:* 0.4%-0.25% (Flurate), 0.4%-0.25% (Flurox, Fluress).

INDICATIONS AND DOSAGES

Removal of foreign bodies and sutures, and for tonometry

Ophthalmic

Adults, Elderly, Children. Instill 1-2 drops in each eye before operating.

Deep ophthalmic anesthesia

Ophthalmic

Adults, Elderly, Children. 2 drops in each eye at 90-second intervals for 3 instillations.

CONTRAINDICATIONS: Hypersensitivity to benoxinate, fluorescein, or any component of the formulation

INTERACTIONS

Drug

None known.

Herbal

None known.

Food

None known.

DIAGNOSTIC TEST EFFECTS: *None known.*

SIDE EFFECTS

Occasional

Stinging, burning, redness

SERIOUS REACTIONS

- Hyperallergic corneal reaction with acute, intense and diffuse epithelial keratitis, a gray, ground glass appearance, sloughing or large areas of necrotic epithelium, corneal filaments and iritis with descemetitis occurs rarely.
- Allergic contact dermatitis with fissuring and dryness of the fingertips has been reported.

SPECIAL CONSIDERATIONS

PATIENT INFORMATION

- Prolonged use of a topical ocular anesthetic is not recommended. It may produce permanent corneal opacification with accompanying visual loss.

bepridil

(beh'prih-dill)

Rx: Vascor

Drug Class: Calcium channel blockers

Pregnancy Category: C

CLINICAL PHARMACOLOGY

Mechanism of Action: A calcium channel blocker that inhibits calcium ion entry across cell membranes of cardiac and vascular smooth muscle; decreases heart rate, myocardial contractility, slows SA and AV conduction. *Therapeutic Effect:* Dilates coronary arteries, peripheral arteries/arterioles.

Pharmacokinetics

Rapidly, completely absorbed from GI tract. Undergoes first-pass metabolism in liver to active metabolite. Primarily excreted in urine. Not removed by hemodialysis. **Half-life:** less than 24 hrs.

AVAILABLE FORMS

- *Tablets:* 200 mg, 300 mg (Vascor).

INDICATIONS AND DOSAGES

Chronic stable angina

PO

Adults, Elderly: Initially, 200 mg/day; after 10 days, dosage may be adjusted. Maintenance: 200-400 mg/day.

CONTRAINDICATIONS: Sick sinus syndrome/second- or third-degree AV block (except in presence of pacemaker), severe hypotension (<90 mm Hg, systolic), history of serious ventricular arrhythmias, uncompensated cardiac insufficiency, congenital QT interval prolongation, use with other drugs prolonging QT interval

INTERACTIONS

Drug

Beta-blockers: May have additive effect.

Digoxin: May increase digoxin concentration.

Procainamide, quinidine: May increase risk of QT interval prolongation.

Hypokalemia-producing agents: May increase risk of arrhythmias.

Herbal

None known.

Food

None known.

DIAGNOSTIC TEST EFFECTS: QT interval may be increased.

SIDE EFFECTS

Frequent

Dizziness, lightheadedness, nervousness, headache, asthenia (loss of strength), hand tremor, nausea, diarrhea

Occasional

Drowsiness, insomnia, tinnitus, abdominal discomfort, palpitations, dry mouth, shortness of breath, wheezing, anorexia, constipation

Rare

Peripheral edema, anxiety, flatulence, nasal congestion, paresthesia

SERIOUS REACTIONS

- CHF, second- and third-degree AV block occur rarely.
- Serious arrhythmias can be induced.
- Overdosage produces nausea, drowsiness, confusion, slurred speech, profound bradycardia.

SPECIAL CONSIDERATIONS

PRECAUTIONS

- Cases of torsades de pointes have developed in patients with hypokalemia, usually related to diuretic use or significant liver disease. Congestive heart failure has been observed infrequently. Hepatic enzyme elevation has been observed. Bepridil hydrochloride has not been reported to reduce serum potassium levels. Exercise caution when using bepridil hydrochloride in patients with left bundle branch block or sinus bradycardia. The initiation of bepridil hydrochloride therapy in patients with myocardial infarctions within 3 months before initiation of drug treatment cannot be recommended.

PATIENT INFORMATION

• Because Q-T interval prolongation is not associated with defined symptomatology, instruct patients on the importance of maintaining any potassium supplementation or potassium-sparing diuretic and the need for routine electrocardiograms and periodic monitoring of serum potassium. The following patient information is printed on the carton label of each unit or bottle of 30 tablets:

• As with any medication, patients should notify their physician of any changes in their overall condition. Patients should follow their physician's instructions regarding follow-up visits. Patients should notify any physician who treats them for a medical condition that they are taking bepridil hydrochloride, as well as any other medications.

PREGNANCY AND LACTATION

• Pregnancy Category C. Reduced litter size at birth and decreased pup survival during lactation were observed at maternal dosages 37 times the maximum daily recommended therapeutic dosage. Bepridil is excreted in human milk. Bepridil concentration in human milk is estimated to reach about one third the concentration in serum.

betaxolol

(bay-tax'oh-lol)

Rx: Betoptic, Betoptic S, Kerlone

Drug Class: Antiadrenergics, beta blocking; Ophthalmics

Pregnancy Category: C

Do not confuse betaxolol with bethanechol.

CLINICAL PHARMACOLOGY

Mechanism of Action: An antihypertensive and antiglaucoma agent that blocks $beta_1$-adrenergic receptors in cardiac tissue. Reduces aqueous humor production. *Therapeutic Effect:* Slows sinus heart rate, decreases BP and reduces intraocular pressure (IOP).

AVAILABLE FORMS

• *Tablets (Kerlone):* 10 mg, 20 mg.

• *Ophthalmic Solution (Betoptic-S):* 0.5%.

• *Ophthalmic Suspension (Betoptic-S):* 0.25%.

INDICATIONS AND DOSAGES

Hypertension

PO

Adults. Initially, 5-10 mg/day. May increase to 20 mg/day after 7-14 days.

Elderly. Initially, 5 mg/day.

Chronic open-angle glaucoma and ocular hypertension

Ophthalmic (Eye Drops)

Adults, Elderly. 1 drop twice a day.

Dosage in renal impairment

For adult and elderly patients who are on dialysis, initially give 5 mg/day; increase by 5 mg/day q2wk. Maximum: 20 mg/day.

UNLABELED USES: Treatment of angle-closure glaucoma during or after iridectomy, malignant glaucoma, secondary glaucoma; with miotics, to decrease IOP in acute and chronic angle-closure glaucoma

CONTRAINDICATIONS: Cardiogenic shock, overt cardiac failure, second- or third-degree heart block, sinus bradycardia

INTERACTIONS

Drug

Cimetidine: May increase betaxolol blood concentration.

Diuretics, other antihypertensives: May increase hypotensive effect of betaxolol.

Insulin, oral hypoglycemics: May prolong hypoglycemic effect of these drugs.

NSAIDs: May decrease antihypertensive effect.

Sympathomimetics, xanthines: May mutually inhibit hypotensive effects and may mask symptoms of hypoglycemia.

Herbal

None known.

Food

None known.

DIAGNOSTIC TEST EFFECTS: May increase serum antinuclear antibody titer and BUN, serum lipoprotein, creatinine, potassium, uric acid, and triglyceride levels.

SIDE EFFECTS

Betaxolol is generally well tolerated, with mild and transient side effects.

Frequent

Systemic: Hypotension manifested as dizziness, nausea, diaphoresis, headache, fatigue, constipation or diarrhea, dyspnea

Ophthalmic: Eye irritation, visual disturbances

Occasional

Systemic: Insomnia, flatulence, urinary frequency, impotence or decreased libido

Ophthalmic: Increased light sensitivity, watering of eye

Rare

Systemic: Rash, arrhythmias, arthralgia, myalgia, confusion, altered taste, increased urination

Ophthalmic: Dry eye, conjunctivitis, eye pain

SERIOUS REACTIONS

- Overdose may produce profound bradycardia, hypotension, and bronchospasm.
- Abrupt withdrawal may result in diaphoresis, palpitations, headache, and tremors.
- Betaxolol administration may precipitate CHF or MI in patients with cardiac disease; thyroid storm in those with thyrotoxicosis; and peripheral ischemia in those with existing peripheral vascular disease.
- Hypoglycemia may occur in patients with previously controlled diabetes.
- Ophthalmic overdose may produce bradycardia, hypotension, bronchospasm, and acute cardiac failure.

SPECIAL CONSIDERATIONS

PRECAUTIONS

- Diabetes Mellitus: Exercise caution in patients subject to spontaneous hypoglycemia or to diabetic patients (especially those with labile diabetes) who are receiving insulin or oral hypoglycemic agents.
- Thyrotoxicosis: Betaxolol hydrochloride may mask certain clinical signs (e.g., tachycardia) of hyperthyroidism. The drug may precipitate a thyroid storm.
- Muscle Weakness: Betaxolol hydrochloride can potentiate muscle weakness consistent with certain myasthenic symptoms (e.g., diplopia, ptosis, and generalized weakness).

• Major Surgery: Betaxolol hydrochloride reduces the ability of the heart to respond to beta-adrenergically medicated sympathetic reflex stimuli.
• Pulmonary: Asthmatic attacks and pulmonary distress may occur during betaxolol treatment.
• Ocular: For angle-closure glaucoma, betaxolol hydrochloride is used to reopen the angle by constriction of the pupil with a miotic agent. Betaxolol has little or no effect on the pupil.

PATIENT INFORMATION

• Instruct patients not to touch dropper tip to any surface, for this may contaminate the contents. Instruct patients not to use the drug with contact lenses in eyes.

PREGNANCY AND LACTATION

• Pregnancy Category C. Drug-related postimplantation loss has occurred in rabbits and rats. Betaxolol hydrochloride has not been shown to be teratogenic. Excretion into human milk is not known.

bimatoprost

(bi-mat'oh-prost)
Rx: Lumigan
Drug Class: Ophthalmics; Prostaglandins
Pregnancy Category: C

CLINICAL PHARMACOLOGY

Mechanism of Action: A synthetic analog of prostaglandin with ocular hypotensive activity. *Therapeutic Effect:* Reduces intraocular pressure (IOP) by increasing the outflow of aqueous humor.

Pharmacokinetics

Absorbed through the cornea and hydrolyzed to the active free acid form. Protein binding: 88%. Moderately distributed into body tissues. Metabolized in liver. Primarily excreted in urine; some elimination in feces. **Half-life:** 45 min.

AVAILABLE FORMS

• *Ophthalmic Solution:* 0.03% (Lumigan).

INDICATIONS AND DOSAGES

Glaucoma, ocular hypertension

Ophthalmic

Adults, Elderly. 1 drop in affected eye(s) once daily, in the evening.

CONTRAINDICATIONS: Hypersensitivity to bimatoprost or any other component of the formulation

INTERACTIONS

Drug

None known.

Herbal

None known.

Food

None known.

DIAGNOSTIC TEST EFFECTS: *None known.*

SIDE EFFECTS

Frequent

Conjunctival hyperemia, growth of eyelashes, and ocular pruritus

Occasional

Ocular dryness, visual disturbance, ocular burning, foreign body sensation, eye pain, pigmentation of the periocular skin, blepharitis, cataract, superficial punctate keratitis, eyelid erythema, ocular irritation, and eyelash darkening

Rare

Intraocular inflammation (iritis)

SERIOUS REACTIONS

• Systemic adverse events, including infections (colds and upper respiratory tract infections), headaches, asthenia, and hirsutism, have been reported.

SPECIAL CONSIDERATIONS

PRECAUTIONS

• Increased brown pigmentation of the iris may occur. Macular edema, including cystoid macular edema in aphakic and pseudophakic patients, may occur. Exercise caution with active intraocular inflammation (e.g., uveitis). Exercise caution with renal or hepatic impairment. Bimatoprost is not to be administered while the patient is wearing contact lenses.

PATIENT INFORMATION

• Increased growth and darkening of eyelashes and darkening of the iris and skin around the eye may occur in some patients. These changes may be permanent. When only one eye is treated, inform patients of the potential for a cosmetic difference between the eyes in eyelash length, darkness or thickness, and/or color changes of the eyelid skin or iris.

• Instruct patients to remove contact lenses before instillation and to reinsert them 15 minutes following drug administration. Solution contains benzalkonium chloride.

PREGNANCY AND LACTATION

• Pregnancy Category C. In pregnant mice and rats, abortion was observed at oral doses of bimatoprost. Fetal harm is not known with topical administration. In animal studies, bimatoprost has been shown to be excreted in breast milk.

bisoprolol fumarate

(bis-ope′pro-lal)

Rx: Zebeta

Drug Class: Antiadrenergics, beta blocking

Pregnancy Category: C

Do not confuse Zebeta with DiaBeta.

CLINICAL PHARMACOLOGY

Mechanism of Action: An antihypertensive that blocks beta$_1$-adrenergic receptors in cardiac tissue. *Therapeutic Effect:* Slows sinus heart rate and decreases BP.

Pharmacokinetics

Well absorbed from the GI tract. Protein binding: 26%-33%. Metabolized in the liver. Primarily excreted in urine. Not removed by hemodialysis. **Half-life:** 9-12 hr (increased in impaired renal function).

AVAILABLE FORMS

• *Tablets:* 5 mg, 10 mg.

INDICATIONS AND DOSAGES

Hypertension

PO

Adults. Initially, 5 mg/day. May increase up to 20 mg/day.

Elderly. Initially, 2.5-5 mg/day. May increase by 2.5-5 mg/day. Maximum: 20 mg/day.

Dosage in hepatic impairment

For adults and elderly patients with cirrhosis or hepatitis whose creatinine clearance is less than 40 ml/minute, initially give 2.5 mg.

UNLABELED USES: Angina pectoris, premature ventricular contractions, supraventricular arrhythmias

CONTRAINDICATIONS: Cardiogenic shock, overt cardiac failure, second- or third-degree heart block

INTERACTIONS

Drug

Cimetidine: May increase bisoprolol blood concentration.

Diuretics, other antihypertensives: May increase the hypotensive effect of bisoprolol.
Insulin, oral hypoglycemics: May mask symptoms of hypoglycemia and prolong the hypoglycemic effect of these drugs.
NSAIDs: May decrease antihypertensive effect.
Sympathomimetics, xanthines: May mutually inhibit effects.
Herbal
None known.
Food
None known.
DIAGNOSTIC TEST EFFECTS: May increase antinuclear antibody titer and BUN, serum lipoprotein, creatinine, potassium, uric acid, and triglyceride levels.
SIDE EFFECTS
Frequent
Hypotension manifested as dizziness, nausea, diaphoresis, headache, cold extremities, fatigue, constipation or diarrhea
Occasional
Insomnia, flatulence, urinary frequency, impotence or decreased libido
Rare
Rash, arthralgia, myalgia, confusion (especially in the elderly), altered taste
SERIOUS REACTIONS
• Overdose may produce profound bradycardia and hypotension.
• Abrupt withdrawal may result in diaphoresis, palpitations, headache, and tremulousness.
• Bisoprolol administration may precipitate CHF and MI in patients with heart disease; thyroid storm in those with thyrotoxicosis; and peripheral ischemia in those with existing peripheral vascular disease.
• Hypoglycemia may occur in patients with previously controlled diabetes.
• Thrombocytopenia, including unusual bruising and bleeding, occurs rarely.

SPECIAL CONSIDERATIONS

PRECAUTIONS
• Sympathetic stimulation is a vital component supporting circulatory function in the setting of congestive heart failure, and beta-blockade may result in further depression of myocardial contractility and precipitate more severe failure. Continued depression of the myocardium with beta-blockers can precipitate cardiac failure in some patients. Exacerbation of angina pectoris, and in some instances myocardial infarction or ventricular arrhythmia, has been observed in patients with coronary artery disease following abrupt cessation of therapy with beta-blockers. Beta-blockers can precipitate or aggravate symptoms of arterial insufficiency in patients with peripheral vascular disease. Because of its relative beta$_1$-selectivity, bisoprolol fumarate may be used with caution in patients with bronchospastic disease who do not respond to or who cannot tolerate other antihypertensive treatment. Take particular care when using anesthetic agents that depress myocardial function, such as ether, cyclopropane, and trichloroethylene. Beta-blockers may mask some of the manifestations of hypoglycemia, particularly tachycardia. Beta-adrenergic blockade may mask clinical signs of hyperthyroidism, such as tachycardia.
PATIENT INFORMATION
• Warn patients, especially those with coronary artery disease, about discontinuing use of bisoprolol fumarate without a physician's supervision. Also advise patients to consult a physician if any difficulty in

breathing occurs or if they develop signs or symptoms of congestive heart failure or excessive bradycardia.

• Caution patients subject to spontaneous hypoglycemia or diabetic patients receiving insulin or oral hypoglycemic agents that beta-blockers may mask some of the manifestations of hypoglycemia, particularly tachycardia, and to use bisoprolol fumarate with caution. Patients should know how they react to this medicine before they operate automobiles and machinery or engage in other tasks requiring alertness.

PREGNANCY AND LACTATION

• Pregnancy Category C. Fetal harm is not known. Small amounts of bisoprolol fumarate have been detected in the milk of lactating rats. Whether this drug is excreted in human milk is not known.

bisoprolol fumarate; hydrochlorothiazide

(bis-oh'-proe-lol fyoo'-muh-rate; hye-droe-klor-oh-thye'-a-zide)

Rx: Ziac

Drug Class: Antiadrenergics, beta blocking; Diuretics, thiazide and derivatives

Pregnancy Category: C

Do not confuse with Zantac.

CLINICAL PHARMACOLOGY

Mechanism of Action: Bisoprolol is an antihypertensive that blocks $beta_1$-adrenergic receptors in cardiac tissue. Hydrochlorothiazide is a sulfonamide derivative that acts as a thiazide diuretic and antihypertensive. As a diuretic, it blocks reabsorption of water and the electrolytes, sodium and potassium, at cortical diluting segment of distal tubule. As an antihypertensive, it reduces plasma, extracellular fluid volume, decreases peripheral vascular resistance (PVR) by direct effect on blood vessels. *Therapeutic Effect:* Slows sinus heart rate, decreases blood pressure (BP). Promotes diuresis.

Pharmacokinetics

Bisoprolol is well absorbed from the gastrointestinal (GI) tract. Protein binding: 26%-33%. Metabolized in liver. Primarily excreted in urine. Not removed by hemodialysis. **Half-life:** 9-12 hrs (half-life is increased in impaired renal function).

Hydrochlorothiazide is variably absorbed from the gastrointestinal (GI) tract. Primarily excreted unchanged in urine. Not removed by hemodialysis. **Half-life:** 5.6-14.8 hrs.

AVAILABLE FORMS

• *Tablets:* 2.5 mg bisoprolol fumarate/6.25 mg hydrochlorothiazide; 5 mg bisoprolol fumarate/6.25 mg hydrochlorothiazide; 10 mg bisoprolol fumarate/6.25 mg hydrochlorothiazide (Ziac).

INDICATIONS AND DOSAGES

Hypertension

PO

Adults, Elderly. Take 1 tablet daily.

CONTRAINDICATIONS: Cardiogenic shock, overt cardiac failure, second- or third-degree heart block, anuria, history of hypersensitivity to bisoprolol, hydrochlorothiazide, sulfonamides, or thiazide diuretics, renal decompensation

INTERACTIONS

Drug

Cholestyramine, colestipol: May decrease the absorption and effects of hydrochlorothiazide.

Cimetidine: May increase bisoprolol blood concentration.

Digoxin: May increase the risk of toxicity of digoxin caused by hypokalemia.

Diuretics, other hypotensives: May increase the hypotensive effect of bisoprolol.

Insulin, oral hypoglycemics: May mask symptoms of hypoglycemia and prolong the hypoglycemic effect of these drugs.

Lithium: May increase the risk of toxicity of lithium.

NSAIDs: May decrease antihypertensive effect.

Sympathomimetics, xanthines: May mutually inhibit effects.

Herbal

None known.

Food

None known.

DIAGNOSTIC TEST EFFECTS: May increase ANA titer, BUN and serum lipoproteins, creatinine, potassium, uric acid, and triglyceride levels, blood glucose levels, bilirubin, calcium, and triglyceride levels. May decrease urinary calcium, and serum magnesium, potassium, and sodium levels.

SIDE EFFECTS

Frequent

Hypotension manifested as dizziness, nausea, headache, cold extremities, fatigue, constipation or diarrhea, increase in urine frequency and volume, potassium depletion

Occasional

Insomnia, impotence or decreased libido, postural hypotension, headache, gastrointestinal (GI) disturbances, flatulence, photosensitivity reaction

Rare

Rash, arthralgia, myalgia, confusion (especially in the elderly), change in taste

SERIOUS REACTIONS

- Overdosage of bisoprolol may produce profound bradycardia and hypotension.
- Abrupt withdrawal may result in sweating, palpitations, headache, and tremulousness.
- May precipitate congestive heart failure (CHF) and myocardial infarction (MI) in patients with heart disease; thyroid storm in patients with thyrotoxicosis; and peripheral ischemia in patients with existing peripheral vascular disease.
- Overdosage of hydrochlorothiazide can lead to lethargy and coma without changes in electrolytes or hydration.
- Vigorous diuresis may lead to profound water loss and electrolyte depletion, resulting in hypokalemia, hyponatremia, and dehydration.
- Glucose levels may be altered.
- Thrombocytopenia, including unusual bruising and bleeding, occurs rarely.

SPECIAL CONSIDERATIONS

PRECAUTIONS

- Avoid beta-blocking agents in patients with overt congestive heart failure. Bisoprolol fumarate and hydrochlorothiazide may precipitate cardiac failure. Exacerbations of angina pectoris and myocardial infarction or ventricular arrhythmia have been observed in patients with coronary artery disease following abrupt cessation of therapy with beta-blockers. Beta-blockers can precipitate or aggravate symptoms of arterial insufficiency in patients with peripheral vascular disease. Patients with bronchospastic pulmonary disease should not receive beta-blockers. The drug combination may mask some of the manifestations of hypoglycemia, particularly tachycardia. The drug combination may mask signs of hyperthyroidism, such as tachycardia.

• Abrupt withdrawal of beta-blockade may be followed by an exacerbation of the symptoms of hyperthyroidism or may precipitate thyroid storm. Thiazides may precipitate azotemia in patients with impaired renal function. Use bisoprolol fumarate and hydrochlorothiazide with caution in patients with impaired hepatic function or progressive liver disease. Thiazides have been shown to increase the urinary excretion of magnesium; this may result in hypomagnesemia. Hyperuricemia or acute gout may be precipitated in certain patients receiving thiazide diuretics.

PATIENT INFORMATION

• Warn patients, especially those with coronary artery disease, against discontinuing use of bisoprolol fumarate without a physician's supervision. Also advise patients to consult a physician if any difficulty in breathing occurs or if they develop other signs or symptoms of congestive heart failure or excessive bradycardia.

• Caution patients subject to spontaneous hypoglycemia or diabetic patients receiving insulin or oral hypoglycemic agents that beta-blockers may mask some of the manifestations of hypoglycemia, particularly tachycardia, and to use bisoprolol fumarate with caution.

• Patients should know how they react to this medicine before they operate automobiles and machinery or engage in other tasks requiring alertness. Advise patients that photosensitivity reactions have been reported with use of thiazides.

botulinum toxin type A

(botch'-you-lin-em)

CLINICAL PHARMACOLOGY

Mechanism of Action: A neurotoxin that blocks neuromuscular conduction by binding to receptor sites on motor nerve endings, and inhibiting the release of acetylcholine, resulting in muscle denervation. *Therapeutic Effect:* Reduces muscle activity.

AVAILABLE FORMS

• *Injection:* 100 units/vial.

INDICATIONS AND DOSAGES

Cervical dystonia in patients who have previously tolerated botulinum toxin type A

IM

Adults, Elderly. Mean dose of 236 units (range: 198-300 units) divided among the affected muscles, based on patient's head and neck position, localization of pain, muscle hypertrophy, patient response, and adverse reaction history.

Cervical dystonia in patients who have not previously been treated with botulinum toxin type A

IM

Adults, Elderly. Administer at lower dosage than for patients who have previously tolerated the drug.

Strabismus

IM

Adults, Children older then 12 yr. 1.25-2.5 units into any one muscle.

Children 2 mo-12yr. 1-2.5 units into any one muscle.

Blepharospasm

IM

Adults. Initially, 1.25-2.5 units. May increase up to 2.5-5.0 units at repeat treatments. Maximum: 5 units per injection or cumulative dose of 200 units over a 30-day period.

Cerebral palsy spasticity

IM

Children older than 18 mo. 1-6 units/kg. Maximum: 50 units per injection site. No more than 400 units per visit or during a 3-month period.

Improvement of brow furrow

IM

Adults 65 yr and younger. Individualized.

UNLABELED USES: Treatment of dynamic muscle contracture in children with cerebral palsy, focal task-specific dystonia, head and neck tremor unresponsive to drug therapy, hemifacial spasms, laryngeal dystonia, oromandibular dystonia, spasmoditic torticollis, writer's cramp

CONTRAINDICATIONS: Infection at proposed injection sites

INTERACTIONS

Drug

Aminoglycoside antibiotics, other drugs that interfere with neuromuscular transmission (such as curare-like compounds): May potentiate the effects of botulinum toxin type A.

Herbal

None known.

Food

None known.

DIAGNOSTIC TEST EFFECTS: *None known.*

SIDE EFFECTS

Alert Side effects usually occur within the first week after injection.

Frequent (15%-11%)

Localized pain, tenderness, or bruising at injection site; localized weakness in injected muscle; upper respiratory tract infection; neck pain; headache

Occasional (10%-2%)

Increased cough, flu-like symptoms, back pain, rhinitis, dizziness, hypertonia, soreness at injection site, asthenia, dry mouth, nausea, somnolence

Rare

Stiffness, numbness, diplopia, ptosis

SERIOUS REACTIONS

- Mild to moderate dysphagia occurs in approximately 20% of patients.
- Arrhythmias and severe dysphagia (manifested as aspiration, pneumonia, and dyspnea) occur rarely.
- Overdose produces systemic weakness and muscle paralysis.

SPECIAL CONSIDERATIONS

PRECAUTIONS

- During the administration of botulinum toxin type A for the treatment of strabismus, retrobulbar hemorrhages sufficient to compromise retinal circulation have occurred from needle penetrations into the orbit. Having appropriate instruments on hand to decompress the orbit is recommended. Ocular (globe) penetrations by needles also have occurred. An ophthalmoscope to diagnose this condition should be available.
- Reduced blinking from botulinum toxin type A injection of the orbicularis muscle can lead to corneal exposure, persistent epithelial defect, and corneal ulceration, especially in patients with cranial nerve VII disorders. One case of corneal perforation in an aphakic eye requiring corneal grafting has occurred because of this effect. Carefully test corneal sensation in eyes previously operated upon, avoid injection into the lower lid area to avoid ectropion, and vigorously treat any epithelial defect. This may require protective drops, ointment, therapeutic soft

contact lenses, or closure of the eye by patching or other means.

PATIENT INFORMATION

• Patients with blepharospasm may have been extremely sedentary for a long time. Caution sedentary patients to resume activity slowly and carefully following the administration of botulinum toxin type A.

PREGNANCY AND LACTATION

• Pregnancy Category C. Fetal harm is not known. Excretion into human milk is not known.

OCULAR CONSIDERATIONS

• Ocular Adverse Reactions: Seven cases of diffuse skin rash and two cases of local swelling of the eyelid skin lasting for several days following eyelid injection have been reported.

• Strabismus: Inducing paralysis in one or more extraocular muscles may produce spatial disorientation, double vision, or past-pointing. Converting the affected eye may alleviate these symptoms. Extraocular muscles adjacent to the injection site are often affected, causing ptosis or vertical deviation, especially with higher doses of botulinum toxin type A. Incidence rates of these side effects for injections for horizontal strabismus are as follows: ptosis, 15.7%; and vertical deviation, 16.9%. The incidence of ptosis was much less after inferior rectus injection (0.9%) and much greater after superior rectus injection (37.7%).

• Blepharospasm: Incidence rates of adverse reactions per treated eye are as follows: ptosis, 11.0%; irritation/tearing, 10.0% (includes dry eye, lagophthalmos, and photophobia); ectropion, keratitis, diplopia, and entropion, reported rarely (incidence less than 1%).

OCULAR DOSAGE AND ADMINISTRATION

• Strabismus: Botulinum toxin type A is intended for injection into extraocular muscles using the electrical activity recorded from the tip of the injection needle as a guide to placement within the target muscle. An injection of botulinum toxin type A is prepared by drawing into a sterile 1.0-ml tuberculin syringe an amount of the properly diluted toxin slightly greater than the intended dose.

• Strabismus Dosage: The initial doses of diluted botulinum toxin type A typically create paralysis of injected muscles beginning 1 or 2 days after injection and increasing in intensity during the first week. The paralysis lasts for 2 to 6 weeks and gradually resolves over a similar period. Overcorrections lasting more than 6 months have been rare. About one half of patients will require subsequent doses because of the lack of binocular motor fusion to stabilize the alignment.

brimonidine

(bry-mo'nih-deen)

Rx: Alphagan-P

Drug Class: Adrenergic agonists; Ophthalmics

Pregnancy Category: B

Do not confuse with bromocriptine.

CLINICAL PHARMACOLOGY

Mechanism of Action: An ophthalmic agent that is a selective alpha$_2$-adrenergic agonist. *Therapeutic Effect:* Reduces intraocular pressure (IOP).

Pharmacokinetics

Plasma concentrations peak within 0.5 to 2.5 hours after ocular administration. Distributed into aqueous humor. Metabolized in liver. Primarily excreted in urine. **Half-life:** 3 hrs.

AVAILABLE FORMS

• *Ophthalmic Solution:* 0.15% (Alphagan P) [contains Purite 0.005% as preservative].

INDICATIONS AND DOSAGES

Glaucoma, ocular hypertension

Ophthalmic

Adults, Elderly, Children 2 yr and older. 1 drop in affected eye(s) 3 times/day.

CONTRAINDICATIONS: Concurrent use of monoamine oxidase (MAO) inhibitor therapy, hypersensitivity to brimonidine tartrate or any other component of the formulation

INTERACTIONS

Drug

Alcohol, CNS depressants: May increase the effect of brimonidine.

Alpha-agonists: May decrease pulse and blood pressure

Beta-blockers (ophthalmic and systemic), other antihypertensives, cardiac glycosides: May cause adverse effects.

Clonidine, tricyclic antidepressants: May blunt the hypotensive effect of these drugs.

MAOIs: May increase risk of hypertensive urgency or emergency.

Herbal

None known.

Food

None known.

DIAGNOSTIC TEST EFFECTS: *None known.*

SIDE EFFECTS

Occasional

Allergic conjunctivitis, conjunctival hyperemia, eye pruritus, burning sensation, conjunctival folliculosis, oral dryness, visual disturbances

SERIOUS REACTIONS

• Bradycardia, hypotension, iritis, miosis, skin reactions, including erythema, eyelid, pruritus, rash, and vasodilation, and tachycardia have been reported.

SPECIAL CONSIDERATIONS

PRECAUTIONS

• Severe cardiovascular disease is a contraindication. Exercise caution in patients with hepatic or renal impairment and patients with depression, cerebral or coronary insufficiency, Raynaud's phenomenon, orthostatic hypotension, or thromboangiitis obliterans.

PATIENT INFORMATION

• Benzalkonium chloride may be absorbed by soft contact lenses. Instruct patients to wait at least 15 minutes to insert soft contact lenses. Brimonidine tartrate may cause fatigue and/or drowsiness and a decrease in mental alertness.

PREGNANCY AND LACTATION

• Pregnancy Category B. In animal studies, brimonidine tartrate crossed the placenta and entered into the fetal circulation to a limited extent. In animal studies, brimonidine tartrate has been shown to be excreted in breast milk.

brinzolamide

(brin-zol'a-mide)

Rx: Azopt

Drug Class: Carbonic anhydrase inhibitors; Ophthalmics

Pregnancy Category: C

CLINICAL PHARMACOLOGY

Mechanism of Action: An ophthalmic agent that inhibits carbonic anhydrase. Decreases aqueous humor secretion. *Therapeutic Effect:* Reduces intraocular pressure (IOP).

Pharmacokinetics

Systemically absorbed to some degree. Protein binding: 60%. Distributed extensively in red blood cells. Sites of metabolism has not been established. Metabolized to active and inactive metabolites. Primarily excreted unchanged in urine.

AVAILABLE FORMS

- *Ophthalmic suspension:* 1% (Azopt).

INDICATIONS AND DOSAGES

Glaucoma, ocular hypertension

Ophthalmic

Adults, Elderly. Instill 1 drop in affected eye(s) 3 times/day.

CONTRAINDICATIONS: Hypersensitivity to brinzolamide or any other component of the formulation

INTERACTIONS

Drug

None known.

Herbal

None known.

Food

None known.

DIAGNOSTIC TEST EFFECTS: *None known.*

SIDE EFFECTS

Occasional

Blurred vision, bitter taste, dry eye, ocular discharge, ocular discomfort and pain, ocular pruritus, headache, rhinitis

Rare

Allergic reactions, alopecia, chest pain, conjunctivitis, diarrhea, diplopia, dizziness, dry mouth, dyspnea, dyspepsia, eye fatigue, hypertonia, keratoconjunctivitis, keratopathy, kidney pain, lid margin crusting or sticky sensation, nausea, pharyngitis, tearing, urticaria

SERIOUS REACTIONS

- Electrolyte imbalance, development of an acidotic state, and possible CNS effects may occur.

SPECIAL CONSIDERATIONS

PRECAUTIONS

- Brinzolamide is not recommended for severe renal impairment. Exercise caution in patients with hepatic impairment. Additive effects occur with oral carbonic anhydrase inhibitor. Concomitant administration is not recommended.

PATIENT INFORMATION

- Temporarily blurred vision may occur. Instruct patients to exercise care in operating machinery or driving a motor vehicle. Brimonidine tartrate may be absorbed by soft contact lenses. Instruct patients to reinsert contact lenses 15 minutes after instillation.

PREGNANCY AND LACTATION

- Pregnancy Category C. Maternal toxicity in rabbits and a significant increase in the number of fetal variations, such as accessory skull bones, have occurred. In rats, statistically decreased body weights of fetuses has occurred. Following oral administration to pregnant rats, brimonidine tartrate was found to cross the placenta and was present in the fetal tissues and blood. In lactating rats, decreases in body weight gain in offspring occur. Brimonidine tartrate was found in milk.

---

bromocriptine mesylate

(broe-moe-krip'teen)

Rx: Parlodel

Drug Class: Antiparkinson agents; Dopaminergics; Ergot alkaloids and derivatives

Pregnancy Category: B

Do not confuse bromocriptine with benztropine, or Parlodel with pindolol.

CLINICAL PHARMACOLOGY

Mechanism of Action: A dopamine agonist that directly stimulates dopamine receptors in the corpus striatum and inhibits prolactin secretion. Also suppresses secretion of growth hormone. *Therapeutic Effect:* Improves symptoms of parkinsonism, suppresses galactorrhea, and reduces serum growth hormone concentrations in acromegaly.

Pharmacokinetics

Indication	*Onset*	*Peak*	*Duration*
Prolactin lowering	2 hr	8 hr	24 hr
Antiparkinson	0.5-1.5 hr	2 hr	N/A
Growth hormone suppressant	1-2 hr	4-8 wk	4-8 hr

Minimally absorbed from the GI tract. Protein binding: 90%-96%. Metabolized in the liver. Excreted in feces by biliary secretion. **Half-life:** 15 hr.

AVAILABLE FORMS

- *Capsules:* 5 mg.
- *Tablets:* 2.5 mg.

INDICATIONS AND DOSAGES

Hyperprolactinemia

PO

Adults, Elderly. Initially, 1.25-2.5 mg/day. May increase by 2.5 mg/day at 3- to 7-day intervals. Range: 2.5 mg 2-3 times a day.

Parkinson's disease

PO

Adults, Elderly. Initially, 1.25 mg twice a day. May increase by 2.5 mg/day every 14-28 days. Range: 30-90 mg/day.

Acromegaly

PO

Adults, Elderly. Initially, 1.25-2.5 mg. May increase at 3- to 7-day intervals. Usual dose 20-30 mg/day.

UNLABELED USES: Treatment of cocaine addiction, hyperprolactinemia associated with pituitary adenomas, neuroleptic malignant syndrome

CONTRAINDICATIONS: Hypersensitivity to ergot alkaloids, peripheral vascular disease, pregnancy, severe ischemic heart disease, uncontrolled hypertension

INTERACTIONS

Drug

Alcohol: May produce a disulfiram-like reaction (chest pain, confusion, flushed face, nausea, vomiting).

Erythromycin, ritonavir: May increase bromocriptine blood concentration and risk of toxicity.

Estrogens, progestins: May decrease the effects of bromocriptine.

Haloperidol, MAOIs, phenothiazines, risperidone: May decrease bromocriptine's prolactin-lowering effect.

Hypotension-producing medications: May increase hypotension.

Levodopa: May increase the effects of bromocriptine.

Herbal

None known.

Food

None known.

DIAGNOSTIC TEST EFFECTS: May increase plasma growth hormone concentration.

SIDE EFFECTS

Frequent

Nausea (49%), headache (19%), dizziness (17%)

Occasional (7%-3%)

Fatigue, light-headedness, vomiting, abdominal cramps, diarrhea, constipation, nasal congestion, somnolence, dry mouth

Rare

Muscle cramps, urinary hesitancy

SERIOUS REACTIONS

• Visual or auditory hallucinations have been noted in patients with Parkinson's disease.

• Long-term, high-dose therapy may produce continuing rhinorrhea, syncope, GI hemorrhage, peptic ulcer, and severe abdominal pain.

SPECIAL CONSIDERATIONS

PRECAUTIONS

• Symptomatic hypotension can occur in patients treated with bromocriptine mesylate for any indication. Thirty cases of stroke have been reported, mostly in postpartum patients whose prenatal and obstetric courses had been uncomplicated. Many of these patients experienced seizures and/or strokes and were reported to have developed a constant and often progressively severe headache hours to days before the acute event. Some cases of strokes and seizures also were preceded by visual disturbances (blurred vision and transient cortical blindness). Nine cases of acute myocardial infarction have been reported.

• Safety and efficacy of bromocriptine mesylate have not been established in patients with renal or hepatic disease. Exercise care when administering bromocriptine mesylate therapy concomitantly with other medications known to lower blood pressure.

• Hyperprolactinemic States: The relative efficacy of bromocriptine mesylate versus surgery in preserving visual fields is not known. Patients with rapidly progressive visual field loss should be evaluated by a neurosurgeon to help decide on the most appropriate therapy. Because pregnancy is often the therapeutic objective in many hyperprolactinemic patients presenting with amenorrhea/galactorrhea and hypogonadism (infertility), a careful assessment of the pituitary is essential to detect the presence of a prolactin-secreting adenoma.

• Acromegaly: Cold-sensitive digital vasospasm has been observed in some acromegalic patients treated with bromocriptine mesylate. Possible tumor expansion while receiving bromocriptine mesylate therapy has been reported in a few patients.

• Parkinson's disease: Safety during long-term use for more than 2 years at the doses required for parkinsonism has not been established. As with any chronic therapy, periodic evaluation of hepatic, hematopoietic, cardiovascular, and renal function is recommended. Symptomatic hypotension can occur, and therefore caution should be exercised when treating patients receiving antihypertensive drugs. High doses of bromocriptine mesylate may be associated with confusion and mental disturbances. Because patients with parkinsonism may manifest mild degrees of dementia, use caution when treating such patients. Bromocriptine mesylate administered alone or concomitantly with levodopa may cause hallucinations (visual or auditory). As with levodopa, exercise caution when administering bromocriptine mesylate to patients with a history of myocardial infarction who have a residual atrial, nodal, or ventricular arrhythmia. Retroperitoneal fibrosis has been reported in a few patients receiving long-term therapy.

PATIENT INFORMATION

• When initiating therapy, caution all patients receiving bromocriptine mesylate regarding engaging in activities that require rapid and precise responses, such as driving an automobile or operating machinery, because dizziness (8% to 16%), drowsiness (8%), faintness and fainting (8%), and syncope (less than 1%) have been reported early in the course of therapy. Advise patients receiving bromocriptine mesylate for hyperprolactinemic states associated with macroadenoma or those who have had previous transsphenoidal surgery to report any persistent watery nasal discharge to their physician. Advise patients receiving bromocriptine mesylate for treatment of a macroadenoma that discontinuation of drug may be associated with rapid regrowth of the tumor and recurrence of their original symptoms.

PREGNANCY AND LACTATION

• Pregnancy Category B. If pregnancy occurs during bromocriptine mesylate administration, careful observation of these patients is mandatory. Prolactin-secreting adenomas may expand, and compression of the optic or other cranial nerves may occur, emergency pituitary surgery becoming necessary. In most cases, the compression resolves following delivery. Reinitiation of bromocriptine mesylate treatment has been reported to produce improvement in the visual fields of patients in whom nerve compression has occurred during pregnancy. The safety of bromocriptine mesylate treatment during pregnancy to the mother and fetus has not been established. Bromocriptine mesylate should not be used during lactation in postpartum women.

buclizine hydrochloride

(bew'-klih-zeen)

Drug Class: Anticholinergics; Antiemetics/antivertigo

Pregnancy Category: C

CLINICAL PHARMACOLOGY

Mechanism of Action: A centrally-acting agent that suppresses nausea and vomiting. Buclizine is an anticholinergic that reduces labyrinth excitability and diminishes vestibular stimulation of labyrinth, affecting chemoreceptor trigger zone (CTZ). Possesses anticholinergic activity. *Therapeutic Effect:* Reduces nausea, vomiting, vertigo.

Pharmacokinetics

None reported.

AVAILABLE FORMS

• *Tablets (softabs):* 50 mg (Bucladin-S).

INDICATIONS AND DOSAGES

Motion sickness

PO

Adults, Elderly, Children 12 yr and older. 50 mg thirty minutes before travel. Dose may be repeated every 4-6 hours as needed. Maximum: 150 mg/day.

CONTRAINDICATIONS: Early pregnancy, hypersensitivity to buclizine or other components of the formulation including tartrazine

INTERACTIONS

Drug

Alcohol, central nervous system (CNS) depression-producing medications: May increase CNS depressant effect.

Apomorphine: May decrease the emetic response of apomorphine.

Other anticholinergics: May potentiate anticholinergic effects.

Herbal

None known.

Food

None known.

DIAGNOSTIC TEST EFFECTS: May produce false-negative results using allergen extracts for skin tests.

SIDE EFFECTS

Frequent

Drowsiness

Occasional

Dryness of mouth, headache, jitteriness

SERIOUS REACTIONS

• Children may experience dominant paradoxical reaction, including restlessness, insomnia, euphoria, nervousness, and tremors.

• Overdosage in children may result in hallucinations, convulsions, and death.

• Hypersensitivity reaction, marked by eczema, pruritus, rash, cardiac disturbances, and photosensitivity, may occur.

• Overdosage may vary from CNS depression, such as sedation, apnea, cardiovascular collapse, or death, to severe paradoxical reaction, including hallucinations, tremor, or seizures.

SPECIAL CONSIDERATIONS

PRECAUTIONS

• This product contains FD&C yellow No. 5 (tartrazine), which may cause allergic-type reactions (including bronchial asthma) in certain susceptible individuals. Although the overall incidence of FD&C yellow No. 5 (tartrazine) sensitivity in the general population is low, it frequently occurs in patients who also have aspirin hypersensitivity.

PATIENT INFORMATION

• Because drowsiness may occur with use of this drug, warn patients of this possibility and caution them against engaging in activities requiring mental alertness, such as driving a car or operating heavy machinery or appliances. Safe and effective dosage in children has not been established.

PREGNANCY AND LACTATION

• Pregnancy Category C. Buclizine hydrochloride, when administered to the pregnant rat, induced fetal abnormalities at doses above the human therapeutic range.

• Clinical data are not adequate to establish nonteratogenicity in early pregnancy. Until such data are available, buclizine hydrochloride is contraindicated for use in early pregnancy. Fetal harm is not known with topical administration. Excretion into human milk is not known.

bupivacaine hydrochloride; lidocaine hydrochloride

(byoo-piv'a-kane; lye'doe-kane)

Rx: Duocaine

Drug Class: Anesthetics, local

Pregnancy Category: C

CLINICAL PHARMACOLOGY

Mechanism of Action: A combination of anesthetics that inhibits conduction of nerve impulses. *Therapeutic Effect:* Causes temporary loss of feeling and sensation.

Pharmacokinetics

The rate of systemic absorption of local anesthetics is dependent upon the total dose and concentration of drug administered.

AVAILABLE FORMS

• *Injection:* 0.375% bupivacaine hydrochloride/ 1% lidocaine hydrochloride (Duocaine).

INDICATIONS AND DOSAGES

Production of local or regional anesthesia for ophthalmologic surgery by peripheral nerve block techniques

Injection, retrobulbar and facial blocks

Adults, Elderly, Children 12 yr and older. Inject 2-5 ml (20-50 mg of lidocaine and 7-18 mg of bupivacaine). A portion of the dose in injected retrobulbarly and the remainder may be used to block facial nerve.

Injection, peribulbar block

Adults, Elderly, Children 12 yr and older. Inject 6-12 ml (60-120 mg of lidocaine and 22-45 mg of bupivacaine).

CONTRAINDICATIONS: Stokes-Adams syndrome, Wolff-Parkinson-White syndrome, severe degrees of sinoatrial atrioventricular, intraventricular block in the absence of an artificial pacemaker, hypersensitivity to lidocaine or bupivacaine or any local anesthetic agent of the amide type or to other components of lidocaine and/or bupivacaine solutions

INTERACTIONS

Drug

Beta-blockers: May decrease hepatic blood flow and reduce lidocaine clearance.

MAOIs, tricyclic antidepressants: May produce severe, prolonged hypertension.

Phenothiazine, butyrophenone: May decrease or reverse the pressor effect.

Tocainide: May increase risk of adverse reactions, including CNS adverse reactions including seizures.

Vasopressors, ergot-type oxytocic drugs: May cause severe, persistent hypertension or cerebrovascular accidents.

Herbal

None known.

Food

None known.

DIAGNOSTIC TEST EFFECTS: *None known.*

SIDE EFFECTS

Occasional

Anxiety, restlessness, blurred vision, confusion, difficulty breathing, dizziness, drowsiness, irregular heartbeat, nausea, vomiting, seizures, skin rash, itching, swelling of face or mouth, tremors

SERIOUS REACTIONS

• Repeated doses may cause a slow accumulation of the drug and its metabolites.

• Early warning signs of CNS toxicity are blurred vision, tremors, depression or drowsiness, restlessness, anxiety, tinnitus, and dizziness.

SPECIAL CONSIDERATIONS

OCULAR CONSIDERATIONS

• Topical anesthesia with preservative-free 2% lidocaine drops has been used successfully in clear corneal phacoemulsification with intraocular lens implantation. (Chuang LH et al: Efficacy and safety of phacoemulsification with intraocular lens implantation under topical anesthesia, *Chang Gung Med J* 27[8]:609, 2004.)

bupropion

(byoo-proe'pee-on)

Rx: Wellbutrin, Wellbutrin SR, Wellbutrin XL, Zyban SR, Zyban SR Refill

Drug Class: Antidepressants, miscellaneous

Pregnancy Category: B

Do not confuse bupropion with buspirone, Wellbutrin with Wellcovorin or Wellferon, or Zyban with Zagam.

CLINICAL PHARMACOLOGY

Mechanism of Action: An aminoketone that blocks the reuptake of neurotransmitters, including serotonin and norepinephrine at CNS presynaptic membranes, increasing their availability at postsynaptic receptor sites. Also reduces the firing rate of noradrenergic neurons. *Therapeutic Effect:* Relieves depression and nicotine withdrawal symptoms.

Pharmacokinetics

Rapidly absorbed from the GI tract. Protein binding: 84%. Crosses the blood-brain barrier. Undergoes extensive first-pass metabolism in the liver to active metabolite. Primarily excreted in urine. **Half-life:** 14 hr.

AVAILABLE FORMS

- *Tablets (Wellbutrin):* 75 mg, 100 mg.
- *Tablets (Extended-Release [Wellbutrin XL]):* 150 mg, 300 mg.
- *Tablets (Sustained-Release [Wellbutrin SR]):* 100 mg, 150 mg, 200 mg.
- *Tablets (Sustained-Release [Zyban]):* 150 mg.

INDICATIONS AND DOSAGES

Depression

PO (Immediate-Release)

Adults. Initially, 100 mg twice a day. May increase to 100 mg 3 times a day no sooner than 3 days after beginning therapy. Maximum: 450 mg/day.

Elderly. 37.5 mg twice a day. May increase by 37.5 mg q3-4 days. Maintenance: Lowest effective dosage.

PO (Sustained-Release)

Adults. Initially, 150 mg/day as a single dose in the morning. May increase to 150 mg twice a day as early as day 4 after beginning therapy. Maximum: 400 mg/day.

Elderly. 50-100 mg/day. May increase by 50-100 mg/day q3-4 days. Maintenance: Lowest effective dosage.

PO (Extended-Release)

Adults. 150 mg once a day. May increase to 300 mg once a day. Maximum: 450 mg a day.

Smoking cessation

PO

Adults. Initially, 150 mg a day for 3 days; then 150 mg twice a day for 7-12 wk.

UNLABELED USES: Treatment of attention deficit hyperactivity disorder in adults and children

CONTRAINDICATIONS: Current or prior diagnosis of anorexia nervosa or bulimia, seizure disorder, use within 14 days of MAOIs.

INTERACTIONS

Drug

Alcohol, lithium, ritonavir, trazodone, tricyclic antidepressants: May increase the risk of seizures.

MAOIs: May increase the risk of neuroleptic malignant syndrome and acute bupropion toxicity.

Herbal

None known.

Food

None known.

DIAGNOSTIC TEST EFFECTS: May decrease serum WBC count.

SIDE EFFECTS

Frequent (32%-18%)

Constipation, weight gain or loss, nausea, vomiting, anorexia, dry mouth, headache, diaphoresis, tremor, sedation, insomnia, dizziness, agitation

Occasional (10%-5%)

Diarrhea, akinesia, blurred vision, tachycardia, confusion, hostility, fatigue

SERIOUS REACTIONS

• The risk of seizures increases in patients taking more than 150 mg/dose of bupropion, in patients with a history of bulimia or seizure disorders and in patients discontinuing drugs that may lower the seizure threshold.

SPECIAL CONSIDERATIONS

PRECAUTIONS

• Bupropion is associated with a dose-related risk of seizures. Use bupropion with extreme caution in patients with severe hepatic cirrhosis. In rats receiving large doses of bupropion chronically, there was an increase in incidence of hepatic hyperplastic nodules and hepatocellular hypertrophy. A substantial proportion of patients treated with Wellbutrin experience some degree of increased restlessness, agitation, anxiety, and insomnia. Patients treated with Zyban experienced insomnia. Antidepressants can precipitate manic episodes in bipolar manic-depressive patients during the depressed phase of their illness and may activate latent psychosis in other susceptible patients. A weight loss occurred patients receiving Wellbutrin. The possibility of a suicide attempt is inherent in depression and may persist until significant remission occurs. Anaphylactoid/anaphylactic reactions characterized by symptoms such as pruritus, urticaria, angioedema, and dyspnea and requiring medical treatment have been reported. Hypertension has been reported in patients receiving bupropion alone and in combination with nicotine replacement therapy. Use Wellbutrin with extreme caution in patients with severe hepatic cirrhosis.

PATIENT INFORMATION

• Make patients aware that Zyban, used as an aid to smoking cessation, contains the same active ingredient found in Wellbutrin and Wellbutrin SR used to treat depression and that Zyban should not be used along with Wellbutrin, Wellbutrin SR, or any other medications that contain bupropion hydrochloride.

• Instruct patients to take Wellbutrin in equally divided doses 3 or 4 times a day to minimize the risk of seizure. As dose is increased during initial titration to doses greater than 150 mg/day, instruct patients to take Wellbutrin SR tablets in two divided doses, preferably with at least 8 hours between successive doses, to minimize the risk of seizures. Advise patients that any central nervous system–active drug such as bupropion hydrochloride may impair their ability to perform tasks requiring judgment or motor and cognitive skills. Consequently, until patients are reasonably certain that bupropion hydrochloride does not adversely affect their performance, they should refrain from driving an automobile or operating complex, hazardous machinery. Advise patients that the use and the cessation of use of alcohol may alter seizure threshold and therefore to minimize the consumption of alcohol and, if possible, to avoid it completely. Advise patients to inform their physicians if they are taking or plan to take any prescription or over-the-counter drugs. Concern is warranted because bupropion hydrochloride and other drugs may affect each other's metabolism. Advise patients to notify their physicians if they become pregnant or intend to become pregnant during therapy. Advise patients to swallow Wellbutrin SR tablets whole so that the release rate is not altered. Instruct patients not to chew, divide, or crush tablets.

PREGNANCY AND LACTATION

• Pregnancy Category B. Reproduction studies performed in rabbits and rats revealed no definitive evidence of impaired fertility or harm to the fetus from bupropion. Like many other drugs, bupropion and its metabolites are secreted in human milk.

OCULAR CONSIDERATIONS

• Adverse reactions for Wellbutrin include accomodation abnormality and dry eye (infrequent). Also observed were diplopia and mydriasis.

• Adverse reactions for Zyban include amblyopia (frequent) and accomodation abnormality and dry eye (infrequent). Also observed were diplopia and mydriasis.

buspirone hydrochloride

(byoo-spir'own)

Rx: BuSpar, BuSpar Dividose

Drug Class: Anxiolytics

Pregnancy Category: B

Do not confuse buspirone with bupropion.

CLINICAL PHARMACOLOGY

Mechanism of Action: Although its exact mechanism of action is unknown, this nonbarbiturate is thought to bind to serotonin and dopamine receptors in the CNS. The drug may also increase norepinephrine metabolism in the locus ceruleus. *Therapeutic Effect:* Produces anxiolytic effect.

Pharmacokinetics

Rapidly and completely absorbed from the GI tract. Protein binding: 95%. Undergoes extensive first-pass metabolism. Metabolized in the liver to active metabolite. Primarily excreted in urine. Not removed by hemodialysis. **Half-life:** 2-3 hr.

AVAILABLE FORMS

• *Tablets:* 5 mg, 7.5 mg, 10 mg, 15 mg, 30 mg.

INDICATIONS AND DOSAGES

Short-term management (up to 4 weeks) of anxiety disorders

PO

Adults. 5 mg 2-3 times a day or 7.5 mg twice a day. May increase by 5 mg/day every 2-4 days. Maintenance: 15-30 mg/day in 2-3 divided doses. Maximum: 60 mg/day.

Elderly. Initially, 5 mg twice a day. May increase by 5 mg/day every 2-3 days. Maximum: 60 mg/day.

Children. Initially, 5 mg/day. May increase by 5 mg/day at weekly intervals. Maximum: 60 mg/day.

UNLABELED USES: Management of panic attack, premenstrual syndrome (aches, pain, fatigue, irritability)

CONTRAINDICATIONS: Concurrent use of MAOIs, severe hepatic or renal impairment

INTERACTIONS

Drug

Alcohol, other CNS depressants: Potentiates effects of buspirone and may increase sedation.

Erythromycin, itraconazole: May increase buspirone blood concentration and risk of toxicity.

MAOIs: May increase BP.

Herbal

Kava kava: May increase sedation.

Food

Grapefruit, grapefruit juice: May increase buspirone blood concentration and risk of toxicity.

DIAGNOSTIC TEST EFFECTS: *None known.*

SIDE EFFECTS

Frequent (12%-6%)

Dizziness, somnolence, nausea, headache

Occasional (5%-2%)

Nervousness, fatigue, insomnia, dry mouth, lightheadedness, mood swings, blurred vision, poor concentration, diarrhea, paraesthesia

Rare

Muscle pain and stiffness, nightmares, chest pain, involuntary movements

SERIOUS REACTIONS

• Buspirone does not appear to cause drug tolerance, psychological or physical dependence, or withdrawal syndrome.

SPECIAL CONSIDERATIONS

PRECAUTIONS

• Reports indicate elevated blood pressure with use of monoamine oxidase inhibitors. Caution patients about operating an automobile or using complex machinery until they are reasonably certain that buspirone treatment does not affect them adversely.

PATIENT INFORMATION

To ensure safe and effective use of buspirone hydrochloride, give the following information and instructions to patients:

• Inform your physician about any medications, prescription or nonprescription, alcohol, or drugs that you are taking now or plan to take during your treatment with buspirone hydrochloride.

• Inform your physician if you are pregnant, or if you are planning to become pregnant, or if you become pregnant while you are taking buspirone hydrochloride.

• Inform your physician if you are breast-feeding an infant.

• Until you experience how this medication affects you, do not drive a car or operate potentially dangerous machinery.

PREGNANCY AND LACTATION

• Pregnancy Category B. No fertility impairment or fetal damage in rats and rabbits has been observed. Fetal harm is not known. Excretion into human milk is not known.

OCULAR CONSIDERATIONS

• Overdose may produce severe nausea, vomiting, dizziness, drowsiness, abdominal distention, and excessive pupil contraction.

calcipotriene

(kal-sip′oh-tri-een)

Rx: Dovonex

Drug Class: Dermatologics

Pregnancy Category: C

CLINICAL PHARMACOLOGY

Mechanism of Action: A synthetic vitamin D3 analogue that regulates skin cell (keratinocyte) production and development. *Therapeutic Effect:* preventing abnormal growth and production of psoriasis (abnormal keratinocyte growth).

Pharmacokinetics

Minimal absorption through intact skin. Metabolized in liver.

AVAILABLE FORMS

• *Cream:* 0.005% (Dovonex).

• *Ointment:* 0.005% (Dovonex).

• *Topical Solution:* 0.005% (Dovonex).

INDICATIONS AND DOSAGES

Psoriasis

Topical

Adults, Elderly, Children 12 yr and older. Apply thin layer to affected skin twice daily (morning and evening); rub in gently and completely.

Scalp psoriasis

Topical Solution

Adults, Elderly, Children 12 yr and older. Apply to lesions after combing hair.

CONTRAINDICATIONS: Hypercalcemia or evidence of vitamin D toxicity, use on face, hypersensitivity to calcipotriene or any component of the formulation

INTERACTIONS

Drug

None known.

Herbal

None known.

Food

None known.

DIAGNOSTIC TEST EFFECTS: Excessive use may increase serum calcium level.

SIDE EFFECTS

Frequent

Burning, itching, skin irritation

Occasional

Erythema, dry skin, peeling, rash, worsening of psoriasis, dermatitis

Rare

Skin atrophy, hyperpigmentation, folliculitis

SERIOUS REACTIONS

- Potential for hypercalcemia may occur.

SPECIAL CONSIDERATIONS

PRECAUTIONS

- Calcipotriene may cause transient irritation of lesions and surrounding uninvolved skin. Reversible elevation of serum calcium has occurred with use of calcipotriene cream. If elevation in serum calcium outside the normal range should occur, discontinue treatment until normal calcium levels are restored.

PATIENT INFORMATION

Give patients the following instructions:

- This medication is to be used as directed by the physician. It is for external use only. Avoid contact with the face or eyes. As with any topical medication, patients should wash hands after application.
- This medication should not be used for any disorder other than that for which it was prescribed.
- Patients should report to their physician any signs of adverse reactions.

PREGNANCY AND LACTATION

- Pregnancy Category C. In a rat study, oral doses resulted in a significantly higher incidence of skeletal abnormalities consisting primarily of enlarged fontanelles and extra ribs. Fetal harm is not known. Calcipotriene may enter the fetal circulation, but whether it is excreted in human milk is not known.

candesartan cilexetil

(kan-de-sar'-tan)

Rx: Atacand

Drug Class: Angiotensin II receptor antagonists

Pregnancy Category: C, 1st; D, 2nd / 3rd

CLINICAL PHARMACOLOGY

Mechanism of Action: An angiotensin II receptor, type AT_1, antagonist that blocks the vasoconstrictor and aldosterone-secreting effects of angiotensin II, inhibiting the binding of angiotensin II to the AT_1 receptors. *Therapeutic Effect:* Causes vasodilation, decreases peripheral resistance, and decreases BP.

Pharmacokinetics

Route	*Onset*	*Peak*	*Duration*
PO	2-3 hr	6-8 hr	Greater than 24 hr

Rapidly, completely absorbed. Protein binding: greater than 99%. Undergoes minor hepatic metabolism to inactive metabolite. Excreted unchanged in urine and in the feces through the biliary system. Not removed by hemodialysis. **Half-life:** 9 hr.

AVAILABLE FORMS

- *Tablets:* 4 mg, 8 mg, 16 mg, 32 mg.

INDICATIONS AND DOSAGES

Hypertension alone or in combination with other antihypertensives

PO

Adults, Elderly, Patients with mildly impaired liver or renal function. Initially, 16 mg once a day in those who are not volume depleted. Can be given once or twice a day with total daily doses of 8-32 mg. Give lower dosage in those treated with diuretics or with severely impaired renal function.

UNLABELED USES: Treatment of heart failure

CONTRAINDICATIONS: Hypersensitivity to candesartan

INTERACTIONS

Drug

None known.

Herbal

None known.

Food

None known.

DIAGNOSTIC TEST EFFECTS: May increase BUN, serum alkaline phosphatase, serum bilirubin, serum creatinine, AST (SGOT), and ALT (SGPT) levels. May decrease blood Hgb and Hct levels.

SIDE EFFECTS

Occasional (6%-3%)

Upper respiratory tract infection, dizziness, back and leg pain

Rare (2%-1%)

Pharyngitis, rhinitis, headache, fatigue, diarrhea, nausea, dry cough, peripheral edema

SERIOUS REACTIONS

- Overdosage may manifest as hypotension and tachycardia. Bradycardia occurs less often. Institute supportive measures.

SPECIAL CONSIDERATIONS

PRECAUTIONS

- Anticipate changes in renal function in susceptible individuals treated with candesartan cilexetil. In studies of angiotensin-converting enzyme (ACE) inhibitors in patients with unilateral or bilateral renal artery stenosis, increases in serum creatinine or blood urea nitrogen have been reported.

PATIENT INFORMATION

- Pregnancy: Advise female patients of childbearing age about the consequences of second- and third-trimester exposure to drugs that act on the renin-angiotensin system, and advise them that these consequences do not appear to have resulted from intrauterine drug exposure that has been limited to the first trimester. Ask these patients to report pregnancies to their physicians as soon as possible.

PREGNANCY AND LACTATION

- Pregnancy Categories C (first trimester) and D (second and third trimesters). The use of drugs that act directly on the renin-angiotensin system during the second and third trimesters of pregnancy has been associated with fetal and neonatal injury, including hypotension, neonatal skull hypoplasia, anuria, reversible or irreversible renal failure, and death. Whether candesartan is excreted in human milk is not known, but candesartan has been shown to be present in rat milk.

capsaicin

(cap-say'sin)

Drug Class: Analgesics, topical; Dermatologics

Do not confuse with Zovirax.

CLINICAL PHARMACOLOGY

Mechanism of Action: A topical analgesic that depletes and prevents reaccumulation of the chemomediator of pain impulses (substance P) from peripheral sensory neurons to CNS. *Therapeutic Effect:* Relieves pain.

Pharmacokinetics

None reported.

AVAILABLE FORMS

- *Cream:* 0.025%, 0.075% (Zostrix).

INDICATIONS AND DOSAGES

Treatment of neuralgia, osteoarthritis, rheumatoid arthritis

Topical

Adults, Elderly, Children older than 2 yr. Apply directly to affected area 3-4 times/day. Continue for 14 to 28 days for optimal clinical response.

UNLABELED USES: Treatment of neurogenic pain

CONTRAINDICATIONS: Hypersensitivity to capsaicin or any component of the formulation

INTERACTIONS

Drug

Anticoagulants, antiplatelet agents, low molecular weight heparins, thrombolytic agents: May increase risk of bleeding.

Herbal

None known.

Food

None known.

DIAGNOSTIC TEST EFFECTS: *None known.*

SIDE EFFECTS

Frequent

Burning, stinging, erythema at site of application

SERIOUS REACTIONS

- None known.

SPECIAL CONSIDERATIONS

PRECAUTIONS

- Instruct patients that if capsaicin gets into their eyes that it will cause a burning sensation and that they should flush their eyes with water.

PREGNANCY AND LACTATION

- There are no reports of birth defects in human beings. Whether capsaicin passes into breast milk is not known.

OCULAR CONSIDERATIONS

- Capsaicin is used to help relieve neuralgia and pain from osteoarthritis, rheumatoid arthritis, or herpes zoster. (MedlinePlus: Capsaicin [topical]. Retrieved May 16, 2004, from http://www.nlm.nih.gov/medlineplus/druginfo/uspdi/202626.html.)

captopril

(cap'-toe-pril)

Rx: Capoten

Drug Class: Angiotensin converting enzyme inhibitors

Pregnancy Category: C

Do not confuse captopril with Capitrol.

CLINICAL PHARMACOLOGY

Mechanism of Action: An ACE inhibitor that suppresses the renin-angiotensin-aldosterone system and prevents conversion of angiotensin I to angiotensin II, a potent vasoconstrictor; may also inhibit angiotensin II at local vascular and renal sites. Decreases plasma angiotensin

II, increases plasma renin activity, and decreases aldosterone secretion. *Therapeutic Effect:* Reduces peripheral arterial resistance, pulmonary capillary wedge pressure; improves cardiac output and exercise tolerance.

Pharmacokinetics

Route	Onset	Peak	Duration
PO	0.25 hr	0.5-1.5 hr	Dose-related

Rapidly, well absorbed from the GI tract (absorption is decreased in the presence of food). Protein binding: 25%-30%. Metabolized in the liver. Primarily excreted in urine. Removed by hemodialysis. **Half-life:** less than 3 hr (increased in those with impaired renal function).

AVAILABLE FORMS

• *Tablets:* 12.5 mg, 25 mg, 50 mg, 100 mg.

INDICATIONS AND DOSAGES

Hypertension

PO

Adults, Elderly. Initially, 12.5-25 mg 2-3 times a day. After 1-2 wk, may increase to 50 mg 2-3 times a day. Diuretic may be added if no response in additional 1-2 wk. If taken in combination with diuretic, may increase to 100-150 mg 2-3 times a day after 1-2 wk. Maintenance: 25-150 mg 2-3 times a day. Maximum: 450 mg/day.

CHF

PO

Adults, Elderly. Initially, 6.25-25 mg 3 times a day. Increase to 50 mg 3 times a day. After at least 2 wk, may increase to 50-100 mg 3 times a day. Maximum: 450 mg/day.

Post-myocardial infarction, impaired liver function

PO

Adults, Elderly. 6.25 mg a day, then 12.5 mg 3 times a day. Increase to 25 mg 3 times a day over several days up to 50 mg 3 times a day over several weeks.

Diabetic nephropathy prevention of kidney failure

PO

Adults, Elderly. 25 mg 3 times a day.

Children. Initially 0.3-0.5 mg/kg/dose titrated up to a maximum of 6 mg/kg/day in 2-4 divided doses.

Neonates. Initially, 0.05-0.1 mg/kg/dose q8-24h titrated up to 0.5 mg/kg/dose given q6-24h.

Dosage in renal impairment

Creatinine clearance 10-50 ml/min. 75% of normal dosage.

Creatinine clearance less than 10 ml/min. 50% of normal dosage.

UNLABELED USES: Diagnosis of anatomic renal artery stenosis, hypertensive crisis, rheumatoid arthritis

CONTRAINDICATIONS: History of angioedema from previous treatment with ACE inhibitors

INTERACTIONS

Drug

Alcohol, antihypertensives, diuretics: May increase the effects of captopril.

Lithium: May increase lithium blood concentration and risk of lithium toxicity.

NSAIDs: May decrease the effects of captopril.

Potassium-sparing diuretics, potassium supplements: May cause hyperkalemia.

Herbal

None known.

Food

All food: Food significantly reduces drug absorption by 30% to 40%.

DIAGNOSTIC TEST EFFECTS: May increase BUN, serum alkaline phosphatase, serum bilirubin, serum creatinine, serum potassium, AST (SGOT), and ALT (SGPT) levels. May decrease serum sodium levels. May cause positive antinuclear antibody titer.

SIDE EFFECTS

Frequent (7%-4%)

Rash

Occasional (4%-2%)

Pruritus, dysgeusia (altered taste)

Rare (less than 2%-0.5%)

Headache, cough, insomnia, dizziness, fatigue, paraesthesia, malaise, nausea, diarrhea or constipation, dry mouth, tachycardia

SERIOUS REACTIONS

- Excessive hypotension ("first-dose syncope") may occur in patients with CHF and in those who are severely salt and volume depleted.
- Angioedema (swelling of face and lips) and hyperkalemia occur rarely.
- Agranulocytosis and neutropenia may be noted in those with collagen vascular disease, including scleroderma and systemic lupus erythematosus, and impaired renal function.
- Nephrotic syndrome may be noted in those with history of renal disease.

SPECIAL CONSIDERATIONS

PRECAUTIONS

- Patients with renal disease have developed increases in blood urea nitrogen and serum creatinine after reduction of blood pressure with captopril. Patients at risk for the development of hyperkalemia include those with renal insufficiency and diabetes mellitus and those using concomitant potassium-sparing diuretics, potassium supplements or potassium-containing salt substitutes or other drugs associated with increases in serum potassium. Persistent nonproductive cough has been reported with all ACE inhibitors. Patients with aortic stenosis might be at particular risk of decreased coronary perfusion when treated with vasodilators.

PATIENT INFORMATION

- Advise patients to report to their physician immediately any signs or symptoms suggesting angioedema (e.g., swelling of face, eyes, lips, tongue, larynx and extremities; difficulty in swallowing or breathing; hoarseness) and to discontinue therapy. Instruct patients to report promptly any indication of infection (e.g., sore throat, fever), which may be a sign of neutropenia, or of progressive edema, which might be related to proteinuria and nephrotic syndrome. Caution all patients that excessive perspiration and dehydration may lead to an excessive fall in blood pressure because of reduction in fluid volume. Other causes of volume depletion such as vomiting or diarrhea also may lead to a fall in blood pressure; advise patients to consult with the physician. Advise patients not to use potassium-sparing diuretics, potassium supplements, or potassium-containing salt substitutes without consulting their physician. Warn patients against interruption or discontinuation of medication unless instructed by the physician. Caution patients with heart failure or patients receiving captopril therapy against rapid increases in physical activity. Inform patients to take captopril 1 hour before meals.

PREGNANCY AND LACTATION

- Pregnancy Category C (first trimester) and D (second and third trimesters). Advise female patients of childbearing age about the consequences of second- and third-trimester exposure to ACE inhibitors, and advise them that these consequences do not appear to have resulted from intrauterine ACE-inhibitor exposure that has been limited to the first trimester. Concentrations of captopril in human milk are approximately 1% of those in maternal blood.

carbachol

(kar'-ba-kole)

Rx: Carboptic, Isopto Carbachol, Miostat

Drug Class: Cholinergics; Miotics; Ophthalmics

Pregnancy Category: C

CLINICAL PHARMACOLOGY

Mechanism of Action: A direct-acting parasympathomimetic agent that stimulates cholinergic receptors resulting in muscarinic and nicotinic effects. Indirectly promotes release of acetylcholine. *Therapeutic Effect:* Produces contraction of the iris sphincter muscle resulting in miosis, and reduction in intraocular pressure associated with decreased resistance to aqueous humor outflow.

Pharmacokinetics

None reported.

AVAILABLE FORMS

- *Intraocular Solution:* 0.01% (Miostat).
- *Ophthalmic Solution:* 0.75% (Isopto Carbachol), 1.5% (Isopto Carbachol), 3% (Carboptic, Isopto Carbachol).

INDICATIONS AND DOSAGES

Glaucoma

Ophthalmic

Adults, Elderly. Instill 1-2 drops of 0.75-3% solution in affected eye(s) up to 3 times/day.

Miosis, ophthalmic surgery

Ophthalmic

Adults, Elderly. Instill 0.5 ml of 0.01% solution into anterior chamber before or after securing sutures.

UNLABELED USES: Postoperative intraocular pressure

CONTRAINDICATIONS: Acute iritis, hypersensitivity to carbachol or any component of the formulation

INTERACTIONS

Drug

None known.

Herbal

None known.

Food

None known.

DIAGNOSTIC TEST EFFECTS: *None known.*

SIDE EFFECTS

Occasional

Blurred vision, burning/irritation of eye, decreased night vision, headache.

SERIOUS REACTIONS

- Retinal detachment has been reported.
- Systemic absorption which includes arrhythmia, hypotension, syncope, asthma occurs rarely.

SPECIAL CONSIDERATIONS

PRECAUTIONS

- Avoid overdosage.

PATIENT INFORMATION

- Difficulty in dark adaptation may occur. Advise caution in night driving and other hazardous occupations in poor light.

PREGNANCY AND LACTATION

- Pregnancy Category C. Fetal harm is not known with topical administration. Excretion into human milk is not known.

carboxymethylcellulose

(kar-box'ee-meth-ill-sell'yoo-lose)

CLINICAL PHARMACOLOGY

Mechanism of Action: Not reported.

Pharmacokinetics

Not reported.

AVAILABLE FORMS

- *Ophthalmic gel:* 1.5% (Tears Again NIGHT & DAY Gel).
- *Ophthalmic solution:* 0.25% (Theratears [preservative free]), 0.5% (Refresh Tears [preservative free]), 0.5% (Refresh Plus [preservative free], 1% (Refresh Liquigel [preservative free]).

INDICATIONS AND DOSAGES

Mild-to-moderate dry eye

Ophthalmic

Adults, Elderly. Instill 1 or 2 drops in affected eye(s) as needed.

CONTRAINDICATIONS: Hypersensitivity to carboxymethylcellulose or any component of the formulation

INTERACTIONS

Drug

None known.

Herbal

None known.

Food

None known.

DIAGNOSTIC TEST EFFECTS: *None known.*

SIDE EFFECTS

Blurred vision for a short time

SERIOUS REACTIONS

- None reported.

SPECIAL CONSIDERATIONS

PATIENT INFORMATION

- Carboxymethylcellulose OTC is for external use only. Give the patient the following instructions: To avoid contamination, do not touch the tip of the container to any surface. Replace cap after using. Do not use if the solution changes color and becomes cloudy. Stop use and see an eye care practitioner if you experience eye pain, changes in vision, continued redness or irritation of the eye or if the condition worsens or persists for more than 72 hours. Keep out of reach of children.

carteolol

(kar-tee'oh-lole)

Rx: Cartrol, Ocupress

Drug Class: Antiadrenergics, beta blocking; Ophthalmics

Pregnancy Category: C

Do not confuse with carvedilol.

CLINICAL PHARMACOLOGY

Mechanism of Action: An antihypertensive that blocks $beta_1$-adrenergic receptor at normal doses and $beta_2$-adrenergic receptors at large doses. Predominantly blocks $beta_1$-adrenergic receptors in cardiac tissue. Reduces aqueous humor production. *Therapeutic Effect:* Slows sinus heart rate, decreases cardiac output, decreases blood pressure (BP), increases airway resistance, decreases intraocular pressure.

Pharmacokinetics

Well absorbed from the gastrointestinal (GI) tract. Protein binding: unknown. Minimally metabolized in liver. Primarily excreted unchanged in urine. Not removed by hemodialysis. **Half-life:** 6 hrs (increased in decreased renal function).

AVAILABLE FORMS

- *Ophthalmic solution:* 1% (Ocupress).
- *Tablets:* 2.5 mg, 5 mg (Cartrol).

INDICATIONS AND DOSAGES

Hypertension

PO

Adults, Elderly. Initially, 2.5 mg/day as single dose either alone or in combination with diuretic. May increase gradually to 5-10 mg/day as a single dose. Maintenance: 2.5-5 mg/day.

Dosage in renal impairment

Creatinine Clearance	*Dosage Interval*
>60 ml/min	24 hrs
20-60 ml/min	48 hrs
<20 ml/min	72 hrs

Open-angle glaucoma, ocular hypertension

Ophthalmic

Adults, Elderly. 1 drop 2 times/day.

UNLABELED USES: Combination with miotics decreases IOP in acute/chronic angle closure glaucoma, treatment of secondary glaucoma, malignant glaucoma, angle closure glaucoma during/after iridectomy

CONTRAINDICATIONS: Bronchial asthma, COPD, bronchospasm, overt cardiac failure, cardiogenic shock, heart block greater than first degree, persistently severe bradycardia

INTERACTIONS

Drug

Cimetidine: May increase carteolol concentrations.

Diuretics, other hypotensives: May increase hypotensive effect.

Insulin, oral hypoglycemics: May mask symptoms of hypoglycemia and prolong hypoglycemic effect of these drugs.

MAOIs: May produce hypertension.

NSAIDs: May decrease antihypertensive effects.

Sympathomimetics, xanthines: May mutually inhibit effects of carteolol.

Herbal

None known.

Food

None known.

DIAGNOSTIC TEST EFFECTS: May increase serum ANA titer, BUN, serum LDH, lipoprotein, alkaline phosphatase, bilirubin, creatinine, potassium, triglyceride, uric acid, SGOT (AST), and SGPT (ALT) levels.

SIDE EFFECTS

Frequent

Oral: Hypotension manifested as dizziness, nausea, diaphoresis, headache, cold extremities, fatigue, constipation/diarrhea

Ophthalmic: Redness of eye or inside of eyelids, decreased night vision

Occasional

Oral: Insomnia, flatulence, urinary frequency, impotence or decreased libido

Ophthalmic: Blepharoconjunctivitis, edema, droopy eyelid, staining of cornea, blurred vision, brow ache, increased light sensitivity, burning, stinging

Rare

Rash, arthralgia, myalgia, confusion (especially elderly), taste disturbances

SERIOUS REACTIONS

- Abrupt withdrawal (particularly in those with coronary artery disease) may produce angina or precipitate MI.
- May precipitate thyroid crisis in those with thyrotoxicosis.
- Beta-blockers may mask signs and symptoms of acute hypoglycemia (tachycardia, BP changes) in diabetic patients.

SPECIAL CONSIDERATIONS

PRECAUTIONS

- Hypersensitivity to other beta-adrenoceptor blocking agents may occur. Use with caution in patients with known diminished pulmonary function.

- With angle-closure glaucoma, the immediate objective of treatment is to reopen the angle. This requires constricting the pupil with a miotic. Carteolol hydrochloride solution has little or no effect on the pupil.

PATIENT INFORMATION

- Muscle weakness such as diplopia, ptosis, and generalized weakness, may occur.
- Risk from Anaphylactic Reaction: Patients may be more reactive to repeated accidental, diagnostic, or therapeutic challenge with such allergens, causing anaphylactic reaction. Such patients may be unresponsive to the usual doses of epinephrine.

PREGNANCY AND LACTATION

- Pregnancy Category C. Increased resorptions and decreased fetal weights in rabbits and rats at maternally toxic doses have occurred. Fetal harm is not known with topical administration. Studies in lactating rats indicate that carteolol hydrochloride is excreted in milk.

OCULAR CONSIDERATIONS

- Ocular Adverse Reactions: Transient eye irritation, burning, tearing, conjunctival hyperemia and edema occurred in about 1 of 4 patients. Ocular symptoms including blurred and cloudy vision, photophobia, decreased night vision, ptosis, blepharoconjunctivitis, abnormal corneal staining, and corneal sensitivity.

carvedilol

(kar-vea'die-lole)

Rx: Coreg

Drug Class: Antiadrenergics, beta blocking

Pregnancy Category: C

Do not confuse carvedilol with carteolol.

CLINICAL PHARMACOLOGY

Mechanism of Action: An antihypertensive that possesses nonselective beta-blocking and alpha-adrenergic blocking activity. Causes vasodilation. *Therapeutic Effect:* Reduces cardiac output, exercise-induced tachycardia, and reflex orthostatic tachycardia; reduces peripheral vascular resistance.

Pharmacokinetics

Route	*Onset*	*Peak*	*Duration*
PO	30 min	1-2 hr	24 hr

Rapidly and extensively absorbed from the GI tract. Protein binding: 98%. Metabolized in the liver. Excreted primarily via bile into feces. Minimally removed by hemodialysis. **Half-life:** 7-10 hr. Food delays rate of absorption.

AVAILABLE FORMS

- *Tablets:* 3.125 mg, 6.25 mg, 12.5 mg, 25 mg.

INDICATIONS AND DOSAGES

Hypertension

PO

Adults, Elderly. Initially, 6.25 mg twice a day. May double at 7-to 14-day intervals to highest tolerated dosage. Maximum: 50 mg/day.

CHF

PO

Adults, Elderly. Initially, 3.125 mg twice a day. May double at 2-wk intervals to highest tolerated dosage. Maximum: For patients weighing more than 85 kg, give 50 mg twice a day, for those weighing 85 kg or less, give 25 mg twice a day.

Left ventricular dysfunction

PO

Adults, Elderly. Initially, 3.125-6.25 mg twice a day. May increase at intervals of 3-10 days up to 25 mg twice a day.

UNLABELED USES: Treatment of angina pectoris, idiopathic cardiomyopathy

CONTRAINDICATIONS: Bronchial asthma or related bronchospastic conditions, cardiogenic shock, pulmonary edema, second- or third-degree AV block, severe bradycardia

INTERACTIONS

Drug

Calcium blockers: Increase risk of conduction disturbances.

Catapres: May potentiate BP effects.

Cimetidine: May increase carvedilol blood concentration.

Digoxin: Increases concentrations of this drug.

Diuretics, other antihypertensives: May increase hypotensive effect.

Insulin, oral hypoglycemics: May mask symptoms of hypoglycemia and prolong hypoglycemic effect of these drugs.

Rifampin: Decreases carvedilol blood concentration.

Herbal

None known.

Food

None known.

DIAGNOSTIC TEST EFFECTS: *None known.*

SIDE EFFECTS

Carvedilol is generally well tolerated, with mild and transient side effects.

Frequent (6%-4%)

Fatigue, dizziness

Occasional (2%)

Diarrhea, bradycardia, rhinitis, back pain

Rare (less than 2%)

Orthostatic hypotension, somnolence, UTI, viral infection

SERIOUS REACTIONS

- Overdose may produce profound bradycardia, hypotension, bronchospasm, cardiac insufficiency, cardiogenic shock, and cardiac arrest.
- Abrupt withdrawal may result in diaphoresis, palpitations, headache, and tremors.
- Carvedilol administration may precipitate CHF and MI in patients with heart disease; thyroid storm in those with thyrotoxicosis; and peripheral ischemia in those with existing peripheral vascular disease.
- Hypoglycemia may occur in patients with previously controlled diabetes.

SPECIAL CONSIDERATIONS

PRECAUTIONS

- Hypotension and syncope occurred in congestive heart failure and hypertensive patients receiving carvedilol. In patients with pheochromocytoma, initiate an alpha-blocking agent before the use of any beta-blocking agent. Agents with nonselective beta-blocking activity may provoke chest pain in patients with Prinzmetal's variant angina. Patients with bronchospastic disease in general should not receive beta-blockers. Carvedilol may be used with caution, however, in patients who do not respond to, or cannot tolerate, other antihypertensive agents. It is prudent, if carvedilol is used, to use the smallest effective dose, to minimize inhibition of endogenous or exogenous beta-agonists. In patients with congestive heart failure and with diabetes, carvedilol therapy may lead to worsening hyperglycemia.

PATIENT INFORMATION

• Advise patients taking carvedilol of the following: They should not interrupt or discontinue using carvedilol without a physician's advice. Patients with congestive heart failure should consult their physician if they experience signs or symptoms of worsening heart failure such as weight gain or increasing shortness of breath. They may experience a drop in blood pressure when standing, resulting in dizziness and, rarely, fainting. Patients should sit or lie down when these symptoms of lowered blood pressure occur. If patients experience dizziness or fatigue, they should avoid driving or hazardous tasks. They should consult a physician if they experience dizziness or faintness, in case the dosage should be adjusted. They should take carvedilol with food. Diabetic patients should report any changes in blood sugar levels to their physician.

PREGNANCY AND LACTATION

• Pregnancy Category C. Studies performed in pregnant rats and rabbits given carvedilol revealed increased postimplantation loss in rats with oral doses. Fetal harm is not known with topical administration. Excretion into human milk is not known.

OCULAR CONSIDERATIONS

• Contact lens wearers may experience decreased lacrimation.

cefaclor

(sef'a-klor)

Rx: Ceclor, Ceclor CD, Ceclor Pulvules

Drug Class: Antibiotics, cephalosporins

Pregnancy Category: B

CLINICAL PHARMACOLOGY

Mechanism of Action: A second-generation cephalosporin that binds to bacterial cell membranes and inhibits cell wall synthesis. *Therapeutic Effect:* Bactericidal.

Pharmacokinetics

Well absorbed from the GI tract. Protein binding: 25%. Widely distributed. Primarily excreted unchanged in urine. Moderately removed by hemodialysis. **Half-life:** 0.6-0.9 hr (increased in impaired renal function).

AVAILABLE FORMS

• *Capsules (Ceclor):* 250 mg, 500 mg.

• *Oral Suspension (Ceclor):* 125 mg/5 ml, 187 mg/5 ml, 250 mg/5 ml, 375 mg/5 ml.

• *Tablets (Extended-release [Ceclor CD]):* 375 mg, 500 mg.

• *Tablets (Chewable [Raniclor]):* 125 mg, 187 mg, 250 mg, 375 mg.

INDICATIONS AND DOSAGES

Bronchitis

PO (Extended-Release)

Adults, Elderly. 500 mg q12h for 7 days.

Lower respiratory tract infections

PO

Adults, Elderly. 250-500 mg q8h.

Otitis media

PO

Children. 20-40 mg/kg/day in 2-3 divided doses. Maximum: 1 g/day.

Pharyngitis, skin/skin-structure infections, tonsillitis

PO (Extended-Release)

Adults, Elderly. 375 mg q12h.

PO (Regular-Release)

Adults, Elderly. 250-500 mg q8h.

Children. 20-40 mg/kg/day in 2-3 divided doses. Maximum: 1 g/day.

Urinary tract infections

PO

Adults, Elderly. 250-500 mg q8h.

Children. 20-40 mg/kg/day in 2-3 divided doses q8h. Maximum: 1 g/day.

PO (Extended-Release)

Adults, Children older than 16 yr. 375-500 mg q12h.

Otitis media

PO

Children older than 1 mo. 40 mg/kg/day in divided doses q8h. Maximum: 1 g/day.

Dosage in renal impairment

Decreased dosage may be necessary in patients with creatinine clearance less than 40 ml/min.

CONTRAINDICATIONS: History of anaphylactic reaction to penicillins or hypersensitivity to cephalosporins

INTERACTIONS

Drug

Probenecid: May increase cefaclor blood concentration.

Herbal

None known.

Food

None known.

DIAGNOSTIC TEST EFFECTS: May increase BUN level and serum alkaline phosphatase, bilirubin, creatinine, LDH, AST (SGOT), and ALT (SGPT) levels. May cause a positive direct or indirect Coombs' test.

SIDE EFFECTS

Frequent

Oral candidiasis, mild diarrhea, mild abdominal cramping, vaginal candidiasis

Occasional

Nausea, serum sickness–like reaction (marked by fever and joint pain; usually occurs after the second course of therapy and resolves after the drug is discontinued)

Rare

Allergic reaction (pruritus, rash, and urticaria)

SERIOUS REACTIONS

- Antibiotic-associated colitis and other superinfections may result from altered bacterial balance.
- Nephrotoxicity may occur, especially in patients with preexisting renal disease.
- Patients with a history of allergies, especially to penicillin, are at increased risk for developing a severe hypersensitivity reaction, marked by severe pruritus, angioedema, bronchospasm, and anaphylaxis.

SPECIAL CONSIDERATIONS

PRECAUTIONS

- In penicillin-sensitive patients, administer cephalosporin antibiotics cautiously. Clinical and laboratory evidence of partial cross-allergenicity of the penicillins and the cephalosporins exists, and there are instances in which patients have had reactions, including anaphylaxis, to both drug classes. Pseudomembranous colitis has been reported with virtually all broad-spectrum antibiotics; therefore it is important to consider the diagnosis in patients who develop diarrhea in association with the use of antibiotics. Such colitis may range in severity from mild to life threatening. Prolonged use of cefaclor may result in the overgrowth of nonsusceptible organisms. Administer cefaclor with caution in the presence of greatly impaired renal function.

PREGNANCY AND LACTATION

• Pregnancy Category B. Reproduction studies have been performed in mice and rats at doses up to 12 times the human dose and have revealed no evidence of impaired fertility or harm to the fetus from cefaclor. Small amounts of cefaclor have been detected in mother's milk following administration of single 500-mg doses.

cefazolin sodium

(sef-a'zoe-lin)

Rx: Ancef, Kefzol

Drug Class: Antibiotics, cephalosporins

Pregnancy Category: B

Do not confuse cefazolin with cefprozil or Cefzil.

CLINICAL PHARMACOLOGY

Mechanism of Action: A first-generation cephalosporin that binds to bacterial cell membranes and inhibits cell wall synthesis. *Therapeutic Effect:* Bactericidal.

Pharmacokinetics

Widely distributed. Protein binding: 85%. Primarily excreted unchanged in urine. Moderately removed by hemodialysis. **Half-life:** 1.4-1.8 hr (increased in impaired renal function).

AVAILABLE FORMS

• *Injection:* 500 mg, 1 g.

• *Ready-to-Hang Infusion:* 1 g/50 ml, 2 g/100 ml.

INDICATIONS AND DOSAGES

Uncomplicated UTIs

IV, IM

Adults, Elderly. 1 g q12h.

Mild to moderate infections

IV, IM

Adults, Elderly. 250-500 mg q8-12h.

Severe infections

IV, IM

Adults, Elderly. 0.5-1 g q6-8h.

Life-threatening infections

IV, IM

Adults, Elderly. 1-1.5 g q6h. Maximum: 12 g/day.

Perioperative prophylaxis

IV, IM

Adults, Elderly. 1 g 30-60 min before surgery, 0.5-1 g during surgery, and q6-8h for up to 24 hrs postoperatively.

Usual pediatric dosage

Children. 50-100 mg/kg/day in divided doses q8h. Maximum: 6 g/day.

Neonates older than 7 days. 40-60 mg/kg/day in divided doses q8-12h.

Neonates 7 days and younger. 40 mg/kg/day in divided doses q12h.

Dosage in renal impairment

Dosing frequency is modified based on creatinine clearance.

Creatinine Clearance	*Dosage Interval*
10-30 ml/min	Usual dose q12h
less than 10 ml/min	Usual dose q24h

CONTRAINDICATIONS: History of anaphylactic reaction to penicillins or hypersensitivity to cephalosporins

INTERACTIONS

Drug

Probenecid: Increases cefazolin blood concentration.

Herbal

None known.

Food

None known.

DIAGNOSTIC TEST EFFECTS: May increase BUN level and serum alkaline phosphatase, bilirubin, creatinine, LDH, AST (SGOT), and ALT (SGPT) levels. May cause a positive direct or indirect Coombs' test

IV INCOMPATIBILITIES: Amikacin (Amikin), amiodarone (Cordarone), hydromorphone (Dilaudid)

IV COMPATIBILITIES: Calcium gluconate, diltiazem (Cardizem), famotidine (Pepcid), heparin, insulin (regular), lidocaine, magnesium sulfate, midazolam (Versed), morphine, multivitamins, potassium chloride, propofol (Diprivan), vecuronium (Norcuron)

SIDE EFFECTS

Frequent

Discomfort with IM administration, oral candidiasis, mild diarrhea, mild abdominal cramping, vaginal candidiasis

Occasional

Nausea, serum sickness–like reaction (marked by fever and joint pain; usually occurs after the second course of therapy and resolves after the drug is discontinued)

Rare

Allergic reaction (rash, pruritus, urticaria), thrombophlebitis (pain, redness, swelling at injection site)

SERIOUS REACTIONS

• Antibiotic-associated colitis and other superinfections may result from altered bacterial balance.

• Nephrotoxicity may occur, especially in patients with pre-existing renal disease.

• Patients with a history of allergies, especially to penicillin, are at increased risk for developing a severe hypersensitivity reaction, marked by severe pruritus, angioedema, bronchospasm, and anaphylaxis.

SPECIAL CONSIDERATIONS

OCULAR INDICATIONS AND USAGE

• Ruptured globe and penetrating ocular injury; intraocular foreign body

PRECAUTIONS

• Serious and occasionally fatal hypersensitivity (anaphylactic) reactions have been reported in patients taking penicillin therapy. Pseudomembranous colitis has been reported with nearly all antibacterial agents, including cefazolin, and has ranged in severity from mild to life threatening. Prolonged use of cefazolin may result in the overgrowth of nonsusceptible organisms. As with all cephalosporins, prescribe cefazolin with caution in individuals with a history of gastrointestinal disease, particularly colitis.

PREGNANCY AND LACTATION

• Pregnancy Category B. Reproduction studies performed in rats, mice, and rabbits have revealed no evidence of impaired fertility or harm to the fetus from cefazolin. Cefazolin is present in very low concentrations in the milk of nursing mothers.

OCULAR DOSAGE AND ADMINISTRATION

• Ruptured globe and penetrating ocular injury: cefazolin 1 g IV q8h and gentamicin 2 mg/kg IV load, and then gentamicin 1 mg/kg IV q8h (adults); cefazolin 25 to 50 mg/kg per day IV in three divided doses and gentamicin 2 mg/kg IV q8h (children).

• Intraocular foreign body and traumatic optic neuropathy in the presence of sinus wall fracture or penetrating orbital injury: gentamicin 2 mg/kg IV load, and then 1 mg/kg IV q8h and cefazolin 1 g IV q8h or clindamycin 600 mg IV q8h.

cefixime

(sef-ix'-zeem)

Rx: Suprax

Drug Class: Antibiotics, cephalosporins

Pregnancy Category: B

Do not confuse Suprax with Sporanox, Surbex, or Surfak.

CLINICAL PHARMACOLOGY

Mechanism of Action: A third-generation cephalosporin that binds to bacterial cell membranes and inhibits cell wall synthesis. *Therapeutic Effect:* Bactericidal.

Pharmacokinetics

Moderately absorbed from the GI tract. Protein binding: 65%-70%. Widely distributed. Primarily excreted unchanged in urine. Minimally removed by hemodialysis. **Half-life:** 3-4 hr (increased in renal impairment).

AVAILABLE FORMS

- *Oral Suspension:* 100 mg/5 ml.
- *Tablets:* 200 mg, 400 mg.

INDICATIONS AND DOSAGES

Otitis media, acute bronchitis, acute exacerbations of chronic bronchitis, pharyngitis, tonsillitis, and uncomplicated UTIs

PO

Adults, Elderly, Children weighing more than 50 kg. 400 mg/day as a single dose or in 2 divided doses.

Children 6 mo-12 yr weighing less than 50 kg. 8 mg/kg/day as a single dose or in 2 divided doses. Maximum: 400 mg.

Uncomplicated gonorrhea

PO

Adults. 400 mg as a single dose.

Dosage in renal impairment

Dosage is modified based on creatinine clearance.

Creatinine Clearance	*% of Usual Dose*
21-60 ml/min	75%
20 ml/min or less	50%

CONTRAINDICATIONS: History of anaphylactic reaction to penicillins, hypersensitivity to cephalosporins

INTERACTIONS

Drug

Probenecid: Increases serum concentration of cefixime.

Herbal

None known.

Food

None known.

DIAGNOSTIC TEST EFFECTS: May increase BUN and serum alkaline phosphatase, bilirubin, creatinine, AST (SGOT), and ALT (SGPT) levels. May increase LDH level. May cause a positive direct or indirect Coombs' test.

SIDE EFFECTS

Frequent

Oral candidiasis, mild diarrhea, mild abdominal cramping, vaginal candidiasis

Occasional

Nausea, serum sickness–like reaction (marked by arthralgia and fever; usually occurs after second course of therapy and resolves after drug is discontinued)

Rare

Allergic reaction (rash, pruritus, urticaria)

SERIOUS REACTIONS

- Antibiotic-associated colitis and other superinfections may result from altered bacterial balance.
- Nephrotoxicity may occur, especially in patients with pre-existing renal disease.
- Patients with a history of allergies, especially to penicillin, are at increased risk for developing a severe

hypersensitivity reaction, marked by severe pruritus, angioedema, bronchospasm, and anaphylaxis.

SPECIAL CONSIDERATIONS

PRECAUTIONS

- Keep in mind the possibility of the emergence of resistant organisms that might result in overgrowth, particularly during prolonged treatment. In such use, careful observation of the patient is essential. If superinfection occurs during therapy, take appropriate measures.
- Adjust the dose of cefixime in patients with renal impairment and in those undergoing continuous ambulatory peritoneal dialysis and hemodialysis. Monitor patients on dialysis carefully.
- Prescribe cefixime with caution to individuals with a history of gastrointestinal disease, particularly colitis.

PREGNANCY AND LACTATION

- Pregnancy Category B. Reproduction studies have been performed in mice and rats at doses up to 400 times the human dose and have revealed no evidence of harm to the fetus from cefixime. Excretion into human milk is not known.

ceftriaxone sodium

(sef-try-ax'-one)

Rx: Rocephin, Rocephin IM Convenience Kit

Drug Class: Antibiotics, cephalosporins

Pregnancy Category: B

CLINICAL PHARMACOLOGY

Mechanism of Action: A third-generation cephalosporin that binds to bacterial cell membranes and inhibits cell wall synthesis. *Therapeutic Effect:* Bactericidal.

Pharmacokinetics

Widely distributed (including to CSF). Protein binding: 83%-96%. Primarily excreted unchanged in urine. Not removed by hemodialysis. **Half-life:** 4.3-4.6 hr IV; 5.8-8.7 hr IM (increased in impaired renal function).

AVAILABLE FORMS

- *Powder for Injection:* 250 mg, 500 mg, 1 g, 2 g.

INDICATIONS AND DOSAGES

Mild to moderate infections

IV, IM

Adults, Elderly. 1-2 g as a single dose or in 2 divided doses.

Serious infections

IV, IM

Adults, Elderly. Up to 4 g/day in 2 divided doses.

Children. 50-75 mg/kg/day in divided doses q12h. Maximum: 2 g/day.

Skin and skin-structure infections

IV, IM

Children. 50-75 mg/kg/day as a single dose or in 2 divided doses. Maximum: 2 g/day.

Meningitis

IV

Children. Initially, 75 mg/kg, then 100 mg/kg/day as a single dose or in divided doses q12h. Maximum: 4 g/day.

Lyme disease

IV

Adults, Elderly. 2-4 g a day for 10-14 days.

Acute bacterial otitis media

IM

Children. 50 mg/kg once a day for 3 days. Maximum: 1 g/day.

Perioperative prophylaxis

IV, IM

Adults, Elderly. 1 g 0.5-2 hrs before surgery.

Uncomplicated gonorrhea

IM

Adults. 250 mg plus doxycycline one time.

Dosage in renal impairment

Dosage modification is usually unnecessary but liver and renal function test results should be monitored in those with both renal and liver impairment or severe renal impairment.

CONTRAINDICATIONS: History of anaphylactic reaction to penicillins or hypersensitivity to cephalosporins

INTERACTIONS

Drug

None known.

Herbal

None known.

Food

None known.

DIAGNOSTIC TEST EFFECTS: May increase BUN level and serum alkaline phosphatase, bilirubin, creatinine, AST (SGOT), and ALT (SGPT) levels. May produce a positive direct or indirect Coombs' test. Interferes with crossmatching procedures and hematologic tests.

IV INCOMPATIBILITIES: Aminophylline, amphotericin B complex (AmBisome, Amphotec, Abelcet), filgrastim (Neupogen), fluconazole (Diflucan), labetalol (Normodyne), pentamidine (Pentam IV), vancomycin (Vancocin)

IV COMPATIBILITIES: Diltiazem (Cardizem), heparin, lidocaine, morphine, propofol (Diprivan)

SIDE EFFECTS

Frequent

Discomfort with IM administration, oral candidiasis, mild diarrhea, mild abdominal cramping, vaginal candidiasis

Occasional

Nausea, serum sickness–like reaction (marked by fever and joint pain; usually occurs after the second course of therapy and resolves after the drug is discontinued)

Rare

Allergic reaction (rash, pruritus, urticaria), thrombophlebitis (pain, redness, swelling at injection site)

SERIOUS REACTIONS

- Antibiotic-associated colitis and other superinfections may result from altered bacterial balance.
- Nephrotoxicity may occur, especially in patients with pre-existing renal disease.
- Patients with a history of allergies, especially to penicillin, are at increased risk for developing a severe hypersensitivity reaction, marked by severe pruritus, angioedema, bronchospasm, and anaphylaxis.

SPECIAL CONSIDERATIONS

PRECAUTIONS

- Although transient elevations of blood urea nitrogen and serum creatinine have been observed, at the recommended dosages the nephrotoxic potential of ceftrioxone is similar to that of other cephalosporins.
- Ceftriaxone is excreted via biliary and renal excretion. Therefore patients with renal failure normally require no adjustment in dosage when usual doses of ceftrioxone are administered, but concentrations of drug in the serum should be monitored periodically. If evidence of accumulation exists, decrease dosage accordingly. Dosage adjustments should not be necessary in patients with hepatic dysfunction. Alterations in prothrombin times have occurred rarely in patients treated with ceftrioxone. Prolonged use of ceftrioxone may result in overgrowth of

nonsusceptible organisms. Careful observation of the patient is essential. If superinfection occurs during therapy, take appropriate measures. Prescribe ceftrioxone with caution to individuals with a history of gastrointestinal disease, especially colitis. Reports indicate sonographic abnormalities in the gallbladder of patients treated with ceftrioxone; some of these patients also had symptoms of gallbladder disease.

PREGNANCY AND LACTATION

• Pregnancy Category B. Reproductive studies have been performed in mice and rats at doses up to 20 times the usual human dose, and no evidence of embryotoxicity, fetotoxicity, or teratogenicity has been found. Low concentrations of ceftriaxone are excreted in human milk.

OCULAR CONSIDERATIONS

• Gonococcal conjunctivitis; preseptal cellulitis; orbital cellulites

OCULAR DOSAGE AND ADMINISTRATION

• Gonococcal Conjunctivitis: Neonatal, 25 to 50 mg/kg, up to 125 mg IV or IM. American Academy of Ophthalmology practice standards require daily injections for 7 days. Adults, 1 g IV or IM daily, with treatment up to 5 days

• Preseptal Cellulitis: Moderate to severe—adults, 1 to 2 g IV q12h; children, 100 mg/kg per day IV in two divided doses. Ceftriaxone sodium should be administered with vancomycin: adults, 0.5 to 1 g IV q12h; children, 40 mg/kg per day IV in two to three divided doses.

• Orbital Cellulitis: Adults, ceftriaxone 1 to 2 g IV q12h plus vancomycin 1 g IV q12h or nafcillin 1 to 2 g IV q4h; children, vancomycin 40 mg/kg per day IV in two to three divided doses or nafcillin 150 mg/kg per day IV in six divided doses plus ceftriaxone 100 mg/kg per day IV in two divided doses

celecoxib

(sel-eh-cox′ib)

Rx: Celebrex

Drug Class: Analgesics, nonnarcotic; COX-2 inhibitors; Nonsteroidal anti-inflammatory drugs

Pregnancy Category: C

Do not confuse Celebrex with Cerebyx or Celexa.

CLINICAL PHARMACOLOGY

Mechanism of Action: An NSAID that inhibits cyclo-oxygenase-2, the enzyme responsible for prostaglandin synthesis. Mechanism of action in treating familial adenomatous polyposis is unknown. *Therapeutic Effect:* Reduces inflammation and relieves pain.

Pharmacokinetics

Widely distributed. Protein binding: 97%. Metabolized in the liver. Primarily eliminated in feces. **Half-life:** 11.2 hr.

AVAILABLE FORMS

• *Capsules:* 100 mg, 200 mg, 400 mg.

INDICATIONS AND DOSAGES

Osteoarthritis

PO

Adults, Elderly. 200 mg/day as a single dose or 100 mg twice a day.

Rheumatoid arthritis

PO

Adults, Elderly. 100-200 mg twice a day.

Acute pain

PO

Adults, Elderly. Initially, 400 mg with additional 200 mg on day 1, if needed. Maintenance: 200 mg twice a day as needed.

Familial adenomatous polyposis
PO
Adults, Elderly. 400 mg twice daily (with food).

CONTRAINDICATIONS: Hypersensitivity to aspirin, NSAIDs, or sulfonamides

INTERACTIONS

Drug

Fluconazole: May increase celecoxib blood level.

Lithium: May increase lithium blood levels.

Warfarin: May increase the risk of bleeding.

Herbal

None known.

Food

None known.

DIAGNOSTIC TEST EFFECTS: May increase AST (SGOT) and ALT (SGPT) levels.

SIDE EFFECTS

Frequent (greater than 5%)
Diarrhea, dyspepsia, headache, upper respiratory tract infection

Occasional (5%-1%)
Abdominal pain, flatulence, nausea, back pain, peripheral edema, dizziness, rash

SERIOUS REACTIONS

• None known.

SPECIAL CONSIDERATIONS

PRECAUTIONS

• Celecoxib cannot be expected to substitute for corticosteroids or to treat corticosteroid insufficiency. Carefully monitor a patient with symptoms and/or signs suggesting liver dysfunction or in whom an abnormal liver test has occurred for evidence of the development of a more severe hepatic reaction. Long-term administration of nonsteroidal antiinflammatory drugs has resulted in renal papillary necrosis and other renal injury. Exercise caution when initiating treatment with celecoxib in patients with considerable dehydration.

• Rehydration of patients first is advisable before starting therapy with celecoxib. Caution also is recommended in patients with preexisting kidney disease. Anemia sometimes occurs in patients receiving celecoxib. Fluid retention and edema have been observed in some patients taking celecoxib. Patients with asthma may have aspirin-sensitive asthma. The use of aspirin in patients with aspirin-sensitive asthma has been associated with severe bronchospasm, which can be fatal. Use celecoxib with caution in patients with preexisting asthma.

PATIENT INFORMATION

• Celecoxib can cause discomfort and, rarely, more serious side effects, such as gastrointestinal bleeding, which may result in hospitalization and even fatal outcomes. Although serious gastrointestinal tract ulcerations and bleeding can occur without warning symptoms, patients should be alert for the signs and symptoms of ulcerations and bleeding and should ask for medical advice when observing any indicative signs or symptoms. Apprise patients of the importance of this follow-up. Instruct patients promptly to report signs or symptoms of gastrointestinal ulceration or bleeding, skin rash, unexplained weight gain, or edema to their physicians. Inform patients of the warning signs and symptoms of hepatotoxicity (e.g., nausea, fatigue, lethargy, pruritus, jaundice, right upper quadrant tenderness, and flu-like symptoms). If these occur, instruct patients to stop therapy and seek immediate medical therapy. Also instruct patients to seek immediate emergency help in the case of an anaphylactoid reaction. Women should avoid celecoxib in late pregnancy because it may cause premature closure of the ductus arteriosus. Inform patients with familial adenomatous polyposis (FAP) that celecoxib has not been shown to reduce colorectal, duodenal, or other FAP-related cancers, or the need for endoscopic surveillance, prophylactic, or other FAP-related surgery. Therefore, instruct all patients with FAP to continue their usual care while receiving celecoxib.

PREGNANCY AND LACTATION

- Pregnancy Category C. Celecoxib produced preimplantation and postimplantation losses and reduced embryo/fetal survival in rats. Fetal harm is not known. Women should avoid celecoxib in late pregnancy because it may cause premature closure of the ductus arteriosus. Celecoxib is excreted in the milk of lactating rats at concentrations similar to those in plasma. Excretion into human milk is not known.

cephalexin

(sef-a-lex'-in)

Rx: Biocef, Keflex, Keftab
Drug Class: Antibiotics, cephalosporins
Pregnancy Category: B

CLINICAL PHARMACOLOGY

Mechanism of Action: A first-generation cephalosporin that binds to bacterial cell membranes and inhibits cell wall synthesis. *Therapeutic Effect:* Bactericidal.

Pharmacokinetics

Rapidly absorbed from the GI tract. Protein binding: 10%-15%. Widely distributed. Primarily excreted unchanged in urine. Moderately removed by hemodialysis. **Half-life:** 0.9-1.2 hr (increased in impaired renal function).

AVAILABLE FORMS

- *Capsules (Biocef):* 500 mg.
- *Capsules (Keflex):* 250 mg, 500 mg.
- *Powder for Oral Suspension (Biocef):* 125 mg/5 ml, 250 mg/5 ml.
- *Tablets:* 250 mg, 500 mg.
- *Tablets (Keftab):* 500 mg.

INDICATIONS AND DOSAGES

Bone infections, prophylaxis of rheumatic fever, follow-up to parenteral therapy

PO

Adults, Elderly. 250-500 mg q6h up to 4 g/day.

Streptococcal pharyngitis, skin and skin-structure infections, uncomplicated cystitis

PO

Adults, Elderly. 500 mg q12h.

Usual pediatric dosage

Children. 25-100 mg/kg/day in 2-4 divided doses.

Otitis media

PO

Children. 75-100 mg/kg/day in 4 divided doses.

Dosage in renal impairment

After usual initial dose, dosing frequency is modified based on creatinine clearance and the severity of the infection.

Creatinine Clearance	*Dosage Interval*
10-40 ml/min	Usual dose q8-12h
less than 10 ml/min	Usual dose q12-24h

CONTRAINDICATIONS: History of anaphylactic reaction to penicillins or hypersensitivity to cephalosporins

INTERACTIONS

Drug

Probenecid: Increases serum concentration of cephalexin.

Herbal

None known.

Food

None known.

DIAGNOSTIC TEST EFFECTS: May increase serum alkaline phosphatase, AST (SGOT), and ALT (SGPT) levels. May produce a positive direct or indirect Coombs' test. Interferes with crossmatching procedures and hematologic tests.

SIDE EFFECTS

Frequent

Oral candidiasis, mild diarrhea, mild abdominal cramping, vaginal candidiasis

Occasional

Nausea, serum sickness–like reaction (marked by fever and joint pain; ususally occurs after the second course of therapy and resolves after the drug is discontinued)

Rare

Allergic reaction (rash, pruritus, urticaria)

SERIOUS REACTIONS

• Antibiotic-associated colitis and other superinfections may result from altered bacterial balance.

• Nephrotoxicity may occur, especially in patients with preexisting renal disease.

• Patients with a history of allergies, especially to penicillin, are at increased risk for developing a severe hypersensitivity reaction, marked by severe pruritus, angioedema, bronchospasm, and anaphylaxis.

SPECIAL CONSIDERATIONS

PRECAUTIONS

• If an allergic reaction to cephalexin occurs, discontinue the drug and treat the patient with the usual agents (e.g., epinephrine or other pressor amines, antihistamines, or corticosteroids). Prolonged use of cephalexin may result in the overgrowth of nonsusceptible organisms. Careful observation of the patient is essential. If superinfection occurs during therapy, take appropriate measures. Positive direct Coombs' tests have been reported during treatment with the cephalosporin antibiotics. Administer cephalexin with caution in the presence of greatly impaired renal function. Perform indicated surgical procedures along with antibiotic therapy. As a result of administration of cephalexin, a false-positive reaction for glucose in the urine may occur. This reaction has been observed with Benedict's and Fehling's solutions and also with Clinitest tablets. As with other beta-lactams, the renal excretion of cephalexin is inhibited by probenecid. Prescribe broad-spectrum antibiotics with caution in individuals with a history of gastrointestinal disease, particularly colitis.

PREGNANCY AND LACTATION

• Pregnancy Category B. Oral administration to rats and mice had no adverse effect on fertility, fetal viability, fetal weight, or litter size. The excretion of cephalexin in the milk increased up to 4 hours after a 500-mg dose; the drug reached a maximum level of 4 mcg/ml, then decreased gradually, and had disappeared 8 hours after administration.

OCULAR CONSIDERATIONS

• Ocular Indications: Dacryocystitis and orbital blow-out fracture; acute infectious dacryoadenitis

OCULAR DOSAGE AND ADMINISTRATION

• Dacryocystitis: For afebrile, mild adult cases, Keflex 500 mg PO q6h

• Acute Infectious Dacryoadenitis: Mild to moderate—adults, 250 to 500 mg orally q6h; children, 25 to 50 mg/kg per day orally in 4 divided doses

• Orbital Blow-out Fracture: 250 to 500 mg orally qid or erythromycin 250 to 500 mg orally qid for 10 to 14 days

cetirizine

(si-tear'a-zeen)

Rx: Zyrtec

Drug Class: Antihistamines, H1

Pregnancy Category: B

Do not confuse Zyrtec with Zantac or Zyprexa.

CLINICAL PHARMACOLOGY

Mechanism of Action: A second-generation piperazine that competes with histamine for H_1-receptor sites on effector cells in the GI tract, blood vessels, and respiratory tract. *Therapeutic Effect:* Prevents allergic response, produces mild bronchodilation, blocks histamine-induced bronchitis.

Pharmacokinetics

Route	Onset	Peak	Duration
PO	less than 1 hr	4-8 hr	less than 24 hr

Rapidly and almost completely absorbed from the GI tract (absorption not affected by food). Protein binding: 93%. Undergoes low first-pass metabolism; not extensively metabolized. Primarily excreted in urine (more than 80% as unchanged drug). **Half-life:** 6.5-10 hr.

AVAILABLE FORMS

• *Syrup:* 5 mg/5 ml.
• *Tablets:* 5 mg, 10 mg.
• *Tablets (Chewable):* 5 mg, 10 mg.

INDICATIONS AND DOSAGES

Allergic rhinitis, urticaria

PO

Adults, Elderly, Children older than 5 yr. Initially, 5-10 mg/day as a single or in 2 divided doses.

Children 2-5 yr. 2.5 mg/day. May increase up to 5 mg/day as a single or in 2 divided doses.

Children 12-23 mo. Initially, 2.5 mg/day. May increase up to 5 mg/day in 2 divided doses.

Children 6-11 mo. 2.5 mg once a day.

Dosage in renal or hepatic impairment

For adult and elderly patients with renal impairment (creatinine clearance of 11-31 ml/min), those receiving hemodialysis (creatinine clearance of less than 7 ml/min), and those with hepatic impairment, dosage is decreased to 5 mg once a day.

UNLABELED USES: Treatment of bronchial asthma

CONTRAINDICATIONS: Hypersensitivity to cetirizine or hydroxyzine

INTERACTIONS

Drug

Alcohol, other CNS depressants: May increase CNS depression.

Herbal

None known.

Food

None known.

DIAGNOSTIC TEST EFFECTS: May suppress wheal and flare reactions to antigen skin testing, unless drug is discontinued 4 days before testing.

SIDE EFFECTS

Occasional (10%-2%)

Pharyngitis; dry mucous membranes, nose, or throat; nausea and vomiting; abdominal pain; headache; dizziness; fatigue; thickening of mucus; somnolence; photosensitivity; urine retention

SERIOUS REACTIONS

• Children may experience paradoxical reactions, including restlessness, insomnia, euphoria, nervousness, and tremor.

• Dizziness, sedation, and confusion are more likely to occur in elderly patients.

SPECIAL CONSIDERATIONS

PRECAUTIONS

• Occurrence of somnolence has been reported in some patients taking cetirizine; therefore, advise patient to exercise due caution when driving a car or operating potentially dangerous machinery. Advise patient to avoid concurrent use of cetirizine with alcohol or other central nervous system depressants because additional reductions in alertness and additional impairment of central nervous system performance may occur.

PREGNANCY AND LACTATION

• Pregnancy Category B. In mice, rats, and rabbits, cetirizine was not teratogenic at oral doses. In mice, cetirizine caused retarded pup weight gain during lactation at oral doses. Cetirizine has been reported to be excreted in human breast milk.

chlorambucil

(klor-am'-bew-sill)

Rx: Leukeran

Drug Class: Antineoplastics, alkylating agents

Pregnancy Category: D

Do not confuse Leukeran with Alkeran, Chloromycetin, Leukine, or Myleran.

CLINICAL PHARMACOLOGY

Mechanism of Action: An alkylating agent and nitrogen mustard that inhibits DNA and RNA synthesis by cross-linking with DNA and RNA strands. Cell cycle-phase nonspecific. *Therapeutic Effect:* Interferes with nucleic acid function.

Pharmacokinetics

Rapidly and completely absorbed from the GI tract. Protein binding: 99%. Rapidly metabolized in the liver to active metabolite. Not removed by hemodialysis. **Half-life:** 1.5 hr; metabolite 2.5 hr.

AVAILABLE FORMS

• *Tablets:* 2 mg.

INDICATIONS AND DOSAGES

Palliative treatment of advanced Hodgkin's disease, advanced malignant (non-Hodgkin's) lymphoma (including giant follicular lymphoma and lymphosarcoma), chronic lymphocytic leukemia

PO

Adults, Elderly, Children. For initial or short-course therapy, 0.1-0.2 mg/kg/day as a single or in divided doses for 3-6 wk (average dose, 4-10 mg/day). Alternatively, 0.4 mg/kg initially as a single daily dose every 2 wk and increased by 0.1 mg/kg every 2 wk until response and myelosuppression occur. Maintenance: 0.03-0.1 mg/kg/day (average dose, 2-4 mg/day).

UNLABELED USES: Treatment of hairy cell leukemia, nephrotic syndrome, ovarian or testicular carcinoma, polycythemia vera

CONTRAINDICATIONS: Previous allergic reaction or disease resistance to drug

INTERACTIONS

Drug

Antigout medications: May decrease the effect of these drugs.

Bone marrow depressants: May increase bone myelosuppression.

Live-virus vaccines: May potentiate virus replication, increase vaccine side effects and decrease the patient's antibody response to the vaccine.

Other immunosuppressants (including steroids): May increase the risk of infection or development of neoplasms.

Herbal

None known.

Food

None known.

DIAGNOSTIC TEST EFFECTS: May increase serum alkaline phosphatase, serum uric acid, and AST (SGOT) levels.

SIDE EFFECTS

Expected

GI effects such as nausea, vomiting, anorexia, diarrhea, and abdominal distress (generally mild, last less than 24 hr and occur only if single dose exceeds 20 mg).

Occasional

Rash or dermatitis, pruritus, cold sores

Rare

Alopecia, urticaria, erythema, hyperuricemia

SERIOUS REACTIONS

- Hematologic toxicity due to myelosuppression occurs frequently and may include neutropenia, leukopenia, progressive lymphopenia, anemia and thrombocytopenia.
- After discontinuation of short-course therapy, thrombocytopenia and leukopenia usually last for 1 to 2 weeks but may persist for 3 to 4 weeks.
- The neutrophil count may continue to decrease for up to 10 days after the last dose.
- Hematologic toxicity appears to be less severe with intermittent rather than continuous drug administration.
- Overdosage may produce seizures in children.
- Excessive serum uric acid level and hepatotoxicity occur rarely.

SPECIAL CONSIDERATIONS

PRECAUTIONS

- Many patients develop a slowly progressive lymphopenia during treatment. Children with nephrotic syndrome and patients receiving high pulse doses of chlorambucil may have an increased risk of seizures.

PATIENT INFORMATION

- Inform patients that the major toxicities of chlorambucil are related to hypersensitivity, drug fever, myelosuppression, hepatotoxicity, infertility, seizures, gastrointestinal toxicity, and secondary malignancies. Never allow patients to take the drug without medical supervision, and instruct them to consult their physician if they experience skin rash, bleeding, fever, jaundice, persistent cough, seizures, nausea, vomiting, amenorrhea, or unusual lumps/masses. Advise women of childbearing age to avoid becoming pregnant.

PREGNANCY AND LACTATION

- Pregnancy Category D. Chlorambucil can cause fetal harm when administered to a pregnant woman. Excretion into human milk is not known.

chloramphenicol

(klor-am-fen′-i-kole)

Rx: AK-Chlor, Chloromycetin Ophthalmic, Chloromycetin Sodium Succinate, Chloroptic, Chloroptic S.O.P., Ocu-Chlor

Drug Class: Anti-infectives, ophthalmic; Anti-infectives, otic; Antibiotics, chloramphenicol and derivatives; Ophthalmics; Otics

Pregnancy Category: C

Do not confuse chloramphenicol with chlorambucil.

CLINICAL PHARMACOLOGY

Mechanism of Action: A dichloroacetic acid derivative that inhibits bacterial protein synthesis by binding to bacterial ribosomal receptor sites. *Therapeutic Effect:* Bacteriostatic (may be bactericidal in high concentrations).

AVAILABLE FORMS

- *Powder for Injection:* 100 mg/ml.
- *Ophthalmic Ointment:* 10 mg/g.
- *Ophthalmic Solution:* 5 mg/ml.

INDICATIONS AND DOSAGES

Mild to moderate infections caused by organisms resistant to other less toxic antibiotics

IV

Adults, Elderly. 50-100 mg/kg/day in divided doses q6h. Maximum: 4 g/day.

Children older than 1 mo. 50-75 mg/kg/day in divided doses q6h. Maximum: 4 g/day

Meningitis

IV

Children older than 1 mo. 50-100 mg/kg/day in divided doses q6h.

Usual ophthalmic dosage

Adults, Elderly, Children. 1-2 drops 4-6 times/day.

CONTRAINDICATIONS: Hypersensitivity to chloramphenicol

INTERACTIONS

Drug

Anticonvulsants, bone marrow depressants: May increase myelosuppression.

Clindamycin, erythromycin: May antagonize the effects of these drugs.

Oral antidiabetics: May increase the effects of these drugs.

Phenobarbital, phenytoin, warfarin: May increase blood concentrations of these drugs.

Vitamin B_{12}: May decrease the effects of vitamin B_{12} in patients with pernicious anemia.

Herbal

None known.

Food

None known.

DIAGNOSTIC TEST EFFECTS: Therapeutic blood level: 10-20 mcg/ml; toxic blood level: greater than 25 mcg/ml. When administered with iron salts, may increase serum iron levels.

SIDE EFFECTS

Occasional

Systemic: Nausea, vomiting, diarrhea

Ophthalmic: Blurred vision, burning, stinging, hypersensitivity reaction

Otic: Hypersensitivity reaction

Rare

"Gray baby" syndrome in neonates (abdominal distention, blue-gray skin color, cardiovascular collapse, unresponsiveness), rash, shortness of breath, confusion, headache, optic neuritis (blurred vision, eye pain), peripheral neuritis (numbness and weakness in feet and hands)

SERIOUS REACTIONS

- Superinfection due to bacterial or fungal overgrowth may occur.

• There is a narrow margin between effective therapy and toxic levels producing blood dyscrasias.

• Myelosuppression, with resulting aplastic anemia, hypoplastic anemia, and pancytopenia, may occur weeks or months later.

SPECIAL CONSIDERATIONS

PRECAUTIONS

• Fungal infections may occur. In all serious infections, supplement the topical use of chloramphenicol by appropriate systemically effective medication.

OCULAR DOSAGE AND ADMINISTRATION

Solution

• Apply 2 drops to the affected eye every 3 hours. Continue administration day and night for the first 48 hours, after which the interval between applications may be increased. Continue treatment for at least 48 hours after the eye appears normal.

Ointment

• Place a small amount of ointment in the lower conjunctival sac every 3 hours or more frequently if deemed advisable by the prescribing physician. Continue administration day and night for the first 48 hours, after which the interval between applications may be increased. Continue treatment for at least 48 hours after the eye appears normal.

chloramphenicol; hydrocortisone acetate

(klor-am-fen′-ih-call; hye-droe-kor′-ti-sone as′-a-tate)

Drug Class: Anti-infectives, ophthalmic; Antibiotics, chloramphenicol and derivatives; Corticosteroids, ophthalmic; Ophthalmics

Pregnancy Category: C

CLINICAL PHARMACOLOGY

Mechanism of Action: Chloramphenicol is an anti-infective, dichloroacetic acid derivative that acts as a bacteriostatic (may be bactericidal in high concentrations) by binding to bacterial ribosomal receptor sites. Hydrocortisone is an adrenal corticosteroid that inhibits accumulation of inflammatory cells at inflammation sites, phagocytosis, lysosomal enzyme release and synthesis or release of mediators of inflammation.

Therapeutic Effect: Inhibits bacterial protein synthesis. Prevents or suppresses cell-mediated immune reactions. Decreases or prevents tissue response to inflammatory process.

Pharmacokinetics

None reported.

AVAILABLE FORMS

• *Ophthalmic suspension:* 12.5 mg/vial, 25 mg/vial (Chloromycetin hydrocortisone).

INDICATIONS AND DOSAGES

Serious infections

Ophthalmic

Adults, Elderly. Instill 2 drops to affected eye(s) every 3 hours. Continue administration day and night for the first 24 hours. Treatment should be continued for at least 48 hours after the eye appears normal.

CONTRAINDICATIONS: Uncomplicated removal of a corneal foreign body, epithelial herpes simplex keratitis, vaccinia, varicella, and other viral diseases of the cornea and conjunctiva, mycobacterial infection of the eye, fungal diseases of ocular structures and hypersensitivity to a chloramphenicol, hydrocortisone or any component of the formulation.

INTERACTIONS

Drug

None known.

Herbal

None known.

Food

None known.

DIAGNOSTIC TEST EFFECTS: *None known.*

SIDE EFFECTS

Occasional

Blurred vision, burning, stinging, hypersensitivity reaction.

SERIOUS REACTIONS

Alert

Bone marrow hypoplasia, including aplastic anemia and death, has been reported following local application of chloramphenicol.

- Superinfection due to bacterial or fungal overgrowth may occur.

SPECIAL CONSIDERATIONS

PRECAUTIONS

- An eye care practitioner should make the initial prescription and renewal of the medication order beyond 20 ml after fluorescein staining. Consider the possibility of persistent fungal infections of the cornea after prolonged steroid dosing. The prolonged use of antibiotics occasionally may result in overgrowth of nonsusceptible organisms, including fungi. In all serious infections, supplement the topical use of chloramphenicol with appropriate systemically effective medication.

chlordiazepoxide

(klor-dye-az-e-pox'ide)

Rx: Libritabs, Librium

Drug Class: Anxiolytics; Benzodiazepines

Pregnancy Category: D

DEA Class: Schedule IV

Do not confuse Librium with Librax.

CLINICAL PHARMACOLOGY

Mechanism of Action: A benzodiazepine that enhances the action of the inhibitory neurotransmitter gamma-aminobutyric acid in the CNS. *Therapeutic Effect:* Produces anxiolytic effect.

AVAILABLE FORMS

- *Capsules:* 5 mg, 10 mg, 25 mg.
- *Injection Powder for Reconstitution.* 100 mg.

INDICATIONS AND DOSAGES

Alcohol withdrawal symptoms

PO

Adults, Elderly. 50-100 mg. May repeat q2-4h. Maximum: 300 mg/24 hr.

Anxiety

PO

Adults. 15-100 mg/day in 3-4 divided doses.

Elderly. 5 mg 2-4 times a day.

IV, IM

Adults. Initially, 50-100 mg, then 25-50 mg 3-4 times a day as needed.

UNLABELED USES: Treatment of panic disorder, tension headache, tremors

CONTRAINDICATIONS: Acute alcohol intoxication, acute angle-closure glaucoma

INTERACTIONS

Drug

Alcohol, other CNS depressants: May increase CNS depression.

Herbal
Kava kava, valerian: May increase CNS depression.
Food
None known.

DIAGNOSTIC TEST EFFECTS: None known. Therapeutic serum drug level is 1-3 mcg/ml; toxic serum drug level is greater than 5 mcg/ml.

SIDE EFFECTS

Frequent
Pain at IM injection site; somnolence, ataxia, dizziness, confusion with oral dose (particularly in elderly or debilitated patients)
Occasional
Rash, peripheral edema, GI disturbances
Rare
Paradoxical CNS reactions, such as hyperactivity or nervousness in children and excitement or restlessness in the elderly (generally noted during first 2 weeks of therapy, particularly in presence of uncontrolled pain)

SERIOUS REACTIONS

- IV administration may produce pain, swelling, thrombophlebitis, and carpal tunnel syndrome.
- Abrupt or too-rapid withdrawal may result in pronounced restlessness, irritability, insomnia, hand tremors, abdominal or muscle cramps, diaphoresis, vomiting, and seizures.
- Overdose results in somnolence, confusion, diminished reflexes, and coma.

SPECIAL CONSIDERATIONS

PRECAUTIONS

- In general, the concomitant administration of chlordiazepoxide and other psychotropic agents is not recommended. If such combination therapy seems indicated, give careful consideration to the pharmacology of the agents to be used, particularly when the known potentiating compounds such as the monoamine oxidase inhibitors and phenothiazines are to be used. Observe the usual precautions in treating patients with impaired renal or hepatic function. Paradoxical reactions—for example, excitement, stimulation, and acute rage—have been reported in psychiatric patients and in hyperactive, aggressive children and should be watched for during chlordiazepoxide therapy. The usual precautions are indicated when chlordiazepoxide is used to treat anxiety states for which there is any evidence of impending depression; bear in mind that suicidal tendencies may be present and that protective measures may be necessary. Although clinical studies have not established a cause-and-effect relationship, physicians should be aware that variable effects on blood coagulation have been reported rarely in patients receiving oral anticoagulants and chlordiazepoxide. In view of isolated reports associating chlordiazepoxide with exacerbation of porphyria, exercise caution in prescribing chlordiazepoxide to patients suffering from this disease.

PATIENT INFORMATION

- To ensure the safe and effective use of benzodiazepines, inform patients that because benzodiazepines may produce psychological and physical dependence, it is advisable that they consult with their physician before increasing the dose or abruptly discontinuing this drug.

PREGNANCY AND LACTATION

- Pregnancy Category D. An increased risk of congenital malformations associated with the use of minor tranquilizers (chlordiazepoxide, diazepam, and meprobamate) during the first trimester of pregnancy has been suggested in several studies.

OCULAR CONSIDERATIONS

- Cycloplegia can occur.

chloroquine / chloroquine phosphate

(klor'oh-kwin)

Rx: Aralen Phosphate

Drug Class: Antiprotozoals

Pregnancy Category: C

CLINICAL PHARMACOLOGY

Mechanism of Action: An amebecide that concentrates in parasite acid vesicles and may interfere with parasite protein synthesis. *Therapeutic Effect:* Increases pH and inhibits parasite growth.

Pharmacokinetics

Rate of absorption is variable. Chloroquine is almost completely absorbed from the gastrointestinal (GI) tract. Protein binding: 50%-65%. Widely distributed into body tissues such as eyes, heart, kidneys, liver, and lungs. Partially metabolized to active de-ethylated metabolites (principal metabolite is desethylchloroquine). Excreted in urine. Removed by hemodialysis. **Half-life:** 1-2 mos.

AVAILABLE FORMS

- *Tablets:* 250 mg, 500 mg (Aralen).

INDICATIONS AND DOSAGES

Chloroquine Phosphate

Treatment of malaria (acute attack): Dose (mg base)

Dose	*Time*	*Adults*	*Children*
Initial	Day 1	600 mg	10 mg/kg
Second	6 hrs later	300 mg	5 mg/kg
Third	Day 2	300 mg	5 mg/kg
Fourth	Day 3	300 mg	5 mg/kg

Suppression of malaria

PO

Adults. 300 mg (base)/wk on same day each week beginning 2 wks before exposure; continue for 6-8 wks after leaving endemic area.

Children. 5 mg (base)/kg/wk.

Malaria prophylaxis

PO

Adults. 600 mg base initially given in 2 divided doses 6 hrs apart.

Children. 10 mg base/kg.

Amebiasis

PO

Adults. 1 g (600 mg base) daily for 2 days; then, 500 mg (300 mg base)/day for at least 2-3 wks.

Chloroquine HCL

Treatment of malaria

IM

Adults. Initially, 160-200 mg base (4-5 ml), repeat in 6 hrs. Maximum: 800 mg base in first 24 hrs. Begin oral therapy as soon as possible and continue for 3 days until approximately 1.5 g base given.

Children. Initially, 5 mg base/kg, repeat in 6 hrs. Do not exceed 10 mg base/ kg/24 hrs.

Amebiasis

IM

Adults. 160-200 mg base (4-5 ml) daily for 10-12 days. Change to oral therapy as soon as possible.

UNLABELED USES: Treatment of sarcoid-associated hypercalcemia, juvenile arthritis, rheumatoid arthritis, systemic lupus erythematosus, solar urticaria, chronic cutaneous vasculitis

CONTRAINDICATIONS: Hypersensitivity to 4-aminoquinoline compounds, retinal or visual field changes

INTERACTIONS

Drug

Alcohol: May increase GI irritation.

Penicillamine: May increase concentration of penicillamine and increase risk of hematologic, renal or severe skin reaction.
Ampicillin: May reduce the absorption of ampicillin. Separate administration by 2 hours.
Antacids and kaolin: May be decreased due to GI binding with kaolin or magnesium trisilicate.
Cimetidine: May increase levels of chloroquine.
Cyclosporine: May increase cyclosporine concentrations.
CYP2D6 inhibitors (chlorpromazine, delavirdine, fluoxetine, miconazole, paroxetine, pergolide, quinidine, quinine, ritonavir, ropinirole): May increase the levels and effects of chloroquine.
CYP2D6 substrates (amphetamines, selected beta-blockers, dextromethorphan, fluoxetine, lidocaine, mirtazapine, nefazodone, paroxetine, risperidone, ritonavir, thioridazine, tricyclic antidepressants, venlafaxine): May increase the levels and effects of CYP2D6 substrates.
CYP2D6 prodrug substrates: Chloroquine may decrease the levels and effects of CYP2D6 prodrug substrates.
CYP3A4 inducers (aminoglutethimide, carbamazepine, nafcillin, nevirapine, phenobarbital, phenytoin, and rifamycins): CYP3A4 inducers may decrease the levels and effects of chloroquine.
CYP3A4 inhibitors (azole antifungals, ciprofloxacin, clarithromycin, diclofenac, doxycycline, erythromycin, imatinib, isoniazid, nefazodone, nicardipine, propofol, protease inhibitors, quinidine, and verapamil): May increase the levels and effects of chloroquine.
Praziquantel: May decrease praziquantel concentrations.

Herbal
None known.
Food
None known.

DIAGNOSTIC TEST EFFECTS: Acute decrease in Hct, Hgb, RBC count may occur.

SIDE EFFECTS
Frequent
Discomfort with IM administration, mild transient headache, anorexia, nausea, vomiting
Occasional
Nervousness, fatigue, pruritus esp. of palms, soles, scalp; bleaching of hair, irritability, personality changes, diarrhea, skin eruptions
Rare
Phlebitis or thrombophlebitis at IV injection site, abdominal cramps, headache, hypotension

SERIOUS REACTIONS
• Ocular toxicity and ototoxicity have been reported.
• Prolonged therapy: peripheral neuritis and neuromyopathy, hypotension, ECG changes, agranulocytosis, aplastic anemia, thrombocytopenia, convulsions, psychosis.
• Overdosage includes symptoms of headache, vomiting, visual disturbance, drowsiness, convulsions, hypokalemia followed by cardiovascular collapse, and death.

SPECIAL CONSIDERATIONS

PRECAUTIONS
• Generally, if any severe blood disorder appears that is not attributable to the disease under treatment, consider discontinuing the drug. Because this drug is known to concentrate in the liver, use it with caution in patients with hepatic disease or alcoholism or along with known hepatotoxic drugs. Administer the drug

with caution to patients having glucose-6-phosphate dehydrogenase deficiency.

PREGNANCY AND LACTATION

• Pregnancy Category C. For nursing mothers, because of the potential for serious adverse reactions in nursing infants from chloroquine, decide whether to discontinue nursing or to discontinue the drug, taking into account the importance of the drug to the mother.

OCULAR CONSIDERATIONS

• Occasional side effects include visual disturbances (blurring, difficulty focusing).

• Irreversible retinal damage has been observed in some patients who had received long-term or high-dosage 4-aminoquinoline therapy. Retinopathy has been reported to be dose related. When contemplating prolonged therapy with any antimalarial compound, perform initial (baseline) and periodic ocular examinations (including visual acuity, slit-lamp biomicroscopy, retinal exam, and visual field tests).

• If there is any indication (past or present) of abnormality in the visual acuity, visual field, or retinal macular areas (such as pigmentary changes or loss of foveal reflex) or any visual symptoms (such as light flashes and streaks) that are not fully explainable by difficulties of accommodation or corneal opacities, discontinue the drug immediately and observe the patient closely for possible progression. Retinal changes (and visual disturbances) may progress even after cessation of therapy.

• Ocular Reactions: Irreversible retinal damage in patients receiving long-term or high-dosage 4-aminoquinoline therapy; visual disturbances (blurring of vision and difficulty of focusing or accommodation); nyctalopia; scotomatous vision with field defects of paracentral, pericentral ring types, and typically temporal scotomas (e.g., difficulty in reading with words tending to disappear, seeing half an object, misty vision, and fog before the eyes) may occur.

C

chlorpheniramine

(klor-fen-ir'a-meen)

Rx: Chlorate

Drug Class: Antihistamines, H1

Pregnancy Category: C

Do not confuse with chlorpromazine or chlorpropamide.

CLINICAL PHARMACOLOGY

Mechanism of Action: A propylamine derivative antihistamine that competes with histamine for histamine receptor sites on cells in the blood vessels, gastrointestinal (GI) tract, and respiratory tract. *Therapeutic Effect:* Inhibits symptoms associated with seasonal allergic rhinitis such as increased mucus production and sneezing.

Pharmacokinetics

Well absorbed after PO and parenteral administration. Food delays absorption. Widely distributed. Metabolized in liver. Primarily excreted in urine. Not removed by dialysis. **Half-life:** 20 hrs.

AVAILABLE FORMS

• *Injection:* 10 mg/ml, 100 mg/ml.

• *Syrup:* 2 mg/5 ml (Aller-Chlor, Diabetic Tussin Allergy Relief [sugar free]).

• *Tablets:* 4 mg (Aller-Chlor, Chlor-Trimeton, Chlorate, Chlorphen).

• *Tablets (sustained-release):* 8 mg (Chlor-Trimeton Allergy 8 Hour), 12 mg (Chlor-Trimeton Allergy 12 Hour).

INDICATIONS AND DOSAGES

Allergic rhinitis, common cold

PO

Adults, Elderly. 4 mg q6-8h or 8-12 mg (sustained-release) q8-12h. Maximum: 24 mg/day.

Children 12 yr and older. 4 mg q6-8h or 8 mg (sustained-release) q12h. Maximum: 24 mg/day.

Children 6-11 yr. 2 mg q4-6h. Maximum: 12 mg/day.

IM/IV/SC

Adults, Elderly. 5-40 mg as a single dose. Maximum: 40 mg/day.

SC

Children 6 yr and older. 87.5 mcg/kg or 2.5 mg/m^2 4 times/day.

CONTRAINDICATIONS: Hypersensitivity to chlorpheniramine or its components

INTERACTIONS

Drug

Alcohol, central nervous system (CNS) depressants: May increase CNS depressant effects.

Anticholinergics: May increase anticholinergic effects.

MAOIs: May increase anticholinergic and CNS depressant effects.

Phenytoin, fosphenytoin: May increase the risk of phenytoin toxicity.

Procarbazine: May increase CNS depressant effects.

Herbal

None known.

Food

None known.

DIAGNOSTIC TEST EFFECTS: *None known.*

IV INCOMPATIBILITIES: Calcium, iodipamide, kanamycin (Kantrex), norepinephrine (Levophed), pentobarbital (Nembutal)

IV COMPATIBILITIES: Amikacin (Amikin), corticotropin, cortisone, hyaluronidase (Wydase), penicillin G

SIDE EFFECTS

Frequent

Drowsiness, dizziness, muscular weakness, hypotension, dry mouth, nose, throat, and lips, urinary retention, thickening of bronchial secretions

Elderly: Sedation, dizziness, hypotension

Occasional

Epigastric distress, flushing, visual or hearing disturbances, paresthesia, diaphoresis, chills

SERIOUS REACTIONS

- Children may experience dominant paradoxical reactions, including restlessness, insomnia, euphoria, nervousness, and tremors.
- Overdosage in children may result in hallucinations, seizures, and death.
- Hypersensitivity reaction, such as eczema, pruritus, rash, cardiac disturbances, and photosensitivity, may occur.
- Overdosage may vary from CNS depression, including sedation, apnea, hypotension, cardiovascular collapse, or death to severe paradoxical reaction, such as hallucinations, tremor, and seizures.

SPECIAL CONSIDERATIONS

PRECAUTIONS

- Chlorpheniramine maleate has an atropine-like action and should be used with caution in patients who may have increased intraocular pressure, hyperthyroidism, cardiovascular disease, or hypertension or in patients with a history of bronchial asthma.

OCULAR CONSIDERATIONS

- Chlorpheniramine maleate can cause ocular dryness, mydriasis, and cycloplegia.

chlorpromazine

(klor-proe'ma-zeen)

Rx: Thorazine

Drug Class: Antiemetics/antivertigo; Antipsychotics; Phenothiazines

Pregnancy Category: C

Do not confuse chlorpromazine with chlorpropamide, clomipramine, or prochlorperazine, or Thorazine with thiamide or thioridazine.

CLINICAL PHARMACOLOGY

Mechanism of Action: A phenothiazine that blocks dopamine neurotransmission at postsynaptic dopamine receptor sites. Possesses strong anticholinergic, sedative, and antiemetic effects; moderate extrapyramidal effects; and slight antihistamine action. *Therapeutic Effect:* Relieves nausea and vomiting; improves psychotic consitions; controls intractable hiccups and porphyria.

Pharmacokinetics

Rapidly absorbed after oral or IM administration. Protein binding: 92%-97%. Metabolized in the liver. Excreted in urine. **Half-life:** 6 hr.

AVAILABLE FORMS

- *Oral Concentrate:*30 mg/ml, 100 mg/ml.
- *Syrup:* 10 mg/5 ml.
- *Tablets:*10 mg, 25 mg, 50 mg, 100 mg, 200 mg.
- *Capsules (Sustained-Release):* 30 mg, 75 mg, 150 mg.
- *Injection (Thorazine):* 25 mg/ml.
- *Suppositories:* 25 mg, 100 mg.

INDICATIONS AND DOSAGES

Severe nausea or vomiting

PO

Adults, Elderly. 10-25 mg q4-6h.

Children. 0.5-1 mg/kg q4-6h.

IV, IM

Adults, Elderly. 25-50 mg q4-6h.

Children. 0.5-1 mg/kg q6-8h.

Rectal

Adults, Elderly. 50-100 mg q6-8h.

Children. 1 mg/kg q6-8h.

Psychotic disorders

PO

Adults, Elderly. 30-800 mg/day in 1-4 divided doses.

Children older than 6 mo. 0.5-1 mg/kg q4-6h.

IV, IM

Adults, Elderly. Initially, 25 mg; may repeat in 1-4 hr. May gradually increase to 400 mg q4-6h. Maximum: 300-800 mg/day.

Children older than 6 mo. 0.5-1 mg/kg q6-8h. Maximum: 75 mg/day for children 5-12 yr; 40 mg/day for children younger than 5 yr.

Intractable hiccups

PO, IV, IM

Adults. 25-50 mg 3 times a day.

Porphyria

PO

Adults. 25-50 mg 3-4 times a day.

IM

Adults, Elderly. 25 mg 3-4 times a day.

UNLABELED USES: Treatment of choreiform movement of Huntington's disease

CONTRAINDICATIONS: Comatose states, myelosuppression, severe cardiovascular disease, severe CNS depression, subcortical brain damage

INTERACTIONS

Drug

Alcohol, other CNS depressants: May increase respiratory depression and the hypotensive effects of chlorpromazine.

Antithyroid agents: May increase the risk of agranulocytosis.

Extrapyramidal symptom-producing medications: Increased risk of extrapyramidal symptoms.
Hypotensives: May increase hypotension.
Levodopa: May decrease the effects of levodopa.
Lithium: May decrease the absorption of chlorpromazine and produce adverse neurologic effects.
MAOIs, tricyclic antidepressants: May increase the anticholinergic and sedative effects of chlorpromazine.

Herbal

None known.

Food

None known.

DIAGNOSTIC TEST EFFECTS: May produce false-positive pregnancy and phenylketonuria (PKU) test results. May cause EKG changes, including Q- and T-wave disturbances. Therapeutic serum level is 50-300 mcg/ml; toxic serum level is greater than 750 mcg/ml.

SIDE EFFECTS

Frequent

Somnolence, blurred vision, hypotension, color vision or night vision disturbances, dizziness, decreased sweating, constipation, dry mouth, nasal congestion

Occasional

Urinary retention, photosensitivity, rash, decreased sexual function, swelling or pain in breasts, weight gain, nausea, vomiting, abdominal pain, tremors

SERIOUS REACTIONS

• Extrapyramidal symptoms appear to be dose related and are divided into three categories: akathisia (including inability to sit still, tapping of feet), parkinsonian symptoms (such as masklike face, tremors, shuffling gait, hypersalivation), and acute dystonias (including torticollis, opisthotonos, and oculogyric crisis). A dystonic reaction may also produce diaphoresis and pallor.

• Tardive dyskinesia, including tongue protrusion, puffing of the cheeks, and puckering of the mouth is a rare reaction that may be irreversible.

• Abrupt discontinuation after long-term therapy may precipitate nausea, vomiting, gastritis, dizziness, and tremors.

• Blood dyscrasias, particularly agranulocytosis and mild leukopenia, may occur.

• Chlorpromazine may lower the seizure threshold.

SPECIAL CONSIDERATIONS

PRECAUTIONS

• Exercise caution, given the likelihood that some patients exposed chronically to neuroleptics will develop tardive dyskinesia. Administer chlorpromazine cautiously to persons with cardiovascular, liver, or renal disease. Evidence indicates that patients with a history of hepatic encephalopathy caused by cirrhosis have increased sensitivity to the central nervous system effects of chlorpromazine (i.e., impaired cerebration and abnormal slowing of the electroencephalogram).

• Because of its central nervous system depressant effect, use chlorpromazine with caution in patients with chronic respiratory disorders such as severe asthma, emphysema, and acute respiratory infections, particularly in children (1 to 12 years of age). Because chlorpromazine can suppress the cough reflex, aspiration of vomitus is possible.

• Chlorpromazine prolongs and intensifies the action of central nervous system depressants such as anesthetics, barbiturate, and narcotics. NOTE: Chlorpromazine does not intensify the anticonvulsant action of barbiturates. Therefore, do not reduce the dosage of anticonvulsants, including barbiturates, if chlorpromazine is started. Instead, start chlorpromazine at low doses and increase as needed.

• Use chlorpromazine with caution in persons who will be exposed to extreme heat or organophosphorus insecticides and in persons receiving atropine or related drugs.

• Neuroleptic drugs elevate prolactin levels; the elevation persists during chronic administration. Chromosomal aberrations in spermatocytes and abnormal sperm have been demonstrated in rodents treated with certain neuroleptics.

• As with all drugs that exert an anticholinergic effect and/or cause mydriasis, use chlorpromazine with caution in patients with glaucoma.

• Chlorpromazine diminishes the effect of oral anticoagulants. Phenothiazines can produce alpha-adrenergic blockade. Chlorpromazine may lower the convulsive threshold; dosage adjustments of anticonvulsants may be necessary. Concomitant administration with propranolol results in increased plasma levels of both drugs. Thiazide diuretics may accentuate the orthostatic hypotension that may occur with phenothiazines. The presence of phenothiazines may produce false-positive phenylketonuria test results. Do not use drugs that lower the seizure threshold, including phenothiazine derivatives, with metrizamide.

• The antiemetic action of chlorpromazine may mask the signs and symptoms of overdosage of other drugs and may obscure the diagnosis and treatment of other conditions such as intestinal obstruction, brain tumor, and Reye's syndrome. When chlorpromazine is used with cancer chemotherapeutic drugs, vomiting as a sign of the toxicity of these agents may be obscured by the antiemetic effect of chlorpromazine.

• Abrupt Withdrawal: Like other phenothiazines, chlorpromazine is not known to cause psychic dependence and does not produce tolerance or addiction. However, some symptoms resembling those of physical dependence may occur following abrupt withdrawal of high-dose therapy, such as gastritis, nausea and vomiting, dizziness, and tremulousness. These symptoms usually can be avoided or reduced by gradual reduction of the dosage or by continuing concomitant antiparkinsonism agents for several weeks after chlorpromazine is withdrawn.

OCULAR CONSIDERATIONS

• Ocular changes have occurred more frequently than skin pigmentation and have been observed in pigmented and nonpigmented patients receiving chlorpromazine, usually for 2 years or more in dosages of 300 mg daily and higher. Eye changes are characterized by deposition of fine particulate matter in the lens and cornea. In more advanced cases, star-shaped opacities also have been observed in the anterior portion of the lens. The nature of the eye deposits has not yet been determined. A small number of patients with more severe ocular changes have had some visual impairment. In addition to these corneal and lenticular changes, epithelial keratopathy and pigmentary retinopathy have been reported. Reports suggest that the eye lesions may regress after withdrawal of the drug.

• Because the occurrence of eye changes seems to be related to dosage levels and/or duration of therapy, it is suggested that patients taking long-term therapy of moderate to high dosage levels have periodic eye examinations.

• Etiology: The cause is not clear, but exposure to light, along with dosage/duration of therapy, appears to be the most significant factor. If either of these reactions is observed, the physician should weigh the benefits of continued therapy against the possible risks and, on the merits of the individual case, determine whether to continue present therapy, lower the dosage, or withdraw the drug.

chlorpropamide

(klor-pro′pa-mide)

Rx: Diabinese

Drug Class: Antidiabetic agents; Sulfonylureas, first-generation

Pregnancy Category: C

Do not confuse with chlorpromazine.

CLINICAL PHARMACOLOGY

Mechanism of Action: A first-generation sulfonylurea that promotes release of insulin from beta cells of pancreas. *Therapeutic Effect:* Lowers blood glucose concentration.

Pharmacokinetics

Rapidly absorbed from the gastrointestinal (GI) tract. Protein binding: 60%-90%. Extensively metabolized in liver. Excreted primarily urine. Removed by hemodialysis. **Half-life:** 30-42 hrs.

AVAILABLE FORMS

• *Tablets:* 100 mg, 250 mg (Diabenese).

INDICATIONS AND DOSAGES

Diabetes mellitus, combination therapy

PO

Adults. Initially, 250 mg once a day. Maintenance: 250-500 mg once a day. Maximum: 750 mg/day.

Elderly. Initially, 100-125 mg once a day. Maintenance: 100-250 mg once a day. Increase or decrease by 50-125 mg a day for 3- to 5-day intervals.

Renal function impairment

Not recommended.

UNLABELED USES: Neurogenic diabetes insipidus

CONTRAINDICATIONS: Diabetic complications, such as ketosis, acidosis, and diabetic coma, severe liver or renal impairment, sole therapy for type 1 diabetes mellitus, or hypersensitivity to sulfonylureas

INTERACTIONS

Drug

Alcohol: Disulfiram-like reactions may occur. Symptoms of low blood sugar including sweating, shaking, weakness, drowsiness, and trouble concentrating will occur.

Beta-blockers, MAOIs, NSAIDs, salicylates: May increase hypoglycemic effect.

Fluoroquinolone antibiotics: May increase the risk of hypoglycemia.

Glucocorticoids, thiazide diuretics: May increase blood glucose.

Oral contraceptives: May increase blood glucose.

Herbal

Bitter melon: May increase the risk of hypoglycemia.

St. John's wort: May increase the risk of hypoglycemia.

Food

None known.

DIAGNOSTIC TEST EFFECTS: *None known.*

SIDE EFFECTS

Frequent

Headache, upper respiratory tract infection

Occasional

Sinusitis, myalgia (muscle aches), pharyngitis, aggravated diabetes mellitus

SERIOUS REACTIONS

• Possible increased risk of cardiovascular mortality with this class of drugs.

• Overdosage can cause severe hypoglycemia prolonged by extended half-life.

SPECIAL CONSIDERATIONS

PRECAUTIONS

• Chlorpropamide administration is associated with increased cardiovascular mortality compared with treatment with diet alone or diet plus insulin. All sulfonylurea drugs are capable of producing severe hypoglycemia. Proper patient selection, dosage, and instructions are important to avoid hypoglycemic episodes. Renal or hepatic insufficiency may cause elevated blood levels of chlorpropamide, and the latter also may diminish gluconeogenic capacity, both of which increase the risk of serious hypoglycemic reactions. Elderly, debilitated, or malnourished patients and those with adrenal or pituitary insufficiency are particularly susceptible to the hypoglycemic action of glucose-lowering drugs. Hypoglycemia may be difficult to recognize in the elderly and in persons who are taking beta-adrenergic blocking drugs. When a patient stabilized on any diabetic regimen is exposed to stress such as fever, trauma, infection, or surgery, a loss of control may occur. The effectiveness of any oral hypoglycemic drug, including chlorpropamide, in lowering blood glucose to a desired level decreases in many patients over time.

PATIENT INFORMATION

• Inform patients of the potential risks and advantages of chlorpropamide and of alternative modes of therapy. Also inform patients about the importance of adherence to dietary instructions, of a regular exercise program, and of regular testing of urine and/or blood glucose.

• Explain the risks of hypoglycemia, its symptoms and treatment, and conditions that predispose to its development to patients and responsible family members. Also explain primary and secondary failure.

• Instruct patients to contact their physician promptly if they experience symptoms of hypoglycemia or other adverse reactions.

PREGNANCY AND LACTATION

• Pregnancy Category C. Whether chlorpropamide can cause fetal harm when administered to a pregnant woman is not known. An analysis of a composite of two samples of human breast milk, each taken 5 hours after ingestion of 500 mg of chlorpropamide by a patient, revealed a concentration of 5 mcg/ml. For reference, the normal peak blood level of chlorpropamide after a single 250-mg dose is 30 mcg/ml. Therefore breast-feeding while taking this medication is not recommended.

chymotrypsin

(ki-mo-trip′-san)

Rx: Catarase

Drug Class: Ophthalmics

CLINICAL PHARMACOLOGY

Mechanism of Action: A proteolytic enzyme obtained from the pancreas of an ox that facilitates dissection of zonule of lens and intracapsular cataract extraction. *Therapeutic Effect:* Reduces trauma to eye.

Pharmacokinetics

None reported.

AVAILABLE FORMS

• *Powder for intraocular injection:* 300 units/vial (Catarase).

INDICATIONS AND DOSAGES

Enzymatic xonulysis in intracapsular lens extraction

Ophthalmic

Adults 20 yr and older, Elderly. Irrigate posterior chamber with reconstituted cymotrypsin using 0.25 to 0.5 ml evenly around circumference of lens following cataract section. Wait 2-4 minutes, and then irrigate the anterior chamber and corneal wound edges with at leat 1 ml of the diluent of balanced salt solution.

CONTRAINDICATIONS: Significant anterior displacement of the lens iris diaphragm with impending vitreous loss or other conditions in which loss of vitreous is a significant problem, and hypersensitivity to chymotrypsin or any component of the formulation.

INTERACTIONS

Drug

None known.

Herbal

None known.

Food

None known.

DIAGNOSTIC TEST EFFECTS: *None known.*

SIDE EFFECTS

Rare

Increased intraocular pressure, moderate uveitis, corneal edema, and striation.

SERIOUS REACTIONS

• Hypersensitivity reactions have been reported.

SPECIAL CONSIDERATIONS

PRECAUTIONS

• Chymotrypsin may produce an acute rise in intraocular pressure following surgery. Use of chymotrypsin is not advised in patients under 20 years of age.

---

cidofovir

(ci-dah'fo-veer)

Rx: Vistide

Drug Class: Antivirals

Pregnancy Category: C

CLINICAL PHARMACOLOGY

Mechanism of Action: An anti-infective that inhibits viral DNA synthesis by incorporating itself into the growing viral DNA chain. *Therapeutic Effect:* Suppresses replication of cytomegalovirus (CMV).

Pharmacokinetics

Protein binding: less than 6%. Excreted primarily unchanged in urine. Effect of hemodialysis unknown. **Elimination half-life:** 1.4-3.8 hr.

AVAILABLE FORMS

• *Injection:* 75 mg/ml (5-ml ampule).

INDICATIONS AND DOSAGES

CMV retinitis in patients with AIDS (in combination with probenecid)

IV infusion

Adults. Induction: Usual dosage, 5 mg/kg at constant rate over 1 hr once weekly for 2 consecutive wk. Give 2 g of PO probenecid 3 hr before cidofovir dose, and then give 1 g 2 hr and 8 hr after completion of the 1-hr cidofovir infusion (total of 4 g). In addition, give 1 L of 0.9% NaCl over 1-2 hr immediately before the cidofovir infusion. If tolerated, a second liter may be infused over 1-3 hr at the start of the infusion or immediately afterward. Maintenance: 5 mg/kg cidofovir at constant rate over 1 hr once every 2 wk.

Dosage in renal impairment

Dosages are modified based on creatinine clearance.

Creatinine Clearance	*Induction Dose*	*Maintenance Dose*
41-55 ml/min	2 mg/kg	2 mg/kg
30-40 ml/min	1.5 mg/kg	1.5 mg/kg
20-29 ml/min	1 mg/kg	1 mg/kg
19 ml/min or less	0.5 mg/kg	0.5 mg/kg

UNLABELED USES: Treatment of ganciclovir-resistant CMV, foscarnet-resistant CMV, adenovirus, and acyclovir-resistant herpes simplex virus or varicella-zoster virus

CONTRAINDICATIONS: Direct intraocular injection, history of clinically severe hypersensitivity to probenecid or other sulfa-containing drugs, hypersensitivity to cidofovir, renal function impairment (serum creatinine level greater than 1.5 mg/dl, creatinine clearance of 55 ml/min or less, or urine protein level greater than 100 mg/dl)

INTERACTIONS

Drug

Nephrotoxic medications (such as aminoglycosides, amphotericin B, foscarnet, IV pentamidine): Increase the risk of nephrotoxicity.

Herbal

None known.

Food

None known.

DIAGNOSTIC TEST EFFECTS: May decrease neutrophil count and serum bicarbonate, phosphate, and uric acid levels. May elevate serum creatinine levels.

IV INCOMPATIBILITIES: No information available for Y-site administration.

SIDE EFFECTS

Frequent

Nausea, vomiting (65%), fever (57%), asthenia (46%), rash (30%), diarrhea (27%), headache (27%), alopecia (25%), chills (24%), anorexia (22%), dyspnea (22%), abdominal pain (17%)

SERIOUS REACTIONS

- Serious adverse reactions may include proteinuria (80%), nephrotoxicity (53%), neutropenia (31%), elevated serum creatinine levels (29%), infection (24%), anemia (20%), ocular hypotony (a decrease in intraocular pressure,12%), and pneumonia (9%).
- Concurrent use of probenecid may produce a hypersensitivity reaction characterized by a rash, fever, chills, and anaphylaxis.
- Acute renal failure occurs rarely.

SPECIAL CONSIDERATIONS

PRECAUTIONS

- Direct intraocular injection of cidofovir is contraindicated; direct injection may be associated with significant decreases in intraocular pressure and impairment of vision.
- Because of the potential for increased nephrotoxicity, doses greater than the recommended dose should not be administered, and the frequency or rate of administration should not be exceeded. Cidofovir is formulated for intravenous infusion only and must not be administered by intraocular injection. Administration of cidofovir by infusion must be accompanied by oral probenecid administration and intravenous saline prehydration.

PATIENT INFORMATION

- Advise patients cidofovir is not a cure for cytomegalovirus retinitis and that they may continue to experience progression of retinitis during and following treatment. Advise patients receiving cidofovir to have regular follow-up eye examinations. Patients also may experience other manifestations of cytomegalovirus disease despite cidofovir therapy.

• Patients infected with human immunodeficiency virus may continue taking antiretroviral therapy, but advise those taking zidovudine temporarily to discontinue zidovudine administration or decrease their zidovudine dose by 50%, on days of cidofovir administration only, because probenecid reduces metabolic clearance of zidovudine.

• Inform patients of the major toxicity of cidofovir, namely renal impairment, and that dose modification, including reduction, interruption, and possibly discontinuation, may be required. Emphasize close monitoring of renal function (routine urinalysis and serum creatinine) while the patient is receiving therapy.

• Emphasize the importance of completing a full course of probenecid with each cidofovir dose. Warn patients of potential adverse events caused by probenecid (e.g., headache, nausea, vomiting, and hypersensitivity reactions). Hypersensitivity/allergic reactions may include rash, fever, chills and anaphylaxis. Administration of probenecid after a meal or use of antiemetics may decrease the nausea. Prophylactic or therapeutic administration of antihistamines and/or acetaminophen can be used to ameliorate hypersensitivity reactions.

• Advise patients that cidofovir causes tumors, primarily mammary adenocarcinomas, in rats. Consider cidofovir a potential carcinogen in human beings. Advise women of the limited enrollment of women in clinical trials of cidofovir.

• Advise patients that cidofovir caused reduced testes weight and hypospermia in animals. Such changes may occur in human beings and cause infertility. Advise women of childbearing potential that cidofovir is embryotoxic in animals and should not be used during pregnancy. Advise women of childbearing potential to use effective contraception during and for 1 month following treatment with cidofovir.

PREGNANCY AND LACTATION

• Pregnancy Category C. Cidofovir was embryotoxic (reduced fetal body weights) in rats following daily intravenous dosing during the period of organogenesis. Excretion into human milk is not known.

---

ciprofloxacin hydrochloride

(sip-ro-floks'a-sin hye-droe-klor'-ide)

Rx: Ciloxan, Cipro, Cipro I.V., Cipro XR

Drug Class: Anti-infectives, ophthalmic; Antibiotics, quinolones; Ophthalmics

Pregnancy Category: C

Do not confuse ciprofloxacin or Ciproxin with Ciloxan, cinoxacin, or Cytoxan.

CLINICAL PHARMACOLOGY

Mechanism of Action: A fluoroquinolone that inhibits the enzyme DNA gyrase in susceptible bacteria, interfering with bacterial cell replication. *Therapeutic Effect:* Bactericidal.

Pharmacokinetics

Well absorbed from the GI tract (food delays absorption). Protein binding: 20%-40%. Widely distributed (including to CSF). Metabolized in the liver to active metabolite. Primarily excreted in urine. Minimal removal by hemodialysis. **Half-life:** 4-6 hr (increased in impaired renal function and the elderly).

AVAILABLE FORMS

- *Tablets (Cipro):* 100 mg, 250 mg, 500 mg, 750 mg.
- *Tablets (Extended-Release [Cipro XR]):* 500 mg, 1000 mg.
- *Infusion:* 200 mg/100 ml, 400 mg/200 ml.
- *Ophthalmic Ointment (Ciloxan):* 0.3%.
- *Ophthalmic Suspension (Ciloxan):* 0.3%.

INDICATIONS AND DOSAGES

Mild to moderate UTIs

PO

Adults, Elderly. 250 mg q12h.

IV

Adults, Elderly. 200 mg q12h.

Complicated UTIs, mild to moderate respiratory tract, bone, joint, skin and skin-structure infections; infectious diarrhea

PO

Adults, Elderly. 500 mg q12h.

IV

Adults, Elderly. 400 mg q12h.

Severe, complicated infections

PO

Adults, Elderly. 750 mg q12h.

IV

Adults, Elderly. 400 mg q12h.

Prostatitis

PO

Adults, Elderly. 500 mg q12h for 28 days.

Uncomplicated bladder infection

PO

Adults. 100 mg twice a day for 3 days.

Acute sinusitis

PO

Adults. 500 mg q12h.

Uncomplicated gonorrhea

PO

Adults. 250 mg as a single dose.

Cystic fibrosis

IV

Children. 30 mg/kg/day in 2-3 divided doses. Maximum: 1.2 g/day.

PO

Children. 40 mg/kg/day. Maximum: 2 g/day.

Corneal ulcer

Ophthalmic

Adults, Elderly. 2 drops q15min for 6 hr, then 2 drops q30min for the remainder of first day, 2 drops q1h on second day, and 2 drops q4h on days 3-14.

Conjunctivitis

Ophthalmic

Adults, Elderly. 1-2 drops q2h for 2 days, then 2 drops q4h for next 5 days.

Dosage in renal impairment

Dosage and frequency are modified based on creatinine clearance and the severity of the infection.

Creatinine Clearance	*Dosage Interval*
less than 30 ml/min	Usual dose q18-24h

Hemodialysis

Adults, Elderly. 250-500 mg q24h (after dialysis).

Peritoneal Dialysis

Adults, Elderly. 250-500 mg q24h (after dialysis).

UNLABELED USES: Treatment of chancroid

CONTRAINDICATIONS: Hypersensitivity to ciprofloxacin or other quinolones; for ophthalmic administration: vaccinia, varicella, epitherlial herpes simplex, keratitis, mycobacterial infection, fungal disease of ocular structure, use after uncomplicated removal of a foreign body.

INTERACTIONS

Drug

Antacids, iron preparations, sucralfate: May decrease ciprofloxacin absorption.

Caffeine, oral anticoagulants: May increase the effects of these drugs.

Theophylline: Decreases clearance and may increase blood concentration and risk of toxicity of theophylline.

Herbal

None known.

Food

None known.

DIAGNOSTIC TEST EFFECTS: May increase BUN and serum alkaline phosphatase, bilirubin, creatinine, LDH, AST (SGOT), and ALT (SGPT) levels.

IV INCOMPATIBILITIES: Aminophylline, ampicillin and sulbactam (Unasyn), cefepime (Maxipime), dexamethasone (Decadron), furosemide (Lasix), heparin, hydrocortisone (Solu-Cortef), methylprednisolone (Solu-Medrol), phenytoin (Dilantin), sodium bicarbonate

IV COMPATIBILITIES: Calcium gluconate, diltiazem (Cardizem), dobutamine (Dobutrex), dopamine (Intropin), lidocaine, lorazepam (Ativan), magnesium, midazolam (Versed), potassium chloride

SIDE EFFECTS

Frequent (5%-2%)

Nausea, diarrhea, dyspepsia, vomiting, constipation, flatulence, confusion, crystalluria

Ophthalmic: Burning, crusting in corner of eye

Occasional (less than 2%)

Abdominal pain or discomfort, headache, rash

Ophthalmic: Bad taste, sensation of something in eye, eyelid redness or itching

Rare (less than 1%)

Dizziness, confusion, tremors, hallucinations, hypersensitivity reaction, insomnia, dry mouth, paresthesia

SERIOUS REACTIONS

- Superinfection (especially enterococcal or fungal), nephropathy, cardiopulmonary arrest, chest pain, and cerebral thrombosis may occur.
- Hypersensitivity reactions, including photosensitivity (as evidenced by rash, pruritus, blisters, edema, and burning skin), have occurred in patients receiving fluoroquinolones.
- Arthropathy may occur if the drug is given to children younger than 18 years.
- Sensitization to the ophthalmic form of the drug may contraindicate later systemic use of ciprofloxacin.

SPECIAL CONSIDERATIONS

PRECAUTIONS

- Fungal infection may occur. Discontinue use at the first appearance of a skin rash or any other sign of hypersensitivity reaction. White crystalline precipitates in bacterial corneal ulcer may occur.

PATIENT INFORMATION

- Do not touch dropper tip to any surface, for this may contaminate the solution.

PREGNANCY AND LACTATION

- Pregnancy Category C. In rabbits, oral doses produced gastrointestinal disturbances resulting in maternal weight loss and an increased incidence of abortion. Intravenous doses in rabbits showed no maternal toxicity, and no embryotoxicity or teratogenicity was observed. Fetal harm is not known with topical administration. Orally administered ciprofloxacin is excreted in the milk of lactating rats, and oral ciprofloxacin has been reported in human breast milk after a single 500-mg dose.

OCULAR ADVERSE REACTIONS

Burning or discomfort; white crystalline precipitates—approximately 17%; lid margin crusting, crystals/scales, foreign body sensation, itching, conjunctival hyperemia, and a bad taste following instillation—less than 10%; corneal staining, keratopathy/keratitis, allergic reactions, lid edema, tearing, photophobia, corneal infiltrates, nausea, and decreased vision—less than 1%

OCULAR DOSAGE AND ADMINISTRATION

- Corneal Ulcers: Instill 2 drops into the affected eye every 15 minutes for the first 6 hours and then 2 drops into the affected eye every 30 minutes for the remainder of the first day. On the second day, instill 2 drops in the affected eye hourly. On the third to the fourteenth day, place 2 drops in the affected eye every 4 hours. Treatment may be continued after 14 days if corneal reepithelialization has not occurred.
- Bacterial Conjunctivitis: Instill 1 or 2 drops into the conjunctival sac(s) every 2 hours while awake for 2 days and 1 or 2 drops every 4 hours while awake for the next 5 days.
- Gonococcal Conjunctivitis: Administer cefixime 400 mg orally or one dose. Ciprofloxacin 500 mg or ofloxacin 400 mg also is indicated as single-dose treatment.

citalopram hydrobromide

(sy-tal'oh-pram)

Rx: Celexa

Drug Class: Antidepressants, serotonin specific reuptake inhibitors

Pregnancy Category: C

Do not confuse Celexa with Celebrex, Zyprexa, or Cerebyx.

CLINICAL PHARMACOLOGY

Mechanism of Action: A selective serotonin reuptake inhibitor that blocks the uptake of the neurotransmitter serotonin at CNS presynaptic neuronal membranes, increasing its availability at postsynaptic receptor sites. *Therapeutic Effect:* Relieves depression.

Pharmacokinetics

Well absorbed after PO administration. Protein binding: 80%. Primarily metabolized in the liver. Primarily excreted in feces with a lesser amount eliminated in urine. **Half-life:** 35 hr.

AVAILABLE FORMS

- *Oral Solution:* 10 mg/5 ml.
- *Tablets:* 10 mg, 20 mg, 40 mg.

INDICATIONS AND DOSAGES

Depression

PO

Adults. Initially, 20 mg once a day in the morning or evening. May increase in 20-mg increments at intervals of no less than 1 wk. Maximum: 60 mg/day.

Elderly, Patients with hepatic impairment. 20 mg/day. May titrate to 40 mg/day only for nonresponding patients.

UNLABELED USES: Treatment of alcohol abuse, dementia, diabetic neuropathy, obsessive-compulsive disorder, smoking cessation

CONTRAINDICATIONS: Sensitivity to citalopram, use within 14 days of MAOIs

INTERACTIONS

Drug

Antifungals, cimetidine, macrolide antibiotics: May increase the citalopram plasma level.

Carbamazepine: May decrease the citalopram plasma level.

MAOIs: May cause serotonin syndrome, marked by autonomic hyperactivity, coma, diaphoresis, excitement, hyperthermia, and rigidity, and neuroleptic malignant syndrome.

Metoprolol: Increases the metoprolol plasma level.

Herbal

None known.

Food

None known.

DIAGNOSTIC TEST EFFECTS: May reduce serum sodium level.

SIDE EFFECTS

Frequent (21%-11%)

Nausea, dry mouth, somnolence, insomnia, diaphoresis

Occasional (8%-4%)

Tremor, diarrhea, abnormal ejaculation, dyspepsia, fatigue, anxiety, vomiting, anorexia

Rare (3%-2%)

Sinusitis, sexual dysfunction, menstrual disorder, abdominal pain, agitation, decreased libido

SERIOUS REACTIONS

• Overdose is manifested as dizziness, drowsiness, tachycardia, somnolence, confusion, and seizures.

SPECIAL CONSIDERATIONS

PRECAUTIONS

• Hyponatremia, activation of mania/hypomania, seizures, suicide, and interference with cognitive and motor performance has been reported. Caution is advisable when using citalopram hydrobromide in patients with diseases or conditions that produce altered metabolism or hemodynamic responses. Approach the use of citalopram hydrobromide in hepatically impaired patients with caution; a lower maximum dosage is recommended.

PATIENT INFORMATION

• Physicians are advised to discuss the following issues with patients for whom they prescribe citalopram hydrobromide: Although in controlled studies citalopram hydrobromide has not been shown to impair psychomotor performance, any psychoactive drug may impair judgment, thinking, or motor skills, and so physicians should caution patients about operating hazardous machinery, including automobiles, until they are reasonably certain that citalopram hydrobromide therapy does not affect their ability to engage in such activities. Physicians should advise patients that although citalopram hydrobromide has not been shown in experiments with normal subjects to increase the mental and motor skill impairments caused by alcohol, the concomitant use of citalopram hydrobromide and alcohol in depressed patients is not advised. Physicians should advise patients to inform their physician if they are taking, or plan to take, any prescription or over-the-counter drugs, for there is a potential for interactions. Physicians should advise patients to notify their physician if they become pregnant or intend to become pregnant during therapy. Physicians should advise patients to notify their physician if they are breast-feeding an infant. Although patients may notice improvement with citalopram hydrobromide therapy in 1 to 4 weeks, physicians should advise them to continue therapy as directed.

PREGNANCY AND LACTATION

• Pregnancy Category C. In animal reproduction studies, citalopram has been shown to have adverse effects on embryo/fetal and postnatal development, including teratogenic effects, when administered at doses greater than human therapeutic doses. Fetal harm is not known. As has been found to occur with many other drugs, citalopram is excreted in human breast milk.

OCULAR CONSIDERATIONS

• Adverse reactions include abnormal accommodation and taste perversion (frequent); conjunctivitis and eye pain (infrequent); mydriasis, photophobia, diplopia, abnormal lacrimation, and cataract (rare).

• Retinal Changes in Rats: Pathologic changes (degeneration/atrophy) were observed in the retinas of albino rats in the 2-year carcinogenicity study with citalopram. An increase in incidence and severity of retinal pathologic conditions occurred in male and female rats receiving 80 mg/kg per day (13 times the maximum recommended daily human dose of 60 mg on a milligram per meter squared basis). Similar findings were not present in rats receiving 24 mg/kg per day for 2 years, in mice treated for 18 months at doses up to 240 mg/kg per day or in dogs treated for 1 year at doses up to 20 mg/kg per day (4, 20, and 10 times, respectively, the maximum recommended daily human dose on a milligram per meter squared basis). Additional studies to investigate the mechanism for this pathologic finding have not been performed, and the potential significance of this effect in human beings has not been established.

clarithromycin

(clare-i-thro-mye'sin)

Rx: Biaxin, Biaxin XL, Biaxin XL-Pak

Drug Class: Antibiotics, macrolides

Pregnancy Category: C

CLINICAL PHARMACOLOGY

Mechanism of Action: A macrolide that binds to ribosomal receptor sites of susceptible organisms, inhibiting protein synthesis of the bacterial cell wall. *Therapeutic Effect:* Bacteriostatic; may be bactericidal with high dosages or very susceptible microorganisms.

Pharmacokinetics

Well absorbed from the GI tract. Protein binding: 65%-75%. Widely distributed. Metabolized in the liver to active metabolite. Primarily excreted in urine. Not removed by hemodialysis. **Half-life:** 3-7 hr; metabolite 5-7 hr (increased in impaired renal function).

AVAILABLE FORMS

• *Oral Suspension:* 125 mg/5 ml, 250 mg/5 ml.

• *Tablets:* 250 mg, 500 mg.

• *Tablets (Extended-Release):* 500 mg.

INDICATIONS AND DOSAGES

Bronchitis

PO

Adults, Elderly. 500 mg q12h for 7-14 days.

Skin, soft tissue infections

PO

Adults, Elderly. 250 mg q12h for 7-14 days.

Children. 7.5 mg/kg q12h for 10 days.

MAC prophylaxis

PO

Adults, Elderly. 500 mg 2 times/day.

Children. 7.5 mg/kg q12h. Maximum: 500 mg 2 times/day.

MAC treatment

PO

Adults, Elderly. 500 mg 2 times/day in combination.

Children. 7.5 mg/kg q12h in combination. Maximum: 500 mg 2 times/day.

Pharyngitis, tonsillitis

PO

Adults, Elderly. 250 mg q12h for 10 days.

Children. 7.5 mg/kg q12h for 10 days.

Pneumonia

PO

Adults, Elderly. 250 mg q12h for 7-14 days.

Children. 7.5 mg/kg q12h.

Maxillary sinusitis

PO

Adults, Elderly. 500 mg q12h for 14 days.

*Children.*7.5 mg/kg q12h. Maximum: 500 mg 2 times/day.

H. pylori

PO

Adults, Elderly. 500 mg q12h for 10-14 days in combination.

Acute otitis media

PO

Children. 7.5 mg/kg q12h for 10 days.

Dosage in renal impairment

For patients with creatinine clearance less than 30 ml/min, reduce dose by 50% and administer once or twice a day.

CONTRAINDICATIONS: Hypersensitivity to clarithromycin or other macrolide antibiotics

INTERACTIONS

Drug

Carbamazepine, digoxin, theophylline: May increase blood concentration and toxicity of these drugs.

Rifampin: May decrease clarithromycin blood concentration.

Warfarin: May increase warfarin effects.

Zidovudine: May decrease blood concentration of zidovudine.

Herbal

None known.

Food

None known.

DIAGNOSTIC TEST EFFECTS: May (rarely) increase BUN, AST (SGOT), and ALT (SGPT) levels.

SIDE EFFECTS

Occasional (6%-3%)

Diarrhea, nausea, altered taste, abdominal pain

Rare (2%-1%)

Headache, dyspepsia

SERIOUS REACTIONS

- Antibiotic-associated colitis and other superinfections may result from altered bacterial balance.
- Hepatotoxicity and thrombocytopenia occur rarely.

SPECIAL CONSIDERATIONS

PRECAUTIONS

- Pseudomembranous colitis has been reported. Clarithromycin may be administered without dosage adjustment to patients with hepatic impairment and normal renal function. Clarithromycin combined with ranitidine bismuth citrate therapy is not recommended in patients with creatinine clearance less than 25 ml/min and should not be used in patients with a history of acute porphyria.

PATIENT INFORMATION

- Clarithromycin tablets and oral suspension can be taken with or without food and can be taken with milk; however, clarithromycin extended-release tablets should be taken with food. Do not refrigerate the suspension.

PREGNANCY AND LACTATION

• Pregnancy Category C. Clarithromycin should not be used in pregnant women except in clinical circumstances where no alternative therapy is appropriate. If pregnancy occurs while the patient is taking this drug, apprise the patient of the potential hazard to the fetus. Clarithromycin has demonstrated adverse effects of pregnancy outcome and/or embryo/fetal development in monkeys, rats, mice, and rabbits. Excretion into human milk is not known.

clemastine fumarate

(klem'as-teen)

Rx: Tavist

Drug Class: Antihistamines, H1

Pregnancy Category: B

CLINICAL PHARMACOLOGY

Mechanism of Action: An ethanolamine that competes with histamine on effector cells in the GI tract, blood vessels, and respiratory tract. *Therapeutic Effect:* Relieves allergy symptoms, including urticaria, rhinitis, and pruritus.

Pharmacokinetics

Route	*Onset*	*Peak*	*Duration*
PO	15-60 min	5-7 hr	10-12 hr

Well absorbed from the GI tract. Metabolized in the liver. Excreted primarily in urine.

AVAILABLE FORMS

• *Syrup (Dayhist, Tavist):* 0.67 mg/5 ml.

• *Tablets (Dayhist, Tavist):* 1.34 mg, 2.68 mg.

INDICATIONS AND DOSAGES

Allergic rhinitis, urticaria

PO

Adults, Children older than 11 yr. 1.34 mg twice a day up to 2.68 mg 3 times a day. Maximum: 8.04 mg/day.

Children 6-11 yr. 0.67-1.34 mg twice a day. Maximum: 4.02 mg/day.

Children younger than 6 yr. 0.05 mg/kg/day divided into 2-3 doses per day. Maximum: 1.34 mg/day.

Elderly. 1.34 mg 1-2 times a day.

CONTRAINDICATIONS: Angle-closure glaucoma, hypersensitivity to clemastine, use within 14 days of MAOIs

INTERACTIONS

Drug

Alcohol, other CNS depressants: May increase CNS depression.

MAOIs: May increase the anticholinergic and CNS depressant effects of clemastine.

Herbal

None known.

Food

None known.

DIAGNOSTIC TEST EFFECTS: May suppress wheal and flare reactions to antigen skin testing unless drug is discontinued 4 days before testing.

SIDE EFFECTS

Frequent

Somnolence, dizziness, urine retention, thickening of bronchial secretions, dry mouth, nose, or throat; in elderly, sedation, dizziness, hypotension

Occasional

Epigastric distress, flushing, blurred vision, tinnitus, paresthesia, diaphoresis, chills

SERIOUS REACTIONS

• A hypersensitivity reaction, marked by eczema, pruritus, rash, cardiac disturbances, angioedema, and photosensitivity, may occur.

• Overdose symptoms may vary from CNS depression, including sedation, apnea, cardiovascular collapse, and death to severe paradoxical reaction, such as hallucinations, tremor, and seizures.

• Children may experience paradoxical reactions, such as restlessness, insomnia, euphoria, nervousness, and tremors.

• Overdose in children may result in hallucinations, seizures, and death.

SPECIAL CONSIDERATIONS

PRECAUTIONS

• Use clemastine fumarate with caution in patients with a history of bronchial asthma, increased intraocular pressure, hyperthyroidism, cardiovascular disease, and hypertension. Antihistamines are more likely to cause dizziness, sedation, and hypotension in elderly patients.

PATIENT INFORMATION

• Antihistamines are prescribed to reduce allergic symptoms.

• Question patients regarding a history of glaucoma, peptic ulcer, urinary retention, or pregnancy before starting antihistamine therapy.

• Advise patients not to take alcohol, sleeping pills, sedatives, or tranquilizers while taking antihistamines.

• Antihistamines may cause drowsiness, dizziness, dry mouth, blurred vision, weakness, nausea, headache, or nervousness in some patients.

• Instruct patients to avoid driving a car or working with hazardous machinery until they assess the effects of this medicine.

• Advise patients to store this medicine in a tightly closed container in a dry, cool place away from heat or direct sunlight and out of the reach of children.

PREGNANCY AND LACTATION

• Pregnancy Category B. Experience with this drug in pregnant women is inadequate to determine whether a potential for harm to the developing fetus exists. Because of the higher risk of antihistamines for infants generally and for newborns and premature infants in particular, antihistamine therapy is contraindicated in nursing mothers.

clindamycin

(klin-da-mye'sin)

Rx: Cleocin HCl, Cleocin Ovules, Cleocin Pediatric, Cleocin Phosphate, Cleocin T, Cleocin Vaginal, Clinda-Derm, Clindagel, Clindamax, Clindets Pledget

Drug Class: Anti-infectives, topical; Antibiotics, lincosamides; Dermatologics

Pregnancy Category: B

CLINICAL PHARMACOLOGY

Mechanism of Action: A lincosamide antibiotic that inhibits protein synthesis of the bacterial cell wall by binding to bacterial ribosomal receptor sites. Topically, it decreases fatty acid concentration on the skin. *Therapeutic Effect:* Bacteriostatic. Prevents outbreaks of acne vulgaris.

Pharmacokinetics

Rapidly absorbed from the GI tract. Protein binding: 92%-94%. Widely distributed. Metabolized in the liver to some active metabolites. Primarily excreted in urine. Not removed by hemodialysis. **Half-life:** 2.4-3 hr (increased in impaired renal function and premature infants).

AVAILABLE FORMS

- *Capsules:* 75 mg, 150 mg, 300 mg.
- *Oral Solution:* 75 mg/5 ml.
- *Injection:* 150 mg/ml.
- *Topical Gel:* 1%.
- *Topical Solution:* 1%.
- *Vaginal Cream (Clindesse):* 2%.
- *Vaginal Suppository:* 100 mg.

INDICATIONS AND DOSAGES

Chronic bone and joint, respiratory tract, skin and soft-tissue, intra-abdominal, and female GU infections; endocarditis; septicemia

PO

Adults, Elderly. 150-450 mg/dose q6-8h.

Children. 10-30 mg/kg/day in 3-4 divided doses. Maximum: 1.8 g/day.

IV, IM

Adults, Elderly. 1.2-1.8 g/day in 2-4 divided doses.

Children. 25-40 mg/kg/day in 3-4 divided doses. Maximum: 4.8 g/day.

Bacterial vaginosis

PO

Adults, Elderly. 300 mg twice a day for 7 days.

Intravaginal

Adults. One applicatorful at bedtime for 3-7 days or 1 suppository at bedtime for 3 days.

Acne vulgaris

Topical

Adults. Apply thin layer to affected area twice a day.

UNLABELED USES: Treatment of malaria, otitis media, *Pneumocystis carinii* pneumonia, toxoplasmosis

CONTRAINDICATIONS: History of antibiotic-associated colitis, regional enteritis, or ulcerative colitis; hypersensitivity to clindamycin or lincomycin; known allergy to tartrazine dye

INTERACTIONS

Drug

Adsorbent antidiarrheals: May delay absorption of clindamycin.

Chloramphenicol, erythromycin: May antagonize the effects of clindamycin.

Neuromuscular blockers: May increase the effects of these drugs.

Herbal

None known.

Food

None known.

DIAGNOSTIC TEST EFFECTS: May increase serum alkaline phosphatase, AST (SGOT), and ALT (SGPT) levels.

IV INCOMPATIBILITIES: Allopurinol (Aloprim), filgrastim (Neupogen), fluconazole (Diflucan), idarubicin (Idamycin)

IV COMPATIBILITIES: Amiodarone (Cordarone), diltiazem (Cardizem), heparin, hydromorphone (Dilaudid), magnesium sulfate, midazolam (Versed), morphine, multivitamins, propofol (Diprivan)

SIDE EFFECTS

Frequent

Systemic: Abdominal pain, nausea, vomiting, diarrhea

Topical: Dry scaly skin

Vaginal: Vaginitis, pruritus

Occasional

Systemic: Phlebitis or thrombophlebitis with IV administration, pain and induration at IM injection site, allergic reaction, urticaria, pruritus

Topical: Contact dermatitis, abdominal pain, mild diarrhea, burning or stinging

Vaginal: Headache, dizziness, nausea, vomiting, abdominal pain

Rare

Vaginal: Hypersensitivity reaction

SERIOUS REACTIONS

• Antibiotic-associated colitis and other superinfections may occur during and several weeks after clindamycin therapy (including the topical form).

• Blood dyscrasias (leukopenia, thrombocytopenia) and nephrotoxicity (proteinuria, azotemia, oliguria) occur rarely.

SPECIAL CONSIDERATIONS

PRECAUTIONS

• Prescribe clindamycin hydrochloride with caution in individuals with a history of gastrointestinal disease, particularly colitis. Prescribe clindamycin hydrochloride with caution in atopic individuals. The use of clindamycin hydrochloride occasionally results in overgrowth of nonsusceptible organisms, particularly yeasts. Clindamycin dosage modification may not be necessary in patients with renal disease. The 75- and 150-mg capsules contain FD&C yellow No. 5 (tartrazine), which may cause allergic-type reactions (including bronchial asthma) in certain susceptible individuals.

PREGNANCY AND LACTATION

• Pregnancy Category B. Reproduction studies performed in rats and mice revealed no evidence of teratogenicity. Clindamycin has been reported to appear in breast milk.

OCULAR DOSAGE AND ADMINISTRATION

• For intraocular foreign body and traumatic optic neuropathy in the presence of sinus wall fracture or penetrating orbital injury, administer gentamicin 2 mg/kg IV load and then 1 mg/kg q8h and cefazolin 1 g IV q8h or clindamycin 600 mg IV q8h

clonazepam

(kloe-na′zi-pam)

Rx: Klonopin, Klonopin Wafer

Drug Class: Anxiolytics; Benzodiazepines

Pregnancy Category: D

DEA Class: Schedule IV

Do not confuse clonazepam with clonidine or lorazepam.

CLINICAL PHARMACOLOGY

Mechanism of Action: A benzodiazepine that depresses all levels of the CNS; inhibits nerve impulse transmission in the motor cortex and suppresses abnormal discharge in petit mal seizures. *Therapeutic Effect:* Produces anxiolytic and anticonvulsant effects.

Pharmacokinetics

Well absorbed from the GI tract. Protein binding: 85%. Metabolized in the liver. Excreted in urine. Not removed by hemodialysis. **Half-life:** 18-50 hr.

AVAILABLE FORMS

• *Tablets:* 0.5 mg, 1 mg, 2 mg.

• *Tablets (Disintegrating):* 0.125 mg, 0.25 mg, 0.5 mg, 1 mg, 2 mg.

INDICATIONS AND DOSAGES

Adjunctive treatment of Lennox-Gastaut syndrome (petit mal variant) and akinetic, myoclonic, and absence (petit mal) seizures

PO

Adults, Elderly, Children 10 yr and older. 1.5 mg/day; may be increased in 0.5- to 1-mg increments every 3 days until seizures are controlled. Do not exceed maintenance dosage of 20 mg/day.

Infants, Children younger than 10 yr or weighing less than 30 kg. 0.01-0.03 mg/kg/day in 2-3 divided doses; may be increased by up to 0.5

mg every 3 days until seizures are controlled. Don't exceed maintenance dosage of 0.2 mg/kg/day.

Panic disorder

PO

Adults, Elderly. Initially, 0.25 mg twice a day; increased in increments of 0.125-0.25 mg twice a day every 3 days. Maximum: 4 mg/day.

UNLABELED USES: Adjunctive treatment of seizures; treatment of simple, complex partial, and tonic-clonic seizures

CONTRAINDICATIONS: Narrow-angle glaucoma, significant hepatic disease

INTERACTIONS

Drug

Alcohol, other CNS depressants: May increase CNS depressant effect.

Herbal

Kava kava: May increase sedation.

Food

None known.

DIAGNOSTIC TEST EFFECTS: *None known.*

SIDE EFFECTS

Frequent

Mild, transient drowsiness; ataxia; behavioral disturbances (aggression, irritability, agitation), especially in children

Occasional

Rash, ankle or facial edema, nocturia, dysuria, change in appetite or weight, dry mouth, sore gums, nausea, blurred vision

Rare

Paradoxical CNS reactions, including hyperactivity or nervousness in children and excitement or restlessness in the elderly (particularly in the presence of uncontrolled pain).

SERIOUS REACTIONS

- Abrupt withdrawal may result in pronounced restlessness, irritability, insomnia, hand tremors, abdominal or muscle cramps, diaphoresis, vomiting, and status epilepticus.
- Overdose results in somnolence, confusion, diminished reflexes, and coma.

C

SPECIAL CONSIDERATIONS

PRECAUTIONS

- Caution patients against engaging in hazardous occupations requiring mental alertness, such as operating machinery or driving a motor vehicle. Clonazepam may increase tonic-clonic seizures (grand mal). Abrupt withdrawal may precipitate status epilepticus.
- Exercise caution in administering the drug to patients with impaired renal function. Clonazepam may produce an increase in salivation.

PATIENT INFORMATION

- Dose Changes: To ensure the safe and effective use of benzodiazepines, inform patients that because benzodiazepines may produce psychological and physical dependence, consultation with their physician before increasing the dose or abruptly discontinuing this drug is advisable.
- Interference with Cognitive and Motor Performance: Because benzodiazepines have the potential to impair judgment, thinking, or motor skills, caution patients about operating hazardous machinery, including automobiles, until they are reasonably certain that clonazepam therapy does not affect them adversely.
- Pregnancy: Advise patients to notify their physician if they become pregnant or intend to become pregnant during therapy with clonazepam.

• Nursing: Advise patients not to breast-feed an infant if they are taking clonazepam.

• Concomitant Medication: Advise patients to inform their physicians if they are taking, or plan to take, any prescription or over-the-counter drugs because of the potential for interactions.

• Alcohol: Advise patients to avoid alcohol while taking clonazepam.

PREGNANCY AND LACTATION

• Pregnancy Category D. Recent reports suggest an association between the use of anticonvulsant drugs by women with epilepsy and an elevated incidence of birth defects in children born to these women. Mothers receiving clonazepam should not breast-feed their infants.

OCULAR CONSIDERATIONS

• Clonazepam may be used in patients with open-angle glaucoma who are receiving appropriate therapy, but it is contraindicated in acute narrow-angle glaucoma. Adverse reactions include eye irritation, visual disturbance, diplopia, eye twitching, styes, visual field defect, xerophthalmia, abnormal eye movements, aphonia, diplopia, and nystagmus.

clonidine

(klon'ih-deen)

Rx: Catapres, Catapres-TTS-1, Catapres-TTS-2, Catapres-TTS-3, Clonidine TTS-1, Clonidine TTS-2, Clonidine TTS-3, Duraclon

Drug Class: Antiadrenergics, central

Pregnancy Category: C

Do not confuse clonidine with clomiphene, Klonopin, or quinidine, or Catapres with with Cetapred.

CLINICAL PHARMACOLOGY

Mechanism of Action: An antiadrenergic, sympatholytic agent that prevents pain signal transmission to the brain and produces analgesia at pre- and post-alpha-adrenergic receptors in the spinal cord. *Therapeutic Effect:* Reduces peripheral resistance; decreases BP and heart rate.

Pharmacokinetics

Route	*Onset*	*Peak*	*Duration*
PO	0.5-1 hr	2-4 hr	Up to 8 hr

Well absorbed from the GI tract. Transdermal best absorbed from the chest and upper arm; least absorbed from the thigh. Protein binding: 20%-40%. Metabolized in the liver. Primarily excreted in urine. Minimally removed by hemodialysis. **Half-life:** 12-16 hr (increased with impaired renal function).

AVAILABLE FORMS

• *Tablets (Catapres):* 0.1 mg, 0.2 mg, 0.3 mg.

• *Transdermal Patch (Catapres TTS):* 2.5 mg (release at 0.1 mg/24 hr), 5 mg (release at 0.2 mg/24 hr), 7.5 mg (release at 0.3 mg/24 hr).

• *Injection (Duraclon):* 100 mcg/ml, 500 mcg/ml.

INDICATIONS AND DOSAGES

Hypertension

PO

Adults. Initially, 0.1 mg twice a day. Increase by 0.1-0.2 mg q2-4 days. Maintenance: 0.2-1.2 mg/day in 2-4 divided doses up to maximum of 2.4 mg/day.

Elderly. Initially, 0.1 mg at bedtime. May increase gradually.

Children. 5-25 mcg/kg/day in divided doses q6h. Increase at 5- to 7-day intervals. Maximum: 0.9 mg/day.

Transdermal

Adults, Elderly. System delivering 0.1 mg/24 hr up to 0.6 mg/24 hr q7 days.

Attention deficit hyperactivity disorder (ADHD)

PO

Children. Initially 0.05 mg/day. May increase by 0.05 mg/day q3-7 days. Maximum: 0.3-0.4 mg/day.

Severe pain

Epidural

Adults, Elderly. 30-40 mcg/hr.

Children. Initially, 0.5 mcg/kg/hr, not to exceed adult dose.

UNLABELED USES: ADHD, diagnosis of pheochromocytoma, opioid withdrawal, prevention of migraine headaches, treatment of dysmenorrhea, menopausal flushing

CONTRAINDICATIONS: Epidural contraindicated in those patients with bleeding diathesis or infection at the injection site, and in those receiving anticoagulation therapy

INTERACTIONS

Drug

Beta-blockers: Discontinuing these drugs may increase risk of clonidine-withdrawal hypertensive crisis.

Tricyclic antidepressants: May decrease effect of clonidine.

Herbal

None known.

Food

None known.

DIAGNOSTIC TEST EFFECTS: *None known.*

IV INCOMPATIBILITIES: None known.

IV COMPATIBILITIES: Bupivacaine (Marcaine, Sensorcaine), fentanyl (Sublimaze), heparin, ketamine (Ketalar), lidocaine, lorazepam (Ativan)

SIDE EFFECTS

Frequent

Dry mouth (40%), somnolence (33%), dizziness (16%), sedation, constipation (10%)

Occasional (5%-1%)

Tablets, injection: Depression, swelling of feet, loss of appetite, decreased sexual ability, itching eyes, dizziness, nausea, vomiting, nervousness

Transdermal: Itching, reddening or darkening of skin

Rare (less than 1%)

Nightmares, vivid dreams, cold feeling in fingers and toes

SERIOUS REACTIONS

- Overdose produces profound hypotension, irritability, bradycardia, respiratory depression, hypothermia, miosis (pupillary constriction), arrhythmias, and apnea.
- Abrupt withdrawal may result in rebound hypertension associated with nervousness, agitation, anxiety, insomnia, hand tingling, tremor, flushing, and diaphoresis.

SPECIAL CONSIDERATIONS

PRECAUTIONS

- Patients may develop an allergic reaction from clonidine film and oral doses. Use clonidine hydrochloride with caution in patients with severe coronary insufficiency, recent myocardial infarction, cerebrovascular disease, or chronic renal failure. Sudden cessation of clonidine treatment has resulted in subjective symptoms such as nervousness, agitation, and headache, accompanied or followed by a rapid rise in blood pressure and elevated catecholamine concentrations in the plasma, but such occurrences usually have been associated with previous administration of high oral doses and/or with continuation of concomitant beta-blocker therapy. Continue administration of clonidine hydrochloride to within 4 hours of surgery, and resume therapy as soon as possible thereafter.

PATIENT INFORMATION

• Advise patients who engage in potentially hazardous activities, such as operating machinery or driving, of a potential sedative effect of clonidine. Caution patients against interruption of clonidine hydrochloride therapy without a physician's advice.

PREGNANCY AND LACTATION

• Pregnancy Category C. In rats, oral doses were associated with increased resorptions. Fetal harm is not known. Because clonidine hydrochloride is excreted in human milk, exercise caution when administering clonidine hydrochloride to a nursing woman.

OCULAR CONSIDERATIONS

• In several studies, oral clonidine hydrochloride produced a dose-dependent increase in the incidence and severity of spontaneously occurring retinal degeneration in albino rats treated for 6 months or longer. Tissue distribution studies in dogs and monkeys revealed that clonidine hydrochloride was concentrated in the choroid of the eye. In view of the retinal degeneration observed in rats, eye examinations were performed in 908 patients before the start of clonidine hydrochloride therapy, who then were examined periodically thereafter. In 353 of these 908 patients, examinations were performed for periods of 24 months or longer. Except for some dryness of the eyes, no drug-related abnormal ocular findings were recorded, and clonidine hydrochloride did not alter retinal function as shown by specialized tests such as the electroretinogram and macular dazzle. In rats, clonidine hydrochloride in combination with amitriptyline produced corneal lesions within 5 days.

clopidogrel

(clo-pid'o-grill)

Rx: Plavix

Drug Class: Platelet inhibitors

Pregnancy Category: B

Do not confuse Plavix with Paxil.

CLINICAL PHARMACOLOGY

Mechanism of Action: A thienopyridine derivative that inhibits binding of the enzyme adenosine phosphate (ADP) to its platelet receptor and subsequent ADP-mediated activation of a glycoprotein complex. *Therapeutic Effect:* Inhibits platelet aggregation.

Pharmacokinetics

Route	*Onset*	*Peak*	*Duration*
PO	1 hr	2 hr	N/A

Rapidly absorbed. Protein binding: 98%. Extensively metabolized by the liver. Eliminated equally in the urine and feces. **Half-life:** 8 hr.

AVAILABLE FORMS

• *Tablets:* 75 mg.

INDICATIONS AND DOSAGES

Myocardial infarction (MI), stroke reduction

PO

Adults, Elderly. 75 mg once a day.

Acute coronary syndrome

PO

Adults, Elderly. Initially, 300 mg loading dose, then 75 mg once a day (in combination with aspirin).

CONTRAINDICATIONS: Active bleeding, coagulation disorders, severe hepatic disease

INTERACTIONS

Drug

Fluvastatin, other NSAIDs, phenytoin, tamoxifen, tolbutamide, torsemide, warfarin: May interfere with metabolism of these drugs.

Herbal

Ginger, ginkgo biloba: May increase the risk of bleeding.

Food

None known.

DIAGNOSTIC TEST EFFECTS: Prolongs bleeding time.

SIDE EFFECTS

Frequent (15%)

Skin disorders

Occasional (8%-6%)

Upper respiratory tract infection, chest pain, flu-like symptoms, headache, dizziness, arthralgia

Rare (5%-3%)

Fatigue, edema, hypertension, abdominal pain, dyspepsia, diarrhea, nausea, epistaxis, dyspnea, rhinitis

SERIOUS REACTIONS

- None known.

SPECIAL CONSIDERATIONS

PRECAUTIONS

- Use clopidogrel bisulfate with caution in patients who may be at risk of increased bleeding from trauma, surgery, or other pathologic conditions. Clopidogrel bisulfate prolongs the bleeding time and should be used with caution in patients with severe hepatic disease.

PATIENT INFORMATION

- Advise patients that it may take them longer than usual to stop bleeding when they take clopidogrel bisulfate and that they should report any unusual bleeding to their physician. Instruct patients to inform physicians and dentists that they are taking clopidogrel bisulfate before any surgery is scheduled and before taking any new drug.

PREGNANCY AND LACTATION

- Pregnancy Category B. Reproduction studies performed in rats and rabbits revealed no evidence of impaired fertility or fetotoxicity. Studies in rats have shown that clopidogrel and/or its metabolites are excreted in the milk. Whether this drug is excreted in human milk is not known.

clotrimazole

(kloe-try-mah-zole)

Rx: Fungoid (Clotrimazole), Fungoid Solution, Lotrimin, Mycelex, Mycelex-G, Mycelex Troche, Mycelex Twin Pak

Drug Class: Antifungals, topical; Dermatologics

Pregnancy Category: B

CLINICAL PHARMACOLOGY

Mechanism of Action: An antifungal that binds with phospholipids in fungal cell membrane. The altered cell membrane permeability. *Therapeutic Effect:* Inhibits yeast growth.

Pharmacokinetics

Poorly, erratically absorbed from GI tract. Bound to oral mucosa. Absorbed portion metabolized in liver. Eliminated in feces. Topical: Minimal systemic absorption (highest concentration in stratum corneum).

Intravaginal: Small amount systemically absorbed. **Half-life:** 3.5-5 hrs.

AVAILABLE FORMS

- *Combination pack:* Vaginal tablet 100 mg and vaginal cream 1% (Mycelex-7).
- *Lotion:* 1% (Lotrimin).
- *Topical Cream:* 1% (Lotrimin, Lotrimin AF, Mycelex, Mycelex OTC).
- *Topical Solution:* 1% (Lotrimin, Lotrimin AF, Mycelex, Mycelex OTC).
- *Troches:* 10 mg (Mycelex).
- *Vaginal Cream:* 1% (Gyne-Lotrimin, Mycelex-7), 2% (Gyne-Lotrimin 3, Mycelex-3, Trivagizole 3).
- *Vaginal Tablets:* 100 mg, 500 mg (Gyne-Lotrimin, Mycelex-7).

INDICATIONS AND DOSAGES

Oropharyngeal candidiasis treatment

PO

Adults, Elderly. 10 mg 5 times/day for 14 days.

Oropharyngeal candidiasis prophylaxis

PO

Adults, Elderly. 10 mg 3 times/day.

Dermatophytosis, cutaneous candidiasis

Topical

Adults, Elderly. 2 times/day. Therapeutic effect may take up to 8 wks.

Vulvovaginal candidiasis

Vaginal (Tablets)

Adults, Elderly. 1 tablet (100 mg) at bedtime for 7 days; 2 tablets (200 mg) at bedtime for 3 days; or 500 mg tablet one time.

Vaginal (Cream)

Adults, Elderly. 1 applicatorful at bedtime for 7-14 days.

UNLABELED USES: Topical: Treatment of paronychia, tinea barbae, tinea capitas.

CONTRAINDICATIONS: Hypersensitivity to clotrimazole or any component of the formulation, children <3 yrs

INTERACTIONS

Drug

Benzodiazepines: May increase benzodiazepine serum concentrations and increase risk of toxicity.

Ergot derivatives: May increase risk of ergotism (nausea, vomiting, vasospastic ischemia).

Fentanyl: May increase or prolong opioid effects (CNS depression).

Tacrolimus: May increase risk of tacrolimus toxicity.

Trimetrexate: May increase risk of trimetrexate toxicity.

Herbal

None known.

Food

None known.

DIAGNOSTIC TEST EFFECTS: May increase SGOT (AST) levels.

SIDE EFFECTS

Frequent

Oral: Nausea, vomiting, diarrhea, abdominal pain

Occasional

Topical: Itching, burning, stinging, erythema, urticaria

Vaginal: Mild burning (tablets/cream); irritation, cystitis (cream)

Rare

Vaginal: Itching, rash, lower abdominal cramping, headache

SERIOUS REACTIONS

- None reported.

SPECIAL CONSIDERATIONS

PRECAUTIONS

- If irritation or sensitivity develops with the use of clotrimazole, discontinue treatment and institute appropriate therapy.

PATIENT INFORMATION

Give patients the following instructions:

• Use the medication for the full treatment time even though the symptoms may have improved. Notify the physician if there is no improvement after 4 weeks of treatment.

• Inform the physician if the area of application shows signs of increased irritation (redness, itching, burning, blistering, oozing) indicative of possible sensitization.

• Avoid sources of infection or reinfection.

PREGNANCY AND LACTATION

• Pregnancy Category B. In clinical trials, use of vaginally applied clotrimazole in pregnant women in their second and third trimesters has not been associated with ill effects. Whether this drug is excreted in human milk is not known.

cocaine hydrochloride

(koe-kane')

Drug Class: Anesthetics, local; Anesthetics, topical; Dermatologics

Pregnancy Category: C

DEA Class: Schedule II

CLINICAL PHARMACOLOGY

Mechanism of Action: A topical anesthetic that decreases membrane permeability, increases norepinephrine at postsynaptic receptor sites, producing intense vasoconstriction. *Therapeutic Effect:* Blocks conduction of nerve impulses.

Pharmacokinetics

Readily absorbed from all mucous membranes. Cocaine penetrates the CNS but is rapidly metabolized. Rapidly hydrolyzed in blood by serum cholinesterases. Metabolized in liver. Excreted in urine **Half-life:** 1-1.5 hrs.

AVAILABLE FORMS

• *Powder, as hydrochloride:* 5 g, 25 g (Cocaine HCl).

• *Topical solution, as hydrochloride:* 40 mg/ml, 100 mg/ml (Cocaine HCl).

INDICATIONS AND DOSAGES

Anesthesia

Topical

Adults, Elderly, Children. 1-4% to mucous membranes. Maximum: 1-3 mg/kg (400 mg). Dosage varies depending upon the area to be anesthetized, vascularity of the tissues, individual tolerance, and anesthetic technique. Administer lowest effective dose.

UNLABELED USES: Horner's syndrome (diagnosis)

CONTRAINDICATIONS: Hypersensitivity to cocaine or any component of the formulation.

INTERACTIONS

Drug

Alcohol: May increase heart rate and blood pressure.

Beta-blockers: May decrease effects of beta-blockers.

Cholinesterase inhibitors: May increase effects and risk of toxicity.

Sympathomimetics: May increase CNS stimulation and risk of cardiovascular effects.

Tricyclic antidepressants, digoxin, methyldopa: May increase risk of arrhythmias.

Herbal

Hemp: May increase toxic effects of cocaine.

St. John's wort: May increase risk of cardiovascular collapse and/or delayed emergence from anesthesia.

Food

None known.

DIAGNOSTIC TEST EFFECTS: May give false-negative results of scintigraphy.

SIDE EFFECTS

Frequent

Loss of sense of smell and taste.

Occasional

Anxiety, central nervous system stimulation or depression.

SERIOUS REACTIONS

- Repeated nasal application may produce stuffy nose, and chronic rhinitis.
- Early signs of overdosage produces increased blood pressure (BP), increased pulse, irregular heartbeat, chills/fever, agitation, nervousness, confusion, inability to remain still, nausea, vomiting, abdominal pain, increased sweating, rapid breathing, and large pupils.
- Advanced signs of overdosage produces arrhythmias, CNS hemorrhage, CHF, convulsions, delirium, hyperreflexia, loss of bladder/bowel control, and respiratory weakness.
- Late signs of overdosage produces loss of reflexes, muscle paralysis, dilated pupils, LOC, cyanosis, pulmonary edema, cardiac and respiratory failure.

SPECIAL CONSIDERATIONS

INDICATIONS AND USAGE

- Cocaine hydrochloride is indicated for the introduction of local (topical) anesthesia of accessible mucous membranes of the oral, laryngeal, and nasal cavities. Cocaine hydrochloride can be used for corneal anesthesia.

PRECAUTIONS

- The safety and effectiveness of cocaine hydrochloride topical solution depends on proper dosage, correct technique, adequate precautions, and readiness for emergencies. Consult standard textbooks for specific techniques and precautions for various anesthetic procedures. Use cocaine hydrochloride topical solution with caution in patients with severely traumatized mucosa and sepsis in the region of the proposed application. Use the drug with caution in persons with known drug sensitivities.

PREGNANCY AND LACTATION

- Pregnancy Category C. Animal reproduction studies have not been conducted with cocaine. Whether the cocaine can cause fetal harm when administered to a pregnant woman or can affect reproduction capacity is not known. Give cocaine to a pregnant woman only if needed.

OCULAR CONSIDERATIONS

- Cocaine causes sloughing of the corneal epithelium, causing clouding, pitting, and occasionally ulceration of the cornea. Cocaine causes mydriasis.

codeine phosphate/codeine sulfate

(koe'deen)

Drug Class: Analgesics, narcotic; Antitussives

Pregnancy Category: C

DEA Class: Schedule II

Do not confuse codeine with Cardene or Lodine.

CLINICAL PHARMACOLOGY

Mechanism of Action: An opioid agonist that binds to opioid receptors at many sites in the CNS, particularly in the medulla. This action inhibits the ascending pain pathways. *Therapeutic Effect:* Alters the perception of and emotional response to pain, suppresses cough reflex.

AVAILABLE FORMS

- *Tablets:* 15 mg, 30 mg, 60 mg.
- *Oral Solution:* 15 mg/5 ml.
- *Injection:* 15 mg/ml, 30 mg/ml.

INDICATIONS AND DOSAGES

Analgesia

PO, IM, Subcutaneous

Adults, Elderly. 30 mg q4-6h. Range: 15-60 mg.

Children. 0.5-1 mg/kg q4-6h. Maximum: 60 mg/dose.

Cough

PO

Adults, Elderly, Children 12 yr and older. 10-20 mg q4-6h.

Children 6-11 yr. 5-10 mg q4-6h.

Children 2-5 yr. 2.5-5 mg q4-6h.

Dosage in renal impairment

Dosage is modified based on creatinine clearance.

Creatinine Clearance	Dosage
10-50 ml/min	75% of usual dose
less than 10 ml/min	50% of usual dose

UNLABELED USES: Treatment of diarrhea

CONTRAINDICATIONS: None known.

INTERACTIONS

Drug

Alcohol, other CNS depressants: May increase CNS or respiratory depression, and hypotension.

MAOIs: May produce a severe, sometimes fatal reaction; plan to administer a test dose, which is one-quarter of usual codeine dose.

Herbal

None known.

Food

None known.

DIAGNOSTIC TEST EFFECTS: May increase serum amylase and lipase levels.

SIDE EFFECTS

Frequent

Constipation, somnolence, nausea, vomiting

Occasional

Paradoxical excitement, confusion, palpitations, facial flushing, decreased urination, blurred vision, dizziness, dry mouth, headache, hypotension (including orthostatic hypotension), decreased appetite, injection site redness, burning, or pain

Rare

Hallucinations, depression, abdominal pain, insomnia

SERIOUS REACTIONS

- Too-frequent use may result in paralytic ileus.
- Overdose may produce cold and clammy skin, confusion, seizures, decreased BP, restlessness, pinpoint pupils, bradycardia, respiratory depression, decreased LOC, and severe weakness.
- The patient who uses codeine repeatedly may develop a tolerance to the drug's analgesic effect as well as physical dependence.

SPECIAL CONSIDERATIONS

PRECAUTIONS

- The respiratory depressant effects of narcotics and their capacity to elevate cerebrospinal fluid pressure may be exaggerated greatly in the presence of head injury or other intracranial lesions. Codeine phosphate may obscure the diagnosis or clinical course in patients with acute abdominal conditions. Give codeine phosphate with caution to certain patients, such as the elderly or debilitated and those with severe impairment of hepatic or renal function, hypothyroidism, Addison's disease, and prostatic hypertrophy or urethral stricture. Codeine phosphate may have a prolonged cumulative effect in patients with kidney or liver dysfunction.

PATIENT INFORMATION

• Codeine may impair the mental and/or physical abilities required for the performance of potentially hazardous tasks such as driving a car or operating machinery. Codeine in combination with other narcotic analgesics, phenothiazines, sedative hypnotics, and alcohol has additive depressant effects.

PREGNANCY AND LACTATION

• Pregnancy Category C. Fetal harm is not known. Codeine appears in the milk of nursing mothers.

---

colchicine

(kol'chi-seen)

Drug Class: Antigout agents

Pregnancy Category: D

CLINICAL PHARMACOLOGY

Mechanism of Action: An alkaloid that decreases leukocyte motility, phagocytosis, and lactic acid production. *Therapeutic Effect:* Decreases urate crystal deposits and reduces inflammatory process.

Pharmacokinetics

Rapidly absorbed from the GI tract. Highest concentration is in the liver, spleen, and kidney. Protein binding: 30%-50%. Reenters the intestinal tract by biliary secretion and is reabsorbed from the intestines. Partially metabolized in the liver. Eliminated primarily in feces.

AVAILABLE FORMS

• *Tablets:* 0.6 mg.

• *Injection:* 1 mg.

INDICATIONS AND DOSAGES

Acute gouty arthritis

PO

Adults, Elderly. 0.6-1.2 mg; then 0.6 mg q1-2h or 1-1.2 mg q2h, until pain is relieved or nausea, vomiting, or diarrhea occurs. Total dose: 4-8 mg.

IV

Adults, Elderly. Initially, 2 mg; then 0.5 mg q6h until satisfactory response. Maximum: 4 mg/wk or 4 mg/one course of treatment. If pain recurs, may give 1-2 mg/day for several days but no sooner than 7 days after a full course of IV therapy (total of 4 mg).

Chronic gouty arthritis

PO

Adults, Elderly. 0.5-0.6 mg once weekly up to once a day, depending on number of attacks per year.

UNLABELED USES: To reduce frequency of recurrence of familial Mediterranean fever; treatment of acute calcium pyrophosphate deposition, amyloidosis, biliary cirrhosis, recurrent pericarditis, sarcoid arthritis

CONTRAINDICATIONS: Blood dyscrasias; severe cardiac, GI, hepatic, or renal disorders

INTERACTIONS

Drug

Bone marrow depressants: May increase the risk of blood dyscrasias.

NSAIDs: May increase the risk of bone marrow depression, neutropenia, and thrombocytopenia.

Herbal

None known.

Food

None known.

DIAGNOSTIC TEST EFFECTS: May increase serum alkaline phosphatase and AST (SGOT) levels. May decrease platelet count.

IV INCOMPATIBILITIES: No information available via Y-site administration.

SIDE EFFECTS

Frequent

PO: Nausea, vomiting, abdominal discomfort

Occasional

PO: Anorexia

Rare

Hypersensitivity reaction, including angioedema

Parenteral: Nausea, vomiting, diarrhea, abdominal discomfort, pain or redness at injection site, neuritis in injected arm

SERIOUS REACTIONS

• Bone marrow depression, including aplastic anemia, agranulocytosis, and thrombocytopenia, may occur with long-term therapy.

• Overdose initially causes a burning feeling in the skin or throat, severe diarrhea, and abdominal pain. The patient then experiences fever, seizures, delirium, and renal impairment, marked by hematuria and oliguria. The third stage of overdose causes hair loss, leukocytosis, and stomatitis.

SPECIAL CONSIDERATIONS

PRECAUTIONS

• Reduction in dosage is indicated if weakness, anorexia, nausea, vomiting, or diarrhea occurs. Administer colchicine with great caution to aged and debilitated patients, especially those with renal, hepatic, gastrointestinal, or heart disease.

PREGNANCY AND LACTATION

• Pregnancy Category D. Colchicine can cause fetal harm when administered to a pregnant woman. Excretion into human milk is not known.

cromolyn sodium

(kroe'moe-lin)

Rx: Crolom, Gastrocrom, Intal, Intal Inhaler, Opticrom

Drug Class: Mast cell stabilizers; Ophthalmics

Pregnancy Category: B

CLINICAL PHARMACOLOGY

Mechanism of Action: An antiasthmatic and antiallergic agent that prevents mast cell release of histamine, leukotrienes, and slow-reacting substances of anaphylaxis by inhibiting degranulation after contact with antigens. *Therapeutic Effect:* Helps prevent symptoms of asthma, allergic rhinitis, mastocytosis, and exercise-induced bronchospasm.

Pharmacokinetics

Minimal absorption after PO, inhalation, or nasal administration. Absorbed portion excreted in urine or by biliary system. **Half-life:** 80-90 min.

AVAILABLE FORMS

• *Oral Concentrate (Gastrocrom):* 100 mg/5ml.

• *Nasal Spray (Nasalcrom):* 40 mg/ml.

• *Solution for Nebulization (Intal):* 10 mg/ml.

• *Solution for Oral Inhalation (Intal):* 800 mcg/inhalation.

• *Ophthalmic Solution (Crolom, Opticrom):* 4%.

INDICATIONS AND DOSAGES

Asthma

Inhalation (nebulization)

Adults, Elderly, Children older than 2 yr. 20 mg 3-4 times a day.

Aerosol Spray

Adults, Elderly, Children 12 yr and older. Initially, 2 sprays 4 times a day. Maintenance: 2-4 sprays 3-4 times a day.

Children 5-11 yr. Initially, 2 sprays 4 times a day, then 1-2 sprays 3-4 times a day.

Prevention of bronchospasm

Inhalation (nebulization)

Adults, Elderly, Children older than 2 yr. 20 mg within 1 hr before exercise or exposure to allergens.

Aerosol Spray

Adults, Elderly, Children older than 5 yr. 2 sprays within 1 hr before exercise or exposure to allergens.

Food allergy, inflammatory bowel disease

PO

Adults, Elderly, Children older than 12 yr. 200-400 mg 4 times a day.

Children 2-12 yr. 100-200 mg 4 times a day. Maximum: 40 mg/kg/day.

Allergic rhinitis

Intranasal

Adults, Elderly, Children older than 6 yr. 1 spray each nostril 3-4 times a day. May increase up to 6 times a day.

Systemic mastocytosis

PO

Adults, Elderly, Children older than 12 yr. 200 mg 4 times a day.

Children 2-12 yr. 100 mg 4 times a day. Maximum: 40 mg/kg/day.

Children younger than 2 yr. 20 mg/kg/day in 4 divided doses. Maximum: 30 mg/kg/day (children 6 mo-2 yr).

Conjunctivitis

Ophthalmic

Adults, Elderly, Children older than 4 yr. 1-2 drops in both eyes 4-6 times a day.

CONTRAINDICATIONS: Status asthmaticus

INTERACTIONS

Drug

None known.

Herbal

None known.

Food

None known.

DIAGNOSTIC TEST EFFECTS: *None known.*

SIDE EFFECTS

Frequent

PO: Headache, diarrhea

Inhalation: Cough, dry mouth and throat, stuffy nose, throat irritation, unpleasant taste

Nasal: Nasal burning, stinging, or irritation; increased sneezing

Ophthalmic: Eye burning or stinging

Occasional

PO: Rash, abdominal pain, arthralgia, nausea, insomnia

Inhalation: Bronchospasm, hoarseness, lacrimation

Nasal: Cough, headache, unpleasant taste, postnasal drip

Ophthalmic: Lacrimation and itching of eye

Rare

Inhalation: Dizziness, painful urination, arthralgia, myalgia, rash

Nasal: Epistaxis, rash

Ophthalmic: Chemosis or edema of conjunctiva, eye irritation

SERIOUS REACTIONS

- Anaphylaxis occurs rarely when cromolyn is given by the inhalation, nasal, or oral route.

SPECIAL CONSIDERATIONS

PRECAUTIONS

- Transient stinging or burning sensation may occur.

PREGNANCY AND LACTATION

- Pregnancy Category B. Adverse fetal effects (increased resorption and decreased fetal weight) were noted only at the very high parenteral doses that produced maternal toxicity in animal studies. Fetal harm is not known with topical administration. Excretion into human milk is not known.

ADVERSE REACTIONS

• Transient ocular stinging or burning may occur upon instillation. Infrequent events include conjunctival injection, watering, itchiness, dryness, swelling, irritation, and hordeolum.

cyclobenzaprine hydrochloride

(sye-kloe-ben'za-preen)

Rx: Flexeril

Drug Class: Musculoskeletal agents; Relaxants, skeletal muscle

Pregnancy Category: B

Do not confuse cyclobenzaprine with cycloserine or cyproheptadine, or Flexeril with Floxin.

CLINICAL PHARMACOLOGY

Mechanism of Action: A centrally acting skeletal muscle relaxant that reduces tonic somatic muscle activity at the level of the brainstem. *Therapeutic Effect:* Relieves local skeletal muscle spasm.

Pharmacokinetics

Route	Onset	Peak	Duration
PO	1 hr	3-4 hr	12-24 hr

Well but slowly absorbed from the GI tract. Protein binding: 93%. Metabolized in the GI tract and the liver. Primarily excreted in urine. **Half-life:** 1-3 days.

AVAILABLE FORMS

• *Tablets:* 5 mg, 10 mg.

INDICATIONS AND DOSAGES

Acute, painful musculoskeletal conditions

PO

Adults. Initially, 5 mg 3 times a day. May increase to 10 mg 3 times a day.

Elderly. 5 mg 3 times a day.

Dosage in hepatic impairment

Mild: 5 mg 3 times a day.

Moderate and severe: Not recommended.

UNLABELED USES: Treatment of fibromyalgia

CONTRAINDICATIONS: Acute recovery phase of MI, arrhythmias, CHF, heart block, conduction disturbances, hyperthyroidism, use within 14 days of MAOIs

INTERACTIONS

Drug

Alcohol, other CNS depression-producing medications (such as tricyclic antidepressants): May increase CNS depression.

MAOIs: May increase the risk of hypertensive crisis and severe seizures.

Herbal

None known.

Food

None known.

DIAGNOSTIC TEST EFFECTS: *None known.*

SIDE EFFECTS

Frequent

Somnolence (39%), dry mouth (27%), dizziness (11%)

Rare (3%-1%)

Fatigue, asthenia, blurred vision, headache, nervousness, confusion, nausea, constipation, dyspepsia, unpleasant taste

SERIOUS REACTIONS

• Overdose may result in visual hallucinations, hyperactive reflexes, muscle rigidity, vomiting, and hyperpyrexia.

SPECIAL CONSIDERATIONS

PRECAUTIONS

• Cyclobenzaprine hydrochloride may interact with monoamine oxidase inhibitors. Hyperpyretic crisis, severe convulsions, and deaths have occurred in patients receiving tricyclic antidepressants and monoamine oxidase inhibitor drugs. Tricyclic antidepressants have been reported to produce arrhythmias, sinus tachycardia, prolongation of the conduction time leading to myocardial infarction, and stroke. Cyclobenzaprine hydrochloride may enhance the effects of alcohol, barbiturates, and other central nervous system depressants. Use cyclobenzaprine hydrochloride with caution in patients with a history of urinary retention, angle-closure glaucoma, and increased intraocular pressure and in patients taking anticholinergic medication.

PATIENT INFORMATION

- Cyclobenzaprine hydrochloride may impair mental and/or physical abilities required for performance of hazardous tasks such as operating machinery or driving a motor vehicle.

PREGNANCY AND LACTATION

- Pregnancy Category B. Reproduction studies performed in rats, mice, and rabbits revealed no evidence of impaired fertility or harm to the fetus. Fetal harm is not known. Whether this drug is excreted in human milk is not known. Because cyclobenzaprine is related closely to the tricyclic antidepressants, some of which are known to be excreted in human milk, exercise caution when administering cyclobenzaprine hydrochloride to a nursing woman.

OCULAR CONSIDERATIONS

- Use cyclobenzaprine hydrochloride with caution in patients with angle-closure glaucoma and increased intraocular pressure.

cyclopentolate hydrochloride

(sye-kloe-pen'toe-late hye-droe-klor'-ide)

Rx: AK-Pentolate, Cyclogyl, Cylate, Ocu-Pentolate, Pentolair

Drug Class: Anticholinergics; Cycloplegics; Mydriatics; Ophthalmics

Pregnancy Category: C

CLINICAL PHARMACOLOGY

Mechanism of Action: An antimuscarinic similar to atropine that competes with acetylcholine. Blocks the responses of the sphincter muscle of the iris and the accommodative muscle of the ciliary body to cholinergic stimulation. *Therapeutic Effect:* Results in mydriasis and cycloplegia.

Pharmacokinetics

Rapid systemic absorption following ophthalmic administration. Shorter duration of action than atropine. Complete recovery takes 6-24 hours.

AVAILABLE FORMS

- *Ophthalmic Solution:* 0.5% (Cyclogyl), 1% (AK-Pentolate, Cyclogyl, Cylate, Ocu-Pentolate, Pentolair), 2% (AK-Pentolate, Cyclogyl).

INDICATIONS AND DOSAGES

Cycloplegia induction, mydriasis induction

Ophthalmic

Adults, Elderly, Children. Instill 1-2 drops of 0.5%-2% solution in eye(s). May repeat with 0.5% or 1% solution in 5-10 minutes as needed.

Neonates, infants. Instill 1 drop of 0.5%-2% solution in eye(s) followed by 1 drop of 0.5% or 1% in 5 minutes as needed.

CONTRAINDICATIONS: Narrow-angle glaucoma, anatomical narrow angles, hypersensitivity to cyclopentolate or any component of the formulation.

INTERACTIONS

Drug

Belladonna, belladonna alkaloids: May increase anticholinergic effects.

Cisapride: May decrease cisapride efficacy.

Herbal

None known.

Food

None known.

DIAGNOSTIC TEST EFFECTS: *None known.*

SIDE EFFECTS

Occasional

Blurred vision, burning of eye, photophobia.

Rare

Conjunctivitis, increased intraocular pressure.

SERIOUS REACTIONS

• Systemic absorption which includes signs and symptoms of confusion, psychosis, ataxia, tachycardia and vasodilation occur rarely.

SPECIAL CONSIDERATIONS

PRECAUTIONS

• Estimate the depth of the angle of the anterior chamber to avoid angle closure. Compress the lacrimal sac to avoid excessive systemic absorption. Observe caution when considering use of this medication in the presence of Down syndrome and in those predisposed to angle-closure glaucoma.

PATIENT INFORMATION

• Burning sensation may occur upon instillation. Advise patients not to drive or engage in other hazardous activities while pupils are dilated. Photophobia may occur. Warn patients not to get this preparation in their child's mouth and to wash their own hands and the child's hands following administration.

PREGNANCY AND LACTATION

• Pregnancy Category C. Excretion into human milk is not known. Increased susceptibility to cyclopentolate has been reported in infants, young children, and in children with spastic paralysis or brain damage. Therefore, use cyclopentolate with great caution in these patients. Do not use the drug in concentrations higher than 0.5% in small infants.

OCULAR CONSIDERATIONS

• Adverse Reactions: increased intraocular pressure, burning, photophobia, blurred vision, irritation, hyperemia, conjunctivitis, blepharoconjunctivitis, punctate keratitis, and synechiae

cyclopentolate hydrochloride; phenylephrine hydrochloride

(sye-kloe-pen'-toe-late hye-droe-klor'-ide; fen-il-ef'-rin hye-droe-klor'-ide)

Rx: Cyclomydril

Drug Class: Adrenergic agonists; Anticholinergics; Mydriatics; Ophthalmics

CLINICAL PHARMACOLOGY

Mechanism of Action: Cyclopentolate is an antimuscarinic similar to atropine that competes with acetylcholine. Blocks the responses of the sphincter muscle of the iris and the accommodative muscle of the ciliary body to cholinergic stimulation. Phenylephrine is a sympathomimetic agent that directly affects alpha-adrenergic receptors. *Therapeutic Effect:* Induces mydriasis of short duration.

Pharmacokinetics
Rapid systemic absorption following ophthalmic administration. Shorter duration of action than atropine. Complete recovery takes 6-24 hours.

AVAILABLE FORMS

• *Ophthalmic Solution:* 0.2% cyclopentolate hydrochloride and 1% phenylephrine hydrochloride (Cyclomydril).

INDICATIONS AND DOSAGES

Mydriasis induction that cannot be produced with cyclopentolate alone

Ophthalmic

Adults, Elderly, Children, Infants, Neonates. Instill 1 drop into the eye every 5-10 minutes, for up to 3 doses, approximately 40-50 minutes before the examination.

CONTRAINDICATIONS: Narrow-angle glaucoma, anatomical narrow angles, hypersensitivity to cyclopentolate, phenylephrine, or any component of the formulation.

INTERACTIONS

Drug

Guanethidine, reserpine, methyldopa, tricyclic antidepressants: May enhance the effects of phenylephrine.

Herbal

None known.

Food

None known.

DIAGNOSTIC TEST EFFECTS: *None known.*

SIDE EFFECTS

Occasional
Increased intraocular pressure, blurred vision, transient stinging, photophobia

Rare
Conjunctivitis

SERIOUS REACTIONS

• Hypersensitivity as conjunctivitis may occur.

• Toxic manifestations include tachycardia, vasodilation, urinary retention, diminished gastrointestinal motility, and decreased secretion in salivary and sweat glands, pharynx, bronchii, and nasal passages. Severe manifestations of toxicity include coma, medullary paralysis, and death.

SPECIAL CONSIDERATIONS

PRECAUTIONS

• To avoid inducing angle-closure glaucoma, estimate the depth of the angle of the anterior chamber. Compress the lacrimal sac to avoid excessive systemic absorption.

• Patient Warning: Advise patients not to drive or engage in other hazardous activities while pupils are dilated. Patients may experience sensitivity to light and should protect eyes in bright illumination during dilation. Warn parents not to get this preparation in their child's mouth and to wash their own hands and the child's hands following administration.

cyclophosphamide

(sye-kloe-foss'fa-mide)

Rx: Cytoxan, Cytoxan Lyophilized, Neosar

Drug Class: Antineoplastics, alkylating agents; Disease-modifying antirheumatic drugs

Pregnancy Category: D

Do not confuse Cytoxan with cefoxitin, Ciloxan, cyclosporine, or Cytotec.

CLINICAL PHARMACOLOGY

Mechanism of Action: An alkylating agent that inhibits DNA and RNA protein synthesis by cross-linking with DNA and RNA strands, preventing cell growth. Cell cycle-phase nonspecific. *Therapeutic Effect:* Potent immunosuppressant.

Pharmacokinetics

Well absorbed from the GI tract. Protein binding: Low. Crosses the blood-brain barrier. Metabolized in the liver to active metabolites. Primarily excreted in urine. Removed by hemodialysis. **Half-life:** 3-12 hr.

AVAILABLE FORMS

- *Tablets (Cytoxan):* 25 mg, 50 mg.
- *Powder for Injection (Neosar):* 100 mg, 200 mg.
- *Powder for Injection (Cytoxan, Neosar):* 500 mg, 1 g, 2 g.

INDICATIONS AND DOSAGES

Ovarian adenocarcinoma, breast carcinoma, Hodgkin's disease, non-Hodgkin's lymphoma, multiple myeloma, leukemia (acute lymphoblastic, acute myelogenous, acute monocytic, chronic granulocytic, chronic lymphocytic), mycosis fungoides, disseminated neuroblastoma, retinoblastoma

PO

Adults. 1-5 mg/kg/day.

Children. Initially, 2-8 mg/kg/day. Maintenance: 2-5 mg/kg twice a week.

IV

Adults. 40-50 mg/kg in divided doses over 2-5 days; or 10-15 mg/kg every 7-10 days or 3-5 mg/kg twice a week.

Children. 2-8 mg/kg/day for 6 days or total dose for 7 days once a week.

Biopsy-proven minimal-change nephrotic syndrome

PO

Adults, Children. 2.5-3 mg/kg/day for 60-90 days.

UNLABELED USES: Treatment of carcinoma of bladder, cervix, endometrium, lung, prostate, or testicles; germ cell ovarian tumors; osteosarcoma; rheumatoid arthritis; systemic lupus erythematosus

CONTRAINDICATIONS: None known.

INTERACTIONS

Drug

Allopurinol, bone marrow depressants: May increase myelosuppression.

Antigout medications: May decrease the effects of these drugs.

Cytarabine: May increase the risk of cardiomyopathy.

Immunosuppressants: May increase the risk of infection and development of neoplasms.

Live-virus vaccines: May potentiate virus replication, increase vaccine side effects, and decrease the patient's antibody response to the vaccine.

Herbal

None known.

Food

None known.

DIAGNOSTIC TEST EFFECTS: May increase serum uric acid levels.

IV INCOMPATIBILITIES: Amphotericin B complex (Abelcet, AmBisome, Amphotec)

IV COMPATIBILITIES: Granisetron (Kytril), heparin, hydromorphone (Dilaudid), lorazepam (Ativan), morphine, ondansetron (Zofran), propofol (Diprivan)

SIDE EFFECTS

Expected

Marked leukopenia 8-15 days after initial therapy

Frequent

Nausea, vomiting (beginning about 6 hr after administration and lasting about 4 hr); alopecia (33%)

Occasional

Diarrhea, darkening of skin and fingernails, stomatitis, headache, diaphoresis

Rare

Pain or redness at injection site

SERIOUS REACTIONS

• Cyclophosphamide's major toxic effect is myelosuppression resulting in blood dyscrasias, such as leukopenia, anemia, thrombocytopenia, and hypoprothrombinemia.

• Expect leukopenia to resolve in 17 to 28 days. Anemia generally occurs after large doses or prolonged therapy. Thrombocytopenia may occur 10-15 days after drug initiation.

• Hemorrhagic cystitis occurs commonly in long-term therapy, especially in pediatric patients.

• Pulmonary fibrosis and cardiotoxicity have been noted with high doses.

• Amenorrhea, azoospermia, and hyperkalemia may also occur.

SPECIAL CONSIDERATIONS

PRECAUTIONS

• Possible development of toxicity may occur if any of the following conditions are present: leukopenia, thrombocytopenia, tumor cell infiltration of bone marrow, previous x-ray therapy, previous therapy with other cytotoxic agents, impaired hepatic function, or impaired renal function.

PREGNANCY AND LACTATION

• Pregnancy Category D. Cyclophosphamide can cause fetal harm when administered to a pregnant woman. Cyclophosphamide is excreted in breast milk.

cyclosporine

(sye-kloe-spor'in)

Rx: Gengraf, Neoral, Restasis, Sandimmune

Drug Class: Immunosuppressives

Pregnancy Category: C

Do not confuse cyclosporine with cycloserine, cyclophosphamide, or Cyklokapron.

CLINICAL PHARMACOLOGY

Mechanism of Action: A cyclic polypeptide that inhibits both cellular and humoral immune responses by inhibiting interleukin-2, a proliferative factor needed for T-cell activity. *Therapeutic Effect:* Prevents organ rejection and relieves symptoms of psoriasis and arthritis.

Pharmacokinetics

Variably absorbed from the GI tract. Protein binding: 90%. Widely distributed. Metabolized in the liver. Eliminated primarily by biliary or fecal excretion. Not removed by hemodialysis. **Half-life:** Adults, 10-27 hr; children, 7-19 hr.

AVAILABLE FORMS

• *Capsules (Softgel [Gengraf, Neoral, Sandimmune]):* 25 mg, 100 mg.

• *Oral Solution (Sandimmune):* 50-ml bottle with calibrated liquid measuring device.

• *Injection (Sandimmune):* 50 mg/ml.

• *Ophthalmic Emulsion (Restasis):* 0.05%.

INDICATIONS AND DOSAGES

Transplantation, prevention of organ rejection

PO

Adults, Elderly, Children. 10-18 mg/kg/dose given 4-12 hr prior to organ transplantation. Maintenance: 5-15 mg/kg/day in divided doses then tapered to 3-10 mg/kg/day.

IV

Adults, Elderly, Children. Initially, 5-6 mg/kg/dose given 4-12 hr before organ transplantation. Maintenance: 2-10 mg/kg/day in divided doses.

Rheumatoid arthritis

PO

Adults, Elderly. Initially, 2.5 mg/kg a day in 2 divided doses. May increase by 0.5-0.75 mg/kg/day. Maximum: 4 mg/kg/day.

Psoriasis

PO

Adults, Elderly. Initially, 2.5 mg/kg/day in 2 divided doses. May increase by 0.5 mg/kg/day. Maximum: 4 mg/kg/day.

Dry eye

Ophthalmic

Adults, Elderly. Instill 1 drop in each affected eye q12h.

UNLABELED USES: Treatment of alopecia areata, aplastic anemia, atopic dermatitis, Behçet's disease, biliary cirrhosis, prevention of corneal transplant rejection

CONTRAINDICATIONS: History of hypersensitivity to cyclosporine or polyoxyethylated castor oil

INTERACTIONS

Drug

ACE inhibitors, potassium-sparing diuretics, potassium supplements: May cause hyperkalemia.

Cimetidine, danazol, diltiazem, erythromycin, ketoconazole: May increase cyclosporine concentration and risk of hepatotoxicity and nephrotoxicity.

Immunosuppressants: May increase risk of infection and lymphoproliferative disorders.

Live-virus vaccines: May increase vaccine side effects, potentiate virus replication, and decrease the patient's antibody response to the vaccine.

Lovastatin: May increase the risk of acute renal failure and rhabdomyolysis.

Herbal

St. John's wort: May alter cyclosporine absorption.

Food

Grapefruit, grapefruit juice: May increase the absorption and risk of toxicity of cyclosporine.

DIAGNOSTIC TEST EFFECTS: May increase BUN and serum alkaline phosphatase, amylase, bilirubin, creatinine, potassium, uric acid, AST (SGOT), and ALT (SGPT) levels. May decrease serum magnesium level. Therapeutic peak serum level is 50-300 ng/ml; toxic serum level is greater than 400 ng/ml.

IV INCOMPATIBILITIES: Amphotericin B complex (Abelcet, AmBisome, Amphotec), magnesium

IV COMPATIBILITIES: Propofol (Diprivan)

SIDE EFFECTS

Frequent

Mild to moderate hypertension (26%), hirsutism (21%), tremor (12%)

Occasional (4%-2%)

Acne, leg cramps, gingival hyperplasia (marked by red, bleeding, and tender gums), paresthesia, diarrhea, nausea, vomiting, headache

Rare (less than 1%)

Hypersensitivity reaction, abdominal discomfort, gynecomastia, sinusitis

SERIOUS REACTIONS

- Mild nephrotoxicity occurs in 25% of renal transplant patients, 38% of cardiac transplant patients, and 37% of liver transplant patients, generally 2 to 3 months after transplantation (more severe toxicity generally occurs soon after transplantation). Hepatotoxicity occurs in 4% of renal transplant patients, 7% of cardiac transplant patients, and 4% of liver transplant patients, generally within the first month after transplantation. Both toxicities usually respond to dosage reduction.

• Severe hyperkalemia and hyperuricemia occur occasionally.

SPECIAL CONSIDERATIONS

PRECAUTIONS

• Oral and Injectable: Hypertension is a common side effect of cyclosporine therapy that may persist. During treatment with cyclosporine, vaccination may be less effective; avoid the use of live attenuated vaccines. For patients with rheumatoid arthritis, it is advisable to monitor serum creatinine and blood pressure. For patients with psoriasis, perform a careful dermatologic and physical examination, including blood pressure measurements (on at least two occasions). Treat patients with malignant or premalignant changes of the skin only after appropriate treatment of such lesions and if no other treatment option exists. Risk of cyclosporine nephropathy is reduced when the starting dose is low (2.5 mg/kg per day), the maximum dose does not exceed 4.0 mg/kg per day, and serum creatinine is monitored regularly during cyclosporine administration.

• Cyclosporine is contraindicated in patients with active ocular infections and hypersensitivity.

PATIENT INFORMATION

• The emulsion from one vial is to be used immediately after opening. The remaining contents should be discarded. Do not allow the tip of the vial to touch the eye or any surface. Do not administer cyclosporine while patients are wearing contact lenses. Instruct patients to remove contact lenses before administration of the emulsion. Lenses may be reinserted 15 minutes following the administration of the emulsion.

• Oral and Injectable: Advise patients that any change of cyclosporine formulation should be made cautiously and only under physician supervision because it may result in the need for a change in dosage.

• Inform patients of the necessity of repeated laboratory tests while they are receiving the drug. Give patients careful dosage instructions, advise them of the potential risks during pregnancy, and inform them of the increased risk of neoplasia.

• Advise patients that during treatment with cyclosporine, vaccination may be less effective and to avoid the use of live attenuated vaccines.

• Caution patients using cyclosporine oral solution with its accompanying syringe for dosage measurement not to rinse the syringe before or after use. Introduction of water into the product by any means will cause variation in dose.

PREGNANCY AND LACTATION

• Pregnancy Category C. Sandimmune oral solution (cyclosporine oral solution) has been shown to be embryotoxic and fetotoxic in rats and rabbits when given in doses 2 to 5 times the human dose. Sandimmune (cyclosporine) is excreted in human milk. Excretion in milk after topical treatment is not known.

OCULAR CONSIDERATIONS

• Administration of cyclosporine is indicated to increase tear production presumed to be hindered by ocular inflammation associated with dry eyes. Increased tear production was not seen in patients currently taking topical antiinflammatory drugs or using punctual plugs.

• In patients with suppressed tear production caused by ocular inflammation associated with dry eyes, cyclosporine emulsion is thought to act as a partial immunomodulator.

OCULAR DOSAGE AND ADMINISTRATION

• Invert the vial a few times to obtain a uniform, white, opaque emulsion before using. Instill 1 drop twice a day approximately 12 hours apart. Restasis can be used with artificial tears, allowing a 15-minute interval between products.

• Uveitis: Neoral 4 to 5 mg/kg per day orally. Dosage can vary.

cyproheptadine

(si-proe-hep'ta-deen)

Rx: Periactin

Drug Class: Antihistamines, H1

Pregnancy Category: B

CLINICAL PHARMACOLOGY

Mechanism of Action: An antihistamine that competes with histamine at histaminic receptor sites. Anticholinergic effects cause drying of nasal mucosa. *Therapeutic Effect:* Relieves allergic conditions (urticaria, pruritus).

Pharmacokinetics

Well absorbed from GI tract. Metabolized in liver. Primarily eliminated in feces. **Half-life:** 16 hrs.

AVAILABLE FORMS

- *Syrup:* 2 mg/5 ml (Periactin).
- *Tablets:* 4 mg (Periactin).

INDICATIONS AND DOSAGES

Allergic condition

PO

Adults, Children older than 15 yr. 4 mg 3 times/day. May increase dose but do not exceed 0.5 mg/kg/day.

Children 7-14 yr. 4 mg 2-3 times/day, or 0.25 mg/kg daily in divided doses.

Children 2-6 yr. 2 mg 2-3 times/day, or 0.25 mg/kg daily in divided doses.

Usual elderly dosage

PO

Initially, 4 mg 2 times/day.

CONTRAINDICATIONS: Acute asthmatic attack, patients receiving MAO inhibitors, history of hypersensitivity to antihistamines

INTERACTIONS

Drug

Alcohol, central nervous system (CNS) depressants: May increase CNS depression.

Fluoxetine, paroxetine: May decrease fluoxetine efficacy.

MAOIs: May increase anticholinergic and CNS depressant effects.

Protirelin: May decrease TSH response.

Herbal

None known.

Food

None known.

DIAGNOSTIC TEST EFFECTS: May suppress flare and wheal reaction to antigen skin testing unless drug is discontinued 4 days before testing. May increase SGPT (AST) levels.

SIDE EFFECTS

Frequent

Drowsiness, dizziness, muscular weakness, dry mouth/nose/throat/lips, urinary retention, thickening of bronchial secretions

Elderly

Frequent

Sedation, dizziness, hypotension

Occasional

Epigastric distress, flushing, visual disturbances, hearing disturbances, paresthesia, sweating, chills

SERIOUS REACTIONS

• Children may experience dominant paradoxical reaction (restlessness, insomnia, euphoria, nervousness, tremors).

• Overdosage in children may result in hallucinations, convulsions, death.

• Hypersensitivity reaction (eczema, pruritus, rash, cardiac disturbances, angioedema, photosensitivity) may occur.

• Overdosage may vary from CNS depression (sedation, apnea, cardiovascular collapse, death) to severe paradoxical reaction (hallucinations, tremor, seizures).

SPECIAL CONSIDERATIONS

PRECAUTIONS

• With overdosage, cyproheptadine hydrochloride may produce hallucinations, central nervous system depression, convulsions, and death. Cyproheptadine hydrochloride may have additive effects with alcohol and other central nervous system depressants such as hypnotics, sedatives, tranquilizers, and antianxiety agents. Warn patients about engaging in activities requiring mental alertness and motor coordination, such as driving a car or operating machinery. Cyproheptadine hydrochloride is more likely to cause dizziness, sedation, and hypotension in elderly patients.

• Use cyproheptadine hydrochloride with caution in patients with a history of bronchial asthma, increased intraocular pressure, hyperthyroidism, cardiovascular disease, or hypertension.

PATIENT INFORMATION

• Cyproheptadine hydrochloride may diminish mental alertness and occasionally may produce excitation in children. Warn patients about engaging in activities requiring mental alertness and motor coordination, such as driving a car or operating machinery.

PREGNANCY AND LACTATION

• Pregnancy Category B. Reproduction studies in rabbits, mice, and rats at oral or subcutaneous doses revealed no evidence of impaired fertility or harm to the fetus. Because of the higher risk of antihistamines for infants generally and for newborns and prematures in particular, antihistamine therapy is contraindicated in nursing mothers. Whether this drug is excreted in human milk is not known.

---

dapiprazole hydrochloride

(da'pi-prah-zohl hye-droh-klor'-ide)

Rx: Rev-Eyes

Drug Class: Antiadrenergics, alpha blocking; Miotics; Ophthalmics

Pregnancy Category: B

CLINICAL PHARMACOLOGY

Mechanism of Action: An alpha-adrenergic blocker that primarily affects $alpha_1$ adrenoceptors. Does not significantly affect intraocular pressure. *Therapeutic Effect:* Induces miosis via relaxation of the smooth dilator (radial) muscle of the iris, which causes papillary constriction.

Pharmacokinetics

Well absorbed. Mydriasis reversal begins in 1 hour and occurs in about 6 hours.

AVAILABLE FORMS

• *Powder for reconstitution:* 0.5% (Rev-Eyes).

INDICATIONS AND DOSAGES
Drug-induced mydriasis
Ophthalmic
Adults, Elderly, Children. 2 drops applied topically to the conjunctiva of each eye. Repeat after 5 min. Do not use more than once per week.
CONTRAINDICATIONS: Acute iritis, hypersensitivity to dapiprazole or any component of the formulation
INTERACTIONS
Drug
None known.
Herbal
None known.
Food
None known.
DIAGNOSTIC TEST EFFECTS: *None known.*
SIDE EFFECTS
Occasional
Burning, eyelid edema, photophobia
SERIOUS REACTIONS
• None reported.

SPECIAL CONSIDERATIONS

PRECAUTIONS
• Do not touch the dropper up to lids or any surface, for this may contaminate the solution.
PATIENT INFORMATION
• Dapiprazole hydrochloride may cause difficulty in dark adaptation and may reduce the field of vision. Instruct patients to exercise caution in night driving or other activities in poor illumination.
PREGNANCY AND LACTATION
• Pregnancy Category B. Reproduction studies performed in rats and rabbits revealed no evidence of impaired fertility or harm to the fetus from dapiprazole. Excretion into human milk is not known.

dapsone
(dap'sone)
Drug Class: Antimycobacterials
Pregnancy Category: C

D

CLINICAL PHARMACOLOGY
Mechanism of Action: An antibiotic that is a competitive antagonist of para-aminobenzoic acid (PABA); it prevents normal bacterial utilization of PABA for synthesis of folic acid. *Therapeutic Effect:* Inhibits bacterial growth.
AVAILABLE FORMS
• *Tablets:* 25 mg, 100 mg.
INDICATIONS AND DOSAGES
Leprosy
PO
Adults, Elderly. 50-100 mg/day for 3-10 yr.
Children. 1-2 mg/kg/24 hr. Maximum: 100 mg/day.
Dermatitis herpetiformis
PO
Adults, Elderly. Initially, 50 mg/day. May increase up to 300 mg/day.
Pneumocystis carinii *pneumonia (PCP)*
PO
Adults, Elderly. 100 mg/day in combination with trimethoprim for 21 days.
Prevention of PCP
PO
Adults, Elderly. 100 mg/day.
Children older than 1 mo. 2 mg/kg/day. Maximum: 100 mg/day.
UNLABELED USES: Treatment of inflammatory bowel disorders, malaria
CONTRAINDICATIONS: None significant.
INTERACTIONS
Drug
Methotrexate: May increase hematologic reactions.

Probenecid: May decrease the excretion of dapsone.

Protease inhibitors (including ritonavir): May increase dapsone blood concentration.

Rifampin: May decrease rifampin blood concentration.

Trimethoprim: May increase the risk of toxic effects.

Herbal

St. John's wort: May decrease dapsone blood concentration.

Food

None significant.

DIAGNOSTIC TEST EFFECTS: *None significant.*

SIDE EFFECTS

Frequent (greater than 10%)

Hemolytic anemia, methemoglobinemia, rash

Occasional (10%-1%)

Hemolysis, photosensitivity reaction

SERIOUS REACTIONS

• Agranulocytosis and blood dyscrasias may occur.

SPECIAL CONSIDERATIONS

PRECAUTIONS

• Hemolysis and Heinz body formation may be exaggerated in individuals with a glucose-6-phosphate dehydrogenase deficiency. Toxic hepatitis and cholestatic jaundice have been reported early in therapy.

PREGNANCY AND LACTATION

• Pregnancy Category C. Use of dapsone in pregnant women has not shown that dapsone increases the risk of fetal abnormalities if administered during all trimesters of pregnancy or affects reproduction capacity. Dapsone is excreted in breast milk in substantial amounts.

demecarium bromide

(de-mi-kare'ee-um bro'-mide)

Rx: Humorsol Ocumeter

Drug Class: Cholinesterase inhibitors; Miotics; Ophthalmics

Pregnancy Category: X

CLINICAL PHARMACOLOGY

Mechanism of Action: A cholinesterase inhibitor that increases the concentration of acetylcholine at cholinergic receptor sites and produces effects equivalent to excessive stimulation of cholinergic receptors. *Therapeutic Effect:* Reduces intraocular pressure due to facilitation of outflow of aqueous humor.

Pharmacokinetics

Decreases intraocular pressure within in a few hours. The duration is variable among individuals.

AVAILABLE FORMS

• *Ophthalmic solution:* 0.125%, 0.25% (Humorsol).

INDICATIONS AND DOSAGES

Glaucoma

Ophthalmic, topical

Adults, Elderly. 1-2 drops of the 0.125% or 0.25% solution in affected eye(s) twice daily to twice weekly.

Cyclostimulant

Ophthalmic, topical

Adults, Elderly. 1 drop of 0.125% or 0.25% solution in each eye daily for 2 to 3 weeks, followed by 1 drop every 2 days for 4 weeks.

Diagnostic aid (accommodative esotropia)

Ophthalmic, topical

Adults, Elderly. 1 drop of 0.125% or 0.25% solution once a day for 2 weeks, then 1 drop every 2 days for 2-3 weeks.

CONTRAINDICATIONS: Pregnancy, active uveal inflammation and/or glaucoma associated with iridocyclitis, hypersensitivity to demecarium or any component of the formulation.

INTERACTIONS

Drug

Succinylcholine, other anticholinesterase agents: May cause additive effects.

Herbal

None known.

Food

None known.

DIAGNOSTIC TEST EFFECTS: *None known.*

SIDE EFFECTS

Occasional

Browache, nausea, vomiting, abdominal cramps, diarrhea, hypersalivation, urinary incontinence, lid muscle twitching, redness, myopia blurred vision, increase in intraocular pressure, iris cysts, breathing difficulties, increased sweating

SERIOUS REACTIONS

• Systemic absorption has been associated with demecarium resulting in anticholinesterase toxicity.

• Overdosage can produce cholinergic crisis characterized by cardiac arrhythmias, diarrhea, muscle weakness, profuse sweating, respiratory difficulties, urinary incontinence, and shock.

SPECIAL CONSIDERATIONS

PRECAUTIONS

• Gonioscopy is recommended before medication with demecarium. Use this drug with caution in patients with chronic angle-closure (narrow-angle) glaucoma or in patients with narrow angles. Use this drug with caution with intraocular inflammation. Compression of the lacrimal duct for several seconds immediately following instillation minimizes absorption. Discontinue drug use if salivation, urinary incontinence, diarrhea, profuse sweating, muscle weakness, respiratory difficulties, shock, or cardiac irregularities occur.

• Added systemic effects are possible for those exposed to organophosphate-type insecticides and pesticides (gardeners, organophosphate plant or warehouse workers, farmers, residents of communities that are undergoing insecticide spraying or dusting). Use extreme caution with marked vagotonia, bronchial asthma, spastic gastrointestinal disturbances, peptic ulcer, pronounced bradycardia and hypotension, recent myocardial infarction, epilepsy, parkinsonism, and other disorders that may respond adversely to vagotonic effects. Dilation of blood vessels and resulting greater permeability increase the possibility of hyphema during ocular surgery. Therefore, discontinue this drug before surgery. Demecarium bromide may cause depression of the concentration of cholinesterase in the serum and erythrocytes, with resultant systemic effects.

PREGNANCY AND LACTATION

• Pregnancy Category X. Demecarium bromide is contraindicated for pregnant women. If this drug is used during pregnancy or if the patient becomes pregnant while taking this drug, apprise the patient of the potential hazard to the fetus. Excretion into human milk is not known.

OCULAR CONSIDERATIONS

• Demecarium bromide may enhance or increase myopia caused by the strong accommodative effect.

desloratidine

(des-loer-at'ah-deen)

Rx: Clarinex, Clarinex Reditabs

Drug Class: Antihistamines, H1

Pregnancy Category: C

Do not confuse Clarinex with Claritin.

CLINICAL PHARMACOLOGY

Mechanism of Action: A nonsedating antihistamine that exhibits selective peripheral histamine H_1 receptor blocking action. Competes with histamine at receptor sites. *Therapeutic Effect:* Prevents allergic responses mediated by histamine, such as rhinitis and urticaria.

Pharmacokinetics

Rapidly and almost completely absorbed from the GI tract. Distributed mainly in liver, lungs, GI tract, and bile. Metabolized in the liver to active metabolite and undergoes extensive first-pass metabolism. Eliminated in urine and feces. **Half-life:** 27 hr (increased in the elderly and in renal or hepatic impairment).

AVAILABLE FORMS

- *Tablets:* 5 mg.
- *Tablets (Orally Disintegrating [Reditabs]):* 5 mg.
- *Syrup:* 2.5 mg/5 ml.

INDICATIONS AND DOSAGES

Allergic rhinitis, urticaria

PO

Adults, Elderly, Children older than 12 yr. 5 mg once a day.

Dosage in hepatic or renal impairment

Dosage is decreased to 5 mg every other day.

CONTRAINDICATIONS: None known.

INTERACTIONS

Drug

Erythromycin, ketoconazole: May increase desloratidine blood concentration.

Herbal

None known.

Food

None known.

DIAGNOSTIC TEST EFFECTS: May suppress wheal and flare reactions to antigen skin testing unless the drug is discontinued 4 days before testing.

SIDE EFFECTS

Frequent (12%)

Headache

Occasional (3%)

Dry mouth, somnolence

Rare (less than 3%)

Fatigue, dizziness, diarrhea, nausea

SERIOUS REACTIONS

- None known.

SPECIAL CONSIDERATIONS

OCULAR CONSIDERATIONS

- Seasonal allergic rhinitis patients had significantly reduced ocular symptoms with desloratadine. (Bachert C: Therapeutic points of intervention and clinical implications: role of desloratadine, Allergy 57[suppl 75]:13-18, 2002.)
- Ocular itching was significantly reduced for desloratadine in combination with ketotifen compared with desloratadine alone at all time points. (Crampton HJ: Comparison of ketotifen fumarate ophthalmic solution alone, desloratadine alone, and their combination for inhibition of the signs and symptoms of seasonal allergic rhinoconjunctivitis in the conjunctival allergen challenge model: a double-masked, placebo- and active-controlled trial, Clin Ther 25[7]:1975-1987, 2003.)

dexamethasone

(dex-a-meth'a-sone)

Rx: Adrenocot, Cortastat, Cortastat 10, Cortastat LA, Dalalone, Dalalone D.P., Dalalone L.A., Decadron, Decadron 5-12 Pak, Decadron Phosphate, Injectable, Decaject, De-Sone LA, Dexacen-4, Dexamethasone, Dexamethasone Intensol, Dexasone, Dexasone LA, Dexpak Taperpak, Hexadrol, Hexadrol Phosphate, Solurex, Solurex LA

Drug Class: Corticosteroids; Corticosteroids, ophthalmic; Corticosteroids, topical; Dermatologics; Ophthalmics

Pregnancy Category: C

Do not confuse dexamethasone with desoximetasone or dextramethophan, or Maxidex with Maxzide.

CLINICAL PHARMACOLOGY

Mechanism of Action: A long-acting glucocorticoid that inhibits accumulation of inflammatory cells at inflammation sites, phagocytosis, lysosomal enzyme release and synthesis, and release of mediators of inflammation. *Therapeutic Effect:* Prevents and suppresses cell and tissue immune reactions and inflammatory process.

Pharmacokinetics

Rapidly, completely absorbed from the GI tract after oral administration. Widely distributed. Protein binding: High. Metabolized in the liver. Primarily excreted in urine. Minimally removed by hemodialysis. **Half-life:** 3-4.5 hr.

AVAILABLE FORMS

- *Elixir:* 0.5 mg/5 ml, 1 mg/ml.
- *Inhalant Ointment.*
- *Inhalant Solution.*
- *Inhalant Suspension.*
- *Intranasal Ointment.*
- *Intranasal Solution.*
- *Intranasal Suspension.*
- *Ophthalmic Ointment.*
- *Ophthalmic Solution.*
- *Ophthalmic Suspension:* 0.1%.
- *Oral Solution:* 0.5 mg/5 ml, 0.5 mg/0.5 ml.
- *Tablets:* 0.25 mg, 0.5 mg, 0.75 mg, 1 mg, 1.5 mg, 2 mg, 4 mg, 6 mg.
- *Topical Aerosol.*
- *Topical Cream.*
- *Injection:* 4 mg/ml.

INDICATIONS AND DOSAGES

Antiinflammatory

PO, IV, IM

Adults, Elderly. 0.75-9 mg/day in divided doses q6-12h.

Children. 0.08-0.3 mg/kg/day in divided doses q6-12h.

Cerebral edema

IV

Adults, Elderly. Initially, 10 mg, then 4 mg (IV or IM) q6h.

PO, IV, IM

Children. Loading dose of 1-2 mg/kg, then 1-1.5 mg/kg/day in divided doses q4-6h.

Nausea and vomiting in chemotherapy patients

IV

Adults, Elderly. 8-20 mg once, then 4 mg (PO) q4-6h or 8 mg q8h.

Children. 10 mg/m^2/dose (Maximum: 20 mg), then 5 mg/m^2/dose q6h.

Physiologic replacement

PO, IV, IM

Children. 0.03-0.15 mg/kg/day in divided doses q6-12h.

Usual ophthalmic dosage, ocular inflammatory conditions

Ointment

Adults, Elderly, Children. Thin coating 3-4 times/day.

Suspension

Adults, Elderly, Children. Initially, 2 drops q1h while awake and q2h at night for 1 day, then reduce to 3-4 times/day.

CONTRAINDICATIONS: Active untreated infections, fungal, tuberculosis, or viral diseases of the eye

INTERACTIONS

Drug

Amphotericin: May increase hypokalemia.

Digoxin: May increase digoxin toxicity caused by hypokalemia.

Diuretics, insulin, oral hypoglycemics, potassium supplements: May decrease the effects of these drugs.

Hepatic enzyme inducers: May decrease the effects of dexamethasone.

Live-virus vaccines: May decrease the patient's antibody response to vaccine, increase vaccine side effects, and potentiate virus replication.

Herbal

None known.

Food

None known.

DIAGNOSTIC TEST EFFECTS: May increase blood glucose and serum lipid, amylase, and sodium levels. May decrease serum calcium, potassium, and thyroxine levels.

IV INCOMPATIBILITIES: Ciprofloxacin (Cipro), daunorubicin (Cerubidine), idarubicin (Idamycin), midazolam (Versed)

IV COMPATIBILITIES: Aminophylline, cimetidine (Tagamet), cisplatin (Platinol), cyclophosphamide (Cytoxan), cytarabine (Cytosar), docetaxel (Taxotere), doxorubicin (Adriamycin), etoposide (VePesid), granisetron (Kytril), heparin, hydromorphone (Dilaudid), lorazepam (Ativan), morphine, ondansetron (Zofran), paclitaxel (Taxol), potassium chloride, propofol (Diprivan)

SIDE EFFECTS

Frequent

Inhalation: Cough, dry mouth, hoarseness, throat irritation

Intranasal: Burning, mucosal dryness

Ophthalmic: Blurred vision

Systemic: Insomnia, facial swelling or cushingoid appearance, moderate abdominal distention, indigestion, increased appetite, nervousness, facial flushing, diaphoresis

Occasional

Inhalation: Localized fungal infection, such as thrush

Intranasal: Crusting inside nose, nosebleed, sore throat, ulceration of nasal mucosa

Ophthalmic: Decreased vision, watering of eyes, eye pain, burning, stinging, redness of eyes, nausea, vomiting

Systemic: Dizziness, decreased or blurred vision

Topical: Allergic contact dermatitis, purpura or blood-containing blisters, thinning of skin with easy bruising, telangiectasis or raised dark red spots on skin

Rare

Inhalation: Increased bronchospasm, esophageal candidiasis

Intranasal: Nasal and pharyngeal candidiasis, eye pain

Systemic: General allergic reaction (such as rash and hives); pain, redness, or swelling at injection site; psychological changes; false sense of well-being; hallucinations; depression

SERIOUS REACTIONS

• Long-term therapy may cause muscle wasting (especially in the arms and legs), osteoporosis, spontaneous fractures, amenorrhea, cataracts, glaucoma, peptic ulcer disease, and CHF.

• The ophthalmic form may cause glaucoma, ocular hypertension, and cataracts.

• Abrupt withdrawal following long-term therapy may cause severe joint pain, severe headache, anorexia, nausea, fever, rebound inflammation, fatigue, weakness, lethargy, dizziness, and orthostatic hypotension.

SPECIAL CONSIDERATIONS

PRECAUTIONS

• Topical forms: Consider the possibility of fungal infections of the cornea after prolonged corticosteroid dosing. Systemic absorption of topical corticosteroids has produced reversible hypothalamic-pituitary-adrenal axis suppression, manifestations of Cushing's syndrome, hyperglycemia, and glycosuria in some patients. Children may absorb proportionally larger amounts of topical corticosteroids and thus may be more susceptible to systemic toxicity. In the presence of dermatologic infections, institute the use of an appropriate antifungal or antibacterial agent. The topical dermatologic product is not for ocular use. However, if applied to the eyelids or skin near the eyes, the drug may enter the eyes. In patients with a history of herpes simplex keratitis, ocular exposure to corticosteroids may lead to a recurrence. Prolonged ocular exposure may cause steroid glaucoma.

PATIENT INFORMATION

• This medication is to be used as directed by the physician. It is for external use only. Avoid contact with the eyes with topical forms.

• Advise patients not to use this medication for any disorder other than that for which it was prescribed.

• The treated skin area should not be bandaged or otherwise covered or wrapped so as to be occlusive unless directed by the physician.

• Patients should report any signs of local adverse reactions, especially under occlusive dressing.

• Advise parents of pediatric patients not to use tight-fitting diapers or plastic pants on a child being treated in the diaper area because these garments may constitute occlusive dressings.

• Warn susceptible patients who are taking immunosuppressant doses of corticosteroids to avoid exposure to chickenpox or measles. Also advise patients that if they are exposed, they should seek medical advice without delay.

PREGNANCY AND LACTATION

• Pregnancy Category C. Because adequate human reproduction studies have not been done with corticosteroids, use of these drugs in pregnancy or in women of childbearing potential requires that the anticipated benefits be weighed against the possible hazards to the mother and embryo or fetus. Carefully observe infants born of mothers who have received substantial doses of corticosteroids during pregnancy for signs of hypoadrenalism. Fetal harm is not known. Corticosteroids appear in breast milk and could suppress growth, interfere with endogenous corticosteroid production, or cause other unwanted effects. Advise mothers taking pharmacologic doses of corticosteroids not to nurse.

OCULAR CONSIDERATIONS

• Ocular Indications and Usages

• Oral Forms: Dexamethasone is used to treat ocular diseases such as chorioretinitis, diffuse posterior uveitis and choroiditis, optic neuritis, and sympathetic ophthalmia.

• Topical Forms: Dexamethasone is used to treat ocular diseases such as severe acute and chronic allergic and inflammatory processes involving the eye and its adnexa, such as allergic conjunctivitis, keratitis, allergic corneal marginal ulcers, herpes zoster ophthalmicus, iritis and iridocyclitis, anterior segment inflammation, and sympathetic ophthalmia.

dexamethasone sodium phosphate

(dex-a-meth'-a-sone soe'-dee-um foss'-fate)

Rx: AK-Dex, Decadron Phosphate, Ophthalmic, Dexamethasone, Ophthalmic, Maxidex, Ocu-Dex

Drug Class: Corticosteroids; Corticosteroids, inhalation; Corticosteroids, ophthalmic; Corticosteroids, topical; Dermatologics; Ophthalmics

Pregnancy Category: C

Do not confuse with desoximetasone, dextramethophan, or Maxzide.

CLINICAL PHARMACOLOGY

Mechanism of Action: A corticosteroid that inhibits accumulation of inflammatory cells at inflammation sites, phagocytosis, lysosomal enzyme release and synthesis and release of mediators of inflammation. *Therapeutic Effect:* Prevents and suppresses cell and tissue immune reactions, inflammatory process.

Pharmacokinetics

Absorbed into aqueous humor, cornea, iris, choroids, ciliary body, and retina. Systemic absorption may occur and is more likely at higher doses or in pediatric therapy.

AVAILABLE FORMS

• *Ointment, Ophthalmic:* 0.05% (AK-Dex, Decadron Phosphate, Ocu-Dex, Dexamethasone Ophthalmic).

• *Solution, Ophthalmic:* 0.1% (Ocu-Dex, Dexamthasone Ophthalmic)

• *Suspension, Ophthalmic:* 0.1% (Maxidex).

INDICATIONS AND DOSAGES

Ocular inflammatory conditions

Ophthalmic, ointment

Adults, Elderly. Apply thin strip 3- 4 times/day.

Ophthalmic, solution and suspension

Adults, Elderly. Instill 1 or 2 drops up to 6 times/day.

CONTRAINDICATIONS: Epithelial herpes simplex keratitis (dendritic keratitis), vaccinia, varicella or other viral diseases of the cornea and conjunctiva, mycobacterial infection of the eye, fungal diseases of ocular structures, hypersensitivity to any component of the medication.

INTERACTIONS

Drug

None known.

Herbal

None known.

Food

None known.

DIAGNOSTIC TEST EFFECTS: *None known.*

SIDE EFFECTS

Frequent

Blurred vision, increase intraocular pressure

Occasional
Decreased vision, watering of eyes, eye pain, burning, stinging, redness of eyes, nausea, vomiting
Rare
Optic nerve damage, posterior subcapsular cataract formation, delayed wound healing

SERIOUS REACTIONS

- The serious reactions of the ophthalmic form of dexamethasone sodium phosphate are glaucoma, ocular hypertension, and cataracts.
- May promote development and spread of secondary infection (usually fungal).

SPECIAL CONSIDERATIONS

PRECAUTIONS

- Consider the possibility of fungal infections of the cornea after prolonged corticosteroid dosing. Use caution in the following cases: psychosis, cerebral malaria, elderly, acquired immunodeficiency syndrome, latent tuberculosis or amebiasis (reactivation of the disease), diabetes mellitus, glaucoma, osteoporosis, ulcerative colitits (intestinal perforation), congestive heart failure, myasthenia gravis, renal disease, esophagitis, peptic ulcer, hypertension, and fungal infections of the eye.

PATIENT INFORMATION

- Advise patients to wait at least 15 minutes after instillation of the drug before they insert their soft contact lenses.

PREGNANCY AND LACTATION

- Pregnancy Category C. In mice, dexamethasone sodium phosphate produces fetal resorptions and cleft palate. In the rabbit the drug produced fetal resorptions and multiple abnormalities involving the head, ears, limbs, and palate. Excretion into human milk is not known; however, steroids are absorbed systemically. The drug could suppress the infant's growth and interfere with endogenous corticosteroid production.

D

dexamethasone sodium phosphate; neomycin sulfate

(dex-a-meth'-a-sone soe'-dee-um foss'-fate; nee-oh-mye'-sin sul'-fate)

Rx: AK-Neo-Dex, Neo-Decadron Ocumeter, Neo-Dex, Neo-Dexair
Drug Class: Anti-infectives, ophthalmic; Anti-infectives, topical; Corticosteroids, ophthalmic; Corticosteroids, topical; Dermatologics; Ophthalmics
Pregnancy Category: C
Do not confuse with desoximetasone, dextramethophan, or Maxzide.

CLINICAL PHARMACOLOGY

Mechanism of Action: A topical steroid-antibiotic preparation that inhibits accumulation of inflammatory cells at inflammation sites by its steroid properties. Neomycin, an aminoglycoside antibiotic, binds to the 30s subunit of the ribosome. *Therapeutic Effect:* Prevents inflammatory process. Interferes with bacterial protein synthesis.

Pharmacokinetics
None reported.

AVAILABLE FORMS

- *Solution, ophthalmic:* 0.35% neomycin (3.5 mg/ml) and 0.1% dexamethasone sodium phosphate (1 mg/ml)/5 ml (AK-Neo-Dex, Neo-Dexair, Neo-Dex, Neo-Decadron).

INDICATIONS AND DOSAGES

Antiinflammatory conditions of the palpebral and bulbar conjunctiva, lid, cornea, and anterior segment of the globe

Ophthalmic

Adults, Elderly. Instill 1-2 drops in affected eye(s) every 3-4 hours.

CONTRAINDICATIONS: Epithelial herpes simplex keratitis, acute infectious stages of vaccina, varicella and many other viral diseases of the cornea and conjunctiva, mycobacterial infection of the eye, fungal diseases of ocular structures, and hypersensitivity to any component of the formulation including sulfites.

INTERACTIONS

Drug

None known.

Herbal

None known.

Food

None known.

DIAGNOSTIC TEST EFFECTS: *None known.*

SIDE EFFECTS

Occasional

Blurred vision, decreased vision, watering of eyes, eye pain, burning, stinging, redness of eyes, nausea, vomiting

SERIOUS REACTIONS

- Secondary infection such as fungal infections of the cornea occurs rarely.
- The serious reactions of the ophthalmic form of dexamethasone are glaucoma, ocular hypertension, and cataracts.

SPECIAL CONSIDERATIONS

PRECAUTIONS

- Hypersensitivity reactions to neomycin are not uncommon. Consider the possibility of fungal infections of the cornea after prolonged corticosteroid dosing. Hypothalamic-pituitary-adrenal axis suppression, Cushing's syndrome, and intracranial hypertension have been reported in children receiving topical corticosteroids.

PATIENT INFORMATION

- Solution: One of the preservatives in the ocular solution, benzalkonium chloride, may be absorbed by soft contact lenses. Instruct patients wearing soft contact lenses to wait at least 15 minutes after drug instillation before they insert their lenses.

PREGNANCY AND LACTATION

- Pregnancy Category C. Corticosteroids are generally teratogenic in laboratory animals when administered systemically at relatively low dosage levels. Whether topical administration of corticosteroids could result in sufficient systemic absorption to produce detectable quantities in breast milk is not known.

OCULAR CONSIDERATIONS

- Ocular Indications and Usage: Dexamethasone sodium phosphate and neomycin sulfate are indicated for steroid-responsive inflammatory ocular conditions for which a corticosteroid is indicated and where bacterial infection or risk of bacterial ocular infection exists. Ocular steroids are indicated in inflammatory conditions of the palpebral and bulbar conjunctiva, cornea, and anterior segment of the globe. Ocular steroids also are indicated in the chronic anterior uveitis and corneal injury from chemical, radiation, or thermal burns, or penetration of foreign bodies.

OCULAR DOSAGE AND ADMINISTRATION

- Solution: Instill 1 or 2 drops every hour during the day and every 2 hours during the night as therapy. Further reduction in dosage to 1 drop 3 or 4 times daily may suffice to control symptoms. Prescribe no more than 20 ml initially.

dexamethasone; neomycin sulfate; polymyxin B sulfate

(dex-a-meth'-a-sone nee-oh-mye'sin sul'-fate; pol-i-mix'-in B sul'fate)

Rx: AK-Trol, Dexacidin, Dexasporin, Maxitrol, Methadex, Ocu-Trol, Poly-Dex

Drug Class: Anti-infectives, ophthalmic; Corticosteroids, ophthalmic; Ophthalmics

Pregnancy Category: C

Do not confuse with desoximetasone, dextramethophan, or Maxzide.

CLINICAL PHARMACOLOGY

Mechanism of Action: A topical steroid-antibiotic preparation that inhibits accumulation of inflammatory cells at inflammation sites by its steroid properties. Neomycin, an aminoglycoside antibiotic, binds to the 30s subunit of the ribosome. Polymyxin B damages bacterial cytoplasmic membrane which causes leakage of intracellular components. *Therapeutic Effect:* Prevents inflammatory process. Interferes with bacterial protein synthesis.

Pharmacokinetics

None reported.

AVAILABLE FORMS

- *Suspension, ophthalmic:* 3.5 mg neomycin sulfate, 10,000 units polymyxin B sulfate, 1 mg dexamethasone (AK-Trol, Dexacidin, Dexasporin, Maxitrol, Methadex, Poly-Dex).
- *Ointment, ophthalmic:* 3.5 mg neomycin sulfate, 10,000 units polymyxin B sulfate, 1 mg dexamethasone (Dexasporin, Maxitrol, Ocu-Trol, Poly-Dex).

INDICATIONS AND DOSAGES

Steroid-responsive inflammatory ocular conditions in which corticosteroid is indicated and where bacterial infection or a risk of infection exists

Ophthalmic, ointment

Adults, Elderly. Place about ½ inch in the affected eye 3-4 times/day or apply at bedtime as an adjunct with drops.

Ophthalmic, suspension

Adults, Elderly. Instill 1-2 drops into affected eye(s) every 3-4 hours.

CONTRAINDICATIONS: Epithelial herpes simplex keratitis, acute infectious stages of vaccina, varicella and many other viral diseases of the cornea and conjunctiva, mycobacterial infection of the eye, fungal diseases of ocular structures, and hypersensitivity to any component of the formulation

INTERACTIONS

Drug

None known.

Herbal

None known.

Food

None known.

DIAGNOSTIC TEST EFFECTS: *None known.*

SIDE EFFECTS

Occasional

Blurred vision, decreased vision, watering of eyes, eye pain, burning, stinging, redness of eyes, nausea, vomiting, increase of intraocular pressure

SERIOUS REACTIONS

- Secondary infection such as fungal infections of the cornea occurs rarely.

D

• The serious reactions of the ophthalmic form of dexamethasone are glaucoma, ocular hypertension, and cataracts.

SPECIAL CONSIDERATIONS

PRECAUTIONS

• Hypersensitivity reactions to neomycin are not uncommon. Consider the possibility of fungal infections of the cornea after prolonged steroid dosing.

OCULAR CONSIDERATIONS

• Ocular Indications and Usage: Chronic anterior uveitis and corneal injury from chemical, radiation, or thermal burns; or penetration of foreign bodies

• Efficacy: Active against *Staphylococcus aureus, Escherichia coli, Haemophilus influenzae, Klebsiella/Enterobacter* species, *Neisseria* species, and *Pseudomonas aeruginosa;* does not provide adequate coverage against *Serratia marcescens* and streptococci and *Streptococcus pneumoniae.*

dexamethasone; tobramycin

(dex-a-meth'-a-sone; toe-bra-mye'-sin)

Rx: Tobradex

Drug Class: Anti-infectives, ophthalmic; Corticosteroids, ophthalmic; Ophthalmics

Pregnancy Category: C

CLINICAL PHARMACOLOGY

Mechanism of Action: A corticosteroid and antibiotic combination that inhibits accumulation of inflammatory cells at inflammation sites, phagocytosis, lysosomal enzyme release and synthesis and release of mediators of inflammation through its steroid properties; and irreversibly binds to protein on bacterial ribosomes through its antibiotic properties. *Therapeutic Effect:* Prevents and suppresses cell and tissue immune reactions, inflammatory process. Interferes in protein synthesis of susceptible microorganisms.

Pharmacokinetics

None reported.

AVAILABLE FORMS

• *Ointment, ophthalmic:* 0.3% tobramycin and 0.1% dexamethasone (TobraDex).

• *Suspension, ophthalmic:* 0.3% tobramycin and 0.1% dexamethasone (TobraDex).

INDICATIONS AND DOSAGES

Ocular inflammatory conditions

Ophthalmic, suspension

Adults, Elderly, Children. Instill 1-2 drops of solution q4h. For severe infections, instill 2 drops q30-60min initially, then reduce to less frequent intervals.

Ophthalmic, ointment

Adults, Elderly, Children. Apply 2-3 times/day. For severe infections, apply ointment q3-4h.

CONTRAINDICATIONS: Epithelial herpes simplex keratitis (dendritic keratitis), vaccinia, varicella or other viral diseases of the cornea and conjunctiva, mycobacterial infection of eye, fungal disease of ocular structures, hypersensitivity to tobramycin, dexamethasone, or any other component of the formulation.

INTERACTIONS

Drug

Aprepitant: May increase systemic exposure to dexamethasone.

Caspofungin: May decrease caspofungin plasma levels.

Cephalosporins: May increase risk of nephrotoxicity.

Fluoroquinolones: May increase risk of tendon rupture.

Itraconazole: May increase dexamethasone plasma concentrations and increase risk of corticosteroid side effects.

Nondepolarizing neuromuscular blockers: May enhance and/or prolong neuromuscular blockade.

Penicillins: May decrease tobramycin efficacy.

Quetiapine: May decrease quetiapine concentrations.

Rotovirus vaccine: May increase risk of infection by the vaccine.

Herbal

Echinacea, Ma huang: May decrease effectiveness of dexamethasone.

Licorice: May increase risk of corticosteroid adverse effects.

Saiboku-To: May enhance and prolong effect of dexamethasone.

Food

None known.

DIAGNOSTIC TEST EFFECTS: *None known.*

SIDE EFFECTS

Frequent

Blurred vision

Occasional

Decreased vision, watering of eyes, eye pain, burning, stinging, itching, redness of eyes, nausea, vomiting, swelling of eyelid

Rare

Nasal and pharyngeal candidiasis, eye pain

SERIOUS REACTIONS

• Superinfections, particularly with fungi, may result from bacterial imbalance with any route of administration.

• The serious reactions of the ophthalmic form of dexamethasone are glaucoma, ocular hypertension, and cataracts.

SPECIAL CONSIDERATIONS

PRECAUTIONS

• Consider the possibility of fungal infections of the cornea and secondary infection after long-term steroid dosing. Cross-sensitivity to other aminoglycoside antibiotics may occur.

PATIENT INFORMATION

• Pregnancy Category C. Fetal growth retardation and increased mortality rates in pregnant rats has been reported. Systemically effective corticosteroids appear in human milk.

OCULAR CONSIDERATIONS

• Ocular Indications and Usage: Dexamethasone and tobramycin are used to treat chronic anterior uveitis and corneal injury from chemical, radiation, or thermal burns or penetration of foreign bodies. The drug combination is active against staphylococci, including *Staphylococcus aureus* and *S. epidermidis* (coagulase-positive and coagulase-negative), including penicillin-resistant strains; streptococci, including some of the group A beta-hemolytic species, some nonhemolytic species, and some *Streptococcus pneumoniae; Pseudomonas aeruginosa, Escherichia coli, Klebsiella pneumoniae, Enterobacter aerogenes, Proteus mirabilis, Morganella morganii,* most *Proteus vulgaris* strains; and *Haemophilus influenzae, H. aegyptius, Moraxella lacunata, Acinetobacter calcoaceticus,* and some *Neisseria* species.

D

dexchlorpheniramine

(dex'klor-fen-eer'a-meen)

Rx: Polaramine, Polaramine Repetabs

Drug Class: Antihistamines, H1

Pregnancy Category: B

CLINICAL PHARMACOLOGY

Mechanism of Action: A propylamine derivative that competes with histamine for H_1-receptor sites on effector cells in the gastrointestinal (GI) tract, blood vessels, and respiratory tract. Dexchlorpheniramine is the dextro-isomer of chlorpheniramine and is approximately two times more active. *Therapeutic Effect:* Prevents allergic response, produces mild bronchodilation, blocks histamine-induced bronchitis.

Pharmacokinetics

Route	Onset	Peak	Duration
PO	0.5 hr	1-2 hr	3-6 hr

Well absorbed from the gastrointestinal (GI) tract. Protein binding: 70%. Widely distributed. Metabolized in liver to active metabolite, undergoes extensive first-pass metabolism. Excreted primarily in urine. Not removed by hemodialysis. **Half-life:** 20 hrs.

AVAILABLE FORMS

- *Tablets:* 2 mg (Polaramine [DSC]).
- *Extended-Release Tablets:* 4 mg, 6 mg (Polaramine Repetabs).
- *Syrup:* 2 mg/ 5 ml (Polaramine).

INDICATIONS AND DOSAGES

Allergic rhinitis, common cold

PO

Adults, Elderly, Children 12 yr or older. 2 mg q4-6h or 4-6 mg timed release at bedtime or q8-10h.

Children 6-11 yr. 4 mg timed release at bedtime or 1 mg q4-6h.

Children 2-5 yr. 0.5 mg q4-6h. Do not use timed release.

UNLABELED USES: Asthma, chemotherapy-induced stomatitis, dermographia, familial immunodeficiency disease, malaria, mastocytosi, Meniere's disease, nausea, neurocysticercosis, otitis media, psoriasis, radiocontrast media reactions, urticaria

CONTRAINDICATIONS: History of hypersensitivity to antihistamines, newborn or premature infants, nursing mothers, third trimester of pregnancy

INTERACTIONS

Drug

Alcohol, central nervous system (CNS) depressants: May increase CNS depression.

Methacholine: May interfere with interpretation of pulmonary function tests after a methacholine bronchial challenge.

Procarbazine: May increase CNS depression.

Herbal

None known.

Food

None known.

DIAGNOSTIC TEST EFFECTS: May interfere with the interpretation of the pulmonary function tests after a methacholine bronchial challenge test.

SIDE EFFECTS

Frequent

Drowsiness, dizziness, headache, dry mouth, nose, or throat, urinary retention, thickening of bronchial secretions, sedation, hypotension

Occasional

Epigastric distress, flushing, blurred vision, tinnitus, paresthesia, sweating, chills

SERIOUS REACTIONS

• Children may experience dominant paradoxical reactions, including restlessness, insomnia, euphoria, nervousness, and tremors.

• Hypersensitivity reaction, such as eczema, pruritus, rash, cardiac disturbances, and photosensitivity, may occur.

• Overdosage may vary from CNS depression, including sedation, apnea, hypotension, cardiovascular collapse, or death to severe paradoxical reaction, such as hallucinations, tremor, and seizures.

SPECIAL CONSIDERATIONS

PRECAUTIONS

• Use dexchlorpheniramine maleate with caution in patients with narrow-angle glaucoma, stenosing peptic ulcer, pyloroduodenal obstruction, symptomatic prostatic hypertrophy, and bladder neck obstruction. Overdoses of antihistamines may cause hallucinations, convulsions, or death, especially in infants and children. Additive effects may occur with alcohol ingestion and other central nervous system depressants (e.g., hypnotics, sedatives, and tranquilizers). Patients should not engage in activities requiring mental alertness, such as driving a car or operating machinery. Dexchlorpheniramine maleate is more likely to cause dizziness, sedation, and hypotension in elderly patients (approximately 60 years or older). Use dexchlorpheniramine maleate with caution in patients with a history of bronchial asthma; increased intraocular pressure, hyperthyroidism, cardiovascular disease, or hypertension.

PATIENT INFORMATION

• Dexchlorpheniramine may cause slight to moderate drowsiness.

• Patients should not engage in activities requiring mental alertness, such as driving or operating machinery.

• Alcohol or other sedative drugs may enhance the drowsiness caused by antihistamines.

• Patients should not take tablets, syrup, and repeat-action tablets with a monoamine oxidase inhibitor or oral anticoagulant.

PREGNANCY AND LACTATION

• Pregnancy Category B. Reproduction studies performed in rabbits and rats revealed no evidence of harm to the fetus. Excretion into human milk is not known. Because certain other antihistamines are known to be excreted in human milk and because dexchlorpheniramine maleate is contraindicated in newborn and premature infants, exercise caution when administering it to a nursing woman.

dextroamphetamine sulfate

(dex-troe-am-fet'a-meen)

Rx: Dexedrine, Dexedrine Spansule, Dextrostat

Drug Class: Adrenergic agonists; Amphetamines; Stimulants, central nervous system

Pregnancy Category: C

DEA Class: Schedule II

Do not confuse dextroamphetamine with dextromethorphan, or Dexedrine with Dextran or Excedrin.

CLINICAL PHARMACOLOGY

Mechanism of Action: An amphetamine that enhances the action of dopamine and norepinephrine by blocking their reuptake from synapses; also inhibits monoamine oxidase and facilitates the release of catecholamines. *Therapeutic Effect:* Increases motor activity and mental alertness; decreases motor restlessness, drowsiness, and fatigue; suppresses appetite.

AVAILABLE FORMS

- *Capsules (Sustained-Release [Dexedrine, Spansule]):* 5 mg, 10 mg, 15 mg.
- *Tablets (Dexedrine):* 5 mg.
- *Tablets (Dextrostat):* 5 mg, 10 mg.

INDICATIONS AND DOSAGES

Narcolepsy

PO

Adults, Children older than 12 yr. Initially, 10 mg/day. Increase by 10 mg/day at weekly intervals until therapeutic response is achieved.

Children 6-12 yr. Initially, 5 mg/day. Increase by 5 mg/day at weekly intervals until therapeutic response is achieved. Maximum: 60 mg/day.

Attention deficit hyperactivity disorder (ADHD)

PO

Children 6 yr and older. Initially, 5 mg once or twice a day. Increase by 5 mg/day at weekly intervals until therapeutic response is achieved.

Children 3-5 yr. Initially, 2.5 mg/day. Increase by 2.5 mg/day at weekly intervals until therapeutic response is achieved. Maximum: 40 mg/day.

Appetite suppressant

PO

Adults. 5-30 mg daily in divided doses of 5-10 mg each, given 30-60 min before meals; or 1 extended-release capsule in the morning.

CONTRAINDICATIONS: Advanced arteriosclerosis, agitated states, glaucoma, history of drug abuse, hypersensitivity to sympathomimetic amines, hyperthyroidism, moderate to severe hypertension, symptomatic cardiovascular disease, use within 14 days of MAOIs

INTERACTIONS

Drug

Beta-blockers: May increase the risk of bradycardia, heart block, and hypertension.

Digoxin: May increase the risk of arrhythmias.

MAOIs: May prolong and intensify the effects of dextroamphetamine.

Meperidine: May increase the risk of hypotension, respiratory depression, seizures, and vascular collapse.

Other CNS stimulants: May increase the effects of dextroamphetamine.

Thyroid hormones: May increase the effects of either drug.

Tricyclic antidepressants: May increase cardiovascular effects.

Herbal

None known.

Food

None known.

DIAGNOSTIC TEST EFFECTS: May increase plasma corticosteroid concentrations.

SIDE EFFECTS

Frequent

Irregular pulse, increased motor activity, talkativeness, nervousness, mild euphoria, insomnia

Occasional

Headache, chills, dry mouth, GI distress, worsening depression in patients who are clinically depressed, tachycardia, palpitations, chest pain, dizziness, decreased appetite

SERIOUS REACTIONS

- Overdose may produce skin pallor or flushing, arrhythmias, and psychosis.
- Abrupt withdrawal after prolonged use of high doses may produce lethargy lasting for weeks.
- Prolonged administration to children with ADHD may inhibit growth.

SPECIAL CONSIDERATIONS

PRECAUTIONS

- Exercise caution in prescribing amphetamines for patients with even mild hypertension.

PATIENT INFORMATION

- Amphetamines may impair the ability of the patient to engage in potentially hazardous activities such as operating machinery or vehicles; therefore, caution the patient accordingly.

PREGNANCY AND LACTATION

- Pregnancy Category C. Dextroamphetamine sulfate has been shown to have embryotoxic and teratogenic effects when administered to mice in doses approximately 41 times the maximum human dose. Amphetamines are excreted in human milk. Advise mothers taking amphetamines to refrain from nursing.

OCULAR CONSIDERATIONS

- Dextroamphetamine sulfate can cause mydriasis and reduction of intraocular pressure.

D

diclofenac

(dye-kloe'fen-ak)

Rx: Cataflam, Solaraze, Voltaren, Voltaren Ophthalmic, Voltaren-XR

Drug Class: Analgesics, nonnarcotic; Nonsteroidal anti-inflammatory drugs; Ophthalmics

Pregnancy Category: B

Do not confuse diclofenac with Diflucan or Duphalac, or Voltaren with Verelan.

CLINICAL PHARMACOLOGY

Mechanism of Action: An NSAID that inhibits prostaglandin synthesis, reducing the intensity of pain. Also constricts the iris sphincter. May inhibit angiogenesis (the formation of blood vessels) by inhibiting substance P or blocking the angiogenic effects of prostaglandin E. *Therapeutic Effect:* Produces analgesic and anti-inflammatory effects. Prevents miosis during cataract surgery. May reduce angiogenesis in inflammed tissue.

Pharmacokinetics

Route	*Onset*	*Peak*	*Duration*
PO	30 min	2-3 hr	Up to 8 hr

Completely absorbed from the GI tract; penetrates cornea after ophthalmic administration (may be systemically absorbed). Protein binding: greater than 99%. Widely distributed. Metabolized in the liver.

Primarily excreted in urine. Minimally removed by hemodialysis. **Half-life:** 1.2-2 hr.

AVAILABLE FORMS

- *Topical Gel (Solaraze):* 3%.
- *Tablets (Cataflam):* 50 mg.
- *Tablets (Enteric-Coated [Voltaren]):* 25 mg, 50 mg, 75 mg.
- *Tablets (Extended-Release [Voltaren XR]):* 100 mg.
- *Ophthalmic Solution (Voltaren Ophthalmic):* 0.1%.

INDICATIONS AND DOSAGES

Osteoarthritis

PO (Cataflam, Voltaren)

Adults, Elderly. 50 mg 2-3 times a day.

PO (Voltaren XR)

Adults, Elderly. 100 mg/day as a single dose.

Rheumatoid arthritis

PO (Cataflam, Voltaren)

Adults, Elderly. 50 mg 2-4 times a day. Maximum: 225 mg/day.

PO (Voltaren XR)

Adults, Elderly. 100 mg once a day. Maximum: 100 mg twice a day.

Ankylosing spondylitis

PO (Voltaren)

Adults, Elderly. 100-125 mg/day in 4-5 divided doses.

Analgesia, primary dysmenorrhea

PO (Cataflam)

Adults, Elderly. 30 mg 3 times a day.

Usual pediatric dosage

Children. 2-3 mg/kg/day in 2-4 divided doses.

Actinic keratoses

Topical

Adults, Adolescents. Apply twice a day to lesion for 60-90 days.

Cataract surgery

Ophthalmic

Adults, Elderly. Apply 1 drop to eye 4 times a day commencing 24 hr after cataract surgery. Continue for 2 wk afterward.

Pain, relief of photophobia in patients undergoing corneal refractive surgery

Ophthalmic

Adults, Elderly. Apply 1 drop to affected eye 1 hr before surgery, within 15 min after surgery, then 4 times a day for 3 days.

UNLABELED USES: Treatment of vascular headaches (oral); to reduce the occurrence and severity of cystoid macular edema after cataract surgery (ophthalmic form)

CONTRAINDICATIONS: Hypersensitivity to aspirin, diclofenac, and other NSAIDs; porphyria

INTERACTIONS

Drug

Acetylcholine, carbachol: May decrease the effects of these drugs (with ophthalmic diclofenac).

Antihypertensives, diuretics: May decrease the effects of these drugs.

Aspirin, other salicylates: May increase the risk of GI side effects such as bleeding.

Bone marrow depressants: May increase the risk of hematologic reactions.

Epinephrine, other antiglaucoma medications: May decrease the antiglaucoma effect of these drugs.

Heparin, oral anticoagulants, thrombolytics: May increase the effects of these drugs.

Lithium: May increase the blood concentration and risk of toxicity of lithium.

Methotrexate: May increase the risk of methotrexate toxicity.

Probenecid: May increase diclofenac blood concentration.

Herbal

Ginkgo biloba: May increase the risk of bleeding.

Food

None known.

DIAGNOSTIC TEST EFFECTS: May increase BUN level; urine protein level; and serum LDH, potassium, alkaline phosphatase, creatinine, AST (SGOT), and ALT (SGPT) levels. May decrease serum uric acid level.

SIDE EFFECTS

Frequent (9%-4%)

PO: Headache, abdominal cramps, constipation, diarrhea, nausea, dyspepsia

Ophthalmic: Burning or stinging on instillation, ocular discomfort

Occasional (3%-1%)

PO: Flatulence, dizziness, epigastric pain

Ophthalmic: Ocular itching or tearing

Rare (less than 1%)

PO: Rash, peripheral edema or fluid retention, visual disturbances, vomiting, drowsiness

SERIOUS REACTIONS

• Overdose may result in acute renal failure.

• Rare reactions with long-term use include peptic ulcer disease, GI bleeding, gastritis, a severe hepatic reaction (jaundice), nephrotoxicity (hematuria, dysuria, proteinuria), and a severe hypersensitivity reaction (bronchospasm or angioedema).

SPECIAL CONSIDERATIONS

PRECAUTIONS

• Diclofenac may slow or delay healing. Concomitant use with topical steroids may increase the potential for healing problems. Administration of diclofenac may result in keratitis, epithelial breakdown, corneal thinning, corneal infiltrates, corneal erosion, corneal ulceration, and corneal perforation. Patients experiencing complicated ocular surgeries, corneal denervation, corneal epithelial defects, diabetes mellitus, ocular surface disease, rheumatoid arthritis, or repeat ocular surgeries in a short amount of time may be at increased risk for adverse corneal events that may be sight threatening. Usage more than 24 hours before surgery or beyond 14 days after surgery may increase risk for adverse corneal events. Diclofenac has no significant effect on intraocular pressure. The drug should not be used with contact lenses.

PATIENT INFORMATION

• Except for use of bandage contact lenses during the first 3 days following refractive surgery, diclofenac should not be used with soft contact lenses.

PREGNANCY AND LACTATION

• Pregnancy Category C. Diclofenac has been shown to cross the placental barrier in mice and rabbits. Because of the known effects of prostaglandin biosynthesis-inhibiting drugs on fetal cardiovascular system (closure of ductus arteriosus), avoid use in late pregnancy. Because of the potential for serious adverse reactions in nursing infants from diclofenac, decide whether to discontinue nursing or to discontinue the drug, taking into account the importance of the drug to the mother.

OCULAR CONSIDERATIONS

• Off-label uses include inhibition of anterior chamber flare following argon laser trabeculoplasty. Diclofenac was administered once before and after argon laser trabeculoplasty. Diclofenac also been used for treatment of seasonal allergic conjunctivitis and pain associated with corneal refractive surgery.

dicloxacillin

(dye-klox'a-sill-in)

Rx: Dynapen

Drug Class: Antibiotics, penicillins

Pregnancy Category: B

CLINICAL PHARMACOLOGY

Mechanism of Action: A propylamine derivative that competes with histamine for H_1-receptor sites on effector cells in the gastrointestinal (GI) tract, blood vessels, and respiratory tract. Dexchlorpheniramine is the dextro-isomer of chlorpheniramine and is approximately two times more active. *Therapeutic Effect:* Prevents allergic response, produces mild bronchodilation, blocks histamine-induced bronchitis.

Pharmacokinetics

Route	Onset	Peak	Duration
PO	0.5 hr	1-2 hr	3-6 hr

Well absorbed from the gastrointestinal (GI) tract. Protein binding: 70%. Widely distributed. Metabolized in liver to active metabolite, undergoes extensive first-pass metabolism. Excreted primarily in urine. Not removed by hemodialysis. **Half-life:** 20 hrs.

AVAILABLE FORMS

- *Tablets:* 2 mg (Polaramine [DSC]).
- *Extended-Release Tablets:* 4 mg, 6 mg (Polaramine Repetabs).
- *Syrup:* 2 mg/ 5 ml (Polaramine).

INDICATIONS AND DOSAGES

Allergic rhinitis, common cold

PO

Adults, Elderly, Children 12 yr or older. 2 mg q4-6h or 4-6 mg timed release at bedtime or q8-10h.

Children 6-11 yr. 4 mg timed release at bedtime or 1 mg q4-6h.

Children 2-5 yr. 0.5 mg q4-6h. Do not use timed release.

UNLABELED USES: Asthma, chemotherapy-induced stomatitis, dermographia, familial immunodeficiency disease, malaria, mastocytosis, Meniere's disease, nausea, neurocysticercosis, otitis media, psoriasis, radiocontrast media reactions, urticaria

CONTRAINDICATIONS: History of hypersensitivity to antihistamines, newborn or premature infants, nursing mothers, third trimester of pregnancy

INTERACTIONS

Drug

Alcohol, central nervous system (CNS) depressants: May increase CNS depression.

Methacholine: May interfere with interpretation of pulmonary function tests after a methacholine bronchial challenge.

Procarbazine: May increase CNS depression.

Herbal

None known.

Food

None known.

DIAGNOSTIC TEST EFFECTS: May interfere with the interpretation of the pulmonary function tests after a methacholine bronchial challenge test.

SIDE EFFECTS

Frequent

Drowsiness, dizziness, headache, dry mouth, nose, or throat, urinary retention, thickening of bronchial secretions, sedation, hypotension

Occasional

Epigastric distress, flushing, blurred vision, tinnitus, paresthesia, sweating, chills

SERIOUS REACTIONS

• Children may experience dominant paradoxical reactions, including restlessness, insomnia, euphoria, nervousness, and tremors.

• Hypersensitivity reaction, such as eczema, pruritus, rash, cardiac disturbances, and photosensitivity, may occur.

• Overdosage may vary from CNS depression, including sedation, apnea, hypotension, cardiovascular collapse, or death to severe paradoxical reaction, such as hallucinations, tremor, and seizures.

SPECIAL CONSIDERATIONS

PRECAUTIONS

• Generally, do not administer penicillinase-resistant penicillins to patients with a history of sensitivity to any penicillin.

• The use of antibiotics may result in overgrowth of nonsusceptible organisms. If new infections from bacteria or fungi occur, discontinue the drug and take appropriate measures.

PATIENT INFORMATION

• Inform patients that penicillin is an antibacterial agent that will work with the natural defenses of the body to control certain types of infections. Advise patients not to take the drug if they have had an allergic reaction to any form of penicillin previously and to inform the physician of any allergies or previous allergic reactions to any drugs they may have had.

• Instruct patients who previously have experienced an anaphylactic reaction to penicillin to wear a medical identification tag or bracelet.

• Because most antibacterial drugs taken by mouth are absorbed best on an empty stomach, direct patients to take penicillin 1 hour before meals or 2 hours after eating unless circumstances warrant otherwise.

• Advise patients to take the entire course of therapy prescribed, even if fever and other symptoms have stopped.

• If any of the following reactions occur, instruct patients to stop taking their prescription and to notify the physician: shortness of breath, wheezing, skin rash, mouth irritation, black tongue, sore throat, nausea, vomiting, diarrhea, fever, swollen joints, or any unusual bleeding or bruising.

• Instruct patients not to take any additional medications without physician approval, including nonprescription drugs such as antacids, laxatives, or vitamins.

• Instruct patients to discard liquid forms of penicillin after 7 days if stored at room temperature or after 14 days if refrigerated.

PREGNANCY AND LACTATION

• Pregnancy Category B. Reproduction studies performed in the mouse, rat, and rabbit have revealed no evidence of impaired fertility or harm to the fetus caused by the penicillinase-resistant penicillins. Penicillins are excreted in breast milk.

OCULAR CONSIDERATIONS

• Ocular Indications and Usage: Internal hordeolum, acute dacryocystitis, lid trauma/oculoplastic procedures.

OCULAR DOSAGE AND ADMINISTRATION

• Internal hordeolum and acute dacryocystitis: 250 mg PO every 6 hours

• Lid trauma/oculoplastic procedures: 250 to 500 mg PO every 6 hours

digoxin

(di-jox′in)

Rx: Digitek, Lanoxicaps, Lanoxin

Drug Class: Antiarrhythmics; Cardiac glycosides; Inotropes

Pregnancy Category: C

Do not confuse digoxin with Desoxyn or doxepin, or Lanoxin with Levsinex or Lonox.

CLINICAL PHARMACOLOGY

Mechanism of Action: A cardiac glycoside that increases the influx of calcium from extracellular to intracellular cytoplasm. *Therapeutic Effect:* Potentiates the activity of the contractile cardiac muscle fibers and increases the force of myocardial contraction. Slows the heart rate by decreasing conduction through the SA and AV nodes.

Pharmacokinetics

Route	Onset	Peak	Duration
PO	0.5-2 hr	28 hr	3-4 days
IV	5-30 min	1-4 hr	3-4 days

Readily absorbed from the GI tract. Widely distributed. Protein binding: 30%. Partially metabolized in the liver. Primarily excreted in urine. Minimally removed by hemodialysis. **Half-life:** 36-48 hr (increased with impaired renal function and in the elderly).

AVAILABLE FORMS

- *Capsules (Lanoxicaps):* 50 mcg, 100 mcg, 200 mcg.
- *Elixir (Lanoxin):* 50 mcg/ml.
- *Tablets (Digitek, Lanoxin):* 125 mcg, 250 mcg.
- *Injection (Lanoxin):* 250 mcg/ml, 100 mcg/ml.

INDICATIONS AND DOSAGES

Rapid loading dose for the management and treatment of CHF; control of ventricular rate in patients with atrial fibrillation; treatment and prevention of recurrent paroxysmal atrial tachycardia

PO

Adults, Elderly. Initially, 0.5-0.75 mg, additional doses of 0.125-0.375 mg at 6- to 8-hr intervals. Range: 0.75-1.25 mg.

Children 10 yr and older. 10-15 mcg/kg.

Children 5-9 yr. 20-35 mcg/kg.

Children 2-4 yr. 30-40 mcg/kg.

Children 1-23 mo. 35-60 mcg/kg.

Neonates, full-term. 25-35 mcg/kg.

Neonates, premature. 20-30 mcg/kg.

IV

Adults, Elderly. 0.6-1 mg.

Children 10 yr and older. 8-12 mcg/kg.

Children 5-9 yr. 15-30 mcg/kg.

Children 2-4 yr. 25-35 mcg/kg.

Children 1-23 mo. 30-50 mcg/kg.

Neonates, full-term. 20-30 mcg/kg.

Neonates, premature. 15-25 mcg/kg.

Maintenance dosage for CHF; control of ventricular rate in patients with atrial fibrillation; treatment and prevention of recurrent paroxysmal atrial tachycardia

PO, IV

Adults, Elderly. 0.125-0.375 mg/day.

Children. 25%-35% loading dose (20%-30% for premature neonates).

Dosage in renal impairment

Dosage adjustment is based on creatinine clearance. Total digitalizing dose: decrease by 50% in end-stage renal disease.

Creatinine Clearance	*Dosage*
10-50 ml/min	25%-75% usual
less than 10 ml/min	10%-25% usual

CONTRAINDICATIONS: Ventricular fibrillation, ventricular tachycardia unrelated to CHF

INTERACTIONS

Drug

Amiodarone: May increase digoxin blood concentration and risk of toxicity; may have an additive effect on the SA and AV nodes.

Amphotericin, glucocorticoids, potassium-depleting diuretics: May increase risk of toxicity due to hypokalemia.

Antiarrhythmics, parenteral calcium, sympathomimetics: May increase risk of arrhythmias.

Antidiarrheals, cholestyramine, colestipol, sucralfate: May decrease absorption of digoxin.

Diltiazem, fluoxetine, quinidine, verapamil: May increase digoxin blood concentration.

Parenteral magnesium: May cause cardiac conduction changes and heart block.

Herbal

Siberian ginseng: May increase serum digoxin levels.

Food

None known.

DIAGNOSTIC TEST EFFECTS: *None known.*

IV INCOMPATIBILITIES: Amphotericin B complex (Abelcet, Amphotec, AmBisome), fluconazole (Diflucan), foscarnet (Foscavir), propofol (Diprivan)

IV COMPATIBILITIES: Cimetidine (Tagamet), diltiazem (Cardizem), furosemide (Lasix), heparin, insulin (regular), lidocaine, midazolam (Versed), milrinone (Primacor), morphine, potassium chloride, propofol (Diprivan)

SIDE EFFECTS

None known. However, there is a very narrow margin of safety between a therapeutic and toxic result. Long-term therapy may produce mammary gland enlargement in women but is reversible when drug is withdrawn.

SERIOUS REACTIONS

- The most common early manifestations of digoxin toxicity are GI disturbances (anorexia, nausea, vomiting) and neurologic abnormalities (fatigue, headache, depression, weakness, drowsiness, confusion, nightmares).
- Facial pain, personality change, and ocular disturbances (photophobia, light flashes, halos around bright objects, yellow or green color perception) may be noted.

SPECIAL CONSIDERATIONS

PRECAUTIONS

- Digoxin is excreted primarily by the kidneys; therefore patients with impaired renal function require smaller than usual maintenance doses of digoxin. In patients with hypokalemia or hypomagnesemia, toxicity may occur despite serum digoxin concentrations less than 2.0 ng/ml because potassium or magnesium depletion sensitizes the myocardium to digoxin. Therefore it is desirable to maintain normal serum potassium and magnesium concentrations in patients being treated with digoxin. Hypercalcemia from any cause predisposes the patient to digitalis toxicity. Hypothyroidism may reduce the requirements for digoxin. Use digoxin with caution in patients with acute myocardial infarction. Reduction in the dose of digoxin for 1 to 2 days before electrical cardioversion of atrial fibrillation may be desirable to avoid the induction of ventricular arrhythmias.

PREGNANCY AND LACTATION

• Pregnancy Category C. Fetal harm is not known. Studies have shown that digoxin concentrations in the mother's serum and milk are similar. However, the estimated exposure of a nursing infant to digoxin via breast-feeding will be far below the usual infant maintenance dose. Therefore, this amount should have no pharmacologic effect on the infant. Nevertheless, exercise caution when administering digoxin to a nursing woman.

OCULAR CONSIDERATIONS

• Digoxin can produce visual disturbances, such as blurred or yellow vision, dazzle, visual hallucinations, photophobia, reduced visual acuity, and altered color perception.

dihydrotachysterol

(dye-hye-droe-tak-iss'ter-ole)

Rx: DHT, DHT Intensol, Hytakerol

Drug Class: Vitamins/minerals

Pregnancy Category: C

CLINICAL PHARMACOLOGY

Mechanism of Action: A fat-soluble vitamin that is essential for absorption, utilization of calcium phosphate, and normal calcification of bone. *Therapeutic Effect:* Stimulates calcium and phosphate absorption from small intestine, promotes secretion of calcium from bone to blood, promotes renal tubule phosphate resorption, acts on bone cells to stimulate skeletal growth and on parathyroid gland to suppress hormone synthesis and secretion.

Pharmacokinetics

Well absorbed from small intestine. Metabolized in liver. Eliminated via biliary system; excreted in urine. **Half-life:** Unknown.

AVAILABLE FORMS

• *Oral Solution:* 0. 2 mg/ml (DHT Intensol).

• *Capsule:* 0. 125 mg (Hytakerol).

• *Tablets:* 0. 125 mg, 0. 2 mg, 0. 4 mg (DHT).

INDICATIONS AND DOSAGES

Hypoparathyroidism

PO

Adults, Elderly, Older Children. Initially, 0.8-2.4 mg/day for several days. Maintenance: 0.2-1 mg/day.

Infants, Young Children. Initially, 1-5 mg/day for 4 days, then 0.1-0.5 mg/day.

Nutritional rickets

PO

Adults, Elderly, Children. 0.5 mg as a single dose or 13-50 mcg/day until healing occurs.

Renal osteodystorphy

PO

Adults, Elderly. 0.25-0.6 mg/24 hrs adjusted as necessary to achieve normal serum calcium levels and promote bone healing.

CONTRAINDICATIONS: Hypercalcemia, malabsorption syndrome, vitamin D toxicity, hypersensitivity to vitamin D products or analogs

INTERACTIONS

Drug

Aluminum-containing antacid (long-term use): May increase aluminum concentration and aluminum bone toxicity.

Calcium-containing preparations, thiazide diuretics: May increase the risk of hypercalcemia.

Magnesium-containing antacids: May increase magnesium concentration.

Herbal

None known.

Food

None known.

DIAGNOSTIC TEST EFFECTS: May increase serum cholesterol, calcium, magnesium, and phosphate levels. May decrease serum alkaline phosphatase.

SIDE EFFECTS

Occasional

Nausea, vomiting

SERIOUS REACTIONS

- Early signs of overdosage are manifested as weakness, headache, somnolence, nausea, vomiting, dry mouth, constipation, muscle and bone pain, and metallic taste sensation.
- Later signs of overdosage are evidenced by polyuria, polydipsia, anorexia, weight loss, nocturia, photophobia, rhinorrhea, pruritus, disorientation, hallucinations, hyperthermia, hypertension, and cardiac arrhythmias.

SPECIAL CONSIDERATIONS

PRECAUTIONS

- In patients with renal osteodystrophy accompanied by hyperphosphatemia, maintenance of a normal serum phosphorus level by dietary phosphate restriction and/or administration of aluminum gels as intestinal phosphate binders is essential to prevent metastatic calcification. Because of its effect on serum calcium, administer dihydrotachysterol to pregnant patients or to patients with renal stones only when the potential benefits outweigh the possible hazards.

PREGNANCY AND LACTATION

- Pregnancy Category C. Animal reproduction studies have shown fetal abnormalities in several species associated with hypervitaminosis D. Excretion into human milk is not known.

diltiazem hydrochloride

(dil-tye'a-zem)

Rx: Cardizem, Cardizem CD, Cardizem LA, Cardizem SR, Cartia XT, Dilacor XR, Diltia XT, Diltiazem Hydrochloride XT, Taztia, Tiazac

Drug Class: Antiarrhythmics, class IV; Calcium channel blockers

Pregnancy Category: C

Do not confuse Cardizem with Cardene or Cardene SR, or Tiazac with Ziac.

CLINICAL PHARMACOLOGY

Mechanism of Action: An antianginal, antihypertensive, and antiarrhythmic agent that inhibits calcium movement across cardiac and vascular smooth-muscle cell membranes. This action causes the dilation of coronary arteries, peripheral arteries, and arterioles. *Therapeutic Effect:* Decreases heart rate and myocardial contractility, slows SA and AV conduction and decreases total peripheral vascular resistance by vasodilation.

Pharmacokinetics

Route	Onset	Peak	Duration
PO	0.5-1 hr	N/A	N/A
PO (extended-release)	2-3 hr	N/A	N/A
IV	3 min	N/A	N/A

Well absorbed from the GI tract. Protein binding: 70%-80%. Undergoes first-pass metabolism in the liver to active metabolite. Primarily excreted in urine. Not removed by hemodialysis. **Half-life:** 3-8 hr.

AVAILABLE FORMS

- *Capsules (Sustained-Release [Cardizem SR]):* 60 mg, 90 mg, 120 mg.
- *Capsules (Extended-Release [Cardizem CD]):* 120 mg, 180 mg, 240 mg, 300 mg, 360 mg.
- *Capsules (Extended-Release [Cartia XT]):* 120 mg, 180 mg, 240 mg, 300 mg.
- *Capsules (Extended-Release [Dilacor XR]):* 120 mg, 180 mg, 240 mg.
- *Capsules (Extended-Release [Diltia XT]):* 120 mg, 180 mg, 240 mg.
- *Capsules (Extended-Release [Taztia XT]):* 120 mg, 180 mg, 240 mg, 300 mg, 360 mg.
- *Caspules (Extended-Release [Tiazac]):* 120 mg, 180 mg, 240 mg, 300 mg, 360 mg, 420 mg.
- *Tablets (Cardizem):* 30 mg, 60 mg, 90 mg, 120 mg.
- *Tablets (Extended-Release [Cardizem LA]):* 120 mg, 180 mg, 240 mg, 300 mg, 360 mg, 420 mg.
- *Injection (Ready-to-Hang Infusion):* 1 mg/ml.

INDICATIONS AND DOSAGES

Angina related to coronary artery spasm (Prinzmetal's variant), chronic stable angina (effort-associated)

PO

Adults, Elderly. Initially, 30 mg 4 times a day. Increase up to 180-360 mg/day in 3-4 divided doses at 1- to 2-day intervals.

PO (Cardizem LA)

Adults, Elderly. Initially, 180 mg/day. May increase at intervals of 7-14 days up to 360 mg/day.

PO (Cardizem CD)

Adults, Elderly. Initially, 120-180 mg/day; titrate over 7-14 days. Range: Up to 480 mg/day.

Essential hypertension

PO (Cardizem CD, Cartia XT)

Adults, Elderly. Initially, 180-240 mg once a day. May increase at 2-week intervals. Maintenance 240-360 mg/day. Maximum: 480 mg once a day.

PO (Cardizem SR)

Adults, Elderly. Initially, 60-120 mg twice a day. May increase at 2-week intervals. Maintenance: 240-360 mg/day.

PO (Cardizem LA)

Adults, Elderly. Initially, 180-240 mg once a day. May increase at 2-week intervals. Maintenance: 120-540 mg/day.

PO (Dilacor XR)

Adults, Elderly. 180-240 mg once a day.

PO (Dilacor XT)

Adults, Elderly. Initially, 180-240 mg a day. May increase at 2-week intervals. Maximum: 540 mg once a day.

PO (Taztia XT)

Adults, Elderly. Initially, 120-240 mg once a day. May increase at 2 week intervals. Maximum: 540 mg once a day.

Temporary control of rapid ventricular rate in atrial fibrillation or flutter, rapid conversion of paroxysmal supraventricular tachycardia to normal sinus rhythm.

IV push

Adults, Elderly. Initially, 0.25 mg/kg actual body weight over 2 min. May repeat in 15 min at dose of 0.35 mg/kg actual body weight. Subsequent doses individualized.

IV Infusion

Adults, Elderly. After initial bolus injection, may begin infusion at 5-10 mg/hr; may increase by 5 mg/hr up to a maximum of 15 mg/hr. Infusion duration should not exceed 24 hr.

CONTRAINDICATIONS: Acute MI, pulmonary congestion, severe hypotension (less than 90 mm Hg systolic), sick sinus syndrome, second- or third-degree AV block (except in the presence of a pacemaker)

INTERACTIONS

Drug

Beta-blockers: May have additive effect.

Carbamazepine, quinidine, theophylline: May increase diltiazem blood concentration and risk of toxicity.

Digoxin: May increase serum digoxin concentration.

Procainamide, quinidine: May increase risk of QT-interval prolongation.

Herbal

None known.

Food

None known.

DIAGNOSTIC TEST EFFECTS: PR interval may be increased.

IV INCOMPATIBILITIES: Acetazolamide (Diamox), acyclovir (Zovirax), aminophylline, ampicillin, ampicillin/sulbactam (Unasyn), cefoperazone (Cefobid), diazepam (Valium), furosemide (Lasix), heparin, insulin, nafcillin, phenytoin (Dilantin), rifampin (Rifadin), sodium bicarbonate

IV COMPATIBILITIES: Albumin, aztreonam (Azactam), bumetanide (Bumex), cefazolin (Ancef), cefotaxime (Claforan), ceftazidime (Fortaz), ceftriaxone (Rocephin), cefuroxime (Zinacef), cimetidine (Tagamet), ciprofloxacin (Cipro), clindamycin (Cleocin), digoxin (Lanoxin), dobutamine (Dobutrex), dopamine (Intropin), gentamicin (Garamycin), hydromorphone (Dilaudid), lidocaine, lorazepam (Ativan), metoclopramide (Reglan), metronidazole (Flagyl), midazolam (Versed), morphine, multivitamins, nitroglycerin, norepinephrine (Levophed), potassium chloride, potassium phosphate, tobramycin (Nebcin), vancomycin (Vancocin)

SIDE EFFECTS

Frequent (10%-5%)

Peripheral edema, dizziness, lightheadedness, headache, bradycardia, asthenia (loss of strength, weakness)

Occasional (5%-2%)

Nausea, constipation, flushing, EKG changes

Rare (less than 2%)

Rash, micturition disorder (polyuria, nocturia, dysuria, frequency of urination), abdominal discomfort, somnolence

SERIOUS REACTIONS

- Abrupt withdrawal may increase frequency or duration of angina.
- CHF and second- and third-degree AV block occur rarely.
- Overdose produces nausea, somnolence, confusion, slurred speech, and profound bradycardia.

SPECIAL CONSIDERATIONS

PRECAUTIONS

- Use diltiazem hydrochloride with caution in patients with impaired renal or hepatic function. Dermatologic events may be transient and may disappear despite continued use of diltiazem hydrochloride.

PREGNANCY AND LACTATION

- Pregnancy Category C. Administration of doses to animals ranging from 5 to 10 times greater than the daily recommended oral antianginal therapeutic dose has resulted in embryo and fetal lethality. Fetal harm is not known. Diltiazem is excreted in human milk. One report suggests that concentrations in breast milk may approximate serum levels.

OCULAR CONSIDERATIONS

• Cyclosporine: A pharmacokinetic interaction between diltiazem and cyclosporine has been observed during studies involving renal and cardiac transplant patients. In renal and cardiac transplant recipients, a reduction of cyclosporine trough dose ranging from 15% to 48% was necessary to maintain cyclosporine trough concentrations similar to those seen before the addition of diltiazem. If these agents are to be administered concurrently, cyclosporine concentrations should be monitored, especially when diltiazem therapy is initiated, adjusted, or discontinued. The effect of cyclosporine on diltiazem plasma concentrations has not been evaluated.

diphenhydramine

(dye-fen-hye'dra-meen)

Rx: Antihistamine, Banaril, Benadryl, Diphedryl, Dytan, Hyrexin, Q-Dryl, Trux-adryl, Valu-Dryl

Drug Class: Antihistamines, H1

Pregnancy Category: B

Do not confuse diphenhydramine with dimenhydrinate, or Benadryl with benazepril, Bentyl, or Benylin, or Banophen with baclofen.

CLINICAL PHARMACOLOGY

Mechanism of Action: An ethanolamine that competitively blocks the effects of histamine at peripheral H_1 receptor sites. *Therapeutic Effect:* Produces anticholinergic, antipruritic, antitussive, antiemetic, antidyskinetic, and sedative effects.

Pharmacokinetics

Route	Onset	Peak	Duration
PO	15-30 min	1-4 hr	4-6 hr
IV, IM	less than 15 min	1-4 hr	4-6 hr

Well absorbed after PO or parenteral administration. Protein binding: 98%-99%. Widely distributed. Metabolized in the liver. Primarily excreted in urine. **Half-life:** 1-4 hr.

AVAILABLE FORMS

• *Capsules (Banophen, Diphen, Genahist):* 25 mg.

• *Capsules (Nytol):* 50 mg.

• *Syrup (Diphen, Diphenhist):* 12.5 mg/5 ml.

• *Tablets (Banophen, Benadryl, Genahist, Nytol):* 25 mg, 50 mg.

• *Injection (Benadryl):* 50 mg/ml.

• *Cream (Benadryl):* 1%, 2%.

• *Spray:* 1%, 2%.

INDICATIONS AND DOSAGES

Moderate to severe allergic reaction, dystonic reaction

PO, IV, IM

Adults, Elderly. 25-50 mg q4h. Maximum: 400 mg/day.

Children. 5 mg/kg/day in divided doses q6-8h. Maximum: 300 mg/day.

Motion sickness, minor allergic rhinitis

PO, IV, IM

Adults, Elderly, Children 12 yr and older. 25-50 mg q4-6h. Maximum: 300 mg/day.

Children 6-11 yr. 12.5-25 mg q4-6h. Maximum: 150 mg/day.

Children 2-5 yr. 6.25 mg q4-6h. Maximum: 37.5 mg/day.

Antitussive

PO

Adults, Elderly, Children 12 yr and older. 25 mg q4h. Maximum: 150 mg/day.

Children 6-11 yr. 12.5 mg q4h. Maximum: 75 mg/day.
Children 2-5 yr. 6.25 mg q4h. Maximum: 37.5 mg/day.

Nighttime sleep aid

PO

Adults, Elderly, Children 12 yr and older. 50 mg at bedtime.
Children 2-11 yr. 1 mg/kg/dose. Maximum: 50 mg.

Pruritus

Topical

Adults, Elderly, Children 12 yr and older. Apply 1% or 2% cream or spray 3-4 times a day.
Children 2-11 yr. Apply 1% cream or spray 3-4 times a day.

CONTRAINDICATIONS: Acute exacerbation of asthma, use within 14 days of MAOIs

INTERACTIONS

Drug

Alcohol, other CNS depressants: May increase CNS depressant effects.
Anticholinergics: May increase anticholinergic effects.
MAOIs: May increase the anticholinergic and CNS depressant effects of diphenhydramine.

Herbal

None known.

Food

None known.

DIAGNOSTIC TEST EFFECTS: May suppress wheal and flare reactions to antigen skin testing unless the drug is discontinued 4 days before testing.

IV INCOMPATIBILITIES: Allopurinol (Aloprim), amphotericin B complex (Abelcet, AmBisome, Amphotec), cefepime (Maxipime), dexamethasone (Decadron), foscarnet (Foscavir)

IV COMPATIBILITIES: Atropine, cisplatin (Platinol), cyclophosphamide (Cytoxan), cytarabine (Ara-C), droperidol (Inapsine), fentanyl, glycopyrrolate (Robinul), heparin, hydrocortisone (Solu-Cortef), hydromorphone (Dilaudid), hydroxyzine (Vistaril), lidocaine, metoclopramide (Reglan), ondansetron (Zofran), promethazine (Phenergan), potassium chloride, propofol (Diprivan)

SIDE EFFECTS

Frequent

Somnolence, dizziness, muscle weakness, hypotension, urine retention, thickening of bronchial secretions, dry mouth, nose, throat, or lips; in elderly, sedation, dizziness, hypotension

Occasional

Epigastric distress, flushing, visual or hearing disturbances, paresthesia, diaphoresis, chills

SERIOUS REACTIONS

- Hypersensitivity reactions, such as eczema, pruritus, rash, cardiac disturbances, and photosensitivity, may occur.
- Overdose symptoms may vary from CNS depression, including sedation, apnea, hypotension, cardiovascular collapse, and death, to severe paradoxical reactions, such as hallucinations, tremor, and seizures.
- Children and neonates may experience paradoxical reactions, including restlessness, insomnia, euphoria, nervousness, and tremors.
- Overdosage in children may result in hallucinations, seizures, and death.

SPECIAL CONSIDERATIONS

PRECAUTIONS

- Diphenhydramine hydrochloride has an atropine-like action and therefore should be used with caution in patients with a history of lower respiratory disease including asthma, increased intraocular pressure, hyperthyroidism, cardiovascular disease, or hypertension.

• Use diphenhydramine hydrochloride with considerable caution in patients with stenosing peptic ulcer, pyloroduodenal obstruction, symptomatic prostatic hypertrophy, or bladder-neck obstruction. In infants and children, overdosage may cause hallucinations, convulsions, or death. Diphenhydramine hydrochloride may diminish mental alertness in children. In the young child, the drug may produce excitation. Diphenhydramine hydrochloride is more likely to cause dizziness, sedation, and hypotension in elderly patients. Use diphenhydramine hydrochloride with caution in patients with a history of lower respiratory disease including asthma, increased intraocular pressure, hyperthyroidism, cardiovascular disease, or hypertension.

PATIENT INFORMATION

• Advise patients taking diphenhydramine hydrochloride that this drug may cause drowsiness and has an additive effect with alcohol. Warn patients about engaging in activities requiring mental alertness, such as driving a car or operating appliances and machinery.

PREGNANCY AND LACTATION

• Pregnancy Category B. Reproduction studies have been performed in rats and rabbits at doses up to 5 times the human dose and have revealed no evidence of impaired fertility or harm to the fetus from diphenhydramine hydrochloride. However, no adequate and well-controlled studies have been performed in pregnant women. Because animal reproduction studies are not always predictive of human response, use this drug during pregnancy only if clearly needed. Because of the higher risk of antihistamines for infants generally, and for newborns and prematures in particular, antihistamine therapy is contraindicated in nursing mothers.

OCULAR CONSIDERATIONS

• Diphenhydramine hydrochloride can cause ocular dryness, mydriasis, and cycloplegia.

• Use diphenhydramine hydrochloride with considerable caution in patients with narrow-angle glaucoma.

---

dipivefrin hydrochloride

(dye-pi′-ve-frin hye-droe-klor′-ide)

Rx: Propine

Drug Class: Adrenergic agonists; Ophthalmics

Pregnancy Category: B

CLINICAL PHARMACOLOGY

Mechanism of Action: A prodrug of epinephrine that penetrates into anterior chamber of the eye through its lipophilic character. *Therapeutic Effect:* Reduces intraocular pressure.

Pharmacokinetics

Onset of action occurs within 30 minutes and peak effect in 1 hour. Dipivefrin is more lipophilic than epinephrine. Distributed to cornea. Dipivefrin is converted to epinephrine inside the eye by enzyme hydrolysis.

AVAILABLE FORMS

• *Ophthalmic solution:* 1 mg/ml (Propine).

INDICATIONS AND DOSAGES

Glaucoma, open-angle

Ophthalmic, topical

Adults, Elderly. Instill 1 drop of 0.1% solution in affected eye(s) q12h.

CONTRAINDICATIONS: Narrow-angle glaucoma, hypersensitivity to dipivefrin or any component of the formulation

INTERACTIONS

Drug

Pilocarpine: May increase myopia.

Herbal

None known.

Food

None known.

DIAGNOSTIC TEST EFFECTS: *None known.*

SIDE EFFECTS

Occasional

Blurred vision, burning or stinging of eye, mydriasis, headache

Rare

Follicular conjunctivitis

SERIOUS REACTIONS

• Signs of systemic absorption include hypertension, arrhythmias, and tachycardia.

• Follicular conjunctivitis has been reported.

SPECIAL CONSIDERATIONS

PRECAUTIONS

• Macular edema has occurred in aphakic patients treated with epinephrine. Administration of dipivefrin hydrochloride is contraindicated in narrow-angle glaucoma because of the potential for angle closure.

PREGNANCY AND LACTATION

• Pregnancy Category B. Studies in rats and rabbits revealed no evidence of impaired fertility or harm to the fetus. Excretion into human milk is not known.

divalproex sodium

(dye-val'-proe-eks soe'-dee-um)

Rx: Depakote, Depakote ER, Depakote Sprinkles

Drug Class: Anticonvulsants

Pregnancy Category: D

CLINICAL PHARMACOLOGY

Mechanism of Action: An anticonvulsant, antimanic, and antimigraine agent that directly increases concentration of the inhibitory neurotransmitter gamma-aminobutyric acid (GABA). *Therapeutic Effect:* Produces anticonvulsant effect.

Pharmacokinetics

Well absorbed from the gastrointestinal (GI) tract. Protein binding: 80%-90%. Metabolized in liver. Primarily excreted in urine. Not removed by hemodialysis. **Half-life:** 6-16 hrs, half-life may be increased with impaired liver function, elderly, children younger than 18 mos.

AVAILABLE FORMS

• *Capsules (enteric-coated):* 125 mg (Depakote Sprinkles).

• *Tablets (enteric-coated):* 125 mg, 250 mg, 500 mg (Depakote).

• *Tablets (extended-release):* 250 mg, 500 mg (Depakote ER).

INDICATIONS AND DOSAGES

Seizures

PO

Adults, Elderly, Children older than 10 yr. Initially, 10-15 mg/kg/day in 1-3 divided doses. May increase by 5-10 mg/kg/day at weekly intervals up to 30-60 mg/kg/day (usual adult dosage: 1000-2500 mg/day).

IV

Adults, Elderly, Children. IV dose equal to oral dose but given at a frequency of q6h.

Manic episodes
PO
Adults, Elderly. Initially, 750 mg/day in divided doses. Maximum: 60 mg/kg/day.

Migraine prophylaxis
PO (extended-release tablets)
Adults, Elderly. Initially, 500 mg/day for 7 days. May increase up to 1000 mg/day.
PO (delayed-release tablets)
Adults, Elderly. Initially, 250 mg 2 times/day. May increase up to 1000 mg/day.

UNLABELED USES: Treatment of myoclonic, simple partial, tonic-clonic seizures

CONTRAINDICATIONS: Active liver disease, hypersensitivity to divalproex or any component of the formulation

INTERACTIONS

Drug
Alcohol, central nervous system (CNS) depressants: May increase CNS depressant effects.
Amitriptyline, primidone: May increase the concentration of amitriptyline and primidone.
Anticoagulants, heparin, platelet aggregation inhibitors, thrombolytics: May increase the risk of bleeding.
Carbamazepine: May decrease divalproex blood concentration.
Liver toxic medications: May increase risk of liver toxicity.
Phenytoin: May alter phenytoin protein binding, increasing the risk of toxicity. Phenytoin may decrease the effects of divalproex.

Herbal
None known.

Food
None known.

DIAGNOSTIC TEST EFFECTS: May increase LDH concentrations, serum bilirubin, SGOT (AST), and SGPT (ALT) levels. Therapeutic serum level is 50-100 mcg/ml; toxic serum level is greater than 100 mcg/ml.

IV INCOMPATIBILITIES: Do not mix with any other medications.

SIDE EFFECTS

Frequent
Epilepsy: Abdominal pain, irregular menses, diarrhea, transient alopecia, indigestion, nausea, vomiting, trembling, weight change
Mania (22%-19%): Nausea, somnolence

Occasional
Epilepsy: Constipation, dizziness, drowsiness, headache, skin rash, unusual excitement, restlessness
Mania (12%-6%): Asthenia, abdominal pain, dyspepsia (heartburn, indigestion, epigastric distress), rash

Rare
Epilepsy: Mood changes, double vision, nystagmus, spots before eyes, unusual bleeding or bruising

SERIOUS REACTIONS

• Liver toxicity may occur, particularly in the first 6 months of divalproex therapy. Liver toxicity may not be preceded by abnormal liver function tests but may be noted as loss of seizure control, malaise, weakness, lethargy, anorexia, and vomiting.
• Blood dyscrasias may occur.

SPECIAL CONSIDERATIONS

PRECAUTIONS

• Hepatic failure resulting in fatalities has occurred in patients receiving valproic acid. Because of reports of thrombocytopenia, inhibition of the secondary phase of platelet aggregation, and abnormal coagulation parameters (e.g., low fibrinogen), platelet counts and coagulation tests are recommended before initiating therapy and at periodic intervals.

PATIENT INFORMATION

• Because divalproex sodium products may produce central nervous system depression, especially when combined with another central nervous system depressant (e.g., alcohol), advise patients not to engage in hazardous activities, such as driving an automobile or operating dangerous machinery, until they are certain they will not become drowsy from the drug.

PREGNANCY AND LACTATION

• Pregnancy Category D. Divalproex sodium has been associated with certain types of birth defects. Valproate is excreted in breast milk.

dorzolamide hydrochloride

(door-zol'-a-mide hye-droe-klor'-ide)

Rx: Trusopt

Drug Class: Carbonic anhydrase inhibitors; Ophthalmics

Pregnancy Category: C

CLINICAL PHARMACOLOGY

Mechanism of Action: An ophthalmic agent that inhibits carbonic anhydrase. Therapeutic Effect: Reduces intraocular pressure (IOP).

Pharmacokinetics

Peak response occurs in 2 hours and the duration of action is 8 to 12 hours. Systemically absorbed to some degree. Protein binding: 33%. Distributed in red blood cells. Sites of metabolism have not been established. Metabolized to active metabolite, N-desethyldorzolamide. Excreted in urine. **Half-life:** unknown; 147 days (terminal red blood cell).

AVAILABLE FORMS

• *Ophthalmic Solution:* 2% (Trusopt).

INDICATIONS AND DOSAGES

Glaucoma, ocular hypertension

Ophthalmic

Adults, Elderly. 1 drop in affected eye(s) 3 times/day.

CONTRAINDICATIONS: Hypersensitivity to dorzolamide or any other component of the formulation

INTERACTIONS

Drug

Topiramate: May increase risk of nephrolithiasis.

Herbal

None known.

Food

None known.

DIAGNOSTIC TEST EFFECTS: *None known.*

SIDE EFFECTS

Frequent

Ocular burning, bitter taste

Occasional

Superficial punctuate keratitis, ocular allergic reaction

SERIOUS REACTIONS

• Iridocyclitis, skin rash, and urolithiasis occur rarely.

• Electrolyte imbalance, development of an acidotic state, and possible CNS effects may occur.

SPECIAL CONSIDERATIONS

PRECAUTIONS

• Dorzolamide hydrochloride is not recommended in patients with severe renal impairment. Exercise caution in patients with hepatic impairment. Conjunctivitis and lid reactions were reported with chronic administration. Concomitant administration of dorzolamide hydrochloride and oral carbonic anhydrase inhibitors is not recommended. Choroidal detachment has been reported after filtration procedures.

PATIENT INFORMATION

• If serious or unusual reactions or signs of hypersensitivity occur, discontinue use of the product. If patients develop any ocular reactions, particularly conjunctivitis and lid reactions, instruct them to discontinue use and seek their eye care practitioner's advice. Dorzolamide hydrochloride contains benzalkonium chloride, which may be absorbed by soft contact lenses. Lenses may be reinserted 15 minutes following drug administration.

PREGNANCY AND LACTATION

• Pregnancy Category C. Rabbit studies revealed malformations of the vertebral bodies. In lactating rats, decreases in body weight gain occurred. Excretion into human milk is not known.

dorzolamide hydrochloride; timolol maleate

(door-zol'a-mide hye-droe-klor'ide; tim'oh-lol mal'ee-ate)

Rx: Cosopt

Drug Class: Antiadrenergics, beta blocking; Carbonic anhydrase inhibitors; Ophthalmics

Pregnancy Category: C

CLINICAL PHARMACOLOGY

Mechanism of Action: A combination ophthalmic agent that inhibits carbonic anhydrase and blocks beta-adrenergic receptors. Reduces aqueous humor production. *Therapeutic Effect:* Reduces intraocular pressure (IOP).

Pharmacokinetics

None reported.

AVAILABLE FORMS

• *Ophthalmic Solution:* 2% dorzolamide hydrochloride and 0.5% timolol maleate (Cosopt).

INDICATIONS AND DOSAGES

Glaucoma, ocular hypertension

Ophthalmic

Adults, Elderly. 1 drop in affected eye(s) twice daily.

CONTRAINDICATIONS: Bronchial asthma or chronic obstructive pulomonary disease, cardiogenic shock, overt cardiac failure, second- and third-degree AV block, severe sinus bradycardia, hypersensitivity to dorzolamide, timolol, or any other component of the formulation

INTERACTIONS

Drug

Carbonic anhydrase inhibitors: May increase the risk of systemic effects.

Beta-blockers: May increase the effects of beta blockers.

Calcium channel blockers: May increase the risk of hypotension, bradycardia, and AV conduction disturbances.

Catecholamine-depleting drugs (e.g. reserpine): May increase risk of hypotension and bradycardia.

Digitalis, calcium antagonists: May increase the risk of AV block and possible digoxin toxicity.

Quinidine: May increase beta-blocker blockade.

Clonidine: May exaggerate clonidine withdrawal response.

Herbal

None known.

Food

None known.

DIAGNOSTIC TEST EFFECTS: *None known.*

SIDE EFFECTS

Frequent

Conjunctival hyperemia, growth of eyelashes, ocular pruritus, taste perversion

Occasional

Ocular dryness and itching, visual disturbance, ocular burning, foreign body sensation, eye pain, pigmentation of the periocular skin, blepharitis, cataract, superficial punctate keratitis, eyelid erythema, ocular irritation, eyelash darkening

Rare

Intraocular inflammation (iritis), hypotension, depression, dizziness, dry mouth, nausea, vomiting, tearing

SERIOUS REACTIONS

- Systemic adverse events, including infections (colds and upper respiratory tract infections), headaches, asthenia, and hirsutism, have been reported.
- Bronchospasm and myocardial infarction have also been reported.

SPECIAL CONSIDERATIONS

PRECAUTIONS

- Cosopt is not recommended for patients with severe renal impairment and history of severe anaphylactic reactions. Adverse ocular effects include conjunctivitis and lid reactions and choroidal detachment after filtration procedures. Timolol has been reported rarely to increase muscle weakness in some patients with myasthenia gravis or myasthenic symptoms.

PATIENT INFORMATION

- Advise patients with bronchial asthma, a history of bronchial asthma, severe chronic obstructive pulmonary disease, sinus bradycardia, second- or third-degree atrioventricular block, or cardiac failure not to take this product. Advise patients that if they develop any ocular reactions, particularly conjunctivitis and lid reactions, they should discontinue use and seek their eye care practitioner's advice. This drug combination contains benzalkonium chloride. Soft lenses may be reinserted 15 minutes following administration of Cosopt.

PREGNANCY AND LACTATION

- Pregnancy Category C. Rabbit studies revealed decreased body weight gain in dams and decreased fetal weights. Timolol maleate has been detected in human milk following oral and ocular drug administration.

doxazosin mesylate

(dox-ay'zoe-sin)

Rx: Cardura

Drug Class: Antiadrenergics, alpha blocking; Antiadrenergics, peripheral

Pregnancy Category: B

Do not confuse doxazosin with doxapram, doxepin, or doxorubicin, or Cardura with Cardene, Cordarone, Coumadin, K-Dur, or Ridaura.

CLINICAL PHARMACOLOGY

Mechanism of Action: An antihypertensive that selectively blocks alpha$_1$-adrenergic receptors, decreasing peripheral vascular resistance. *Therapeutic Effect:* Causes peripheral vasodilation and lowers of BP. Also relaxes smooth muscle of bladder and prostate.

Pharmacokinetics

Route	*Onset*	*Peak*	*Duration*
PO	N/A	2-6 hr	24 hr

Well absorbed from the GI tract. Protein binding: 98%-99%. Metabolized in the liver. Primarily eliminated in feces. Not removed by hemodialysis. **Half-life:** 19-22 hr.

AVAILABLE FORMS

- *Tablets:* 1 mg, 2 mg, 4 mg, 8 mg.

INDICATIONS AND DOSAGES
Mild to moderate hypertension
PO
Adults. Initially, 1 mg once a day. May increase to a maximum of 16 mg/day.
Elderly. Initially, 0.5 mg once a day.
Benign prostatic hyperplasia, alone or in combination with finasteride (Proscar)
PO
Adults, Elderly. Initially, 1 mg/day. May increase q1-2 wk. Maximum: 8 mg/day.
CONTRAINDICATIONS: None known.
INTERACTIONS
Drug
Estrogen, NSAIDs: May decrease the effect of doxazosin.
Hypotension-producing medications, such as antihypertensives and diuretics: May increase the effect of doxazosin.
Herbal
None known.
Food
None known.
DIAGNOSTIC TEST EFFECTS: *None known.*
SIDE EFFECTS
Frequent (20%-10%)
Dizziness, asthenia, headache, edema
Occasional (9%-3%)
Nausea, pharyngitis, rhinitis, pain in extremities, somnolence
Rare (3%-1%)
Palpitations, diarrhea, constipation, dyspnea, myalgia, altered vision, dizziness, nervousness
SERIOUS REACTIONS
• First-dose syncope (hypotension with sudden loss of consciousness) may occur 30 to 90 minutes following initial dose of 2 mg or greater, a too-rapid increase in dosage, or addition of another antihypertensive agent to therapy. First-dose syncope may be preceded by tachycardia (pulse rate of 120-160 beats/minute).

SPECIAL CONSIDERATIONS

PRECAUTIONS
• Carcinoma of the prostate causes many of the symptoms associated with benign prostatic hypertrophy, and the two disorders frequently coexist. Although syncope is the most severe orthostatic effect of doxazosin mesylate, other symptoms of lowered blood pressure such as dizziness, light-headedness, or vertigo can occur. Administer doxazosin mesylate with caution to patients with evidence of impaired hepatic function or to patients receiving drugs known to influence hepatic metabolism. Mean white blood cell and neutrophil counts are decreased. Increased incidence of myocardial necrosis or fibrosis is displayed by rats.
PATIENT INFORMATION
• Refer to the patient instructions that are distributed with the prescription for complete instructions. Make patients aware of the possibility of syncopal and orthostatic symptoms, especially at the initiation of therapy, and urge them to avoid driving or hazardous tasks for 24 hours after the first dose, after a dosage increase, and after interruption of therapy when treatment is resumed. Caution patients to avoid situations where injury could result should syncope occur during initiation of doxazosin therapy. Also advise patients of the need to sit or lie down when symptoms of lowered blood pressure occur, although these symptoms are not always orthostatic, and to be careful when rising from a sitting or lying position. If dizziness, light-headedness, or palpitations are bothersome, advise pa-

tients to report them to the physician so that dose adjustment can be considered. Also advise patients that drowsiness or somnolence can occur with doxazosin mesylate or any selective $alpha_1$-adrenoceptor antagonist, requiring caution in persons who must drive or operate heavy machinery. Advise patients about the possibility of priapism as a result of treatment with $alpha_1$-antagonists. Patients should know that this adverse event is rare. If patients experience priapism, instruct them to bring it to immediate medical attention, for if not treated promptly, priapism can lead to permanent erectile dysfunction (impotence).

PREGNANCY AND LACTATION

- Pregnancy Category B. Studies in pregnant rabbits and rats at oral doses have revealed no evidence of harm to the fetus. Studies in lactating rats indicate that doxazosin accumulates in rat breast milk. Excretion into human milk is not known.

doxercalciferol

(dox-er-cal-sif′-er-ol)

Rx: Hectorol

Drug Class: Vitamins/minerals

Pregnancy Category: B

CLINICAL PHARMACOLOGY

Mechanism of Action: A fat-soluble vitamin that is essential for absorption, utilization of calcium phosphate, and normal calcification of bone. *Therapeutic Effect:* Stimulates calcium and phosphate absorption from small intestine, promotes secretion of calcium from bone to blood, promotes renal tubule phosphate resorption, acts on bone cells to stimulate skeletal growth and on parathyroid gland to suppress hormone synthesis and secretion.

Pharmacokinetics

Readily absorbed from small intestine. Metabolized in liver. Partially eliminated in urine. Not removed by hemodialysis. **Half-life:** up to 96 hrs.

AVAILABLE FORMS

- *Capsule:* 2.5 mcg (Hectorol).
- *Injection:* 2 mcg/ml (Hectorol).

INDICATIONS AND DOSAGES

Secondary hyperparathyroidism, dialysis patients

IV

Adults, Elderly. Titrate dose to lower iPTH to 150-300 pg/ml. Adjust dose at 8-week intervals to a maximum dose of 18 mcg/week. Initially, if iPTH level is more than 400 pg/ml, give 4 mcg 3 times/week after dialysis, administered as a bolus dose.

Dose titration:

iPTH level decreased by 50% and more than 300 pg/ml: Dose may be increased by 1-2 mcg at 8-week intervals as needed.

iPTH level 150-300 pg/ml: Maintain the current dose.

iPTH level <100 pg/ml: Suspend drug for 1 week and resume at a reduced dose of at least 1 mcg lower.

PO

Adults, Elderly. Dialysis patients: Titrate dose to lower iPTH to 150-300 pg/ml. Adjust dose at 8-week intervals to a maximum dose of 20 mcg 3 times/week. Initially, if iPTH is more than 400 pg/ml, give 10 mcg 3 times/week at dialysis.

Dose titration:

iPTH level decreased by 50% and more than 300 pg/ml: Increase dose to 12.5 mcg 3 times/week for 8 more weeks. This titration process may continue at 8-week intervals. Each increase should be by 2.5 mcg/dose.

iPTH level 150-300 pg/ml: Maintain current dose.

iPTH level less than 100 pg/ml: Suspend drug for 1 week and resume at a reduced dose. Decrease each dose by at least 2.5 mcg.

Secondary hyperparathyroidism, predialysis patients

PO

Adults, Elderly. Titrate dose to lower iPTH to 35-70 pg/ml with stage 3 disease or to 70-110 pg/ml with stage 4 disease. Dose may be adjusted at 2-week intervals with a maximum dose of 3.5 mcg/day. Begin with 1 mcg/day.

Dose titration:

iPTH level more than 70 pg/ml with stage 3 disease or more than 110 pg/ml with stage 4 disease: Increase dose by 0.5 mcg every 2 weeks as needed.

iPTH level 35-70 pg/ml with stage 3 disease or 70-110 pg/ml with stage 4 disease: Maintain current dose.

iPTH level is less than 35 pg/ml with stage 3 disease or less than 70 pg/ml with stage 4 disease: Suspend drug for 1 week, then resume at a reduced dose of at least 0.5 mcg lower.

CONTRAINDICATIONS: Hypercalcemia, malabsorption syndrome, vitamin D toxicity, hypersensitivity to doxercalciferol or other vitamin D analogs

INTERACTIONS

Drug

Aluminum-containing antacid (long-term use): May increase aluminum concentration and aluminum bone toxicity.

Calcium-containing preparations, thiazide diuretics: May increase the risk of hypercalcemia.

Magnesium-containing antacids: May increase magnesium concentration.

Herbal

None known.

Food

None known.

DIAGNOSTIC TEST EFFECTS: May increase serum cholesterol, calcium, magnesium, and phosphate levels. May decrease serum alkaline phosphatase.

SIDE EFFECTS

Occasional

Edema, headache, malaise, dizziness, nausea, vomiting, dyspnea

Rare

Bradycardia, sleep disorder, pruritus, anorexia, constipation

SERIOUS REACTIONS

- Early signs of overdosage are manifested as weakness, headache, somnolence, nausea, vomiting, dry mouth, constipation, muscle and bone pain, and metallic taste sensation.
- Later signs of overdosage are evidenced by polyuria, polydipsia, anorexia, weight loss, nocturia, photophobia, rhinorrhea, pruritus, disorientation, hallucinations, hyperthermia, hypertension, and cardiac arrhythmias.

SPECIAL CONSIDERATIONS

PRECAUTIONS

- Use doxercalciferol with caution in patients with impaired hepatic function. Overdosage of any form of vitamin D, including doxercalciferol, is dangerous. Pharmacologic doses of vitamin D and its derivatives should be withheld during doxercalciferol treatment to avoid possible additive effects and hypercalcemia. Magnesium-containing antacids and doxercalciferol should not be used concomitantly in patients on chronic renal dialysis. The principal adverse effects of treatment with doxercalciferol are hypercalcemia, hyperphosphatemia, and oversuppression of immunoreactive parathyroid hormone (less than 150 pg/ml).

PATIENT INFORMATION

• Inform the patient, spouse, or guardian about compliance with instructions about diet, calcium supplementation, and avoidance of the use of nonprescription drugs without prior approval from the physician. Also carefully inform patients about the symptoms of hypercalcemia.

PREGNANCY AND LACTATION

• Pregnancy Category B. Reproduction studies in rat and rabbits have revealed no teratogenic or fetotoxic effects from doxercalciferol. Because animal reproduction studies are not always predictive of human response, use this drug during pregnancy only if clearly needed. Excretion into human milk is not known.

doxycycline

(dox-i-sye'kleen)

Rx: Adoxa, Atridox, Doryx, Doxy-Caps, Monodox, Vibramycin, Vibramycin Calcium, Vibramycin Hyclate, Vibramycin Monohydrate

Drug Class: Antibiotics, tetracyclines

Pregnancy Category: D

Do not confuse doxycycline with Dicyclomine or doxylamine, or Monodox with Monopril.

CLINICAL PHARMACOLOGY

Mechanism of Action: A tetracycline antibiotic that inhibits bacterial protein synthesis by binding to ribosomes. *Therapeutic Effect:* Bacteriostatic.

AVAILABLE FORMS

• *Capsules (Doryx):* 75 mg, 100 mg.
• *Capsules (Monodox):* 50 mg, 100 mg.
• *Capsules (Vibramycin):* 100 mg.
• *Oral Suspension (Vibramycin):* 25 mg/5 ml.
• *Syrup (Vibramycin):* 50 mg/5 ml.
• *Tablets (Adoxa):* 50 mg, 75 mg, 100 mg.
• *Tablets (Periostat):* 20 mg.
• *Tablets (Vibra-Tabs):* 100 mg.
• *Injection, Powder for Reconstitution (Doxy-100):* 100 mg.

INDICATIONS AND DOSAGES

Respiratory, skin, and soft-tissue infections; UTIs; pelvic inflammatory disease (PID); brucellosis; trachoma; Rocky Mountain spotted fever; typhus; Q fever; rickettsia; severe acne (Adoxa); smallpox; psittacosis; ornithosis; granuloma inguinale; lymphogranuloma venereum; intestinal amebiasis (adjunctive treatment); prevention of rheumatic fever

PO

Adults, Elderly. Initially, 100 mg q12h, then 100 mg/day as single dose or 50 mg q12h for severe infections.

Children 8 yr and older and weighing more than 45 kg. 2-4 mg/kg/day divided q12-24h. Maximum: 200 mg/day.

IV

Adults, Elderly. Initially, 200 mg as 1-2 infusions; then 100-200 mg/day in 1-2 divided doses.

Children 8 yr and older. 2-4 mg/kg/day divided q12-24h. Maximum: 200 mg/day.

Acute gonococcal infections

PO

Adults. Initially, 200 mg, then 100 mg at bedtime on first day; then 100 mg twice a day for 14 days.

Syphilis

PO, IV

Adults. 200 mg/day in divided doses for 14-28 days.

Traveler's diarrhea

PO

Adults, Elderly. 100 mg/day during a period of risk (up to 14 days) and for 2 days after returning home.

Periodontitis

PO

Adults. 20 mg twice a day.

UNLABELED USES: Treatment of atypical mycobacterial infections, rheumatoid arthritis, gonorrhea and malaria; prevention of Lyme disease; prevention or treatment of traveler's diarrhea.

CONTRAINDICATIONS: Children 8 years and younger, hypersensitivity to tetracyclines or sulfites, last half of pregnancy, severe hepatic dysfunction

INTERACTIONS

Drug

Antacids containing aluminum, calcium, or magnesium; laxatives containing magnesium: Decrease doxycycline absorption.

Barbiturates, carbamazepine, phenytoin: May decrease doxycycline blood concentrations.

Cholestyramine, colestipol: May decrease doxycycline absorption.

Oral contraceptives: May decrease the effects of oral contraceptives.

Oral iron preparations: Impair absorption of doxycycline.

Herbal

None known.

Food

None known.

DIAGNOSTIC TEST EFFECTS: May increase serum alkaline phosphatase, amylase, bilirubin, AST (SGOT), and ALT (SGPT) levels. May alter CBC.

IV INCOMPATIBILITIES: Allopurinol (Aloprim), heparin, piperacillin and tazobactam (Zosyn)

IV COMPATIBILITIES: Amiodarone (Cordarone), diltiazem (Cardizem), hydromorphone (Dilaudid), magnesium sulfate, morphine, propofol (Diprivan)

SIDE EFFECTS

Frequent

Anorexia, nausea, vomiting, diarrhea, dysphagia, possibly severe photosensitivity

Occasional

Rash, urticaria

SERIOUS REACTIONS

- Superinfection (especially fungal) and benign intracranial hypertension (headache, visual changes) may occur.
- Hepatotoxicity, fatty degeneration of the liver, and pancreatitis occur rarely.

SPECIAL CONSIDERATIONS

PRECAUTIONS

- As with other antibiotic preparations, use of this drug may result in overgrowth of nonsusceptible organisms, including fungi. If superinfection occurs, discontinue the antibiotic and institute appropriate therapy. Bulging fontanels in infants and benign intracranial hypertension in adults have been reported in individuals receiving tetracyclines.
- Doxycycline offers substantial but not complete suppression of the asexual blood stages of *Plasmodium* strains. Doxycycline does not suppress *P. falciparum* sexual blood stage gamocytes. Subjects completing this prophylactic regimen still may transmit the infection to mosquitoes outside endemic areas.

PATIENT INFORMATION

- Inform patients that no present-day antimalarial agent, including doxycycline, guarantees protection against malaria. Instruct patients to avoid excessive sunlight or artificial ultraviolet light while receiving doxycycline and to discontinue therapy if phototoxicity (e.g., skin eruption) occurs. Sunscreen or sunblock should be considered. Advise patients to drink fluids liberally along with doxycycline to reduce the risk of esophageal irritation and ulceration. Absorption of tetracyclines is reduced when taken with foods, especially those that contain calcium. However, the absorption of doxycycline is not influenced greatly by simultaneous ingestion of food or milk. Absorption of tetracyclines is reduced when the patient is taking bismuth subsalicylate. Use of doxycycline might increase the incidence of vaginal candidiasis.

PREGNANCY AND LACTATION

- Pregnancy Category D. Results of animal studies indicate that tetracyclines cross the placenta, are found in fetal tissues, and can have toxic effects on the developing fetus (often related to retardation of skeletal development). Evidence of embryotoxicity also has been noted in animals treated early in pregnancy. If any tetracycline is used during pregnancy or if the patient becomes pregnant while taking this drug, apprise the patient of the potential hazard to the fetus. Tetracyclines are excreted in human milk.

OCULAR CONSIDERATIONS

- Ocular Indications and Usage: Lid disease, meibomian gland dysfunction, meibomitis, blepharitis, and acne rosacea

OCULAR DOSAGE AND ADMINISTRATION

- 50 to 100 mg PO bid for 4 weeks, qd 4 to 8 weeks.

echothiophate iodide

(ek-oh-thye′oh-fate eye′-oh-dide)

Rx: Phospholine Iodide

Drug Class: Cholinesterase inhibitors; Miotics; Ophthalmics

Pregnancy Category: C

CLINICAL PHARMACOLOGY

Mechanism of Action: A cholinesterase inhibitor that causes acetylcholine to accumulate at cholinergic receptor sites and produce effects like excessive stimulation of cholinergic receptors. *Therapeutic Effect:* Causes conjunctival hyperemia and constriction of the sphincter pupillae and ciliary muscles, which results in miosis and paralysis of accommodation.

Pharmacokinetics

None reported.

AVAILABLE FORMS

- *Powder for reconstitution, ophthalmic:* 6.25 mg [0.125%] (Phospholine Iodide).

INDICATIONS AND DOSAGES

Glaucoma

Ophthalmic

Adults, Elderly. Instill 1 drop twice daily into eyes with 1 dose prior to bedtime.

Accommodative esotropia, diagnosis

Ophthalmic

Children. Instill 1 drop once daily into both eyes at bedtime for 2-3 weeks.

Accommodative esotropia, treatment

Ophthalmic

Children. Instill 1 drop once daily.

CONTRAINDICATIONS: Active uveal inflammation, angle-closure glaucoma, hypersensitivity to echothiophate products

E

INTERACTIONS

Drug

Succinylcholine: May increase neuromuscular blockade.

Herbal

None known.

Food

None known.

DIAGNOSTIC TEST EFFECTS: *None known.*

SIDE EFFECTS

Occasional

Headache, browache, blurred vision, burning and stinging of eyes, decreased night vision, intraocular pressure changes, iritis, uveitis

SERIOUS REACTIONS

• Cardiac irregularities have been reported.

SPECIAL CONSIDERATIONS

PRECAUTIONS

• Gonioscopy is recommended. Routine examination is needed to detect lens opacity. Avoid use with uveitis. Digital compression of the nasolacrimal ducts minimizes drainage into the nasal chamber. Temporary discontinuance of medication is necessary if cardiac irregularities occur. Use anticholinesterase drugs with extreme caution in patients with marked vagotonia, bronchial asthma, spastic gastrointestinal disturbances, peptic ulcer, pronounced bradycardia and hypotension, recent myocardial infarction, epilepsy, and parkinsonism. Hyphema is possible with ocular surgery. Exercise great caution in patients with a history of retinal detachment. Temporary discontinuance is necessary if salivation, urinary incontinence, diarrhea, profuse sweating, muscle weakness, or respiratory difficulties occur. Additive systemic effects may occur in patients exposed to carbamate- or organophosphate-type insecticides and pesticides (professional gardeners, farmers, workers in plants manufacturing or formulating such products). During periods of exposure to such pesticides, advise patients to wear respiratory masks and to wash and change clothing frequently.

PREGNANCY AND LACTATION

• Pregnancy Category C. Fetal harm is not known. Potential exists for serious adverse reactions in nursing infants.

---

emedastine

(e-med'a-steen)

Rx: Emadine

Drug Class: Antihistamines, H_1; Antihistamines, ophthalmic; Ophthalmics

Pregnancy Category: B

CLINICAL PHARMACOLOGY

Mechanism of Action: An ophthalmic H_1-receptor antagonist that inhibits histamine-stimulated vascular permeability in the conjunctiva. *Therapeutic Effect:* Relieves ocular itching associated with allergic conjunctivitis.

Pharmacokinetics

Negligible absorption after ophthalmic administration. Metabolized into inactive metabolites. Excreted in urine. **Half-life:** 6.6 hr

AVAILABLE FORMS

• *Ophthalmic Solution:* 0.05% (Emadine).

INDICATIONS AND DOSAGES

Allergic conjunctivitis

Ophthalmic

Adults, Elderly, Children 3 yr and older. 1-2 drops in affected eye(s) twice daily.

CONTRAINDICATIONS: Hypersensitivity to emedastine or any other component of the formulation

INTERACTIONS

Drug

None known.

Herbal

None known.

Food

None known.

DIAGNOSTIC TEST EFFECTS: *None known.*

SIDE EFFECTS

Frequent (11%)

Headache

Occasional (less than 5%)

Abnormal dreams, asthenia (loss of strength, energy) bad taste, blurred vision, burning or stinging, dry eyes, foreign body sensation, tearing

SERIOUS REACTIONS

• Somnolence and malaise occurs rarely.

SPECIAL CONSIDERATIONS

PATIENT INFORMATION

• Advise patients not to wear a contact lens if their eye is red. Instruct them to wait at least 10 minutes after drug instillation before they insert their soft contact lenses.

PREGNANCY AND LACTATION

• Pregnancy Category B. Studies showed increase in external, visceral, and skeletal anomalies in rats. Emedastine difumarate was identified in breast milk in rats following oral administration. Excretion into human milk is not known.

enalapril maleate

(en-al'a-pril)

Rx: Vasotec

Drug Class: Angiotensin converting enzyme inhibitors

Pregnancy Category: C

Do not confuse enalapril with Anafranil, Eldepryl, or ramipril.

CLINICAL PHARMACOLOGY

Mechanism of Action: This angiotensin-converting enzyme (ACE) inhibitor suppresses the renin-angiotensin-aldosterone system, and prevents conversion of angiotensin I to angiotensin II, a potent vasoconstrictor; may inhibit angiotensin II at local vascular, renal sites. Decreases plasma angiotensin II, increases plasma renin activity, decreases aldosterone secretion. *Therapeutic Effect:* In hypertension, reduces peripheral arterial resistance. In congestive heart failure (CHF), increases cardiac output; decreases peripheral vascular resistance, BP, pulmonary capillary wedge pressure, heart size.

Pharmacokinetics

Route	Onset	Peak	Duration
PO	1 hr	4-6 hr	24 hr
IV	15 min	1-4 hr	6 hr

Readily absorbed from the GI tract (not affected by food). Protein binding: 50%-60%. Converted to active metabolite. Primarily excreted in urine. Removed by hemodialysis. **Half-life:** 11 hr (half-life is increased in those with impaired renal function).

AVAILABLE FORMS

• *Tablets:* 2.5 mg, 5 mg, 10 mg, 20 mg.

• *Injection:* 1.25 mg/ml.

INDICATIONS AND DOSAGES

Hypertension alone or in combination with other antihypertensives

PO

Adults, Elderly. Initially, 2.5-5 mg/day. Range: 10-40 mg/day in 1-2 divided doses.

Children. 0.1 mg/kg/day in 1-2 divided doses. Maximum: 0.5 mg/kg/day.

Neonates. 0.1 mg/kg/day q24h.

IV

Adults, Elderly. 0.625-1.25 mg q6h up to 5 mg q6h.

Children, Neonates. 5-10 mcg/kg/dose q8-24h.

Adjunctive therapy for CHF

PO

Adults, Elderly. Initially, 2.5-5 mg/day. Range: 5-20 mg/day in 2 divided doses.

Dosage in renal impairment

Dosage is modified based on creatinine clearance.

Creatinine Clearance	*% Usual Dose*
10-50 ml/min	75-100
less than 10 ml/min	50

UNLABELED USES: Treatment of diabetic nephropathy or renal crisis in scleroderma

CONTRAINDICATIONS: History of angioedema from previous treatment with ACE inhibitors

INTERACTIONS

Drug

Alcohol, antihypertensives, diuretics: May increase the effects of enalapril.

Herbal

None known.

Food

None known.

DIAGNOSTIC TEST EFFECTS: May increase BUN and serum alkaline phosphatase, serum bilirubin, serum creatinine, serum potassium, AST (SGOT), and ALT (SGPT) levels. May decrease serum sodium levels. May cause positive ANA titer.

IV INCOMPATIBILITIES: Amphotericin B (Fungizone), amphotericin B complex (Abelcet, AmBisome, Amphotec), cefepime (Maxipime), phenytoin (Dilantin)

IV COMPATIBILITIES: Calcium gluconate, dobutamine (Dobutrex), dopamine (Inotropin), fentanyl (Sublimaze), heparin, lidocaine, magnesium sulfate, morphine, nitroglycerin, potassium chloride, potassium phosphate, propofol (Diprivan)

SIDE EFFECTS

Frequent (7%-5%)

Headache, dizziness

Occasional (3%-2%)

Orthostatic hypotension, fatigue, diarrhea, cough, syncope

Rare (less than 2%)

Angina, abdominal pain, vomiting, nausea, rash, asthenia (loss of strength, energy), syncope

SERIOUS REACTIONS

- Excessive hypotension ("first-dose syncope") may occur in patients with CHF and in those who are severely salt or volume depleted.
- Angioedema (swelling of face, lips) and hyperkalemia occur rarely.
- Agranulocytosis and neutropenia may be noted in patients with collagen vascular diseases, including scleroderma and systemic lupus erythematosus, and impaired renal function.
- Nephrotic syndrome may be noted in those with history of renal disease.

SPECIAL CONSIDERATIONS

PRECAUTIONS

- Give enalapril maleate with caution to patients with obstruction in the outflow tract of the left ventricle. Anticipate changes in renal function in susceptible individuals. Elevated serum potassium was observed in approximately 1% of hypertensive patients in clinical trials. Cough has been reported with all angiotensin-converting enzyme (ACE) inhibitors. In patients undergoing major surgery or during anesthesia with agents that produce hypotension, enalapril may block angiotensin II formation following compensatory renin release.

PATIENT INFORMATION

• Angioedema: Angioedema, including laryngeal edema, may occur at any time during treatment with ACE inhibitors, including enalapril. Advise patients to report immediately any signs or symptoms suggesting angioedema (swelling of face, extremities, eyes, lips, tongue, difficulty in swallowing or breathing) and to take no more drug until they have consulted with the prescribing physician.

• Hypotension: Caution patients to report light-headedness, especially during the first few days of therapy. If actual syncope occurs, instruct patients to discontinue the drug until they have consulted with the prescribing physician.

• Caution all patients that excessive perspiration and dehydration may lead to an excessive fall in blood pressure because of reduction in fluid volume. Other causes of volume depletion such as vomiting or diarrhea also may lead to a fall in blood pressure; advise patients to consult with their physician.

• Hyperkalemia: Advise patients not to use salt substitutes containing potassium without consulting their physician.

• Neutropenia: Advise patients to report promptly any indication of infection (e.g., sore throat or fever) that may be a sign of neutropenia.

• Pregnancy: Advise female patients of childbearing age about the consequences of second- and third-trimester exposure to ACE inhibitors, and advise them also that these consequences do not appear to have resulted from intrauterine ACE-inhibitor exposure that has been limited to the first trimester. Ask these patients to report pregnancies to their physicians as soon as possible.

• NOTE: As with many other drugs, certain advice to patients being treated with enalapril is warranted. This information is intended to aid in the safe and effective use of this medication. Such advice is not a disclosure of all possible adverse or intended effects.

PREGNANCY AND LACTATION

• Pregnancy Categories C (first trimester) and D (second and third trimesters). The use of ACE inhibitors during the second and third trimesters of pregnancy has been associated with fetal and neonatal injury, including hypotension, neonatal skull hypoplasia, anuria, reversible or irreversible renal failure, and death. Enalapril and enalaprilat have been detected in human breast milk.

epinastine

(eh-pin-ass'-teen)

Rx: Elestat

Drug Class: Antihistamines, H1; Antihistamines, ophthalmic; Ophthalmics

Pregnancy Category: C

CLINICAL PHARMACOLOGY

Mechanism of Action: An ophthalmic H_1 receptor antagonist that inhibits the release of histamine from the mast cell. *Therapeutic Effect:* Prevents pruritus associated with allergic conjunctivitis.

Pharmacokinetics

Low systemic exposure. Protein binding: 64%. Less than 10% is metabolized. Excreted primarily in urine and, to a lesser extent, in feces. **Half-life:** 12 hr.

AVAILABLE FORMS

• *Ophthalmic Solution:* 0.05%.

INDICATIONS AND DOSAGES

Allergic conjunctivitis

Ophthalmic

Adults, Elderly, Children 3 yr and older. 1 drop in each eye twice a day. Continue treatment until period of exposure (pollen season, exposure to offending allergen) is over.

CONTRAINDICATIONS: None known.

INTERACTIONS

Drug

None known.

Herbal

None known.

Food

None known.

DIAGNOSTIC TEST EFFECTS: *None known.*

SIDE EFFECTS

Occasional

Ocular (10%-1%): Burning sensation in the eye, hyperemia, pruritus

Non-ocular (10%): Cold symptoms, upper respiratory tract infection

Rare (3%-1%)

Headache, rhinitis, sinusitis, increased cough, pharyngitis

SERIOUS REACTIONS

• None known.

epinephrine; lidocaine hydrochloride

(eh-pih-nef'-rin; lye'-doe-kane hye-droh-klor'-ide)

Rx: Xylocaine HCl with Epinephrine, Xylocaine-MPF-Epinephrine, Xylocaine with Epinephrine Dental Cartridges

Drug Class: Anesthetics, local

Pregnancy Category: B

Do not confuse with ephedrine.

CLINICAL PHARMACOLOGY

Mechanism of Action: Lidocaine blocks the initiation and conduction of nerve impulses via decreased permeability of sodium ions. Epinephrine increases the duration of action of lidocaine by causing vasoconstriction (via alpha effects) which slows the vascular absorption of lidocaine. *Therapeutic Effect:* Causes a local anesthetic effect.

Pharmacokinetics

Minimal absorption after topical administration.

AVAILABLE FORMS

• *Injection solution:* Epinephrine 1:50,000; Lidocaine 2% (Xylocaine with Epinephrine Dental Cartridges), Epinephrine 1:100,000; Lidocaine 1% (Xylocaine HCl with Epinephrine), Epinephrine 1:100,000; Lidocaine 2% (Xylocaine HCl with Epinephrine,

Xylocaine with Epinephrine Dental Cartridges), Epinephrine 1:200,000; Lidocaine 0.5% (Xylocaine HCl with Epinephrine), Epinephrine 1:200,000; Lidocaine 1% (Xylocaine-MPF-Epinephrine), Epinephrine 1:200,000; Lidocaine 1.5%, Epinephrine 1:200,000; Lidocaine 2% (Xylocaine-MPF-Epinephrine).

• *Injectable kit:* Epinephrine 200,000; Lidocaine 1.5%.

INDICATIONS AND DOSAGES

Dental anesthesia, infiltration, or conduction block

Injection

Adults, Elderly, Children 10 yr and older. The effective anesthetic dose varies with procedure, intensity of anesthesia needed, duration of anesthesia required, and physical condition of the patient. Always use the lowest effective dose along with careful aspiration. Do not exceed 6.6 mg/kg body weight or 300 mg of lidocaine hydrochloride and 3 mcg (0.003 mg) of epinephrine/kg of body weight or 0.2 mg epinephrine per dental appointment.

Children less than 10 yr. 20-30 mg (1-1.5 ml) of lidocaine hydrochloride as a 2% solution with epinephrine 1:100,000; maximum: 4-5 mg of lidocaine hydrochloride/kg of body weight or 100-150 mg as a single dose.

CONTRAINDICATIONS: Myasthenia gravis, shock, cardiac conduction disease, angle-closure glaucoma, hypersensitivity to lidocaine, epinephrine, or any component of the formulation, hypersensitivity to other local anesthetics of the amide type

INTERACTIONS

Drug

Beta-blockers: May increase blood pressure.

General anesthetics: May increase sensitivity of myocardium to dysrhythmic effects of epinephrine.

MAOIs, tricyclic antidepressants: May increase cardiovascular effects.

Herbal

None known.

Food

None known.

DIAGNOSTIC TEST EFFECTS: *None known.*

SIDE EFFECTS

Occasional

Nausea, vomiting, anxiety, restlessness, disorientation, confusion, dizziness, tremor

Rare

Bradycardia, somnolence

SERIOUS REACTIONS

• Hypersensitivity reactions rarely occur. Asthmatic syndromes have been reported.

• High blood levels may result in CNS depression, unconsciousness, and possible respiratory arrest.

SPECIAL CONSIDERATIONS

PRECAUTIONS

• Instruct patients not to use this preparation while wearing soft contact lenses.

PREGNANCY AND LACTATION

• Pregnancy Category C. Fetal harm is not known. Excretion into human milk is not known.

epinephrine; pilocarpine

(eh-pih-nef'rin; pye-loe-kar'peen)

Drug Class: Adrenergic agonists; Cholinergics; Miotics; Ophthalmics

Pregnancy Category: C

Do not confuse with ephedrine.

CLINICAL PHARMACOLOGY

Mechanism of Action: Epinephrine is a sympathomimetic, adrenergic agonist that stimulates alpha-adrenergic receptors, $beta_1$-adrenergic receptors and $beta_2$-adrenergic receptors and decreases production of aqueous humor and increases aqueous outflow. Pilocarpine is a parasympathomimetic that directly stimulates cholinergic receptors resulting in pupilary constriction (miosis), constriction of ciliary muscle, resulting in increased accommodation, and reduced intraocular pressure with an increase in the outflow and decrease in the inflow of aqueous humor. *Therapeutic Effect:* Increases aqueous outflow. Lowers intraocular pressure and aqueous humor.

Pharmacokinetics

May have systemic absorption from drainage into nasal pharyngeal passages. Mydriasis occurs within several minutes, persists several hours; vasoconstriction occurs within 5 min, lasts less than 1 hr.

AVAILABLE FORMS

• *Ophthalmic Solution:* Epinephrine bitartrate 1% and pilocarpine hydrochloride 1%, 2%, 3%, 4%, 6%.

INDICATIONS AND DOSAGES

Glaucoma

Ophthalmic

Adults, Elderly. Instill 1-2 drops up to 6 times/day.

CONTRAINDICATIONS: Acute iritis or glaucoma after cataract extraction, narrow-angle glaucoma, hypersensitivity to epinephrine, pilocarpine or any component of the formulation

INTERACTIONS

Drug

Dipivefrin: May increase myopia.

Latanoprost: May reduce latanoprost efficacy.

Herbal

None known.

Food

None known.

DIAGNOSTIC TEST EFFECTS: *None known.*

SIDE EFFECTS

Frequent

Headache, stinging, burning or other eye irritation, watering of eyes

Occasional

Blurred or decreased vision, eye pain

Rare

Retinal detachment

SERIOUS REACTIONS

• Retinal detachment has been reported in susceptible eyes.

SPECIAL CONSIDERATIONS

PRECAUTIONS

• Use with caution in patients with unverified glaucoma, hypertension, diabetes, hyperthyroidism, cardiac disease, or cerebral arteriosclerosis. Rare cases of retinal detachment have occurred.

PATIENT INFORMATION

• Instruct patients not to use this drug while wearing soft contact lenses.

PREGNANCY AND LACTATION

- Pregnancy Category C. Fetal harm is not known. Excretion into human milk is not known.

---

epinephryl borate

(ep-i-nef'-rill bor'-ate)

Rx: Epifrin, Epinal, Eppy/N

Drug Class: Adrenergic agonists; Ophthalmics

Pregnancy Category: C

CLINICAL PHARMACOLOGY

Mechanism of Action: A direct-acting sympathomimetic amine whose mechanism of action is unknown. *Therapeutic Effect:* Increases outflow of aqueous humor from anterior eye chamber.

Pharmacokinetics

May have systemic absorption from drainage into nasal pharyngeal passages. Mydriasis occurs within several minutes, persists several hours; vasoconstriction occurs within 5 min, lasts less than 1 hr.

AVAILABLE FORMS

- *Ophthalmic solution:* 0.5%, 1%, 2% (Epifrin).
- *Ophthalmic solution (borate):* 0.5% (Epinal), 1% (Epinal, Eppy/N), 2% (Eppy/N).

INDICATIONS AND DOSAGES

Glaucoma

Ophthalmic

Adults, Elderly. Instill 1 drop 1-2 times/day.

UNLABELED USES: Ophthalmic: Treatment of conjunctival congestion during surgery, secondary glaucoma

CONTRAINDICATIONS: Cardiac arrhythmias, cerebrovascular insufficiency, hypertension, hyperthyroidism, ischemic heart disease, narrow-angle glaucoma, shock, hypersensitivity to epinephryl borate or any component of the formulation

INTERACTIONS

Drug

Beta-blockers: May decrease the effects of beta-blockers.

Digoxin, sympathomimetics: May increase risk of arrhythmias.

Ergonovine, methergine, oxytocin: May increase vasoconstriction.

MAOIs, tricyclic antidepressants: May increase cardiovascular effects.

Herbal

None known.

Food

None known.

DIAGNOSTIC TEST EFFECTS: *None known.*

SIDE EFFECTS

Frequent

Headache, stinging, burning or other eye irritation, watering of eyes

Occasional

Blurred or decreased vision, eye pain

SERIOUS REACTIONS

- Systemic absorption occurs rarely. These effects include fast, irregular, or pounding heartbeat, feeling faint, increased sweating, paleness, trembling, and increased blood pressure.

SPECIAL CONSIDERATIONS

PRECAUTIONS

- Instruct patients not to use this preparation on soft contact lenses. Instruct patients immediately to report any decrease in visual acuity. If a general anesthetic is to be used, consult the anesthesiologist. Patient should not use if solution is brown.

eprosartan

(eh-pro-sar'tan)

Rx: Teveten

Drug Class: Angiotensin II receptor antagonists

Pregnancy Category: C, 1st; D, 2nd / 3rd

CLINICAL PHARMACOLOGY

Mechanism of Action: An angiotensin II receptor antagonist that blocks the vasoconstrictor and aldosterone-secreting effects of angiotensin II, inhibiting the binding of angiotensin II to the AT_1 receptors. *Therapeutic Effect:* Causes vasodilation, decreases peripheral resistance, and decreases BP.

Pharmacokinetics

Rapidly absorbed after PO administration. Protein binding: 98%. Undergoes first-pass metabolism in the liver to active metabolites. Excreted in urine and biliary system. Minimally removed by hemodialysis. **Half-life:** 5-9 hr.

AVAILABLE FORMS

- *Tablets:* 400 mg, 600 mg.

INDICATIONS AND DOSAGES

Hypertension

PO

Adults, Elderly. Initially, 600 mg/day. Range: 400-800 mg/day.

CONTRAINDICATIONS: Bilateral renal artery stenosis, hyperaldosteronism

INTERACTIONS

Drug

None known.

Herbal

None known.

Food

None known.

DIAGNOSTIC TEST EFFECTS: May increase BUN, serum alkaline phosphatase, serum bilirubin, serum creatinine, AST (SGOT), and ALT (SGPT) levels. May decrease blood Hgb and Hgb levels.

SIDE EFFECTS

Occasional (5%-2%)

Headache, cough, dizziness

Rare (less than 2%)

Muscle pain, fatigue, diarrhea, upper respiratory tract infection, dyspepsia

SERIOUS REACTIONS

- Overdosage may manifest as hypotension and tachycardia. Bradycardia occurs less often.

SPECIAL CONSIDERATIONS

PRECAUTIONS

- Anticipate changes in renal function in susceptible individuals. In studies of angiotensin-converting enzyme inhibitors in patients with unilateral or bilateral renal artery stenosis, increases in serum creatinine or blood urea nitrogen have been reported.

PATIENT INFORMATION

- Pregnancy: Advise female patients of childbearing age about the consequences of second- and third-trimester exposure to drugs that act on the renin-angiotensin system, and advise them that these consequences do not appear to have resulted from intrauterine drug exposure that has been limited to the first trimester. Ask these patients to report pregnancies to their physicians as soon as possible so that treatment may be discontinued under medical supervision.

PREGNANCY AND LACTATION

- Pregnancy Categories C (first trimester) and D (second and third trimesters). The use of drugs that act directly on the renin-angiotensin system during the second and third trimesters of pregnancy has been associated with fetal and neonatal injury, including hypotension, neonatal skull hypoplasia, anuria, reversible or irreversible renal failure, and death. Eprosartan is excreted in animal milk; whether eprosartan is excreted in human milk is not known.

erythromycin

(er-ith-roe-mye'sin)

Rx: A/T/S, Akne-Mycin, Emgel, E-Mycin, Eryc, Erycette, Erygel, Erymax, Ery-Tab, Erythra-Derm, PCE Dispertab, Romycin, Roymicin, Staticin, Theramycin, Theramycin Z, T-Stat

Drug Class: Anti-infectives, ophthalmic; Anti-infectives, topical; Antibiotics, macrolides; Ophthalmics

Pregnancy Category: B

Do not confuse erythromycin with azithromycin or Ethmozine, or Eryc with Emct.

CLINICAL PHARMACOLOGY

Mechanism of Action: A macrolide that reversibly binds to bacterial ribosomes, inhibiting bacterial protein synthesis. *Therapeutic Effect:* Bacteriostatic.

Pharmacokinetics

Variably absorbed from the GI tract (depending on dosage form used). Protein binding: 70%-90%. Widely distributed. Metabolized in the liver. Primarily eliminated in feces by bile. Not removed by hemodialysis. **Half-life:** 1.4-2 hr (increased in impaired renal function).

AVAILABLE FORMS

- *Topical Gel (A/T/S, Emgel, Erygel):* 2%.
- *Injection Powder for Reconstitution (Erythrocin):*500 mg, 1 g.
- *Ophthalmic Ointment:* 5 mg/g.
- *Topical Ointment (Akne-Mycin):* 2%.
- *Oral Suspension (EryPed, EES):* 200 mg/5 ml, 400 mg/5 ml.
- *Topical Solution (Staticin):* 1.5%.
- *Topical Solution (A/T/S, Ery-Derm, Erythra-Derm):* 2%.
- *Tablet (Chewable [Ery-Ped]):* 200 mg.
- *Tablets (Ery-Tab):* 250 mg, 333 mg, 500 mg.
- *Tablets (EES):* 400 mg.
- *Tablets (Erythrocin):* 250 mg, 500 mg.
- *Tablets (PCE):* 333 mg, 500 mg.

INDICATIONS AND DOSAGES

Mild to moderate infections of the upper and lower respiratory tract, pharyngitis, skin infections

PO

Adults, Elderly. 250 mg q6h, 500 mg q12h, or 333 mg q8h. Maximum: 4 g/day.

Children. 30-50 mg/kg/day in divided doses up to 60-100 mg/kg/day for severe infections.

Neonates. 20-40 mg/kg/day in divided doses q6-12h.

IV

Adults, Elderly, Children. 15-20 mg/kg/day in divided doses. Maximum: 4 g/day.

Preoperative intestinal antisepsis

PO

Adults, Elderly. 1 g at 1 pm, 2 pm, and 11 pm on day before surgery (with neomycin).

Children. 20 mg/kg at 1 pm, 2 pm, and 11 pm on day before surgery (with neomycin).

Acne vulgaris

Topical

Adults. Apply thin layer to affected area twice a day.

E

Gonococcal ophthalmia neonatorum
Ophthalmic
Neonates. 0.5-2 cm no later than 1 hr after delivery.
UNLABELED USES: Systemic: Treatment of acne vulgaris, chancroid, *Campylobacter* enteritis, gastroparesis, Lyme disease
Topical: Treatment of minor bacterial skin infections
Ophthalmic: Treatment of blepharitis, conjunctivitis, keratitis, chlamydial trachoma
CONTRAINDICATIONS: Administration of fixed-combination product, Pediazole, to infants younger than 2 months; history of hepatitis due to macrolides; hypersensitivity to macrolides; preexisting hepatic disease.
INTERACTIONS
Drug
Buspirone, cyclosporine, felodipine, lovastatin, simvastatin: May increase the blood concentration and toxicity of these drugs.
Carbamazepine: May inhibit the metabolism of carbamazepine.
Chloramphenicol, clindamycin: May decrease the effects of these drugs.
Hepatotoxic medications: May increase the risk of hepatotoxicity.
Theophylline: May increase the risk of theophylline toxicity.
Warfarin: May increase warfarin's effects.
Herbal
None known.
Food
None known.
DIAGNOSTIC TEST EFFECTS: May increase serum alkaline phosphatase, bilirubin, AST (SGOT), and ALT (SGPT) levels.
IV INCOMPATIBILITIES: Fluconazole (Diflucan)
IV COMPATIBILITIES: Aminophylline, amiodarone (Cordarone), diltiazem (Cardizem), heparin, hydromorphone (Dilaudid), lidocaine, lorazepam (Ativan), magnesium sulfate, midazolam (Versed), morphine, multivitamins, potassium chloride
SIDE EFFECTS
Frequent
IV: Abdominal cramping or discomfort, phlebitis or thrombophlebitis
Topical: Dry skin (50%)
Occasional
Nausea, vomiting, diarrhea, rash, urticaria
Rare
Ophthalmic: Sensitivity reaction with increased irritation, burning, itching, and inflammation
Topical: Urticaria
SERIOUS REACTIONS
- Antibiotic-associated colitis and other superinfections may occur.
- High dosages in patients with renal impairment may lead to reversible hearing loss.
- Anaphylaxis and hepatotoxicity occur rarely.
- Ventricular arrhythmias and prolonged QT interval occur rarely with the IV drug form.

SPECIAL CONSIDERATIONS

PRECAUTIONS
- Exercise caution when administering erythromycin to patients with impaired hepatic function. Reports indicate that erythromycin may aggravate the weakness of patients with myasthenia gravis. Prolonged or repeated use of erythromycin may result in an overgrowth of nonsusceptible bacteria or fungi. When indicated, incision and drainage or other surgical procedures should be performed along with antibiotic therapy.

PATIENT INFORMATION

• Topical: This form of erythromycin is for external use only and should be kept away from the eyes, nose, mouth, and other mucous membranes. Use concomitant topical acne therapy with caution because a cumulative irritant effect may occur, especially with the use of peeling, desquamating, or abrasive agents.

• Pledgets: Patients using Ery 2% pads should receive the following information and instructions:

• This medication is to be used as directed by the physician. It is for external use only. Avoid contact with eyes, nose, mouth, and all mucous membranes.

• This medication should not be used for any disorder other than that for which it was prescribed.

• Patients should not use any other topical acne medication unless otherwise directed by their physician.

• Patients should report to their physician any signs of local adverse reactions.

PREGNANCY AND LACTATION

• Pregnancy Category B. No evidence of teratogenicity or any other adverse effect on reproduction was found in female rats fed erythromycin base. Fetal harm is not known. Erythromycin is excreted in breast milk.

OCULAR CONSIDERATIONS

• When tetracyclines are contraindicated or not tolerated, erythromycin is indicated for the treatment of uncomplicated urethral, endocervical, or rectal infections in adults caused by *Chlamydia trachomatis*. Erythromycin also is indicated for conjunctivitis of the newborn, pneumonia of infancy, and urogenital infections during pregnancy.

• Irritation of the eyes and tenderness of the skin also have been reported with topical use of erythromycin.

• Erythromycin is indicated for chlamydial and gonococcal conjunctivitis in newborns.

estrogens, conjugated

(ess'-troe-jenz)

Rx: Cenestin, Enjuvia, Premarin, Premarin Intravenous, Premarin Vaginal

Drug Class: Estrogens; Hormones/hormone modifiers

Pregnancy Category: X

Do not confuse Premarin with Primaxin or Remeron.

CLINICAL PHARMACOLOGY

Mechanism of Action: An estrogen that increases synthesis of DNA, RNA, and various proteins in target tissues; reduces release of gonadotropin-releasing hormone from the hypothalamus; and reducies follicle-stimulating hormone (FSH) and leuteinizing hormone (LH) release from the pituitary gland. *Therapeutic Effect:* Promotes normal growth, promotes development of femal sex organs, and maintains GU function and vasomotor stability. Prevents accelerated bone loss by inhibiting bone resorption, restoring balance of bone resorption and formation. Inhibits LH and decreases serum concentration of testosterone.

Pharmacokinetics

Well absorbed from the GI tract. Widely distributed. Protein binding: 50%-80%. Metabolized in the liver. Primarily excreted in urine.

AVAILABLE FORMS

• *Tablets (Cenestin, Premarin):* 0.3 mg, 0.45 mg, 0.625 mg, 0.9 mg, 1.25 mg.
• *Tablets (Enjuvia):* 0.625 mg, 1.25 mg.
• *Injection:* 25 mg.
• *Vaginal Cream.* 0.625 mg/g.

INDICATIONS AND DOSAGES

Vasomotor symptoms associated with menopause, atrophic vaginitis, kraurosis vulvae

PO

Adults, Elderly. 0.3-0.625 mg/day cyclically (21 days on, 7 days off) or continuously.

Intravaginal

Adults, Elderly. 0.5-2 g/day cyclically, such as 21 days on and 7 days off.

Female hypogonadism

PO

Adults. 0.3-0.625 mg/day in divided doses for 20 days; then a rest period of 10 days.

Female castration, primary ovarian failure

PO

Adults. Initially, 1.25 mg/day cyclically. Adjust dosage, upward or downward, according to severity of symptoms and patient response. For maintenance, adjust dosage to lowest level that will provide effective control.

Osteoporosis

PO

Adults, Elderly. 0.3-0.625 mg/day, cyclically, such as 25 days on and 5 days off.

Breast cancer

PO

Adults, Elderly. 10 mg 3 times a day for at least 3 mo.

Prostate cancer

PO

Adults, Elderly. 1.25-2.5 mg 3 times a day.

Abnormal uterine bleeding

PO

Adults. 1.25 mg q4h for 24 hr, then 1.25 mg/day for 7-10 days.

IV, IM

Adults. 25 mg; may repeat once in 6-12 hr.

UNLABELED USES: Prevention of estrogen deficiency–induced premenopausal osteoporosis

Cream: Prevention of nosebleeds

CONTRAINDICATIONS: Breast cancer with some exceptions, hepatic disease, thrombophlebitis, undiagnosed vaginal bleeding

INTERACTIONS

Drug

Bromocriptine: May interfere with the effects of bromocriptine.

Cyclosporine: May increase blood cyclosporine concentration and the risk of hepatotoxicity and nephrotoxicity.

Hepatotoxic medications: May increase the risk of hepatotoxicity.

Herbal

None known.

Food

None known.

DIAGNOSTIC TEST EFFECTS: May increase blood glucose, HDL, serum calcium, and triglyceride levels. May decrease serum cholesterol levels and LDH concentrations. May affect serum metapyrone testing and thyroid function tests.

IV INCOMPATIBILITIES: No information available via Y-site administration.

SIDE EFFECTS

Frequent

Vaginal bleeding, such as spotting or breakthrough bleeding; breast pain or tenderness; gynecomastia

Occasional

Headache, hypertension, intolerance to contact lenses

High doses: Anorexia, nausea

Rare
Loss of scalp hair, depression

SERIOUS REACTIONS

• Prolonged administration may increase the risk of gallbladder disease, thromboembolic disease, and breast, cervical, vaginal, endometrial, and hepatic carcinoma.

SPECIAL CONSIDERATIONS

PRECAUTIONS

• Estrogens, with the addition of a progestin, has a lower reported incidence of endometrial hyperplasia than would be induced by estrogen treatment alone. The relationship between estrogen replacement therapy and reduction of cardiovascular disease in postmenopausal women has not been proved. Obtain a complete medical and family history before the initiation of any estrogen therapy. Some studies have shown that women taking estrogen replacement therapy have hypercoagulability, primarily related to decreased antithrombin activity. Estrogen therapy may be associated with massive elevations of plasma triglycerides, leading to pancreatitis in patients with familial defects of lipoprotein metabolism. Because estrogens may cause some degree of fluid retention, patients with asthma, epilepsy, migraine, and cardiac or renal dysfunction require careful observation.

• Endometriosis may be exacerbated with administration of estrogen therapy. Certain patients may develop abnormal uterine bleeding and mastodynia. Administer estrogens with caution to patients with impaired liver function. Preexisting uterine leiomyomas may increase in size during estrogen use. Use estrogens with caution in individuals with metabolic bone disease associated with severe hypocalcemia.

PREGNANCY AND LACTATION

• Pregnancy Category X. Do not use estrogens during pregnancy. Estrogen administration to nursing mothers has been shown to decrease the quantity and quality of the milk.

OCULAR CONSIDERATIONS

• Adverse reactions include steepening of corneal curvature and intolerance to contact lenses.

E

estrogens, conjugated; medroxyprogesterone acetate

(ess′-troe-jens, kon′-joo-gay-ted; me-drox′-ee-proe-jes′-ter-rone ass′-eh-tayte)

Rx: Premphase, Prempro

Drug Class: Estrogens; Hormones/hormone modifiers; Progestins

Pregnancy Category: X

CLINICAL PHARMACOLOGY

Mechanism of Action: Conjugated estrogens are estrogens that increase synthesis of DNA, RNA, and various proteins in responsive tissues; reduces release of gonadotropin-releasing hormone, reducing follicle-stimulating hormone (FSH) and leuteinizing hormone (LH). Medroxyprogesterone acetate is a hormone that transforms endometrium from proliferative to secretory in an estrogen-primed endometrium; inhibits secretion of pituitary gonadotropins. *Therapeutic Effect:* Conjugated estrogens promote vasomotor stability, maintain genitourinary (GU) function, normal growth, development of female sex organs; prevents accelerated bone loss by inhibiting bone resorption, restoring balance of bone resorption and formation; inhibits LH, decreases serum concentration of testosterone. Medroxyprogesterone acetate prevents follicular maturation and ovulation; stimulates growth of mammary alveolar tissue; relaxes uterine smooth muscle; restores hormonal imbalance.

Pharmacokinetics

Conjugated estrogens are well absorbed from the gastrointestinal (GI) tract. Widely distributed. Protein binding: 50%-80%. Metabolized in liver. Primarily excreted in urine. **Half-life:** 4-10 hrs.

Medroxyprogesterone's absorption varies depending on the patient but is generally low. Binds mainly to albumin or other plasma proteins. Metabolized in liver. Primarily excreted in urine. **Half-life:** 2-4 hrs.

AVAILABLE FORMS

- *Tablets:* 0.3 mg of conjugated estrogens and 1.5 mg of medroxyprogesterone acetate (Prempro Low Dose), 0.45 mg of conjugated estrogens and 1.5 mg of medroxyprogesterone acetate (Prempro), 0.625 mg of conjugated estrogens and 2.5 mg of medroxyprogesterone acetate (Prempro), 0.625 mg of conjugated estrogens and 5 mg of medroxyprogesterone acetate (Prempro), and 0.625 mg of conjugated estrogens and 5 mg of medroxyprogesterone acetate (Premphase).

INDICATIONS AND DOSAGES

Menopausal symptoms, osteoporosis, vulvar/vaginal atrophy

PO

(Prempro) Adults, Elderly. 1 tablet once daily.

Menopausal symptoms, osteoporosis, vulvar/vaginal atrophy

PO

(Premphase) Adults, Elderly. 1 maroon conjugated estrogen tablet on days 1 through 14 and 1 light blue conjugated estrogens/medroxyprogesterone tablet on days 15 through 28.

CONTRAINDICATIONS: Breast cancer with some exceptions, liver disease, thrombophlebitis, undiagnosed vaginal bleeding, estrogen-dependent neoplasia (known or suspected), pregnancy (known or suspected), hypersensitivity to conjugated estrogens, medroxyprogesterone acetate or any component of the formulation.

INTERACTIONS

Drug

Bromocriptine: May interfere with the effects of bromocriptine.

Cyclosporine: May increase the blood concentration and liver and nephrotoxicity of cyclosporine.

Liver toxic medications: May increase the risk of liver toxicity.

Phenobarbital, carbamazepine, and rifampin: May reduce plasma concentrations of estrogens.

Erythromycin, clarithromycin, ketoconazole, itraconazole, ritonavir: May increase plasma concentrations of estrogens.

Herbal

St. John's wort: May reduce plasma concentrations of estrogens.

Food

Grapefruit juice: May increase plasma concentration of estrogens.

DIAGNOSTIC TEST EFFECTS: Conjugated estrogens may affect metapyrone testing, thyroid function tests. May decrease serum cholesterol levels, and LDH concentrations. May increase blood glucose levels, HDL concentrations, serum calcium, and triglyceride levels.

Medroxyprogesterone may alter thyroid and liver function tests, prothrombin time, and metapyrone test.

SIDE EFFECTS

Frequent

Change in vaginal bleeding, such as spotting or breakthrough bleeding, breast pain or tenderness, gynecomastia

Occasional

Headache, increased blood pressure (BP), intolerance to contact lenses, nausea, edema, weight change, breast tenderness, nervousness, insomnia, fatigue, dizziness

Rare

Loss of scalp hair, mental depression, dermatologic changes, headache, fever

SERIOUS REACTIONS

• Prolonged administration may increase risk of gallbladder, thromboembolic disease, or breast, cervical, vaginal, endometrial, and liver carcinoma.

SPECIAL CONSIDERATIONS

PRECAUTIONS

• Possible induction of endometrial cancer and breast cancer may occur. Increased risk of thrombophlebitis and/or thromboembolic disease is possible. Increased risk of surgically confirmed gallbladder disease is possible. Occasional blood pressure increases during estrogen replacement therapy have been reported. Administration of estrogens may lead to severe hypercalcemia in patients with breast cancer and bone metastases. Discontinue medication pending examination if there is sudden partial or complete loss of vision or a sudden onset of proptosis, diplopia, or migraine. If examination reveals papilledema or retinal vascular lesions, withdraw medication. A causal relationship between estrogen replacement therapy and reduction of cardiovascular disease in postmenopausal women has not been proved. Existing data do not support the use of the combination of estrogen and progestin in postmenopausal women without a uterus. Certain patients may develop abnormal uterine bleeding.

PREGNANCY AND LACTATION

• Pregnancy Category X. Do not use estrogens and progestins during pregnancy. Estrogen administration to nursing mothers has been shown to decrease the quantity and quality of the milk. Detectable amounts of progestin have been identified in the milk of mothers receiving the drug.

OCULAR CONSIDERATIONS

• Adverse reactions include neuroocular lesions such as retinal thrombosis and optic neuritis, steepening of corneal curvature, and intolerance of contact lenses. Discontinue medication pending examination if there is sudden partial or complete loss of vision or a sudden onset of proptosis, diplopia, or migraine. If examination reveals papilledema or retinal vascular lesions, withdraw medication.

ethambutol

(e-tham′byoo-tole)

Rx: Myambutol

Drug Class: Antimycobacterials

Pregnancy Category: B

Do not confuse ethambutol or Myambutol with Nembutal.

CLINICAL PHARMACOLOGY

Mechanism of Action: An isonicotinic acid derivative that interferes with RNA synthesis. *Therapeutic Effect:* Suppresses the multiplication of mycobacteria.

Pharmacokinetics

Rapidly and well absorbed from the GI tract. Protein binding: 20%-30%.

Widely distributed. Metabolized in the liver. Primarily excreted in urine. Removed by hemodialysis. **Half-life:** 3-4 hr (increased in impaired renal function).

AVAILABLE FORMS

• *Tablets:* 100 mg, 400 mg.

INDICATIONS AND DOSAGES

Tuberculosis

PO

Adults, Elderly, Children. 15-25 mg/kg/day as a single dose or 50 mg/kg 2 times/wk. Maximum: 2.5 g/dose.

Atypical mycobacterial infections

PO

Adults, Elderly, Children. 15 mg/kg/day. Maximum: 1 g/day.

Dosage in renal impairment

Dosage interval is modified based on creatinine clearance.

Creatinine Clearance	*Dosage Interval*
10-50 ml/min	q24-36h
less than 10 ml/min	q48h

UNLABELED USES: Treatment of atypical mycobacterial infections

CONTRAINDICATIONS: Optic neuritis

INTERACTIONS

Drug

Neurotoxic medications: May increase the risk of neurotoxicity.

Herbal

None known.

Food

None known.

DIAGNOSTIC TEST EFFECTS: May increase serum uric acid levels.

SIDE EFFECTS

Occasional

Acute gouty arthritis (chills, pain, swelling of joints with hot skin), confusion, abdominal pain, nausea, vomiting, anorexia, headache

Rare

Rash, fever, blurred vision, eye pain, red-green color blindness

SERIOUS REACTIONS

• Optic neuritis (more common with high-dosage or long-term ethambutol therapy), peripheral neuritis, thrombocytopenia, and an anaphylactoid reaction occur rarely.

SPECIAL CONSIDERATIONS

PREGNANCY AND LACTATION

• Pregnancy Category B. Administration of this drug to pregnant human patients has produced no detectable effect upon the fetus. Carefully weigh the possible teratogenic potential in women capable of bearing children against the benefits of therapy. Published reports indicate that five women received the drug during pregnancy without apparent adverse effect upon the fetus. Excretion into human milk is not known.

PRECAUTIONS

• Because this drug may have adverse effects on vision, physical examination should include ophthalmoscopy, finger perimetry, and testing of color discrimination. In patients with visual defects such as cataracts, recurrent inflammatory conditions of the eye, optic neuritis, and diabetic retinopathy, the evaluation of changes in visual acuity is more difficult, and one should take care to be sure the variations in vision are not due to the underlying disease conditions. In such patients, consider the relationship between benefits expected and possible visual deterioration, because evaluation of visual changes is difficult.

• Ethambutol hydrochloride is not recommended for use in children under 13 years of age because safe conditions for use have not been established. Patients with decreased renal function need the dosage reduced as determined by serum levels of ethambutol hydrochloride because the main path of excretion of this drug is by the kidneys.

OCULAR CONSIDERATIONS

• Ethambutol hydrochloride may produce decreases in visual acuity that appear to be due to optic neuritis and to be related to dose and duration of treatment. The effects are generally reversible when administration of the drug is discontinued promptly. In rare cases, recovery may be delayed for up to 1 year or more, and the effect possibly may be irreversible in these cases.

• Advise patients to report promptly to their eye care practitioner in any change of visual acuity.

• The change in visual acuity may be unilateral or bilateral, and hence each eye must be tested separately and both eyes tested together. Testing of visual acuity should be performed before beginning ethambutol hydrochloride therapy and periodically during drug administration, except that it should be done monthly when a patient is on a dosage of more than 15 mg/kg per day. Studies have shown that there are definite fluctuations of one or two lines of the Snellen chart in the visual acuity of many tuberculous patients not receiving ethambutol hydrochloride.

• If corrective glasses are used before treatment, these must be worn during visual acuity testing. During 1 to 2 years of therapy, a refractive error may develop that must be corrected to obtain accurate test results. Patients developing visual abnormality during ethambutol hydrochloride treatment may show subjective visual symptoms before, or simultaneously with, the demonstration of decreases in visual acuity and other subjective eye symptoms.

• Recovery of visual acuity generally occurs over a period of weeks to months after the drug has been discontinued. Patients then have received ethambutol hydrochloride again without recurrence of loss of visual acuity.

E

ethinyl estradiol; norethindrone

(eth'i-nil ess-tra-dye'ole; nor-eth'in-drone)

Rx: Brevicon, Estrostep Fe, femhrt 1/5, Genora 1/35, Jenest, Junel, Loestrin 21 1/20, Loestrin 21 1.5/30, Loestrin FE 1/20, Loestrin FE 1.5/30, Microgestin FE 1/20, Microgestin FE 1.5/30, Modicon, Necon 0.5/35, Necon 1/35, Necon 10/11, Necon 7/7/7, Nelova 1/35, Norethin 1/35 E, Norinyl 1/35, Nortrel, Nortrel 7/7/7, Ortho-Novum 1/35, Ortho-Novum 10/11, Ortho-Novum 7/7/7, Ovcon 35, Ovcon 50, Tri-Norinyl

Drug Class: Contraceptives; Estrogens; Hormones/hormone modifiers; Progestins

Pregnancy Category: X

CLINICAL PHARMACOLOGY

Mechanism of Action: A combination oral contraceptive that inhibits ovulation by a negative feedback mechanism on the hypothalamus, which alters the normal pattern of gonadotropin secretion of a follicle-stimulating hormone (FSH) and luteinizing hormone by the anterior pituitary. In postmenopausal women, exogenous estrogen is used to replace decreased endogenous production. *Therapeutic Effect:* Prevents conception.

Pharmacokinetics

Well absorbed. Protein binding: more than 95%. Widely distributed. Primarily excreted in urine. **Half-life:** 24 hours (ethinyl estradiol), 8-13 hours (norethindrone).

AVAILABLE FORMS

• *Tablets, monophasic formulations:* 0.02 mg ethinyl estradiol and 1 mg norethindrone (Loestrin 21 1/20), 0.02 mg ethinyl estradiol and 1 mg norethindrone and 75 mg ferrous fumarate (Junel, Loestrin FE 1.5/30, Microgestin FE 1.5/30), 0.03 mg ethinyl estradiol and 1.5 mg norethindrone (Loestrin 21 1.5/30, Microgestin 1.5/30), 0.03 mg ethinyl estradiol and 1.5 mg norethindrone and 75 mg ferrous fumarate (Loestrin FE 1.5/30), 0.035 mg ethinyl estradiol and 0.5 mg norethindrone (Brevicon, Modicon 28, Necon 0.5/35, Nortrel), 0.035 mg ethinyl estradiol and 1 mg norethindrone (Necon 1/35-28, Norinyl 1+35, Nortrel 1/35, Ortho-Novum 1/35), 0.035 mg ethinyl estradiol and 0.4 mg norethindrone (Ovcon 35 21-day, Ovcon 35 28-day), 0.05 ethinyl estradiol and 1 mg norethindrone (Ovcon 50).

• *Tablets, biphasic formulations:* 0.035 mg ethinyl estradiol and 0.5 mg norethindrone/ 0.035 mg ethinyl estradiol and 1 mg norethindrone (Jenest, Necon 10/11, Ortho-Novum 10/11).

• *Tablets, triphasic formulations:* 0.035 mg ethinyl estradiol and 0.5 mg norethindrone/ 0.035 mg ethinyl estradiol and 1 mg norethindrone/ 0.035 mg ethinyl estradiol and 0.5 mg norethindrone (Tri-Norinyl), 0.02 mg ethinyl estradiol and 1 mg norethindrone/ 0.03 mg ethinyl estradiol and 1 mg norethindrone/ 0.035 mg ethinyl estradiol and 1 mg norethindrone/ 75 mg ferrous fumarate (Estrostep Fe), 0.035 mg ethinyl estradiol and 0.5 mg norethindrone/ 0.035 mg ethinyl estradiol and 0.75 mg norethindrone/0.035 mg ethinyl estradiol and 1 mg norethindrone (Necon 7/7/7, Nortrel 7/7/7, Ortho-Novum 7/7/7).

• *Tablets:* 5 mcg ethinyl estradiol and 1 mg norethindrone acetate (femhrt 1/5).

INDICATIONS AND DOSAGES

Prevention of pregnancy

PO

Adults. 1 tablet daily for 21 days followed by 1 inactive tablet daily for 7 days; repeat regimen.

UNLABELED USES: Acne, treatment of hypermenorrhea, endometriosis, female hypogonadism

CONTRAINDICATIONS: History of or current thrombophlebitis or venous thromboembolic disorders (including DVT and PE), active or recent (within 1 year) arterial thromboembolic disease (e.g., stroke, MI), cerebral vascular disease, coronary artery disease, severe hypertension, diabetes mellitus with vascular involvement, severe headache with focal neurological symptoms, known or suspected breast carcinoma, endometrial cancer, estrogen-dependent neoplasms, undiagnosed abnormal genital bleeding, hepatic dysfunction or tumor, cholestatic jaundice of pregnancy, jaundice with prior combination hormonal contraceptive use, major surgery with prolonged immobilization, heavy smoking (15 cigarettes/ day) in patients >35 years of age, pregnancy, hypersensitivity to ethinyl estradiol, norethindrone, norethindrone acetate, or any component of the formulation

INTERACTIONS

Drug

Acetaminophen: May increase plasma concentration of synthetic estrogens, possibly by inhibiting conjugation; may also decrease the plasma concentration of acetaminophen.
Acitretin: May interfere with the contraceptive effect.
Aminoglutethimide: May increase CYP metabolism of progestins leading to possible decrease in contraceptive effectiveness.
Antibiotics (e.g. ampicillin, tetracycline): May increase risk of pregnancy.
Anticoagulants: May increase or decrease the effects of coumarin derivatives.
Anticonvulsants (e.g. carbamazepine, felbamate, phenobarbital, phenytoin, topiramate): May increase the metabolism of ethinyl estradiol and/or some progestins, leading to possible decrease in contraceptive effectiveness.
Atorvastatin: Atorvastatin increases the area-under-curve (AUC) for norethindrone and ethinyl estradiol.
Benzodiazepines: May decrease the clearance of some benzodiazepines (e.g. alprazolam, chlordiazepoxide, diazepam) and increase the clearance of others (e.g., lorazepam, oxazepam, temazepam)
Clofibric acid: Combination hormonal contraceptives may increase the clearance of clofibric acid.
Cyclosporine: May inhibit the metabolism of cyclosporine, leading to increased plasma concentrations.
CYP3A4 inducers: May decrease the levels/effects of ethinyl estradiol and norethindrone.
Griseofulvin: May induce the metabolism of combination hormonal contraceptives causing menstrual changes.
Morphine: May increase the clearance of morphine.
Non-nucleoside reverse transcriptase inhibitors (NNRTIs): May decrease plasma levels of combination hormonal contraceptives.
Prednisolone: May inhibit the metabolism of prednisolone, leading to increased plasma concentrations.
Protease inhibitors: Amprenavir, lopinavir, nelfinavir, and ritonavir may decrease plasma levels of combination hormonal contraceptives. Indinavir may increase plasma levels of combination hormonal contraceptives.
Rifampin: May increase the metabolism of ethinyl estradiol and norethindrone resulting in decreased contraceptive effectiveness and increased menstrual irregularities.
Salicylic acid: May increase the clearance of salicylic acid. Selegiline: May increase the serum concentration of selegiline.
Theophylline: May inhibit the metabolism of theophylline, leading to increased plasma concentrations.
Tricyclic antidepressants (amitriptyline, imipramine, nortriptyline): May increase plasma levels of TCA antidepressants by inhibiting metabolism.

Herbal

St. John's wort: May decrease the effectiveness of combination hormonal contraceptives.
Black cohosh, dong quai: May increase estrogenic activity.
Red clover, saw palmetto, ginseng: May increase hormonal effects.

Food

None known.

DIAGNOSTIC TEST EFFECTS: *None known.*

SIDE EFFECTS

Frequent

Abdominal cramping, bloating, nausea, swelling of breasts, peripheral edema, evidenced by swollen ankles, feet

Occasional

Vomiting, amenorrhea, breakthrough bleeding, depression, weight changes, temporary infertility after discontinuation of use

Rare

Hypertension

SERIOUS REACTIONS

• Arterial thromboembolism, pulmonary embolism, thrombophlebitis, venous thrombosis, cerebral hemorrhage, cerebral thrombosis, gallbladder disease, hepatic adenomas or benign liver tumors, myocardial infarction, and retinal thrombosis occur rarely.

SPECIAL CONSIDERATIONS

PRECAUTIONS

• Use of oral contraceptives is associated with increased risks of several serious conditions, including myocardial infarction, thromboembolism, stroke, hepatic neoplasia, and gallbladder disease. Risk of morbidity increases in the presence of hypertension, hyperlipidemias, hypercholesterolemia, obesity, and diabetes.

• An increased risk of myocardial infarction, thromboembolic and thrombotic disease, thrombotic and hemorrhagic strokes, vascular disease, and gallbladder surgery may occur. Benign hepatic adenomas, glucose intolerance, increased blood pressure, headaches, breakthrough bleeding and spotting, ectopic and intrauterine pregnancy are associated with oral contraceptive use.

• Women who are being treated for hyperlipidemia should be followed closely. If jaundice develops in any woman receiving such drugs, discontinue the medication. Ethinyl estradiol and norethindrone may cause some degree of fluid retention.

PREGNANCY AND LACTATION

• Pregnancy Category X. Small amounts of oral contraceptive steroids have been identified in the milk of nursing mothers, and a few adverse effects on the child have been reported, including jaundice and breast enlargement. In addition, oral contraceptives given in the postpartum period may interfere with lactation by decreasing the quantity and quality of breast milk. If possible, advise the nursing mother not to use oral contraceptives but to use other forms of contraception until she has weaned her child completely.

OCULAR CONSIDERATIONS

• Clinical case reports have been made of retinal thrombosis associated with the use of oral contraceptives. Discontinue oral contraceptive use if there is unexplained partial or complete loss of vision, onset of proptosis or diplopia, papilledema, or retinal vascular lesions. Undertake appropriate diagnostic and therapeutic measures immediately. An eye care practitioner should assess contact lens wearers who develop visual changes or contact lens intolerance.

etidronate disodium

(ee-tid'roe-nate)

Rx: Didronel, Didronel I.V.

Drug Class: Bisphosphonates

Pregnancy Category: B

Do not confuse etidronate with etidocaine or etomidate.

CLINICAL PHARMACOLOGY

Mechanism of Action: A bisphosphonate that decreases mineral release and matrix in bone and inhibits osteocytic osteolysis. *Therapeutic Effect:* Decreases bone resorption.

AVAILABLE FORMS

- *Tablets:* 200 mg, 400 mg.
- *Injection:* 300-mg ampule (50 mg/ml).

INDICATIONS AND DOSAGES

Paget's disease

PO

Adults, Elderly. Initially, 5-10 mg/kg/day not to exceed 6 mo, or 11-20 mg/kg/day not to exceed 3 mo. Repeat only after drug-free period of at least 90 days.

Heterotopic ossification caused by spinal cord injury

PO

Adult, Elderly. 20 mg/kg/day for 2 wk; then 10 mg/kg/day for 10 wks.

Heterotopic ossification complicating total hip replacement

PO

Adults, Elderly. 20 mg/kg/day for 1 mo before surgery; then 20 mg/kg/day for 3 mo after surgery.

Hypercalcemia associated with malignancy

IV

Adults, Elderly. 7.5 mg/kg/day for 3 days. For retreatment, allow 7 days between treatment courses. Follow with oral therapy on day after last infusion. Begin with 20 mg/kg/day for 30 days; may extend up to 90 days.

CONTRAINDICATIONS: Clinically overt osteomalacia

INTERACTIONS

Drug

Antacids containing aluminum, calcium, magnesium mineral supplements: May decrease the absorption of etidronate.

Herbal

None known.

Food

Foods with calcium: May decrease the absorption of etidronate.

DIAGNOSTIC TEST EFFECTS: *None known.*

IV INCOMPATIBILITIES: Do not mix with other medications.

SIDE EFFECTS

Frequent

Nausea; diarrhea; continuing or more frequent bone pain in patients with Paget's disease

Occasional

Bone fractures, especially of the femur

Parenteral: Metallic, altered taste

Rare

Hypersensitivity reaction

SERIOUS REACTIONS

- Nephrotoxicity, including hematuria, dysuria, and proteinuria, has occurred with parenteral route.

SPECIAL CONSIDERATIONS

PRECAUTIONS

- Amblyopia was reported as an adverse reaction in 3.3% of the patients.

famciclovir

(fam-si'klo-veer)

Rx: Famvir

Drug Class: Antivirals

Pregnancy Category: B

Do not confuse Famvir with Femhrt.

CLINICAL PHARMACOLOGY

Mechanism of Action: A synthetic nucleoside that inhibits viral DNA synthesis. *Therapeutic Effect:* Suppresses replication of herpes simplex virus and varicella-zoster virus.

Pharmacokinetics

Rapidly and extensively absorbed after PO administration. Protein binding: 20%-25%. Rapidly metabolized to penciclovir by enzymes in the GI wall, liver, and plasma. Eliminated unchanged in urine. Removed by hemodialysis. **Half-life:** 2 hr.

AVAILABLE FORMS

- *Tablets:* 125 mg, 250 mg, 500 mg.

INDICATIONS AND DOSAGES

Herpes zoster

PO

Adults. 500 mg q8h for 7 days.

Recurrent genital herpes

PO

Adults. 125 mg twice a day for 5 days.

Suppression of recurrent genital herpes

PO

Adults. 250 mg twice a day for up to 1 yr.

Recurrent herpes simplex

PO

Adults. 500 mg twice a day for 7 days.

Dosage in renal impairment

Dosage and frequency are modified based on creatinine clearance.

Creatinine Clearance	*Herpes Zoster*	*Genital Herpes*
40-59 ml/min	500 mg q12h	125 mg q12h
20-39 ml/min	500 mg q24h	125 mg q24h
less than 20 ml/min	250 mg q24h	125 mg q24h

Dosage in hemodialysis patients

For adults with herpes zoster, give 250 mg after each dialysis treatment; for adults with genital herpes, give 125 mg after each dialysis treatment.

CONTRAINDICATIONS: None known.

INTERACTIONS

Drug

None known.

Herbal

None known.

Food

None known.

DIAGNOSTIC TEST EFFECTS: *None known.*

SIDE EFFECTS

Frequent

Headache (23%), nausea (12%)

Occasional (10%-2%)

Dizziness, somnolence, numbness of feet, diarrhea, vomiting, constipation, decreased appetite, fatigue, fever, pharyngitis, sinusitis, pruritus

Rare (less than 2%)

Insomnia, abdominal pain, dyspepsia, flatulence, back pain, arthralgia

SERIOUS REACTIONS

- None known.

SPECIAL CONSIDERATIONS

PRECAUTIONS

- The efficacy of famciclovir has not been established for initial episode genital herpes infection, ocular zoster, or disseminated zoster or in immunocompromised patients with herpes zoster. Dosage adjustment is recommended when administering famciclovir to patients with creatinine clearance values less than 60 ml/min. In patients with underlying renal disease who have received inappropriately high doses of famciclovir for their level of renal function, acute renal failure has been reported.

PATIENT INFORMATION

• Inform patients that famciclovir is not a cure for genital herpes. No data exist that evaluate whether famciclovir will prevent transmission of infection to others. Because genital herpes is a sexually transmitted disease, patients should avoid contact with lesions or intercourse when lesions and/or symptoms are present to avoid infecting partners. Genital herpes also can be transmitted in the absence of symptoms through asymptomatic viral shedding. If medical management of recurrent episodes is indicated, advise patients to initiate therapy at the first sign or symptom.

PREGNANCY AND LACTATION

• Pregnancy Category B. Famciclovir was tested for effects on embryo-fetal development in rats and rabbits at oral doses. No adverse effects were observed on embryo-fetal development. Following oral administration of famciclovir to lactating rats, penciclovir was excreted in breast milk at concentrations higher than those seen in the plasma. Whether famciclovir is excreted in human milk is not known.

OCULAR CONSIDERATIONS

Ocular Dosing

For ophthalmic zoster, famciclovir 500 mg 3 times/day for 7 days was well tolerated and demonstrated efficacy similar to acyclovir 800 mg 5 times/day for 7 days. (Tyring S, Engst R, Corriveau C, et al: Famciclovir for ophthalmic zoster: a randomised acyclovir controlled study, *Br J Ophthalmol* 85(5)576, 2001.)

famotidine

(fam-o'tah-deen)

Rx: Pepcid, Pepcid RPD

Drug Class: Antihistamines, H2; Gastrointestinals

Pregnancy Category: B

CLINICAL PHARMACOLOGY

Mechanism of Action: An antiulcer agent and gastric acid secretion inhibitor that inhibits histamine action at histamine 2 receptors of parietal cells. *Therapeutic Effect:* Inhibits gastric acid secretion when fasting, at night, or when stimulated by food, caffeine, or insulin.

Pharmacokinetics

Route	*Onset*	*Peak*	*Duration*
PO	1 hr	1-4 hr	10-12 hr
IV	1 hr	0.5-3 hr	10-12 hr

Rapidly, incompletely absorbed from the GI tract. Protein binding: 15%-20%. Partially metabolized in the liver. Primarily excreted in urine. Not removed by hemodialysis. **Half-life:** 2.5-3.5 hr (increased with impaired renal function).

AVAILABLE FORMS

• *Oral Suspension (Pepcid):* 40 mg/5 ml.

• *Tablets (Pepcid):* 20 mg, 40 mg.

• *Tablets (Pepcid AC):* 10 mg, 20 mg.

• *Tablets (Chewable [Pepcid AC]):* 10 mg.

• *Capsules (Pepcid AC):* 10 mg.

• *Injection (Pepcid):* 10 mg/ml.

INDICATIONS AND DOSAGES

Acute treatment of duodenal and gastric ulcers

PO

Adults, Elderly, Children 12 yr and older. 40 mg/day at bedtime.

Children 1-11 yr. 0.5 mg/kg/day at bedtime. Maximum: 40 mg/day.

Duodenal ulcer maintenance
PO
Adults, Elderly. 20 mg/day at bedtime.
Gastroesophageal reflux disease
PO
Adults, Elderly, Children 12 yr and older. 20 mg twice a day.
Children 1-11 yr. 1 mg/kg/day in 2 divided doses.
Children 3 mo to 11 mo. 0.5 mg/kg/dose twice a day.
Children younger than 3 mo. 0.5 mg/kg/dose once a day.
Esophagitis
PO
Adults, Elderly, Children 12 yr and older. 2-40 mg twice a day.
Hypersecretory conditions
PO
Adults, Elderly, Children 12 yr and older. Initially, 20 mg q6h. May increase up to 160 mg q6h.
Acid indigestion, heartburn (over-the-counter)
PO
Adults, Elderly, Children 12 yr and older. 10-20 mg 15-60 min before eating. Maximum: 2 doses per day.
Usual Parenteral Dosage
IV
Adults, Elderly, Children 12 yr and older. 20 mg q12h.
Dosage in renal impairment
Dosing frequency is modified based on creatinine clearance.

Creatinine Clearance	Dosing Frequency
10-50 ml/min	q24h
less than 10 ml/min	q36-48h

UNLABELED USES: Autism, prevention of aspiration pneumonitis
CONTRAINDICATIONS: None known.
INTERACTIONS
Drug
Antacids: May decrease the absorption of famotidine.
Ketoconazole: May decrease the absorption of ketoconazole.
Herbal
None known.
Food
None known.
DIAGNOSTIC TEST EFFECTS: Interferes with skin tests using allergen extracts. May increase liver enzyme levels.
IV INCOMPATIBILITIES: Amphotericin B complex (Abelcet, Amphotec, AmBisome), cefepime (Maxipime), furosemide (Lasix), piperacillin/tazobactam (Zosyn)
IV COMPATIBILITIES: Calcium gluconate, dobutamine (Dobutrex), dopamine (Intropin), heparin, hydromorphone (Dilaudid), insulin (regular), lidocaine, lorazepam (Ativan), magnesium sulfate, midazolam (Versed), morphine, nitroglycerin, norepinephrine (Levophed), potassium chloride, potassium phosphate, propofol (Diprivan)
SIDE EFFECTS
Occasional (5%)
Headache
Rare (2% or less)
Constipation, diarrhea, dizziness
SERIOUS REACTIONS
- None known.

SPECIAL CONSIDERATIONS

PRECAUTIONS
- Lower doses may need to be used in patients with renal insufficiency.

PATIENT INFORMATION
- Instruct the patient to shake the oral suspension vigorously for 5 to 10 seconds before each use. Unused constituted oral suspension should be discarded after 30 days.
- Instruct patients to leave the orally disintegrating famotidine tablet in the unopened package until the time of use. Instruct patients then to open the tablet blister pack with dry hands

and to place the tablet on the tongue to dissolve and to be swallowed with saliva. No water is needed for taking the tablet. Inform phenylketonuric patients that famotidine contains phenylalanine.

PREGNANCY AND LACTATION

• Pregnancy Category B. Reproduction studies performed in rats and rabbits have revealed no evidence of impaired fertility or harm to the fetus from famotidine. Studies performed in lactating rats have shown that famotidine is secreted into breast milk. Famotidine is detectable in human milk.

felodipine

(fell-o'da-peen)

Rx: Plendil

Drug Class: Calcium channel blockers

Pregnancy Category: C

Do not confuse Plendil with Pletal, or Renedil with Prinivil.

CLINICAL PHARMACOLOGY

Mechanism of Action: An antihypertensive and antianginal agent that inhibits calcium movement across cardiac and vascular smooth-muscle cell membranes. Potent peripheral vasodilator (does not depress SA or AV nodes). *Therapeutic Effect:* Increases myocardial contractility, heart rate, and cardiac output; decreases peripheral vascular resistance and BP.

Pharmacokinetics

Route	*Onset*	*Peak*	*Duration*
PO	2-5 hr	N/A	N/A

Rapidly, completely absorbed from the GI tract. Protein binding: greater than 99%. Undergoes first-pass metabolism in the liver. Primarily excreted in urine. Not removed by hemodialysis. **Half-life:** 11-16 hr.

AVAILABLE FORMS

• *Tablets (Extended-Release):* 2.5 mg, 5 mg, 10 mg.

INDICATIONS AND DOSAGES

Hypertension

PO

Adults. Initially, 5 mg/day as single dose.

Elderly, Patients with impaired hepatic function. Initially, 2.5 mg/day. Adjust dosage at no less than 2-wk intervals. Maintenance: 2.5-10 mg/day.

UNLABELED USES: Treatment of CHF, chronic angina pectoris, Raynaud's phenomenon

CONTRAINDICATIONS: None known.

INTERACTIONS

Drug

Beta-blockers: May have additive effect.

Digoxin: May increase digoxin blood concentration.

Erythromycin: May increase felodipine blood concentration and risk of toxicity.

Hypokalemia-producing agents (such as fursosemide and certain other diuretics): May increase risk of arrhythmias.

Procainamide, quinidine: May increase risk of QT-interval prolongation.

Herbal

DHEA: May increase felodipine blood concentration.

Food

Grapefruit, grapefruit juice: May increase the absorption and blood concentration of felodipine.

DIAGNOSTIC TEST EFFECTS: *None known.*

SIDE EFFECTS

Frequent (22%-18%)

Headache, peripheral edema

Occasional (6%-4%)

Flushing, respiratory infection, dizziness, light-headedness, asthenia (loss of strength, weakness)

Rare (less than 3%)

Paresthesia, abdominal discomfort, nervousness, muscle cramping, cough, diarrhea, constipation

SERIOUS REACTIONS

• Overdose produces nausea, somnolence, confusion, slurred speech, hypotension, and bradycardia.

SPECIAL CONSIDERATIONS

PRECAUTIONS

• Felodipine occasionally may precipitate hypotension. Exercise caution when using felodipine in patients with heart failure or compromised ventricular function, particularly in combination with a beta-blocker. Patients with impaired liver function may have elevated plasma concentrations of felodipine. Peripheral edema was the most common adverse event in the clinical trials.

PATIENT INFORMATION

• Instruct patients to take felodipine whole and not to crush or chew the tablets. Advise patients that mild gingival hyperplasia (gum swelling) has been reported. Good dental hygiene decreases the incidence and severity of gingival hyperplasia.

• NOTE: As with many other drugs, certain advice to patients being treated with felodipine is warranted. This information is intended to aid in the safe and effective use of this medication. Such advice is not a disclosure of all possible adverse or intended effects.

PREGNANCY AND LACTATION

• Pregnancy Category C. Studies in pregnant rabbits showed digital anomalies consisting of reduction in size and degree of ossification of the terminal phalanges in the fetuses. Fetal harm is not known. Excretion into human milk is not known.

fexofenadine hydrochloride

(fex-oh-fen'eh-deen)

Rx: Allegra

Drug Class: Antihistamines, H1

Pregnancy Category: C

CLINICAL PHARMACOLOGY

Mechanism of Action: A piperidine that competes with histamine for H_1-receptor sites on effector cells. *Therapeutic Effect:* Relieves allergic rhinitis symptoms.

Pharmacokinetics

Rapidly absorbed after PO administration. Protein binding: 60%-70%. Does not cross the blood-brain barrier. Minimally metabolized. Eliminated in feces and urine. Not removed by hemodialysis. **Half-life:** 14.4 hr (increased in renal impairment).

AVAILABLE FORMS

• *Tablets:* 30 mg, 60 mg, 180 mg.

INDICATIONS AND DOSAGES

Allergic rhinitis, urticaria

PO

Adults, Elderly, Children 12 yr and older. 60 mg twice a day or 180 mg once a day.

Children 6-11 yr. 30 mg twice a day.

Dosage in renal impairment

For adults, elderly, and children 12 years and older, dosage is reduced to 60 mg once a day. For children 6-11 years, dosage is reduced to 30 mg once a day.

CONTRAINDICATIONS: None known.

INTERACTIONS

Drug

Antacids: May decrease fexofenadine absorption if given within 15 minutes of a fexofenadine dose.

Herbal

None known.

Food

None known.

DIAGNOSTIC TEST EFFECTS: May suppress wheal and flare reactions to antigen skin testing unless drug is discontinued at least 4 days before testing.

SIDE EFFECTS

Rare (less than 2%)

Somnolence, headache, fatigue, nausea, vomiting, abdominal distress, dysmenorrhea

SERIOUS REACTIONS

- None known.

SPECIAL CONSIDERATIONS

PREGNANCY AND LACTATION

- Pregnancy Category C. No evidence of teratogenicity in rats or rabbits at oral terfenadine doses has been found. Excretion into human milk is not known.

fluconazole

(floo-con'a-zole)

Rx: Diflucan
Drug Class: Antifungals
Pregnancy Category: C
Do not confuse Diflucan with diclofenac.

CLINICAL PHARMACOLOGY

Mechanism of Action: A fungistatic antifungal that interferes with cytochrome P-450, an enzyme necessary for ergosterol formation. *Therapeutic Effect:* Directly damages fungal membrane, altering its function.

Pharmacokinetics

Well absorbed from GI tract. Widely distributed, including to CSF. Protein binding: 11%. Partially metabolized in liver. Excreted unchanged primarily in urine. Partially removed by hemodialysis. **Half-life:** 20-30 hr (increased in impaired renal function).

AVAILABLE FORMS

- *Tablets:* 50 mg, 100 mg, 150 mg, 200 mg.
- *Powder for Oral Suspension:* 10 mg/ml, 40 mg/ml.
- *Injection:* 2 mg/ml (in 100- or 200-ml containers).

INDICATIONS AND DOSAGES

Oropharyngeal candidiasis

PO, IV

Adults, Elderly. 200 mg once, then 100 mg/day for at least 14 days.

Children. 6 mg/kg/day once, then 3 mg/kg/day.

Esophageal candidiasis

PO, IV

Adults, Elderly. 200 mg once, then 100 mg/day (up to 400 mg/day) for 21 days and at least 14 days following resolution of symptoms.

Children. 6 mg/kg/day once, then 3 mg/kg/day (up to 12 mg/kg/day) for 21 days at at least 14 days following resolution of symptoms.

Vaginal candidiasis

PO

Adults. 150 mg once.

Prevention of candidiasis in patients undergoing bone marrow transplantation

PO

Adults. 400 mg/day.

Systemic candidiasis

PO, IV

Adults, Elderly. 400 mg once, then 200 mg/day (up to 400 mg/day) for at least 28 days and at least 14 days following resolution of symptoms.

Children. 6-12 mg/kg/day.

Cryptococcal meningitis
PO, IV
Adults, Elderly. 400 mg once, then 200 mg/day (up to 800 mg/day) for 10-12 wk after CSF becomes negative (200 mg/day for suppression of relapse in patients with AIDS).
Children. 12 mg/kg/day once, then 6-12 mg/kg/day (6 mg/kg/day for suppression of relapse in patients with AIDS).
Onychomycosis
PO
Adults. 150 mg/wk.
Dosage in renal impairment
After a loading dose of 400 mg, the daily dosage is based on creatinine clearance:

Creatinine Clearance	*% of Recommended Dose*
greater than 50 ml/min	100
21-50 ml/min	50
11-20 ml/min	25
Dialysis	Dose after dialysis

UNLABELED USES: Treatment of coccidioidomycosis, cryptococcosis, fungal pneumonia, onychomycosis, ringworm of the hand, septicemia
CONTRAINDICATIONS: None known.
INTERACTIONS
Drug
Cyclosporine: High fluconazole doses increase cyclosporine blood concentration.
Oral antidiabetics: May increase blood concentration and effects of oral antidiabetics.
Phenytoin, warfarin: May decrease the metabolism of these drugs.
Rifampin: May increase fluconazole metabolism.
Herbal
None known.
Food
None known.
DIAGNOSTIC TEST EFFECTS: May increase serum alkaline phosphatase, serum bilirubin, AST (SGOT), and ALT (SGPT) levels.
IV INCOMPATIBILITIES: Amphotericin B (Fungizone), amphotericin B complex (Abelcet, Ambisome, Amphotec), ampicillin (Polycillin), calcium gluconate, cefotaxime (Claforan), ceftazidime (Fortaz), ceftriaxone (Rocephin), cefuroxime (Zinacef), chloramphenicol (Chloromycetin), clindamycin (Cleocin), co-trimoxazole (Bactrim), diazepam (Valium), digoxin (Lanoxin), erythromycin (Erythrocin), furosemide (Lasix), haloperidol (Haldol), hydroxyzine (Vistaril), imipenem and cilastatin (Primaxin)
IV COMPATIBILITIES: Diltiazem (Cardizem), dobutamine (Dobutrex), dopamine (Intropin), heparin, lorazepam (Ativan), midazolam (Versed), propofol (Diprivan)
SIDE EFFECTS
Occasional (4%-1%)
Hypersensitivity reaction (including chills, fever, pruritus, and rash), dizziness, drowsiness, headache, constipation, diarrhea, nausea, vomiting, abdominal pain
SERIOUS REACTIONS
• Exfoliative skin disorders, serious hepatic effects, and blood dyscrasias (such as eosinophilia, thrombocytopenia, anemia, and leukopenia) have been reported rarely.

SPECIAL CONSIDERATIONS

PREGNANCY AND LACTATION
• Pregnancy Category C. Fluconazole was administered orally to pregnant rabbits during organogenesis. Maternal weight gain was impaired at all dose levels, and abortions occurred. Fluconazole is secreted in human milk at concentra-

tions similar to plasma. Therefore the use of fluconazole in nursing mothers is not recommended.

OCULAR CONSIDERATIONS

• Cyclosporine AUC and maximum concentration (Cmax) were determined before and after the administration of fluconazole 200 mg daily for 14 days in eight renal transplant patients who had been on cyclosporine therapy for at least 6 months and on a stable cyclosporine dose for at least 6 weeks. A significant increase in cyclosporine AUC, Cmax, and Cmin (24-hour concentration) and a significant reduction in apparent oral clearance occurred following the administration of fluconazole. The mean ±SD increase in AUC was 92% ± 43% (range: 18% to 147%). The Cmax increased 60% ± 48% (range: –5% to 133%). The Cmin increased 157% ± 96% (range: 33% to 360%). The apparent oral clearance decreased 45% ± 15% (range: –15% to –60%).

flucytosine

(floo-sye′-toe-seen)

Rx: Ancobon

Drug Class: Antifungals

Pregnancy Category: C

CLINICAL PHARMACOLOGY

Mechanism of Action: An antifungal that penetrates fungal cells and is converted to fluorouracil which competes with uracil interfering with fungal RNA and protein synthesis. *Therapeutic Effect:* Damages fungal membrane.

Pharmacokinetics

Well absorbed from gastrointestinal (GI) tract. Widely distributed, including cerebrospinal fluid (CSF). Protein binding: 2%-4%. Metabolized in liver. Partially removed by hemodialysis. **Half-life:** 3-8 hrs (half-life is increased with impaired renal function).

AVAILABLE FORMS

• *Capsule:* 250 mg, 500 mg.

INDICATIONS AND DOSAGES

Fungal infections, candidiasis, cryptococcosis

PO

Adults, Elderly, Children. 50 to 150 mg/kg/day in 4 equally divided doses.

Dosage in renal function impairment

Based on creatinine clearance:

Creatinine Clearance	*Dosage Interval*
20-40 ml/min	q12h
10-20 ml/min	q24h
0-10 ml/min	q24-48h

CONTRAINDICATIONS: Hypersensitivity to flucytosine.

INTERACTIONS

Drug

Amphotericin B: May increase the effects of flucytosine.

Levomethadyl: May increase risk of cardiotoxicity.

Zidovudine: May increase the risk of hematologic toxicity.

Herbal

None known.

Food

None known.

DIAGNOSTIC TEST EFFECTS: May increase creatinine values if determined by the ektachem method.

SIDE EFFECTS

Occasional

Pruritus, rash, photosensitivity, dizziness, drowsiness, headache, diarrhea, nausea, vomiting, abdominal pain, increased liver enzymes, jaundice, increased BUN and creatinine, weakness, hearing loss

SERIOUS REACTIONS

• Hepatic dysfunction and severe bone marrow suppression occur rarely.

SPECIAL CONSIDERATIONS

PRECAUTIONS

• Before instituting therapy with flucytosine, determine electrolytes (because of hypokalemia) and the hematologic and renal status of the patient. Close monitoring of the patient during therapy is essential.

PREGNANCY AND LACTATION

• Pregnancy Category C. Flucytosine has been shown to be teratogenic in the rat and mouse. Excretion into human milk is not known.

fluorescein

(flure'-e-seen sow-dee-um)

Rx: AK-Fluor, Angioscein, Fluorescite, Fluorets, Fluor-I-Strip, Fluor-I-Strip-A.T., Ful-Glo, Funduscein, Ocu-Flur 10

Drug Class: Diagnostics, nonradioactive

Do not confuse with fluoride.

CLINICAL PHARMACOLOGY

Mechanism of Action: An indicator dye used as a diagnostic agent with a low molecular weight, high water solubility, and fluorescence that penetrates any break in epithelial barrier to permit rapid penetration. Emits light at a wavelength of 520 to 530 nanometers (green-yellow) when exposed to light in the blue wavelength (465 to 490 nanometers). *Therapeutic Effect:* Diagnosis of corneal and conjunctival abnormalities.

Pharmacokinetics

Rapidly absorbed. Protein binding: 85%. Widely distributed. Metabolized in liver to an active metabolite, fluorescein monoglucuronide. Primarily excreted in urine. **Half-life:** 24 min (parent compound), 4 hrs (metabolite).

AVAILABLE FORMS

• *Injection, solution:* 10% (AK-Fluor, Angiscein, Fluorescite), 25% (AK-Fluor, Fluorescite).

• *Strip, ophthalmic:* 0.6 mg (Ful-Glo), 1 mg (Fluorets, Fluor-I-Strip-AT), 9 mg (Fluor-I-Strip).

INDICATIONS AND DOSAGES

Retinal angiography

Injection

Adults, Elderly. Inject contents of ampule or vial of 10% or 25% solution rapidly into the antecubital vein

Applanation tonometry

Ophthlalmic strips

Adults, Elderly. Place strip, which has been moistened with a drop of sterile water, at the fornix in the lower cul-de-sac close to the punctum. Patient should close lid tightly over strip until desired amount of staining is observed or retract upper lid and touch tip of strip to the bulbar conjunctiva on the temporal side until adequate staining is achieved.

CONTRAINDICATIONS: Concomitant soft contact lens use (ophthalmic strips), hypersensitivity to fluorescein or any component of the formulation

INTERACTIONS

Drug

None known.

Herbal

None known.

Food

None known.

DIAGNOSTIC TEST EFFECTS: May interfere with digoxin assay results.

SIDE EFFECTS

Occasional

Ophthalmic: Burning sensation in the eye

Injection: Stinging, bronchospasm, generalized hives and itching, hypersensitivity, headache gastrointestinal distress, nausea, strong taste, vomiting, hypotension, syncope

Rare

Injection: anaphylaxis, basilar artery ischemia, cardiac arrest, severe shock, convulsions, thrombophlebitis at injection site

SERIOUS REACTIONS

• Anaphylactic reactions have occurred leading to laryngeal edema, bronchospasm, shock and even death.

SPECIAL CONSIDERATIONS

INDICATIONS AND USAGE

• Use of fluorescein sodium is indicated by diagnostic fluorescein angiography or angioscopy of the fundus and of the iris vasculature.

PRECAUTIONS

• Exercise caution in patients with a history of allergy or bronchial asthma. An emergency tray including items such as 0.1% epinephrine for intravenous or intramuscular use; an antihistamine, soluble steroid, and aminophylline for intravenous use; and oxygen should always be available in the event of possible reaction to fluorescein injection.

• Patient Warning: Skin will attain a temporary yellowish discoloration. Urine attains a bright yellow color. Discoloration of the skin fades in 6 to 12 hours; urine fluorescein concentration decreases in 24 to 36 hours. Generalized hives and itching, bronchospasm, and anaphylaxis have been reported but are rare. A strong taste may develop after injection.

PREGNANCY AND LACTATION

• Avoid angiography on patients who are pregnant, especially those in first trimester. No reports have indicated fetal complications from fluorescein injection during pregnancy. Excretion into human milk is not known.

CONSIDERATIONS

• Off-label uses include oral fluorography. The dosage is 1000 to 1500 mg of fluorescein sodium mixed with a citrus drink and crushed ice.

fluorescein sodium; proparacaine hydrochloride

(flure'e-seen sow'dee-um; proe-par'a-kane hye-droe-klor'ide)

Rx: Flucaine, Fluoracaine

Drug Class: Anesthetics, ophthalmic; Diagnostics, nonradioactive; Ophthalmics

CLINICAL PHARMACOLOGY

Mechanism of Action: A diagnostic agent and local anesthetics that prevents initiation and transmission of impulses at nerve cell membranes by decreasing ion permeability through stabilizing. *Therapeutic Effect:* Local anesthetic effect.

Pharmacokinetics

None reported.

AVAILABLE FORMS

• *Ophthalmic Solution:* 0.25% fluorescein sodium and 0.5% proparacaine hydrochloride (Flucaine, Fluoracaine).

INDICATIONS AND DOSAGES

Ophthalmic surgery

Ophthalmic

Adults, Elderly, Children. Instill 1 drop in each eye every 5-10 minutes for 5-7 doses.

Tonometry, gonioscopy, suture removal

Ophthalmic

Adults, Elderly. Instill 1-2 drops in each eye just prior to procedure.

CONTRAINDICATIONS: Hypersensitivity to fluorescein, proparacaine, or any component of the formulation or ester-type local anesthetics

INTERACTIONS

Drug

None known.

Herbal

None known.

Food

None known.

DIAGNOSTIC TEST EFFECTS: *None known.*

SIDE EFFECTS

Occasional

Burning, stinging of the eye

Rare

Allergic contact dermatitis

SERIOUS REACTIONS

• Allergic contact dermatitis, conjunctival congestion and hemorrhage, corneal opacification, erosion of the corneal epithelium, iritis, irritation, keratitis, and sensitization have been reported.

SPECIAL CONSIDERATIONS

INDICATIONS AND USAGE

• Tonometry, gonioscopy, and removal of corneal foreign bodies

PRECAUTIONS

• Use fluorescein sodium and proparacaine hydrochloride cautiously in patients with known allergies, cardiac disease, or hyperthyroidism. Prolonged use possibly may delay wound healing. Rare systemic toxicity (manifested by central nervous system simulation followed by depression) may occur. Protection of the eye from irritating chemicals, foreign bodies, and rubbing during the period of anesthesia is important. Thoroughly rinse tonometers soaked in sterilizing or detergent solutions with sterile distilled water before use. Advise patients to avoid touching the eye until the anesthesia has worn off.

fluorometholone

(flure-oh-meth'oh-lone)

Rx: Eflone, Flarex, Fluor-Op, FML Forte Liquifilm, FML Liquifilm, FML S.O.P.

Drug Class: Corticosteroids, ophthalmic; Ophthalmics

Pregnancy Category: C

CLINICAL PHARMACOLOGY

Mechanism of Action: An ophthalmic corticosteroid that decreases inflammation by suppression of migration of polymorphonuclear leukocytes and reversal of increased capillary permeability. *Therapeutic Effect:* Decrease ocular inflammation.

Pharmacokinetics

Absorbed into aqueous humor with slight systemic absorption.

AVAILABLE FORMS

• *Ophthalmic Suspension, as base:* 0.1% (Eflone, FML Liquifilm, Flarex, Fluor-Op), 0.25% (FML Forte Liquifilm).

• *Ophthalmic Ointment:* 0.1% (FML S.O.P).

INDICATIONS AND DOSAGES

Treatment of steroid-responsive inflammatory conditions of the eye

Ophthalmic Ointment

Adults, Elderly. Apply thin strip to conjunctival sac every 4 hours in severe cases or 1-3 times per day in mild to moderate cases.

Ophthalmic Solution

Adults, Elderly, Children 2 yr and older. Instill 1-2 drops into conjunctival sac every hour during the day, every 2 hours at night until favorable response is obtained. Then use 1

drop every 4 hours. For mild to moderate inflammation, instill 1-2 drops into conjunctival sac 2-4 times/day.
CONTRAINDICATIONS: Viral diseases of the cornea and conjunctiva, mycobacterial or fungal infections of the eye, untreated eye infections which may be masked or enhanced by steroids, hypersensitivity to fluorometholone or any component of the formulation

INTERACTIONS

Drug

None known.

Herbal

None known.

Food

None known.

DIAGNOSTIC TEST EFFECTS: *None known.*

SIDE EFFECTS

Occasional

Burning, tearing, itching, blurred vision

Rare

Cataract formation, corneal ulcers, glaucoma with optic nerve damage

SERIOUS REACTIONS

- Hypercorticoidism and taste perversion occurs rarely.
- Superinfections, particularly with fungi, may result from bacterial imbalance via any route of administration.

SPECIAL CONSIDERATIONS

PRECAUTIONS

- Renewal of the medication order beyond 20 ml should be made by an eye care practitioner only after examination of the patient with fluorescein staining. If signs and symptoms fail to improve after 2 days, reevaluate the patient. Suspect fungal invasion in any persistent corneal ulceration where a corticosteroid has been used or is in use. Take fungal cultures when appropriate. If this product is used for 10 days or longer, monitor intraocular pressure.

PATIENT INFORMATION

- If inflammation or pain persists longer than 48 hours or becomes aggravated, advise patients to discontinue the use of the medication and consult a physician. This product is sterile when packaged. To prevent contamination, instruct patients to avoid touching the bottle tip to eyelids or to any other surface. The use of this bottle by more than one person may spread infection. Instruct patients to keep the bottle tightly closed when not in use and to keep the drug out of reach of children.

PREGNANCY AND LACTATION

- Pregnancy Category C. Fluorometholone has been shown to be embryocidal and teratogenic in rabbits when administered at low multiples of the human ocular dose. Fetal harm is not known with topical administration. Excretion into human milk is not known.

fluorometholone acetate

(flure-oh-meth'-oh-lone ass'-eh-tate)

Drug Class: Corticosteroids, ophthalmic; Ophthalmics
Pregnancy Category: C

CLINICAL PHARMACOLOGY

Mechanism of Action: An ophthalmic corticosteroid that decreases inflammation by suppression of migration of polymorphonuclear leukocytes and reversal of increased capillary permeability. *Therapeutic Effect:* Decrease ocular inflammation.

Pharmacokinetics

Absorbed into aqueous humor with slight systemic absorption.

AVAILABLE FORMS

- *Ophthalmic Suspension:* 5 ml and 10 ml plastic Drop-Tainer dispensers.

INDICATIONS AND DOSAGES

Treatment of steroid-responsive inflammatory conditions of the eye

Ophthalmic

Adults, Elderly, Children 2 yr and older. Instill 1-2 drops every hour during the day, every 2 hours at night until favorable response is obtained. Then use 1 drop every 4 hours. For mild to moderate inflammation, instill 1-2 drops 2-4 times/day.

CONTRAINDICATIONS: Viral diseases of the cornea and conjunctiva, mycobacterial or fungal infections of the eye, untreated eye infections which may be masked or enhanced by steroids, hypersensitivity to fluorometholone acetate or any component of the formulation

INTERACTIONS

Drug

None known.

Herbal

None known.

Food

None known.

DIAGNOSTIC TEST EFFECTS: *None known.*

SIDE EFFECTS

Occasional

Burning, tearing, itching, blurred vision

Rare

Cataract formation, corneal ulcers, glaucoma with optic nerve damage

SERIOUS REACTIONS

- Hypercorticoidism and taste perversion occurs rarely.
- Superinfections, particularly with fungi, may result from bacterial imbalance via any route of administration.

SPECIAL CONSIDERATIONS

PRECAUTIONS

- Consider fungus invasion in any persistent corneal ulceration where a steroid has been used or is in use.

PREGNANCY AND LACTATION

- Pregnancy Category C. Fluorometholone has been shown to be embryocidal and teratogenic in rabbits when administered at low multiples of the human ocular dose. Fetal harm is not known with topical administration. Excretion into human milk is not known.

fluorometholone; sulfacetamide sodium

(flure-oh-meth'oh-lone; sul-fa-set'a-mide soe'dee-um)

Rx: FML-S Liquifilm

Drug Class: Anti-infectives, ophthalmic; Antibiotics, sulfonamides; Corticosteroids, ophthalmic; Ophthalmics

Pregnancy Category: C

CLINICAL PHARMACOLOGY

Mechanism of Action: Fluorometholone is an ophthalmic corticosteroid that decreases inflammation by suppression of migration of polymorphonuclear leukocytes and reversal of increased capillary permeability. Sulfacetamide sodium interferes with synthesis of folic acid that bacteria require for growth. *Therapeutic Effect:* Decrease ocular inflammation. Prevents further bacterial growth. Bacteriostatic.

Pharmacokinetics

Absorbed into aqueous humor with slight systemic absorption.

AVAILABLE FORMS

• *Ophthalmic Suspension:* 0.1% fluorometholone and 10% sulfacetamide sodium (FML-S).

INDICATIONS AND DOSAGES

Treatment of steroid-responsive inflammatory conditions of the eye

Ophthalmic

Adults, Elderly, Children older than 2 months. Instill 1-3 drops every 2-3 hours while awake.

INTERACTIONS

Drug

None known.

Herbal

None known.

Food

None known.

DIAGNOSTIC TEST EFFECTS: *None known.*

SIDE EFFECTS

Occasional

Burning, tearing, itching, blurred vision

Rare

Cataract formation, corneal ulcers, glaucoma with optic nerve damage

SERIOUS REACTIONS

• Superinfections, particularly with fungi, may result from bacterial imbalance via any route of administration.

SPECIAL CONSIDERATIONS

PRECAUTIONS

• Renewal of the medication order beyond 20 ml should be made only by an eye care practitioner after evaluation of the patient's intraocular pressure; examination of the patient with fluorescein staining.

PREGNANCY AND LACTATION

• Pregnancy Category C. Fluorometholone has been shown to be embryocidal and teratogenic in rabbits when administered at low multiples of the human dose. Fetal harm is not known with topical administration. Excretion into human milk is not known.

---

fluoxetine hydrochloride

(floo-ox'e-teen)

Rx: Prozac, Prozac Weekly, Rapiflux, Sarafem

Drug Class: Antidepressants, serotonin specific reuptake inhibitors

Pregnancy Category: C

Do not confuse fluoxetine with fluvastatin, Prozac with Prilosec, Proscar, or ProSom; or Sarafem with Serophene.

CLINICAL PHARMACOLOGY

Mechanism of Action: A psychotherapeutic agent that selectively inhibits serotonin uptake in the CNS, enhancing serotonergic function. *Therapeutic Effect:* Relieves depression; reduces obsessive-compulsive and bulimic behavior.

Pharmacokinetics

Well absorbed from the GI tract. Crosses the blood-brain barrier. Protein binding: 94%. Metabolized in the liver to active metabolite. Primarily excreted in urine. Not removed by hemodialysis. **Half-life:** 2-3 days; metabolite 7-9 days.

AVAILABLE FORMS

• *Capsules (Prozac):* 10 mg, 20 mg, 40 mg.

• *Capsules (Sarafem):* 10 mg, 20 mg.

• *Capsules (Delayed-Release [Prozac Weekly]):* 90 mg.

• *Oral Solution (Prozac):* 20 mg/5 ml.

• *Tablets (Prozac):* 10 mg, 20 mg.

INDICATIONS AND DOSAGES

Depression, obsessive-compulsive disorder

PO

Adults. Initially, 20 mg each morning. If therapeutic improvement does not occur after 2 wk, gradually increase to maximum of 80 mg/day in 2 equally divided doses in morning and at noon. Prozac Weekly: 90 mg/wk, begin 7 days after last dose of 20 mg.

Elderly. Initially, 10 mg/day. May increase by 10-20 mg q2wk.

Children 7-17 yr. Initially, 5-10 mg/day. Titrate upward as needed. Usual dosage is 20 mg/day.

Panic disorder

PO

Adults, Elderly. Initially, 10 mg/day. May increase to 20 mg/day after 1 week. Maximum: 60 mg/day.

Bulimia nervosa

PO

Adults. 60 mg each morning.

Premenstrual dysphoric disorder

PO

Adults. 20 mg/day.

UNLABELED USES: Treatment of hot flashes

CONTRAINDICATIONS: Use within 14 days of MAOIs

INTERACTIONS

Drug

Alcohol, other CNS depressants: May increase CNS depression.

Highly protein-bound medications (including oral anticoagulants): May increase adverse effects.

MAOIs: May produce serotonin syndrome and neuroleptic malignant syndrome.

Phenytoin: May increase phenytoin blood concentration and risk of toxicity.

Herbal

St. John's wort: May increase fluoxetine's pharmacologic effects and risk of toxicity.

Food

None known.

DIAGNOSTIC TEST EFFECTS: *None known.*

SIDE EFFECTS

Frequent (more than 10%)

Headache, asthenia, insomnia, anxiety, nervousness, somnolence, nausea, diarrhea, decreased appetite

Occasional (9%-2%)

Dizziness, tremor, fatigue, vomiting, constipation, dry mouth, abdominal pain, nasal congestion, diaphoresis, rash

Rare (less than 2%)

Flushed skin, light-headedness, impaired concentration

SERIOUS REACTIONS

- Overdose may produce seizures, nausea, vomiting, agitation, and restlessness.

SPECIAL CONSIDERATIONS

PRECAUTIONS

- Anxiety and insomnia and altered appetite and weight have been reported.
- Mania/hypomania, seizures, suicide, and hyponatremia has been reported. Caution patients about operating hazardous machinery, including automobiles.

PATIENT INFORMATION

- Because fluoxetine may impair judgment, thinking, or motor skills, advise patients to avoid driving a car or operating hazardous machinery until they are reasonably certain that their performance is not affected.
- Advise patients to inform their physician if they are taking or plan to

take any prescription or over-the-counter drugs or alcohol.

- Advise patients to notify their physician if they become pregnant or intend to become pregnant during therapy.
- Advise patients to notify their physician if they are breast-feeding an infant.
- Advise patients to notify their physician if they develop a rash or hives.

PREGNANCY AND LACTATION

- Pregnancy Category B. Fetal harm is not known. Because fluoxetine is excreted in human milk, nursing while taking fluoxetine is not recommended.

flurbiprofen

(flure-bi'proe-fen)

Rx: Ansaid, Ocufen

Drug Class: Analgesics, non-narcotic; Nonsteroidal anti-inflammatory drugs; Ophthalmics

Pregnancy Category: B

Do not confuse Ocufen with Ocuflox.

CLINICAL PHARMACOLOGY

Mechanism of Action: A phenylalkanoic acid that produces analgesic and antiinflammatory effect by inhibiting prostaglandin synthesis. Also relaxes the iris sphincter. *Therapeutic Effect:* Reduces the inflammatory response and intensity of pain. Prevents or decreases miosis during cataract surgery.

Pharmacokinetics

Well absorbed from the GI tract; ophthalmic solution penetrates cornea after administration, and may be systemically absorbed. Protein binding: 99%. Widely distributed. Metabolized in the liver. Primarily excreted in urine. **Half-life:** 3-4 hr.

AVAILABLE FORMS

- *Tablets (Ansaid):* 50 mg, 100 mg.
- *Ophthalmic Solution (Ocufen):* 0.03%.

INDICATIONS AND DOSAGES

Rheumatoid arthritis, osteoarthritis

PO

Adults, Elderly. 200-300 mg/day in 2-4 divided doses. Maximum: 100 mg/dose or 300 mg/day.

Dysmenorrhea, pain

PO

Adults. 50 mg 4 times a day

Usual ophthalmic dosage

Adults, Elderly, Children. Apply 1 drop q30min starting 2 hr before surgery for total of 4 doses.

CONTRAINDICATIONS: Active peptic ulcer, chronic inflammation of GI tract, GI bleeding or ulceration, history of hypersensitivity to aspirin or NSAIDs

INTERACTIONS

Drug

Acetylcholine, carbachol: May decrease the effects of these drugs (with ophthalmic flurbiprofen).

Antihypertensives, diuretics: May decrease the effects of these drugs.

Aspirin, other salicylates: May increase the risk of GI side effects such as bleeding.

Bone marrow depressants: May increase the risk of hematologic reactions.

Epinephrine, other antiglaucoma medications: May decrease the antiglaucoma effect of these drugs.

Heparin, oral anticoagulants, thrombolytics: May increase the effects of these drugs.

Lithium: May increase the blood concentration and risk of toxicity of lithium.

Methotrexate: May increase the risk of methotrexate toxicity.
Probenecid: May increase the flurbiprofen blood concentration.

Herbal

Feverfew: May decrease the effects of feverfew.
Ginkgo biloba: May increase the risk of bleeding.

Food

None known.

DIAGNOSTIC TEST EFFECTS: May increase bleeding time and serum LDH, alkaline phosphatase, AST (SGOT), and ALT (SGPT) levels.

SIDE EFFECTS

Occasional

PO (9%-3%): Headache, abdominal pain, diarrhea, indigestion, nausea, fluid retention

Ophthalmic: Burning or stinging on instillation, keratitis, elevated intraocular pressure

Rare (less than 3%)

PO: Blurred vision, flushed skin, dizziness, somnolence, nervousness, insomnia, unusual fatigue, constipation, decreased appetite, vomiting, confusion

SERIOUS REACTIONS

- Overdose may result in acute renal failure.
- Rare reactions with long-term use include peptic ulcer disease, GI bleeding, gastritis, severe hepatic reaction (jaundice), nephrotoxicity (hematuria, dysuria, proteinuria), a severe hypersensitivity reaction (angioedema, bronchospasm) and cardiac arrhythmias.

SPECIAL CONSIDERATIONS

PRECAUTIONS

- Wound healing may be delayed with the use of flurbiprofen sodium. Cautious use of flurbiprofen sodium 0.03% liquifilm sterile ocular solution is recommended in surgical patients with known bleeding tendencies or who are receiving other medications that may prolong bleeding time.

PREGNANCY AND LACTATION

- Pregnancy Category C. Flurbiprofen has been shown to be embryocidal, to delay parturition, to prolong gestation, to reduce weight, and/or slightly to retard growth of fetuses when given to rats in oral doses. Fetal harm is not known with topical administration. Excretion into human milk is not known.

fluticasone propionate

(flu-tic'a-zone)

Rx: Cutivate, Flonase, Flovent, Flovent Rotadisk

Drug Class: Corticosteroids, inhalation; Corticosteroids, topical; Dermatologics

Pregnancy Category: C

CLINICAL PHARMACOLOGY

Mechanism of Action: A corticosteroid that controls the rate of protein synthesis, depresses migration of polymorphonuclear leukocytes, reverses capillary permeability, and stabilizes lysosomal membranes. *Therapeutic Effect:* Prevents or controls inflammation.

Pharmacokinetics

Inhalation/intranasal: Protein binding: 91%. Undergoes extensive first-pass metabolism in liver. Excreted in urine. **Half-life:** 3-7.8 hrs. Topical: Amount absorbed depends on affected area and skin condition (absorption increased with fever, hydration, inflamed or denuded skin).

AVAILABLE FORMS

- *Aerosol for Oral Inhalation (Flovent, Flovent HFA):* 44 mcg/inhalation, 110 mcg/inhalation, 220 mcg/ inhalation.
- *Powder for Oral Inhalation (Flovent Diskus):* 50 mcg, 100 mcg, 250 mcg.
- *Intranasal Spray (Flonase):* 50 mcg/inhalation.
- *Topical Cream (Cutivate):* 0.05%.
- *Topical Ointment (Cutivate):* 0.005%.

INDICATIONS AND DOSAGES

Allergic Rhinitis

Intranasal

Adults, Elderly. Initially, 200 mcg (2 sprays in each nostril once daily or 1 spray in each nostril q12h). Maintenance: 1 spray in each nostril once daily. Maximum: 200 mcg/day.

Children older than 4 yr. Initially, 100 mcg (1 spray in each nostril once daily). Maximum: 200 mcg/day.

Relief of inflammation and pruritus associated with steroid-responsive disorders, such as contact dermatitis and eczema

Topical

Adults, Elderly, Children older than 3 mo. Apply sparingly to affected area once or twice a day.

Maintenance treatment for asthma for those previously treated with bronchodilators

Inhalation Powder (Flovent Diskus)

Adults, Elderly, Children 12 yr and older. Initially, 100 mcg q12h. Maximum: 500 mcg/day.

Inhalation (Oral [Flovent])

Adults, Elderly, Children 12 yr and older. 88 mcg twice a day. Maximum: 440 mcg twice a day.

Maintenance treatment for asthma for those previously treated with inhaled steroids

Inhalation Powder (Flovent Diskus)

Adults, Elderly, Children 12 yr and older. Initially, 100-250 mcg q12h. Maximum: 500 mcg q12h.

Inhalation (Oral [Flovent])

Adults, Elderly, Children 12 yr and older. 88-220 mcg twice a day. Maximum: 440 mcg twice a day.

Maintenance treatment for asthma for those previously treated with oral steroids

Inhalation Powder (Flovent Diskus)

Adults, Elderly, Children 12 yr and older. 500-1000 mcg twice a day.

Inhalation (Oral [Flovent])

*Adults, Elderly, Children 12 yr and older.*880 mcg twice a day.

CONTRAINDICATIONS: Primary treatment of status asthmaticus or other acute asthma episodes (inhalation); untreated localized infection of nasal mucosa

INTERACTIONS

Drug

None known.

Herbal

None known.

Food

None known.

DIAGNOSTIC TEST EFFECTS: *None known.*

SIDE EFFECTS

Frequent

Inhalation: Throat irritation, hoarseness, dry mouth, cough, temporary wheezing, oropharyngeal candidiasis (particularly if mouth is not rinsed with water after each administration)

Intranasal: Mild nasopharyngeal irritation; nasal burning, stinging, or dryness; rebound congestion; rhinorrhea; loss of taste

Occasional

Inhalation: Oral candidiasis

Intranasal: Nasal and pharyngeal candidiasis, headache

Topical: Skin burning, pruritus

SERIOUS REACTIONS

- None known.

SPECIAL CONSIDERATIONS

PRECAUTIONS

• Some patients may experience symptoms of systemically active corticosteroid withdrawal—for example, joint and/or muscular pain, lassitude, and depression—despite maintenance or even improvement of respiratory function. Hypercorticism and adrenal suppression may appear in a small number of patients. A reduction of growth velocity in children or teenagers may occur as a result of inadequate control of chronic diseases such as asthma or from use of corticosteroids for treatment. Use fluticasone propionate with caution in patients with tuberculous infection of the respiratory tract; untreated systemic fungal, bacterial, viral, or parasitic infections; or ocular herpes simplex.

PATIENT INFORMATION

• Patients being treated with fluticasone propionate should receive the following information and instructions. This information is intended to aid them in the safe and effective use of this medication. This information is not a disclosure of all possible adverse or intended effects.

• Patients should use fluticasone propionate at regular intervals as directed. Results of clinical trials indicated significant improvement may occur within the first 1 or 2 days of treatment; however, the full benefit may not be achieved until treatment has been administered for 1 to 2 weeks or longer. The patient should not increase the prescribed dosage but should contact the physician if symptoms do not improve or if the condition worsens.

• Warn patients to avoid exposure to chickenpox or measles and, if they are exposed, to consult their physicians without delay.

• For the proper use of fluticasone propionate inhalation powder or aerosol and to attain maximum improvement, the patient should read and follow carefully the accompanying patient's instructions for use.

PREGNANCY AND LACTATION

• Pregnancy Category C. Subcutaneous studies in the mouse and rat revealed fetal toxicity including embryonic growth retardation, omphalocele, cleft palate, and retarded cranial ossification. Fetal harm is not known. Excretion into human milk is not known.

OCULAR CONSIDERATIONS

• Adverse reactions include dryness and irritation, conjunctivitis, and blurred vision. Rare instances of glaucoma, increased intraocular pressure, and cataracts have been reported following the inhaled administration of corticosteroids, including fluticasone propionate.

fluvastatin

(floo'va-sta-tin)

Rx: Lescol, Lescol XL

Drug Class: Antihyperlipidemics; HMG CoA reductase inhibitors

Pregnancy Category: X

Do not confuse fluvastatin with fluoxetine.

CLINICAL PHARMACOLOGY

Mechanism of Action: An antihyperlipidemic that inhibits HMG-CoA reductase, the enzyme that catalyzes the early step in cholesterol synthesis. *Therapeutic Effect:* Decreases LDL cholesterol, VLDL, and plasma triglyceride levels. Slightly increases HDL cholesterol concentration.

Pharmacokinetics

Well absorbed from the GI tract and is unaffected by food. Does not cross the blood-brain barrier. Protein binding: greater than 98%. Primarily eliminated in feces. **Half-life:** 1.2 hr.

AVAILABLE FORMS

- *Capsules (Lescol):* 20 mg, 40 mg.
- *Tablets (Extended-Release [Lescol XL]):* 80 mg.

INDICATIONS AND DOSAGES

Hyperlipoproteinemia

PO

Adults, Elderly. Initially, 20 mg/day (capsule) in the evening. May increase up to 40 mg/day. Maintenance: 20-40 mg/day in a single dose or divided doses.

Patients requiring more than a 25% decrease in LDL cholesterol. 40 mg (capsule) 1-2 times a day. Or 80-mg tablet once a day.

CONTRAINDICATIONS: Active hepatic disease, unexplained increased serum transaminase levels

INTERACTIONS

Drug

Cyclosporine, erythromycin, gemfibrozil, immunosuppressants, niacin: Increases the risk of acute renal failure and rhabdomyolysis with these drugs.

Herbal

None known.

Food

None known.

DIAGNOSTIC TEST EFFECTS: May increase serum CK and transaminase concentrations

SIDE EFFECTS

Frequent (8%-5%)

Headache, dyspepsia, back pain, myalgia, arthralgia, diarrhea, abdominal cramping, rhinitis

Occasional (4%-2%)

Nausea, vomiting, insomnia, constipation, flatulence, rash, pruritus, fatigue, cough, dizziness

SERIOUS REACTIONS

- Myositis (inflammation of voluntary muscle) with or without increased CK, and muscle weakness, occur rarely. These conditions may progress to frank rhabdomyolysis and renal impairment.

SPECIAL CONSIDERATIONS

PRECAUTIONS

- The 3-hydroxy-3-methylglutaryl–coenzyme A (HMG-CoA) reductase inhibitors may cause elevation of creatine phosphokinase and transaminase levels. These inhibitors theoretically might blunt adrenal or gonadal steroid hormone production.

PATIENT INFORMATION

- Advise patients to report promptly unexplained muscle pain, tenderness, or weakness, particularly if accompanied by malaise or fever. Inform women that if they become pregnant while receiving fluvastatin sodium, they should discontinue the drug immediately to avoid possible harmful effects on a developing fetus from a relative deficit of cholesterol and biological products derived from cholesterol.
- In addition, advise female patients not to take fluvastatin sodium during nursing.

PREGNANCY AND LACTATION

- Pregnancy Category X. The HMG-CoA reductase inhibitors are contraindicated during pregnancy and in nursing mothers. Administer fluvastatin sodium to women of childbearing age only when such patients are highly unlikely to conceive and have been informed of the potential hazards. If the patient becomes pregnant while taking this class of drug, discontinue therapy and apprise the patient of the potential hazard to the fetus. Based on preclinical data, the drug is present in breast milk in a 2:1 ratio (milk:plasma). Because of the potential for serious adverse reactions in nursing infants, nursing women should not take fluvastatin sodium.

folic acid/sodium folate (vitamin B_9)

(foe'lik)

Drug Class: Hematinics; Vitamins/minerals

Pregnancy Category: A

Do not confuse Folvite with Florvite.

CLINICAL PHARMACOLOGY

Mechanism of Action: A coenzyme that stimulates production of platelets, RBCs, and WBCs. *Therapeutic Effect:* Essential for nucleoprotein synthesis and maintenance of normal erythropoiesis.

Pharmacokinetics

PO form almost completely absorbed from the GI tract (upper duodenum). Protein binding: High. Metabolized in the liver and plasma to active form. Excreted in urine. Removed by hemodialysis.

AVAILABLE FORMS

- *Tablets:* 0.4 mg, 0.8 mg, 1 mg.
- *Injection:* 5 mg/ml.

INDICATIONS AND DOSAGES

Vitamin B_9 deficiency

PO, IV, IM, Subcutaneous

Adults, Elderly, Children 12 yr and older. Initially, 1 mg/day. Maintenance: 0.5 mg/day.

Children 1-11 yr. Initially 1 mg/day. Maintenance: 0.1-0.4 mg/day.

Infants. 50 mcg/day.

Dietary supplement

PO, IV, IM, Subcutaneous

Adults, Elderly, Children 4 yr and older. 0.4 mg/day.

Children 1-younger than 4 yr. 0.3 mg/day.

Children younger than 1 yr. 0.1 mg/day.

Pregnant women. 0.8 mg/day.

UNLABELED USES: To decrease the risk of colon cancer

CONTRAINDICATIONS: Anemias (aplastic, normocytic, pernicious, refractory)

INTERACTIONS

Drug

Analgesics, carbamazepine, estrogens: May increase folic acid requirements.

Antacids, cholestyramine: May decrease the absorption of folic acid.

Hydantoin anticonvulsants: May decrease the effects of these drugs.

Methotrexate, triamterene, trimethoprim: May antagonize the effects of folic acid.

Herbal

None known.

Food

None known.

DIAGNOSTIC TEST EFFECTS: May decrease vitamin B_{12} concentration.

SIDE EFFECTS

None known.

SERIOUS REACTIONS

- Allergic hypersensitivity occurs rarely with parenteral form. Oral folic acid is nontoxic.

SPECIAL CONSIDERATIONS

PRECAUTIONS

- Folic acid may obscure pernicious anemia in that hematologic remission can occur while neurologic manifestations remain progressive.

PREGNANCY AND LACTATION

- Pregnancy Category A.

fomivirsen

(foh-mih-ver'-sen)

Rx: Vitravene

Drug Class: Antivirals; Ophthalmics

Pregnancy Category: C

CLINICAL PHARMACOLOGY

Mechanism of Action: An antiviral that binds to messenger RNA, inhibiting the synthesis of viral proteins. *Therapeutic Effect:* Blocks replication of cytomegalovirus (CMV).

AVAILABLE FORMS

- *Intravitreal Injection:* 6.6 mg/ml.

INDICATIONS AND DOSAGES

CMV retinitis

Intravitreal injection

Adults. 330 mcg (0.05 ml) every other week for 2 doses, then 330 mcg every 4 weeks.

CONTRAINDICATIONS: None significant.

INTERACTIONS

Drug

None significant.

Herbal

None significant.

Food

None significant.

DIAGNOSTIC TEST EFFECTS: May alter liver function test results and serum alkaline phosphatase level. May decrease blood Hgb levels and neutrophil and platelet counts.

SIDE EFFECTS

Frequent (10%-5%)

Fever, headache, nausea, diarrhea, vomiting, abdominal pain, anemia, uveitis, abnormal vision

Occasional (5%-2%)

Chest pain, confusion, dizziness, depression, neuropathy, anorexia, weight loss, pancreatitis, dyspnea, cough

SERIOUS REACTIONS

- Thrombocytopenia may occur.

SPECIAL CONSIDERATIONS

PRECAUTIONS

- Ocular inflammation (uveitis) including iritis and vitritis occurs in approximately 1 in 4 patients. Inflammatory reactions are more common during induction dosing. Topical corticosteroids have been useful in the medical management of inflammatory changes, and with medical management and time, patients may be able to continue to receive intravitreal injections of fomivirsen sodium after the inflammation has resolved.
- Increased intraocular pressure has been commonly reported. The increase is usually a transient event, and in most cases the pressure returns to the normal range without any treatment or with temporary use of topical medications. Monitor intraocular pressure at each visit and manage elevations of intraocular pressure, if sustained, with medications to lower intraocular pressure.

PATIENT INFORMATION

- Fomivirsen sodium intravitreal injection is not a cure for cytomegalovirus (CMV) retinitis, and some immunocompromised patients may continue to experience progression of retinitis during and following treatment. Advise patients receiving fomivirse sodium to have regular follow-up ocular examinations. Infection with CMV may exist as a systemic disease, in addition to CMV retinitis. Therefore, monitor patients for extraocular CMV infections (e.g., pneumonitis and colitis) and retinitis in the opposite eye, if only one infected eye is being treated. Patients infected with human immunodeficiency virus should continue taking antiretroviral therapy as otherwise indicated.

PREGNANCY AND LACTATION

• Pregnancy Category C. Fetal harm is not known with topical administration. Excretion into human milk is not known.

foscarnet sodium

(foss-car'net)

Rx: Foscavir

Drug Class: Antivirals

Pregnancy Category: C

CLINICAL PHARMACOLOGY

Mechanism of Action: An antiviral that selectively inhibits binding sites on virus-specific DNA polymerase and reverse transcriptase. *Therapeutic Effect:* Inhibits replication of herpes virus.

Pharmacokinetics

Sequestered into bone and cartilage. Protein binding: 14%-17%. Primarily excreted unchanged in urine. Removed by hemodialysis. **Half-life:** 3.3-6.8 hr (increased in impaired renal function).

AVAILABLE FORMS

• *Injection:* 24 mg/ml.

INDICATIONS AND DOSAGES

Cytomegalovirus (CMV) retinitis

IV

Adults, Elderly. Initially, 60 mg/kg q8h or 100 mg/kg q12h for 2-3 wk. Maintenance: 90-120 mg/kg/day as a single IV infusion.

Herpes infection

IV

Adults. 40 mg/kg q8-12h for 2-3 wk or until healed.

Dosage in renal impairment

Dosages are individualized based on creatinine clearance. Refer to the dosing guide provided by the manufacturer.

CONTRAINDICATIONS: None known.

INTERACTIONS

Drug

Nephrotoxic medications: May increase the risk of nephrotoxicity.

Pentamidine (IV): May cause reversible hypocalcemia, hypomagnesemia, and nephrotoxicity.

Zidovudine (AZT): May increase the risk of anemia.

Herbal

None known.

Food

None known.

DIAGNOSTIC TEST EFFECTS: May increase serum alkaline phosphatase, bilirubin, creatinine, AST (SGOT), and ALT (SGPT) levels. May decrease serum magnesium and potassium levels. May alter serum calcium and phosphate concentrations.

IV INCOMPATIBILITIES: Acyclovir (Zovirax), amphotericin B (Fungizone), co-trimoxazole (Bactrim), diazepam (Valium), digoxin (Lanoxin), diphenhydramine (Benadryl), dobutamine (Dobutrex), droperidol (Inapsine), ganciclovir (Cytovene), haloperidol (Haldol), leucovorin, midazolam (Versed), pentamidine (Pentam IV), prochlorperazine (Compazine), vancomycin (Vancocin)

IV COMPATIBILITIES: Dopamine (Intropin), heparin, hydromorphone (Dilaudid), lorazepam (Ativan), morphine, potassium chloride

SIDE EFFECTS

Frequent

Fever (65%); nausea (47%); vomiting, diarrhea (30%)

Occasional (5% or greater)

Anorexia, pain and inflammation at injection site, fever, rigors, malaise, headache, paresthesia, dizziness, rash, diaphoresis, abdominal pain

Rare (5%-1%)
Back or chest pain, edema, flushing, pruritus, constipation, dry mouth

SERIOUS REACTIONS

• Nephrotoxicity occurs to some extent in most patients.

• Seizures and serum mineral or electrolyte imbalances may be life-threatening.

SPECIAL CONSIDERATIONS

PRECAUTIONS

• Take care to infuse solutions containing foscarnet sodium only into veins with adequate blood flow to permit rapid dilution and distribution to avoid local irritation. Local irritation and ulcerations of penile epithelium have been reported in male patients receiving foscarnet sodium, possibly related to the presence of drug in the urine. One case of vulvovaginal ulcerations in a female receiving foscarnet sodium has been reported. Adequate hydration with close attention to personal hygiene may minimize the occurrence of such events. Anemia has been reported in 33% of patients receiving foscarnet sodium in controlled studies. Granulocytopenia has been reported in 17% of patients receiving foscarnet sodium in controlled studies.

PATIENT INFORMATION

• Mucocutaneous Acyclovir-Resistant Herpes Simplex Virus Infections: Advise patients that foscarnet sodium is not a cure for herpes simplex virus infections. Although complete healing is possible, relapse occurs in most patients. Because relapse may be due to acyclovir-sensitive herpes simplex virus, sensitivity testing of the viral isolate is advised. In addition, repeated treatment with foscarnet sodium has led to the development of resistance associated with poorer response. In the case of poor therapeutic response, sensitivity testing of the viral isolate also is advised. Inform patients that the major toxicities of foscarnet are renal impairment, electrolyte disturbances, and seizures and that dose modifications and possibly discontinuation may be required.

PREGNANCY AND LACTATION

• Pregnancy Category C. Daily subcutaneous doses administered to rabbits and rats during gestation caused an increase in the frequency of skeletal anomalies/variations. Foscarnet sodium was excreted in maternal milk at concentrations 3 times higher than peak maternal blood concentrations.

OCULAR CONSIDERATIONS

• CMV Retinitis: A prospective, randomized, controlled clinical trial (FOS-03) was conducted in 24 patients with acquired immunodeficiency syndrome (AIDS) and CMV retinitis comparing treatment with foscarnet sodium to no treatment. Patients received induction treatment of foscarnet sodium, 60 mg/kg every 8 hours for 3 weeks, followed by maintenance treatment with 90 mg/kg per day until retinitis progression (appearance of a new lesion or advancement of the border of a posterior lesion greater than 750 μm in diameter). All diagnoses and determinations of retinitis progression were made from masked reading of retinal photographs. The 13 patients randomized to treatment with foscarnet sodium had a significant delay in progression of CMV retinitis compared with untreated controls. Median times to retinitis progression from study entry were 93 days (range 21 to more than 364) and 22 days (range 7 to 42), respectively.

• In another prospective clinical trial of CMV retinitis in patients with AIDS (ACTG-915), 33 patients were treated with 2 to 3 weeks of foscarnet sodium induction (60 mg/kg tid) and then randomized to 90 mg/kg per day or 120 mg/kg per day maintenance therapy. The median times from study entry to retinitis progression were not significantly different between the treatment groups, 96 (range 14 to more than 176) days and 140 (range 16 to more than 233) days, respectively.

• In study ACTG 129/FGCRT SOCA, 107 patients with newly diagnosed CMV retinitis were randomized to treatment with foscarnet sodium (induction: 60 mg/kg tid for 2 weeks; maintenance: 90 mg/kg qd), and 127 were randomized to treatment with ganciclovir (induction: 5 mg/kg bid; maintenance: 5 mg/kg qd). The median time to progression on the two drugs was similar (foscarnet = 59, and ganciclovir = 56 days).

• Relapsed CMV Retinitis: The CMV Retinitis Retreatment Trial (ACTG 228/SOCA CRRT) was a randomized, open-label comparison of foscarnet sodium or ganciclovir monotherapy to the combination of both drugs for the treatment of persistently active or relapsed CMV retinitis in patients with AIDS. Subjects were randomized to one of the three treatments: foscarnet sodium 90 mg/kg bid induction followed by 120 mg/kg qd maintenance; ganciclovir 5 mg/kg bid induction followed by 10 mg/kg qd maintenance; or the combination of the two drugs, consisting of continuation of the subject's current therapy and induction dosing of the other drug (as given), followed by maintenance with foscarnet sodium 90 mg/kg qd plus ganciclovir 5 mg/kg qd. Assessment of retinitis progression was performed by masked evaluation of retinal photographs. The median times to retinitis progression or death were 39 days for the foscarnet sodium group, 61 days for the ganciclovir group, and 105 days for the combination group. For the alternative endpoint of retinitis progression (censoring on death), the median times were 39 days for the foscarnet sodium group, 61 days for the ganciclovir group, and 132 days for the combination group. Because of censoring on death, the latter analysis may overestimate the treatment effect. Treatment modifications because of toxicity were more common in the combination group than in the foscarnet sodium or ganciclovir monotherapy groups.

PATIENT INFORMATION

• CMV Retinitis: Advise patients that foscarnet sodium is not a cure for CMV retinitis and that they may continue to experience progression of retinitis during or following treatment. Advise patients to have regular eye examinations.

---

fosinopril

(fo-sin'o-pril)

Rx: Monopril

Drug Class: Angiotensin converting enzyme inhibitors

Pregnancy Category: D

Do not confuse Monopril with Monurol.

CLINICAL PHARMACOLOGY

Mechanism of Action: An ACE inhibitor that suppresses the renin-angiotensin-aldosterone system and prevents conversion of angiotensin I to angiotensin II, a potent vasoconstrictor; may also inhibit angiotensin II at local vascular and renal sites. Decreases plasma angiotensin II, increases plasma renin activity, and decreases aldosterone secretion. *Therapeutic Effect:* Reduces peripheral arterial resistance, pulmonary capillary wedge pressure; improves cardiac output, and exercise tolerance.

Pharmacokinetics

Route	Onset	Peak	Duration
PO	1 hr	2-6 hr	24 hr

Slowly absorbed from the GI tract. Protein binding: 97%-98%. Metabolized in the liver and GI mucosa to active metabolite. Primarily excreted in urine. Minimal removal by hemodialysis. **Half-life:** 11.5 hr.

AVAILABLE FORMS

- *Tablets:* 10 mg, 20 mg, 40 mg.

INDICATIONS AND DOSAGES

Hypertension (monotherapy)

PO

Adults, Elderly. Initially, 10 mg/day. Maintenance: 20-40 mg/day. Maximum: 80 mg/day.

Hypertension (with diuretic)

PO

Adults, Elderly. Initially, 10 mg/day titrated to patient's needs.

Heart failure

PO

Adults, Elderly. Initially, 5-10 mg. Maintenance: 20-40 mg/day.

UNLABELED USES: Treatment of diabetic and nondiabetic nephropathy, post-myocardial infarction left ventricular dysfunction, renal crisis in scleroderma

CONTRAINDICATIONS: History of angioedema from previous treatment with ACE inhibitors

INTERACTIONS

Drug

Alcohol, antihypertensives, diuretics: May increase the effects of fosinopril.

Lithium: May increase lithium blood concentration and risk of lithium toxicity.

NSAIDs: May decrease the effects of fosinopril.

Potassium-sparing diuretics, potassium supplements: May cause hyperkalemia.

Herbal

None known.

Food

None known.

DIAGNOSTIC TEST EFFECTS: May increase BUN, serum alkaline phosphatase, serum bilirubin, serum creatinine, serum potassium, AST (SGOT), and ALT (SGPT) levels. May decrease serum sodium levels. May cause positive antinuclear antibody titer.

SIDE EFFECTS

Frequent (12%-9%)

Dizziness, cough

Occasional (4%-2%)

Hypotension, nausea, vomiting, upper respiratory tract infection

SERIOUS REACTIONS

- Excessive hypotension ("first-dose syncope") may occur in patients with CHF and in those who are severely salt and volume depleted.
- Angioedema (swelling of face and lips) and hyperkalemia occur rarely.
- Agranulocytosis and neutropenia may be noted in those with collagen vascular disease, including scleroderma and systemic lupus erythematosus, and impaired renal function.
- Nephrotic syndrome may be noted in those with history of renal disease.

SPECIAL CONSIDERATIONS

PRECAUTIONS

- Give fosinopril sodium with caution to patients with obstruction in the outflow tract of the left ventricle. Anticipate changes in renal function in susceptible individuals. Elevated serum potassium was observed in hypertensive patients in clinical trials. Cough has been reported with all angiotensin-converting enzyme (ACE) inhibitors. In patients undergoing major surgery or during anesthesia with agents that produce hypotension, enalapril may block angiotensin II formation following compensatory renin release.

PATIENT INFORMATION

• Angioedema: Angioedema, including laryngeal edema, can occur with treatment with ACE inhibitors, especially following the first dose. Advise patients immediately to report to their physician any signs or symptoms suggesting angioedema (e.g., swelling of face, eyes, lips, tongue, larynx, mucous membranes, and extremities; difficulty in swallowing or breathing; or hoarseness) and to discontinue therapy.

• Symptomatic Hypotension: Caution patients that light-headedness can occur, especially during the first days of therapy, and to report it to a physician. Advise patients that if syncope occurs, they should discontinue fosinopril sodium until they have consulted the physician.

• Caution all patients that inadequate fluid intake or excessive perspiration, diarrhea, or vomiting can lead to an excessive fall in blood pressure, with the same consequences of light-headedness and possible syncope.

• Hyperkalemia: Advise patients not to use potassium supplements or salt substitutes containing potassium without consulting the physician.

• Neutropenia: Advise patients to report promptly any indication of infection (e.g., sore throat or fever), which could be a sign of neutropenia.

• Pregnancy: Advise female patients of childbearing age about the consequences of second- and third-trimester exposure to ACE inhibitors, and inform them that these consequences do not appear to have resulted from intrauterine ACE inhibitor exposure that has been limited to the first trimester. Ask these patients to report pregnancies to their physicians as soon as possible.

PREGNANCY AND LACTATION

• Pregnancy Category C (first trimester) and D (second and third trimesters). Angiotensin-converting enzyme inhibitors can cause fetal and neonatal morbidity and death when administered to pregnant women. Ingestion of 20 mg daily for 3 days resulted in detectable levels of fosinoprilat in breast milk. Do not administer fosinopril sodium to nursing mothers.

furosemide

(fur-oh'se-mide)

Rx: Lasix

Drug Class: Diuretics, loop

Pregnancy Category: C

Do not confuse Lasix with Lidex, Luvox, or Luxiq, or furosemide with Torsemide.

CLINICAL PHARMACOLOGY

Mechanism of Action: A loop diuretic that enhances excretion of sodium, chloride, and potassium by direct action at the ascending limb of the loop of Henle. *Therapeutic Effect:* Produces diuresis and lower BP.

Pharmacokinetics

Route	Onset	Peak	Duration
PO	30-60 min	1-2 hr	6-8 hr
IV	5 min	20-60 min	2 hr
IM	30 min	N/A	N/A

Well absorbed from the GI tract. Protein binding: 91%-97%. Partially metabolized in the liver. Primarily excreted in urine (nonrenal clearance increases in severe renal impairment). Not removed by hemodialysis. **Half-life:** 30-90 min (increased in renal or hepatic impairment, and in neonates).

AVAILABLE FORMS

- *Oral Solution:* 10 mg/ml, 40 mg/5 ml.
- *Tablets:* 20 mg, 40 mg, 80 mg.
- *Injection:* 10 mg/ml.

INDICATIONS AND DOSAGES

Edema, hypertension

PO

Adults, Elderly. Initially, 20-80 mg/dose; may increase by 20-40 mg/dose q6-8h. May titrate up to 600 mg/day in severe edematous states.

Children. 1-6 mg/kg/day in divided doses q6-12h.

IV, IM

Adults, Elderly. 20-40 mg/dose; may increase by 20 mg/dose q1-2h.

Children. 1-2 mg/kg/dose q6-12h.

Neonates. 1-2 mg/kg/dose q12-24h.

IV Infusion

Adults, Elderly. Bolus of 0.1 mg/kg, followed by infusion of 0.1 mg/kg/hr; may double q2h. Maximum: 0.4 mg/kg/hr.

Children. 0.05 mg/kg/hr; titrate to desired effect.

UNLABELED USES: Hypercalcemia

CONTRAINDICATIONS: Anuria, hepatic coma, severe electrolyte depletion

INTERACTIONS

Drug

Amphotericin B, nephrotoxic and ototoxic medications: May increase the risk of nephrotoxicity and ototoxicity.

Anticoagulants, heparin: May decrease the effects of these drugs.

Lithium: May increase the risk of lithium toxicity.

Other hypokalemia-causing medications: May increase the risk of hypokalemia.

Probenecid: May increase furosemide blood concentration.

Herbal

None known.

Food

None known.

DIAGNOSTIC TEST EFFECTS: May increase blood glucose, BUN, and serum uric acid levels. May decrease serum calcium, chloride, magnesium, potassium, and sodium levels.

IV INCOMPATIBILITIES: Ciprofloxacin (Cipro), diltiazem (Cardizem), dobutamine (Dobutrex), dopamine (Intropin), doxorubicin (Adriamycin), droperidol (Inapsine), esmolol (Brevibloc), famotidine (Pepcid), filgrastim (Neupogen), fluconazole (Diflucan), gemcitabine (Gemzar), gentamicin (Garamycin), idarubicin (Idamycin), labetalol (Trandate), meperidine (Demerol), metoclopramide (Reglan), midazolam (Versed), milrinone (Primacor), nicardipine (Cardene), ondansetron (Zofran), quinidine, thiopental (Pentothal), vecuronium (Norcuron), vinblastine (Velban), vincristine (Oncovin), vinorelbine (Navelbine)

IV COMPATIBILITIES: Aminophylline, amiodarone (Cordarone), bumetanide (Bumex), calcium gluconate, cimetidine (Tagamet), heparin, hydromorphone (Dilaudid), lidocaine, morphine, nitroglycerin, norepinephrine (Levophed), potassium chloride, propofol (Diprivan)

SIDE EFFECTS

Expected

Increased urinary frequency and urine volume

Frequent

Nausea, dyspepsia, abdominal cramps, diarrhea or constipation, electrolyte disturbances

Occasional

Dizziness, light-headedness, headache, blurred vision, paresthesia, photosensitivity, rash, fatigue, bladder spasm, restlessness, diaphoresis

Rare

Flank pain

SERIOUS REACTIONS

- Vigorous diuresis may lead to profound water loss and electrolyte depletion, resulting in hypokalemia, hyponatremia, and dehydration.
- Sudden volume depletion may result in increased risk of thrombosis, circulatory collapse, and sudden death.
- Acute hypotensive episodes may occur, sometimes several days after beginning therapy.
- Ototoxicity—manifested as deafness, vertigo, or tinnitus—may occur, especially in patients with severe renal impairment.
- Furosemide use can exacerbate diabetes mellitus, systemic lupus erythematosus, gout, and pancreatitis.
- Blood dyscrasias have been reported.

SPECIAL CONSIDERATIONS

PRECAUTIONS

- Excessive diuresis may cause dehydration and blood volume reduction with circulatory collapse and possibly vascular thrombosis and embolism, particularly in elderly patients. Hypokalemia may develop with furosemide use. Sorbitol present in oral solution may cause diarrhea (especially in children). Patients allergic to sulfonamides also may be allergic to furosemide. Observe patients regularly for the possible occurrence of blood dyscrasias, liver or kidney damage, or other idiosyncratic reactions.

PATIENT INFORMATION

- Advise patients receiving furosemide that they may experience symptoms from excessive fluid and/or electrolyte losses. The postural hypotension that sometimes occurs usually can be managed by getting up slowly. Potassium supplements and/or dietary measures may be needed to control or avoid hypokalemia.
- Inform patients with diabetes mellitus that furosemide may increase blood glucose levels and thereby affect urine glucose tests. The skin of some patients may be more sensitive to the effects of sunlight during furosemide use.
- Hypertensive patients should avoid medications that may increase blood pressure, including over-the-counter products for appetite suppression and cold symptoms.

PREGNANCY AND LACTATION

- Pregnancy Category C. Furosemide has been shown to cause unexplained maternal deaths and abortions in rabbits. Fetal harm is not known. Because furosemide appears in breast milk, exercise caution when administering furosemide to a nursing mother. Excretion into human milk is not known.

OCULAR CONSIDERATIONS

- Adverse reactions include blurred vision and xanthopsia.

gabapentin

(ga'ba-pen-tin)

Rx: Neurontin

Drug Class: Anticonvulsants

Pregnancy Category: C

Do not confuse Neurontin with Noroxin.

CLINICAL PHARMACOLOGY

Mechanism of Action: An anticonvulsant and antineuralgic agent whose exact mechanism unknown. May increase the synthesis or accumulation of gamma-aminobutyric acid by binding to as-yet-undefined receptor sites in brain tissue. *Therapeutic Effect:* Reduces seizure activity and neuropathic pain.

Pharmacokinetics

Well absorbed from the GI tract (not affected by food). Protein binding: less than 5%. Widely distributed. Crosses the blood-brain barrier. Primarily excreted unchanged in urine. Removed by hemodialysis. **Half-life:** 5-7 hr (increased in impaired renal function and the elderly).

AVAILABLE FORMS

- *Capsules:* 100 mg, 300 mg, 400 mg.
- *Oral Solution:* 250 mg/5 ml.
- *Tablets:* 600 mg, 800 mg.

INDICATIONS AND DOSAGES

Adjunctive therapy for seizure control

PO

Adults, Elderly, Children older than 12 yr. Initially, 300 mg 3 times a day. May titrate dosage. Range: 900-1800 mg/day in 3 divided doses. Maximum: 3,600 mg/day.

Children 3-12 yr. Initially, 10-15 mg/kg/day in 3 divided doses. May titrate up to 25-35 mg/kg/day (for children 5-12 yr) and 40 mg/kg/day (for children 3-4 yr) Maximum: 50 mg/kg/day.

Adjunctive therapy for neuropathic pain

PO

Adults, Elderly. Initially, 100 mg 3 times a day; may increase by 300 mg/day at weekly intervals. Maximum: 3600 mg/day in 3 divided doses.

Children. Initially, 5 mg/kg/dose at bedtime, followed by 5 mg/kg/dose for 2 doses on day 2, then 5 mg/kg/dose for 3 doses on day 3. Range: 8-35 mg/kg/day in 3 divided doses.

Postherpetic neuralgia

PO

Adults, Elderly. 300 mg on day 1, 300 mg twice a day on day 2, and 300 mg 3 times a day on day 3. Titrate up to 1,800 mg/day.

Dosage in renal impairment

Dosage and frequency are modified based on creatinine clearance:

Creatinine Clearance	*Dosage*
60 ml/min or higher	400 mg q8h
30-59 ml/min	300 mg q12h
16-29 ml/min	300 mg daily
less than 16 ml/min	300 mg every other day
Hemodialysis	200-300 mg after each 4-hr hemodialysis session

UNLABELED USES: Treatment of essential tremor, hot flashes, hyperhidrosis, migraines, psychiatric disorders

G

CONTRAINDICATIONS: None known.

INTERACTIONS

Drug

None known.

Herbal

None known.

Food

None known.

DIAGNOSTIC TEST EFFECTS: May decrease serum WBC count.

SIDE EFFECTS

Frequent (19%-10%)

Fatigue, somnolence, dizziness, ataxia

Occasional (8%-3%)

Nystagmus, tremor, diplopia, rhinitis, weight gain

Rare (less than 2%)

Nervousness, dysarthria, memory loss, dyspepsia, pharyngitis, myalgia

SERIOUS REACTIONS

- Abrupt withdrawal may increase seizure frequency.
- Overdosage may result in diplopia, slurred speech, drowsiness, lethargy, and diarrhea.

SPECIAL CONSIDERATIONS

PATIENT INFORMATION

- Instruct patients to take gabapentin only as prescribed. Advise patients that gabapentin may cause dizziness, somnolence, and other symptoms and signs of central nervous system depression. Accordingly, advise patients not to drive a car or operate other complex machinery until they have gained sufficient experience on gabapentin to gauge whether it affects their mental and/or motor performance adversely. Blurred vision often is reported as a side effect.

PREGNANCY AND LACTATION

- Pregnancy Category C. Gabapentin has been shown to be fetotoxic in rodents, causing delayed ossification of several bones in the skull, vertebrae, forelimbs, and hindlimbs. Fetal harm is not known. Gabapentin is secreted into human milk following oral administration.

ganciclovir sodium

(gan-sy'clo-ver)

Rx: Cytovene, Vitrasert

Drug Class: Antivirals

Pregnancy Category: C

Do not confuse Cytovene with Cytosar.

CLINICAL PHARMACOLOGY

Mechanism of Action: This synthetic nucleoside competes with viral DNA polymerase and is incorporated into growing viral DNA chains. *Therapeutic Effect:* Interferes with synthesis and replication of viral DNA.

Pharmacokinetics

Widely distributed. Protein binding: 1%-2%. Undergoes minimal metabolism. Excreted unchanged primarily in urine. Removed by hemodialysis. **Half-life:** 2.5-3.6 hr (increased in impaired renal function).

AVAILABLE FORMS

- *Capsules (Cytovene):* 250 mg, 500 mg.
- *Powder for Injection (Cytovene):* 500 mg.
- *Implant (Vitrasert):* 4.5 mg.

INDICATIONS AND DOSAGES

Cytomegalovirus (CMV) retinitis

IV

Adults, Children 3 mo and older. 10 mg/kg/day in divided doses q12h for 14-21 days, then 5 mg/kg/day as a single daily dose.

Prevention of CMV disease in transplant patients

IV

Adults, Children. 10 mg/kg/day in divided doses q12h for 7-14 days, then 5 mg/kg/day as a single daily dose.

Other CMV infections

IV

Adults. Initially, 10 mg/kg/day in divided doses q12h for 14-21 days, then 5 mg/kg/day as a single daily dose. Maintenance: 1000 mg 3 times a day or 500 mg q3h (6 times a day).

Children. Initially, 10 mg/kg/day in divided doses q12h for 14-21 days, then 5 mg/kg/day as a single daily dose. Maintenance: 30 mg/kg/dose q8h.

Intravitreal implant

Adults. 1 implant q6-9mo plus oral ganciclovir.

Children 9 yr and older. 1 implant q6-9mo plus oral ganciclovir (30 mg/dose q8h).

Adult dosage in renal impairment

Dosage and frequency are modified based on CrCl.

CrCl	*Induction Dosage*	*Maintenance Dosage*	*Oral*
50-69 ml/ min	2.5 mg/kg q12h	2.5 mg/kg q24h	1500 mg/ day
25-49 ml/ min	2.5 mg/kg q24h	1.25 mg/ kg q24h	1000 mg/ day
10-24 ml/ min	1.25 mg/kg q24h	0.625 mg/ kg q24h	500 mg/ day
less than 10 ml/ min	1.25 mg/kg 3 times/ wk	0.625 mg/kg 3 times/ wk	500 mg 3 times/ wk

CrCl = creatinine clearance

UNLABELED USES: Treatment of other CMV infections, such as gastroenteritis, hepatitis, and pneumonitis

CONTRAINDICATIONS: Absolute neutrophil count less than 500/mm^3, platelet count less than 25,000/mm^3, hypersensitivity to acyclovir or ganciclovir, immunocompetent patients, patients with congenital or neonatal CMV disease.

INTERACTIONS

Drug

Bone marrow depressants: May increase bone marrow depression.

Imipenem and cilastatin: May increase the risk of seizures.

Zidovudine (AZT): May increase the risk of hepatotoxicity.

Herbal

None known.

Food

None known.

DIAGNOSTIC TEST EFFECTS: May increase serum alkaline phosphatase, bilirubin, AST (SGOT), and ALT (SGPT) levels.

IV INCOMPATIBILITIES: Aldesleukin (Proleukin), amifostine (Ethyol), aztreonam (Azactam), cefepime (Maxipime), cytarabine (ARA-C), doxorubicin (Adriamycin), fludarabine (Fludara), foscarnet (Foscavir), gemcitabine (Gemzar), ondansetron (Zofran), piperacillin and tazobactam (Zosyn), sargramostim (Leukine), vinorelbine (Navelbine)

IV COMPATIBILITIES: Amphotericin B, enalapril (Vasotec), filgrastim (Neupogen), fluconazole (Diflucan), propofol (Diprivan)

SIDE EFFECTS

Frequent

Diarrhea (41%), fever (40%), nausea (25%), abdominal pain (17%), vomiting (13%)

Occasional (11%-6%)

Diaphoresis, infection, paresthesia, flatulence, pruritus

Rare (4%-2%)

Headache, stomatitis, dyspepsia, phlebitis

SERIOUS REACTIONS

• Hematologic toxicity occurs commonly: leukopenia in 41%-29% of patients and anemia in 25%-19%.

• Intraocular insertion occasionally results in visual acuity loss, vitreous hemorrhage, and retinal detachment.

• GI hemorrhage occurs rarely.

gatifloxacin

(gah-tee-floks'a-sin)

Rx: Tequin, Tequin Teqpaq, Zymar

Drug Class: Antibiotics, quinolones

Pregnancy Category: C

CLINICAL PHARMACOLOGY

Mechanism of Action: A fluoroquinolone that inhibits two enzymes, topoisomerase II and IV, in susceptible microorganisms. *Therapeutic Effect:* Interferes with bacterial DNA replication. Prevents or delays resistance emergence. Bactericidal.

Pharmacokinetics

Well absorbed from the GI tract after PO administration. Protein binding: 20%. Widely distributed. Metabolized in liver. Primarily excreted in urine. **Half-life:** 7-14 hr.

AVAILABLE FORMS

• *Tablets (Tequin):* 200 mg, 400 mg.

• *Injection (Tequin):* 200-mg, 400-mg vials.

• *Ophthalmic Solution (Zymar):* 0.3%.

INDICATIONS AND DOSAGES

Chronic bronchitis, complicated urinary tract infections, pyelonephritis, skin infections

PO, IV

Adults, Elderly. 400 mg/day for 7-10 days (5 days for chronic bronchitis).

Sinusitis

PO, IV

Adults, Elderly. 400 mg/day for 10 days.

Pneumonia

PO, IV

Adults, Elderly. 400 mg/day for 7-14 days.

Cystitis

PO, IV

Adults, Elderly. 400 mg as a single dose or 200 mg/day for 3 days.

Urethral gonorrhea in men and women, endocervical and rectal gonorrhea in women

PO, IV

Adults, Elderly. 400 mg as a single dose.

Topical treatment of bacterial conjunctivitis due to susceptible strains of bacteria

Ophthalmic

Adults, Elderly, Children 1 yr and older. 1 drop q2h while awake for 2 days, then 1 drop up to 4 times/day for days 3-7.

Dosage in renal impairment

Creatinine Clearance	*Dosage*
40 ml/min	400 mg/day
Less than 40 ml/min	Initially, 400 mg/day then 200 mg/day
Hemodialysis	Initially, 400 mg/day then 200 mg/day
Peritoneal dialysis	Initially, 400 mg/day then 200 mg/day

CONTRAINDICATIONS: Hypersensitivity to quinolones

INTERACTIONS

Drug

Antacids, digoxin, iron preparations: May decrease gatifloxacin plasma concentration and half-life.

Probenecid: May increase gatifloxacin plasma concentration and half-life.

Herbal

None known.

Food

None known.

DIAGNOSTIC TEST EFFECTS: *None known.*

IV INCOMPATIBILITIES: Amphotericin (Fungizone), potassium phosphate

IV COMPATIBILITIES: Aminophylline, calcium gluconate, hydromorphone (Dilaudid), lidocaine, lorazepam (Ativan), magnesium sulfate, methylprednisolone (Solu-Medrol), metoclopramide (Reglan), midazolam (Versed), morphine, nitroglycerin, potassium chloride, sodium phosphate

SIDE EFFECTS

Occasional (8%-3%)

Nausea, vaginitis, diarrhea, headache, dizziness

Ophthalmic: conjunctival irritation, increased tearing, corneal inflammation

Rare (3%-0.1%)

Abdominal pain, constipation, dyspepsia, stomatitis, edema, insomnia, abnormal dreams, diaphoresis, altered taste, rash

Ophthalmic: corneal swelling, dry eye, eye pain, eyelid swelling, headache, red eye, reduced visual acuity, altered taste

SERIOUS REACTIONS

- Pseudomembranous colitis, as evidenced by severe abdominal pain and cramps, severe watery diarrhea, and fever, may occur.
- Superinfection, manifested as genital or anal pruritus, ulceration or changes in oral mucosa, and moderate to severe diarrhea, may occur.

gentamicin sulfate

(jen-ta-mye'sin)

Rx: Garamycin, Garamycin Ophthalmic, Garamycin Topical, Genoptic, Gentacidin, Gentak, Gentasol, Ocu-Mycin

Drug Class: Anti-infectives, ophthalmic; Anti-infectives, otic; Anti-infectives, topical; Antibiotics, aminoglycosides; Dermatologics; Ophthalmics; Otics

Pregnancy Category: C

CLINICAL PHARMACOLOGY

Mechanism of Action: An aminoglycoside antibiotic that irreversibly binds to the protein of bacterial ribosomes. *Therapeutic Effect:* Interferes with protein synthesis of susceptible microorganisms. Bactericidal.

Pharmacokinetics

Rapid, complete absorption after IM administration. Protein binding: less than 30%. Widely distributed (does not cross the blood-brain barrier, low concentrations in CSF). Excreted unchanged in urine. Removed by hemodialysis. **Half-life:** 2-4 hr (increased in impaired renal function and neonates; decreased in cystic fibrosis and burn or febrile patients).

AVAILABLE FORMS

- *Injection (Garamycin):* 10 mg/ml, 40 mg/ml.
- *Ophthalmic Solution (Gentacidin, Genoptic, Gentak):* 0.3%.
- *Ophthalmic Ointment (Gentak):* 0.3%.
- *Cream (Garamycin):* 0.1%.
- *Ointment:* 0.1%.

INDICATIONS AND DOSAGES

Acute pelvic, bone, intra-abdominal, joint, respiratory tract, burn wound, postoperative, and skin or skin-structure infections; complicated UTIs; septicemia; meningitis

IV, IM

Adults, Elderly. Usual dosage, 3-6 mg/kg/day in divided doses q8h or 4-6.6 mg/kg once a day.

Children 5-12 yr. Usual dosage 2-2.5 mg/kg/dose q8h.

Children younger than 5 yr. Usual dosage, 2.5 mg/kg/dose q8h.

Neonates. Usual dosage 2.5-3.5 mg/kg/dose q8-12h.

Hemodialysis

IV, IM

Adults, Elderly. 0.5-0.7 mg/kg/dose after dialysis.

Children. 1.25-1.75 mg/kg/dose after dialysis.

Intrathecal

Adults. 4-8 mg/day.

Children 3 mo-12 yr. 1-2 mg/day.

Neonates. 1 mg/day.

Superficial eye infections

Ophthalmic Ointment

Adults, Elderly. Usual dosage, apply thin strip to conjunctiva 2-3 times a day.

Ophthalmic Solution

Adults, Elderly, Children. Usual dosage, 1-2 drops q2-4h up to 2 drops/hr.

Superficial skin infections

Topical

Adults, Elderly. Usual dosage, apply 3-4 times/day.

Dosage in renal impairment

Creatinine clearance greater than 41-60 ml/min. Dosage interval q12h.

Creatinine clearance 20-40 ml/min. Dosage interval q24h.

Creatinine clearance less than 20 ml/min. Monitor levels to determine dosage interval.

UNLABELED USES: Topical: Prophylaxis of minor bacterial skin infections, treatment of dermal ulcer

CONTRAINDICATIONS: Hypersensitivity to gentamicin, other aminoglycosides (cross-sensitivity), or their components. Sulfite sensitivity may result in anaphylaxis, especially in asthmatic patients.

INTERACTIONS

Drug

Nephrotoxic mediations, other aminoglycosides, ototoxic medications: May increase the risk of nephrotoxicity or ototoxicity.

Neuromuscular blockers: May increase neuromuscular blockade.

Herbal

None known.

Food

None known.

DIAGNOSTIC TEST EFFECTS: May increase serum creatinine, serum bilirubin, BUN, serum LDH, AST (SGOT), and ALT (SGPT) levels. May decrease serum calcium, magnesium, potassium, and sodium concentrations. Therapeutic peak serum level is 6-10 mcg/ml and trough is 0.5-2 mcg/ml. Toxic peak serum level is greater than 10 mcg/ml, and trough is greater than 2 mcg/ml.

IV INCOMPATIBILITIES: Allopurinol (Aloprim), amphotericin B complex (Abelcet, AmBisome, Amphotec), furosemide (Lasix), heparin, hetastarch (Hespan), idarubicin (Idamycin), indomethacin (Indocin), propofol (Diprivan)

IV COMPATIBILITIES: Amiodarone (Cordarone), diltiazem (Cardizem), enalapril (Vasotec), filgrastim (Neupogen), hydromorphone (Dilaudid), insulin, lorazepam (Ativan), magnesium sulfate, midazolam (Versed), morphine, multivitamins

SIDE EFFECTS

Occasional

IM: Pain, induration

IV: Phlebitis, thrombophlebitis, hypersensitivity reactions (fever, pruritus, rash, urticaria)

Ophthalmic: Burning, tearing, itching, blurred vision

Topical: Redness, itching

Rare

Alopecia, hypertension, weakness

SERIOUS REACTIONS

- Nephrotoxicity (as evidenced by increased BUN and serum creatinine levels and decreased creatinine clearance) may be reversible if the drug is stopped at the first sign of symptoms.
- Irreversible ototoxicity (manifested as tinnitus, dizziness, ringing or roaring in the ears, and diminished hearing), and neurotoxicity (as evidenced by headache, dizziness, lethargy, tremor, and visual disturbances) occur occasionally. The risk of these effects increases with higher dosages or prolonged therapy and when the solution is applied directly to the mucosa.
- Superinfections, particularly with fungal infections, may result from bacterial imbalance no matter which administration route is used.
- Ophthalmic application may cause paresthesia of conjunctiva or mydriasis.

SPECIAL CONSIDERATIONS

PRECAUTIONS

- Prolonged use of topical antibiotics may give rise to overgrowth of nonsusceptible organisms including fungi. Bacterial resistance to gentamicin also may develop. If purulent discharge, inflammation, or pain becomes aggravated, the patient should discontinue use of the medication and consult a physician. If irritation or hypersensitivity to any component of the drug develops, instruct the patient to discontinue use of this preparation, and institute appropriate therapy. Ocular ointments may retard corneal healing.

PATIENT INFORMATION

- To avoid contamination, instruct the patient not to touch tip of container to the eye, eyelid, or any surface.

PREGNANCY AND LACTATION

- Pregnancy Category C. Gentamicin has been shown to depress body weights, kidney weights, and median glomerular counts in newborn rats when administered systemically to pregnant rats. Fetal harm is not known with topical administration.

---

gentamicin sulfate; prednisolone acetate

Rx: Pred-G, Pred-G S.O.P.

Drug Class: Anti-infectives, ophthalmic; Antibiotics, aminoglycosides; Corticosteroids, ophthalmic; Ophthalmics

Pregnancy Category: C

CLINICAL PHARMACOLOGY

Mechanism of Action: Gentamicin is an aminoglycoside that irreversibly binds to the protein of bacterial ribosomes. Prednisolone is an adrenal corticosteroid that inhibits accumulation of inflammatory cells at inflammation sites, phagocytosis, lysosomal enzyme release and synthesis, and release of mediators of inflammation. *Therapeutic Effect:* Interferes in protein synthesis of susceptible microorganisms. Prevents or suppresses cell-mediated immune reactions; decreases or prevents tissue response to inflammatory process.

Pharmacokinetics

None reported.

AVAILABLE FORMS

• *Ophthalmic Suspension:* 0.3 % gentamicin sulfate and 0.6% prednisolone acetate (Pred-G S.O.P.).

• *Ophthalmic Ointment:* 0.3% gentamicin sulfate and 1% prednisolone acetate (Pred-G).

INDICATIONS AND DOSAGES

Treatment of steroid responsive inflammatory conditions, superficial ocular infections

Ophthalmic Ointment

Adults, Elderly. Apply ½ inch ribbon in the conjunctival sac 1-3 times/day.

Ophthalmic Suspension

Adults, Elderly. Instill 1 drop 2-4 times/day. During the initial 24-48 hours, the dosing frequency may be increased if necessary up to 1 drop every hour.

CONTRAINDICATIONS: Viral disease of the cornea and conjunctiva (including epithelia herpes simplex keratitis, vaccinia, varicella), mycobacterial or fungal infection of the eye, uncomplicated removal of a corneal foreign body, hypersensitivity to gentamicin, prednisolone, other aminoglycosides or corticosteroids, or any component of the formulation

INTERACTIONS

Drug

None known.

Herbal

None known.

Food

None known.

DIAGNOSTIC TEST EFFECTS: *None known.*

SIDE EFFECTS

Occasional

Burning, tearing, itching, blurred vision

Rare

Delayed wound healing, secondary infection, intraocular pressure increased, glaucoma

SERIOUS REACTIONS

• Optic nerve damage occurs rarely.

SPECIAL CONSIDERATIONS

PRECAUTIONS

• Ocular irritation and punctuate keratitis may occur. A physician should renew the medication order beyond 20 ml only after examination of the patient's intraocular pressure; examination of the patient with the aid of magnification such as slit-lamp biomicroscopy; and, where appropriate, fluorescein staining. Suspect fungal invasion in any persistent corneal ulceration where a corticosteroid has been used or is in use.

PATIENT INFORMATION

• If inflammation or pain persists longer than 48 hours or becomes aggravated, advise the patient to discontinue use of the medication and to consult a physician. This product is sterile when packaged. To prevent contamination, instruct the patient to avoid touching the bottle tip to eyelids or to any other surface. The use of this bottle by more than one person may spread infection. Instruct the patient to protect the drug from freezing and from heat of 40° C (104° F) and above. Instruct the patient to keep the drug out of reach of children and to shake it well before using.

PREGNANCY AND LACTATION

• Pregnancy Category C. Gentamicin has been shown to depress body weight, kidney weight, and median glomerular counts in newborn rats when administered systemically to pregnant rats in daily doses. Prednisolone has been shown to be teratogenic in mice when given in doses 1 to 10 times the human ocular dose. Systemically administered corticosteroids appear in human milk and could suppress growth, interfere with endogenous corticosteroid production, or cause other untoward effects. Excretion into human milk with topical administration is not known.

glatiramer

(gla-teer'a-mer)

Rx: Copaxone

Drug Class: Immunosuppressives

Pregnancy Category: B

Do not confuse Copaxone with Compazine.

CLINICAL PHARMACOLOGY

Mechanism of Action: An immunosuppressive whose exact mechanism is unknown. May act by modifying immune processes thought to be responsible for the pathogenesis of multiple sclerosis (MS). *Therapeutic Effect:* Slows progression of MS.

Pharmacokinetics

Substantial fraction of glatiramer is hydrolyzed locally. Some fraction of injected material enters lymphatic circulation, reaching regional lymph nodes; some may enter systemic circulation intact.

AVAILABLE FORMS

- *Injection:* 20 mg/ml in prefilled syringes.

INDICATIONS AND DOSAGES

MS

Subcutaneous

Adults, Elderly. 20 mg once a day.

CONTRAINDICATIONS: Hypersensitivity to glatiramer or mannitol

INTERACTIONS

Drug

None known.

Herbal

None known.

Food

None known.

DIAGNOSTIC TEST EFFECTS: *None known.*

SIDE EFFECTS

Expected (73%-40%)

Pain, erythema, inflammation, or pruritus at injection site; asthenia

Frequent (27%-18%)

Arthralgia, vasodilation, anxiety, hypertonia, nausea, transient chest pain, dyspnea, flu-like symptoms, rash, pruritus

Occasional (17%-10%)

Palpitations, back pain, diaphoresis, rhinitis, diarrhea, urinary urgency

Rare (8%-6%)

Anorexia, fever, neck pain, peripheral edema, ear pain, facial edema, vertigo, vomiting

SERIOUS REACTIONS

- Infection is a common effect.
- Lymphadenopathy occurs occasionally.

SPECIAL CONSIDERATIONS

OCULAR CONSIDERATIONS

- Glatiramer acetate (Copaxone) is being investigated as a possible neuroprotective agent to protect the optic nerve from the effects of glutamate in glaucoma. Glatiramer acetate is a synthetic copolymer with antigenic specificity for the immune mechanism that acts as a neuroprotector of retinal ganglion cells. The drug is designed to protect the optic nerve from the effects of toxic levels of glutamate. (Bonner H: Ocular drug preview: spotlight on emerging pharmaceuticals, Review of Optometry vol 141, issue 12, 2004. http://www.revoptom.com/index.asp?page=2_1309.htm.)

glimepiride

(gly-mep′er-ide)

Rx: Amaryl

Drug Class: Antidiabetic agents; Sulfonylureas, second generation

Pregnancy Category: C

Do not confuse glimepiride with glipizide or glyburide.

CLINICAL PHARMACOLOGY

Mechanism of Action: A second-generation sulfonylurea that promotes release of insulin from beta cells of the pancreas and increases insulin sensitivity at peripheral sites. *Therapeutic Effect:* Lowers blood glucose concentration.

Pharmacokinetics

Route	*Onset*	*Peak*	*Duration*
PO	N/A	2-3 hr	24 hr

Completely absorbed from the GI tract. Protein binding: greater than 99%. Metabolized in the liver. Excreted in urine and eliminated in feces. **Half-life:** 5-9.2 hr.

AVAILABLE FORMS

- *Tablets:* 1 mg, 2 mg, 4 mg.

INDICATIONS AND DOSAGES

Diabetes mellitus

PO

Adults, Elderly. Initially, 1-2 mg once a day, with breakfast or first main meal. Maintenance: 1-4 mg once a day. After dose of 2 mg is reached, dosage should be increased in increments of up to 2 mg q1-2wk, based on blood glucose response. Maximum: 8 mg/day.

Dosage in renal impairment

PO

Adults. 1 mg once/day.

CONTRAINDICATIONS: Diabetic complications, such as ketosis, acidosis, and diabetic coma; severe hepatic or renal impairment; monotherapy for type 1 diabetes mellitus; stress situations, including severe infection, trauma, and surgery

INTERACTIONS

Drug

Beta-blockers: May increase the hypoglycemic effect of glimepiride and mask signs of hypoglycemia.

Cimetidine, ciprofloxacin, fluconazole, MAOIs, quinidine, ranitidine, large doses of salicylates: May increase the effects of glimepiride.

Corticosteroids, lithium, thiazide diuretics: May decrease the effects of glimepiride.

Oral anticoagulants: May increase the effects of oral anticoagulants.

Herbal

None known.

Food

None known.

DIAGNOSTIC TEST EFFECTS: May increase BUN and LDH concentrations and serum alkaline phosphatase, creatinine, and AST (SGOT) levels.

SIDE EFFECTS

Frequent

Altered taste sensation, dizziness, somnolence, weight gain, constipation, diarrhea, heartburn, nausea, vomiting, stomach fullness, headache

Occasional

Increased sensitivity of skin to sunlight, peeling of skin, itching, rash

SERIOUS REACTIONS

- Overdose or insufficient food intake may produce hypoglycemia, especially with increased glucose demands.
- GI hemorrhage, cholestatic hepatic jaundice, leukopenia, thrombocytopenia, pancytopenia, agranulocytosis, and aplastic or hemolytic anemia occur rarely.

SPECIAL CONSIDERATIONS

PRECAUTIONS

• Glimepiride administration is associated with increased cardiovascular mortality compared with treatment with diet alone or diet plus insulin. All sulfonylurea drugs are capable of producing severe hypoglycemia. Patients with impaired renal function may be more sensitive to the glucose-lowering effect of glimepiride. Hypoglycemia may be difficult to recognize in the elderly and in persons who are taking beta-adrenergic blocking drugs or other sympatholytic agents. Hypoglycemia is more likely to occur when caloric intake is deficient, after severe or prolonged exercise, when alcohol is ingested, or when more than one glucose-lowering drug is used. Combined use of glimepiride with insulin or metformin may increase the potential for hypoglycemia. When a patient stabilized on any diabetic regimen is exposed to stress such as fever, trauma, infection, or surgery, a loss of control may occur.

PATIENT INFORMATION

• Inform patients of the potential risks and advantages of glimepiride and of alternative modes of therapy. Also inform patients about the importance of adherence to dietary instructions, of a regular exercise program, and of regular testing of blood glucose. Explain the risks of hypoglycemia, its symptoms and treatment, and conditions that predispose to its development to patients and responsible family members. Also explain the potential for primary and secondary failure.

PREGNANCY AND LACTATION

• Pregnancy Category C. Glimepiride did not produce teratogenic effects in rats with oral doses. In rat reproduction studies, significant concentrations of glimepiride were observed in the serum and breast milk of the dams, as well as in the serum of the pups. Excretion into human milk is not known.

OCULAR CONSIDERATIONS

• Ocular examinations were carried out in more than 500 subjects during long-term studies using the methodology of Taylor and West and Laties et al. No significant differences were seen between glimepiride and glyburide in the number of subjects with clinically important changes in visual acuity, intraocular pressure, or in any of the five lens-related variables examined.

• Eye examinations were carried out during long-term studies using the method of Chylack et al. No significant or clinically meaningful differences were seen between glimepiride and glipizide with respect to cataract progression by subjective LOCS II grading and objective image analysis systems, visual acuity, intraocular pressure, and general eye examination.

glipizide

(glip'i-zide)

Rx: Glucotrol, Glucotrol XL

Drug Class: Antidiabetic agents; Sulfonylureas, second generation

Pregnancy Category: C

Do not confuse glipizide with glimepiride or glyburide.

CLINICAL PHARMACOLOGY

Mechanism of Action: A second-generation sulfonylurea that promotes the release of insulin from beta cells of the pancreas and increases insulin sensitivity at peripheral sites. *Therapeutic Effect:* Lowers blood glucose concentration.

Pharmacokinetics

Route	*Onset*	*Peak*	*Duration*
PO	15-30 min	2-3 hr	12-24 hr
Extended-release	2-3 hr	6-12 hr	24 hr

Well absorbed from the GI tract. Protein binding: 99%. Metabolized in the liver. Excreted in urine. **Half-life:** 2-4 hr.

AVAILABLE FORMS

- *Tablets (Glucotrol):* 5 mg, 10 mg.
- *Tablets (Extended-Release [Glucotrol XL]):* 2.5 mg, 5 mg, 10 mg.

INDICATIONS AND DOSAGES

Diabetes mellitus

PO

Adults. Initially, 5 mg/day or 2.5 mg in the elderly or those with hepatic disease. Adjust dosage in 2.5- to 5-mg increments at intervals of several days. Maximum single dose: 15 mg. Maximum dose/day: 40 mg. Maintenance (extended-release tablet): 20 mg/day.

Elderly. Initially, 2.5-5 mg/day. May increase by 2.5-5 mg/day q1-2wk.

CONTRAINDICATIONS: Diabetic ketoacidosis with or without coma, type 1 diabetes mellitus

INTERACTIONS

Drug

Beta-blockers: May increase the hypoglycemic effect of glipizide and mask signs of hypoglycemia.

Cimetidine, ciprofloxacin, fluconazole, MAOIs, quinidine, ranitidine, large doses of salicylates: May increase the effects of glipizide.

Corticosteroids, lithium, thiazide diuretics: May decrease the effects of glipizide.

Oral anticoagulants: May increase the effects of oral anticoagulants.

Herbal

None known.

Food

None known.

DIAGNOSTIC TEST EFFECTS: May increase BUN and LDH concentrations and serum alkaline phosphatase, creatinine, and AST (SGOT) levels.

SIDE EFFECTS

Frequent

Altered taste sensation, dizziness, somnolence, weight gain, constipation, diarrhea, heartburn, nausea, vomiting, stomach fullness, headache

Occasional

Increased sensitivity of skin to sunlight, peeling of skin, itching, rash

SERIOUS REACTIONS

- Overdose or insufficiet food intake may produce hypoglycemia, especially with increased glucose demands.
- GI hemorrhage, cholestatic hepatic jaundice, leukopenia, thrombocytopenia, pancytopenia, agranulocytosis, and aplastic or hemolytic anemia occurs rarely.

SPECIAL CONSIDERATIONS

PRECAUTIONS

- Glipizide administration is associated with increased cardiovascular mortality compared with treatment with diet alone or diet plus insulin. All sulfonylurea drugs are capable of producing severe hypoglycemia. Patients with impaired renal function may be more sensitive to the glucose-lowering effect of glimepiride. Hypoglycemia may be difficult to recognize in the elderly and in persons who are taking beta-adrenergic blocking drugs or other sympatholytic agents. Hypoglycemia is more likely to occur when caloric intake is deficient, after severe or prolonged exercise, when alcohol is ingested, or when more than one glucose-lowering drug is used. Combined use of glimepiride with insulin or metformin may increase the potential for hypoglycemia. When a patient stabilized on any diabetic regimen is exposed to stress such as fever, trauma, infection, or surgery, a loss of control may occur.

PATIENT INFORMATION

• Inform patients of the potential risks and advantages of glipizide and of alternative modes of therapy. Also inform patients about the importance of adhering to dietary instructions, of a regular exercise program, and of regular testing of urine and/or blood glucose.

• Explain the risks of hypoglycemia, its symptoms and treatment, and conditions that predispose to its development to patients and responsible family members. Also explain primary and secondary failure.

• Inform patients that glipizide extended-release tablets should be swallowed whole. Patients should not chew, divide, or crush tablets. Patients should not be concerned if they occasionally notice in their stool something that looks like a tablet. In the glipizide extended-release tablet, the medication is contained within a shell that has been specially designed to slowly release the drug so the body can absorb it. When this process is completed, the empty tablet is eliminated from the body.

PREGNANCY AND LACTATION

• Pregnancy Category C. Glipizide was found to be mildly fetotoxic in rat reproduction studies at all dose levels. Although whether glipizide is excreted in human milk is not known, some sulfonylurea drugs are known to be excreted in human milk.

glyburide

(glye' byoor-ide)

Rx: DiaBeta, Glycron, Glynase Pres-Tab, Micronase

Drug Class: Antidiabetic agents; Sulfonylureas, second generation

Pregnancy Category: C

Do not confuse glyburide with glimepiride or glipizide, or Micronase with Micro-K, Micronor.

G

CLINICAL PHARMACOLOGY

Mechanism of Action: A second-generation sulfonylurea that promotes release of insulin from beta cells of the pancreas and increases insulin sensitivity at peripheral sites. *Therapeutic Effect:* Lowers blood glucose concentration.

Pharmacokinetics

Route	*Onset*	*Peak*	*Duration*
PO	0.25-1 hr	1-2 hr	12-24 hr

Well absorbed from the GI tract. Protein binding: 99%. Metabolized in the liver to weakly active metabolite. Primarily excreted in urine. Not removed by hemodialysis. **Half-life:** 1.4-1.8 hr.

AVAILABLE FORMS

• *Tablets (DiaBeta, Micronase):* 1.25 mg, 2.5 mg, 5 mg.

• *Tablets (Glynase):* 1.5 mg, 3 mg, 6 mg.

INDICATIONS AND DOSAGES

Diabetes mellitus

PO

Adults. Initially 2.5-5 mg. May increase by 2.5 mg/day at weekly intervals. Maintenance: 1.25-20 mg/day. Maximum: 20 mg/day.

Elderly. Initially, 1.25-2.5 mg/day. May increase by 1.25-2.5 mg/day at 1- to 3-wk intervals.

PO (micronized tablets [Glynase])
Adults, Elderly. Initially 0.75-3 mg/day. May increase by 1.5 mg/day at weekly intervals. Maintenance: 0.75-12 mg/day as a single dose or in divided doses.

Dosage in renal impairment
Glyburide is not recommended in patients with creatinine clearance less than 50 ml/min.

CONTRAINDICATIONS: Diabetic ketoacidosis with or without coma, monotherapy for type 1 diabetes mellitus

INTERACTIONS

Drug
Beta-blockers: May increase the hypoglycemic effect of glyburide and mask signs of hypoglycemia.
Cimetidine, ciprofloxacin, fluconazole, MAOIs, quinidine, ranitidine, large doses of salicylates: May increase the effects of glyburide.
Corticosteroids, lithium, thiazide diuretics: May decrease the effects of glyburide.
Oral anticoagulants: May increase the effects of oral anticoagulants.

Herbal
None known.

Food
None known.

DIAGNOSTIC TEST EFFECTS: May increase BUN and LDH concentrations and serum alkaline phosphatase, creatinine, and AST (SGOT) levels.

SIDE EFFECTS

Frequent
Altered taste sensation, dizziness, somnolence, weight gain, constipation, diarrhea, heartburn, nausea, vomiting, stomach fullness, headache

Occasional
Increased sensitivity of skin to sunlight, peeling of skin, itching, rash

SERIOUS REACTIONS
• Overdose or insufficient food intake may produce hypoglycemia, especially in patients with increased glucose demands.
• Cholestatic jaundice, leukopenia, thrombocytopenia, pancytopenia, agranulocytosis, and aplastic or hemolytic anemia occur rarely.

SPECIAL CONSIDERATIONS

PRECAUTIONS
• Glyburide administration is associated with increased cardiovascular mortality compared with treatment with diet alone or diet plus insulin. All sulfonylurea drugs are capable of producing severe hypoglycemia. Patients with impaired renal function may be more sensitive to the glucose-lowering effect of glyburide. Hypoglycemia may be difficult to recognize in the elderly and in persons who are taking beta-adrenergic blocking drugs or other sympatholytic agents. Hypoglycemia is more likely to occur when caloric intake is deficient, after severe or prolonged exercise, when alcohol is ingested, or when more than one glucose-lowering drug is used. When a patient stabilized on any diabetic regimen is exposed to stress such as fever, trauma, infection, or surgery, a loss of control may occur.

PATIENT INFORMATION
• Inform patients of the potential risks and advantages of glyburide and of alternative modes of therapy. Also inform patients about the importance of adherence to dietary instructions, of a regular exercise program, and of regular testing of urine and/or blood glucose.
• Explain the risks of hypoglycemia, its symptoms and treatment, and conditions that predispose to its

development to patients and responsible family members. Also explain primary and secondary failure.

PREGNANCY AND LACTATION

• Pregnancy Category B. Reproduction studies have been performed in rats and rabbits at doses up to 500 times the human dose and have revealed no evidence of impaired fertility or harm to the fetus from glyburide. Because recent information suggests that abnormal blood glucose levels during pregnancy are associated with a higher incidence of congenital abnormalities, many experts recommend that insulin be used during pregnancy to maintain blood glucose as close to normal as possible. Excretion into human milk is not known.

OCULAR CONSIDERATIONS

• Changes in accommodation and/or blurred vision have been reported with glyburide and other sulfonylureas. These changes are thought to be related to fluctuation in glucose levels.

glycerin

(gli'ser-in)

Rx: Osmoglyn

Drug Class: Ophthalmics

Pregnancy Category: C

CLINICAL PHARMACOLOGY

Mechanism of Action: An osmotic dehydrating agent that increases osmotic pressure and draws fluid into colon and stimulates evaulcation of inspissated feces. Lowers both intraocular and intracranial pressure by osmotic dehydrating effects. Increases blood flow to ischemic areas, decreases serum free fatty acids, and increases synthesis of glycerides in the brain. *Therapeutic Effect:* Aids in fecal evacuation.

Pharmacokinetics

Well absorbed after PO administration but poorly absorbed after rectal administration. Widely distributed to extracellular space. Rapidly metabolized in liver. Primarily excreted in urine. **Half-life:** 30-45 min.

AVAILABLE FORMS

• *Ophthalmic solution:* 1% (Bausch & Lomb Computer Eye Drops).

• *Oral Solution:* 50% (Osmoglyn).

• *Rectal Solution:* 2.3 g (Fleet Babylax), 5.6 g (Fleet Liquid Glycerin Suppositories).

• *Suppositories:* 1 g (Fleet Glycerin Suppositories for Children), 2 g (Fleet Glycerin Suppositories), 3 g (Fleet Maximum-Strength Glycerin Suppositories), 82.5% (Sani-Supp).

INDICATIONS AND DOSAGES

Constipation

Rectal

Adults, Elderly, Children 6 yr and older. 3 g/day.

Children younger than 6 yr. 1-1.5 g/day.

Ophthalmologic procedures

Ophthalmic

Adults, Elderly Children. 1 or 2 drops before examination q3-4h.

Reduction of intracranial pressure

PO

Adults, Elderly, Children. 1.5 g/kg/day q4h or 1 g/kg/dose q6h.

Reduction of intraocular pressure

PO

Adults, Elderly, Children. 1-1.8 g/kg 1-1.5 hrs preoperatively.

UNLABELED USES: Viral meningoencephalitis

CONTRAINDICATIONS: Hypersensitivity to any component in the preparation, well-established anuria, severe dehydration, frank or impending acute pulmonary edema, severe cardiac decompensation

G

INTERACTIONS

Drug

PO medications: May decrease transit time of concurrently administered oral medication, decreasing absorption.

Herbal

Licorice: May increase risk of hypokalemia

Food

None known.

DIAGNOSTIC TEST EFFECTS: May suppress wheal and flare reactions to antigen skin testing unless antihistamines are discontinued 4 days before testing.

SIDE EFFECTS

Frequent

Oral: Nausea, headache,vomiting

Rectal: Some degree of abdominal discomfort, nausea, mild cramps, headache, vomiting

Occasional

Oral: Diarrhea, dizziness, dry mouth or increased thirst

Ophthalmic: pain and irritation may occur upon instillation

Rectal: faintness, weakness, abdominal pain, bloating

SERIOUS REACTIONS

- Laxative abuse includes symptoms of abdominal pain, weakness, fatigue, thirst, vomiting, edema, bone pain, fluid and electrolyte imbalance, hypoalbuminemia, and syndromes that mimic colitis.

SPECIAL CONSIDERATIONS

PRECAUTIONS

- Because glycerin is an irritant and may cause pain, instill a local anesthetic shortly before its use.

PATIENT INFORMATION

Give patients the following instructions:

- Computer Eye Drops: To avoid contamination, do not touch the tip of the container to any surface. Replace cap after using. If solution changes color or becomes cloudy, do not use. If you experience eye pain, changes in vision, or continued redness or irritation of the eye, or if the condition worsens or persists for more than 72 hours, discontinue use and consult an eye care practitioner. Keep this and all drugs out of the reach of children. Keep container tightly closed. Remove contact lenses before using.

PREGNANCY AND LACTATION

- Pregnancy Category C. Fetal harm is not known with topical administration. Excretion into human milk is not known.

glycerin; polysorbate 80

(gli'ser-in; pol-ee-sor'bate)

CLINICAL PHARMACOLOGY

Mechanism of Action: Not reported.

Pharmacokinetics

Not reported.

AVAILABLE FORMS

- *Ophthalmic solution:* 20 single-use vial pack [preservative free] (Refresh Endura).

INDICATIONS AND DOSAGES

Relief of dry eye and eye irritation

Ophthalmic

Adults, Elderly. Instill 1 or 2 drops in affected eye(s) as needed.

CONTRAINDICATIONS: Hypersensitivity to glycerin, polysorbate 80, or any component of the formulation

INTERACTIONS

Drug

None known.

Herbal

None known.

Food

None known.

DIAGNOSTIC TEST EFFECTS: *None known.*

SIDE EFFECTS

Blurred vision for a short time

SERIOUS REACTIONS

- None reported.

SPECIAL CONSIDERATIONS

PATIENT INFORMATION

Give patients the following instructions:

- For external use only. To avoid contamination, do not touch the tip of the container to any surface. Do not reuse. Once opened, discard. Do not touch unit-dose tip to eye. Do not use if solution changes color. Stop use and ask a doctor if you experience eye pain, changes in vision, or continued redness or irritation of the eye, or if the condition worsens or persists for more than 72 hours. Keep out of the reach of children.

gold sodium thiomalate

(gold sodium thigh-oh-mal′-ate)

Rx: Myochrysine

Drug Class: Disease modifying antirheumatic drugs; Gold compounds

Pregnancy Category: C

CLINICAL PHARMACOLOGY

Mechanism of Action: A gold compound whose mechanism of action is unknown. May decrease prostaglandin synthesis or alter cellular mechanisms by inhibiting sulfhydryl systems. *Therapeutic Effect:* Decreases synovial inflammation, retards cartilage and bone destruction, suppresses or prevents—but does not cure—arthritis and synovitis.

AVAILABLE FORMS

- *Injection:* 50 mg/ml.

INDICATIONS AND DOSAGES

Rheumatoid arthritis

IM

Adults, Elderly. Initially, 10 mg, followed by 25 mg for second dose, then 25-50 mg/wk until improvement noted or total of 1 g has been administered. Maintenance: 25-50 mg q2wk for 2-20 wk; if stable, may increase intervals to q3-4wk.

Children. Initially, 10 mg, then 1 mg/kg/wk up to a maximum single dose of 50 mg. Maintenance: 1 mg/kg/dose q2-4wk.

Dosage in renal impairment

Dosage is modified based on creatinine clearance.

Creatinine Clearance	*Dosage*
50-80 ml/min	50% of usual dose
less than 50 ml/min	not recommended

UNLABELED USES: Treatment of psoriatic arthritis

CONTRAINDICATIONS: Colitis; concurrent use of antimalarials, immunosuppressive agents, penicillamine, or phenylbutazone; CHF; exfoliative dermatitis; history of blood dyscrasias; severe hepatic or renal impairment; systemic lupus erythematosus

INTERACTIONS

Drug

Bone marrow depressants, hepatotoxic and nephrotoxic medications: May increase the risk of toxicity.

Penicillamine: May increase the risk of adverse hematologic or renal effects.

Herbal

None known.

Food

None known.

DIAGNOSTIC TEST EFFECTS: May decrease Hgb level, Hct, and WBC and platelet counts. May increase urine protein level. May alter liver function test results.

SIDE EFFECTS

Frequent

Pruritic dermatitis, stomatitis, diarrhea, abdominal pain, nausea

Occasional

Vomiting, anorexia, flatulence, dyspepsia, conjunctivitis, photosensitivity

Rare

Constipation, urticaria, rash

SERIOUS REACTIONS

• Signs and symptoms of gold toxicity include decreased Hgb level, decreased granulocyte count (less than 150,000/mm^3), proteinuria, hematuria, blood dyscrasias (anemia, leukopenia [WBC less than 4000 mm^3], thrombocytopenia, and eosinophilia), glomerulonephritis, nephrotic syndrome, and cholestatic jaundice.

SPECIAL CONSIDERATIONS

PRECAUTIONS

• Do not use gold salts concomitantly with penicillamine. The safety of coadministration with cytotoxic drugs has not been established. Use caution in patients with history of blood dyscrasias, hypersensitivity, skin rash, previous kidney or liver disease, marked hypertension, and compromised cerebral or cardiovascular circulation. Diabetes mellitus or congestive heart failure should be under control before gold therapy is instituted.

PREGNANCY AND LACTATION

• Pregnancy Category C. Gold sodium thiomalate has been shown to be teratogenic during the organogenetic period in rats and rabbits. The presence of gold has been demonstrated in the milk of lactating mothers.

OCULAR CONSIDERATIONS

• There have been rare reports of reactions involving the eye such as iritis, corneal ulcers, and gold deposits in ocular tissues.

gramicidin; neomycin sulfate; polymyxin B sulfate

(gram-i-sye'din; nee-oh-mye'sin sul'fate; pol-ee-mix'in bee sul'fate)

Rx: AK-Spore, Neocidin, Neosporin Ophthalmic, Ocu-Spore-G

Drug Class: Anti-infectives, ophthalmic; Ophthalmics

CLINICAL PHARMACOLOGY

Mechanism of Action: An antibiotic that interferes with bacterial protein synthesis by binding to 30S ribosomal subunits. It also binds to phospholipids, alters permeability, and damages the bacterial cytoplasmic membrane permitting leakage of intracellular constituents. *Therapeutic Effect:* Interferes in protein synthesis of susceptible microorganisms.

Pharmacokinetics

None reported.

AVAILABLE FORMS

• *Ophthalmic Solution:* 0.025 mg gramicidin, 1.75 mg neomycin, 10,000 units polymyxin B per ml (AK-Spore, Neocidin, Neosporin Ophthalmic, Ocu-Spore-G).

INDICATIONS AND DOSAGES

Superficial eye infections

Ophthalmic Solution

Adults, Elderly, Children. Instill 1-2 drops 4-6 times/day or more frequently as required for severe infections.

CONTRAINDICATIONS: Hypersensitivity to neomycin, polymyxin B, gramicidin or any component of the formulation

INTERACTIONS

Drug

None known.

Herbal

None known.

Food

None known.

DIAGNOSTIC TEST EFFECTS: *None known.*

SIDE EFFECTS

Occasional

Irritation, burning, stinging, itching, inflammation

SERIOUS REACTIONS

- Angioneurotic edema, urticaria, vesicular and maculopapular dermatitis occurs rarely.
- Symptoms of neomycin sensitization include itching, reddening, edema, and failure to heal.

SPECIAL CONSIDERATIONS

PRECAUTIONS

- As with other antibiotic preparations, prolonged use of gramicidin/neomycin sulfate/polymyxin B sulfate ocular solution may result in overgrowth of nonsusceptible organisms including fungi. If superinfection occurs, initiate appropriate measures. Bacterial resistance also may develop. If purulent discharge, inflammation, or pain becomes aggravated, instruct the patient to discontinue use of the medication and consult a physician. Allergic cross-reactions may occur that could prevent the use of any or all of the following antibiotics for the treatment of future infections: kanamycin, paromomycin, streptomycin, and possibly gentamicin.

PATIENT INFORMATION

- Advise patients not to use this product if they are allergic to any of the listed ingredients. Instruct patients to keep container tightly closed when not in use and to keep the drug out of reach of children.

PREGNANCY AND LACTATION

- Pregnancy Category C. Fetal harm is not known with topical administration. Excretion into human milk is not known.

guanabenz

(gwan'a-benz)

Drug Class: Antiadrenergics, central

Pregnancy Category: C

CLINICAL PHARMACOLOGY

Mechanism of Action: An alpha-adrenergic agonist that stimulates alpha$_2$-adrenergic receptors. Inhibits sympathetic cardioaccelerator and vasoconstrictor center to heart, kidneys, peripheral vasculature. *Therapeutic Effect:* Decreases systolic, diastolic blood pressure (BP). Chronic use decreases peripheral vascular resistance.

Pharmacokinetics

Well absorbed from gastrointestinal (GI) tract. Widely distributed. Protein binding: 90%. Metabolized in liver. Excreted in urine and feces. Not removed by hemodialysis. **Half-life:** 6 hrs.

AVAILABLE FORMS

- *Tablets:* 4 mg, 8 mg (Wytensin).

INDICATIONS AND DOSAGES

Hypertension

PO

Adults. Initially, 4 mg 2 times/day. Increase by 4-8 mg at 1-2 wk intervals. Elderly. Initially, 4 mg/day. May increase q1-2 wks. Maintenance: 8-16 mg/day. Maximum: 32 mg/day.

CONTRAINDICATIONS: History of hypersensitivity to guanabenz or any component of the formulation

INTERACTIONS

Drug

Beta-blockers, hypotensive-producing medications: May increase antihypertensive effect.

Herbal

Licorice, yohimbine: May decrease guanabenz effectiveness.

Food

None known.

DIAGNOSTIC TEST EFFECTS: May decrease cholesterol, total triglyceride concentrations.

SIDE EFFECTS

Frequent

Drowsiness, dry mouth, dizziness

Occasional

Weakness, headache, nausea, decreased sexual ability

Rare

Ataxia, sleep disturbances, rash, itching, diarrhea, constipation, altered taste, muscle aches

SERIOUS REACTIONS

• Abrupt withdrawal may result in rebound hypertension manifested as nervousness, agitation, anxiety, insomnia, hand tingling, tremor, flushing, and sweating.

• Overdosage produces hypotension, somnolence, lethargy, irritability, bradycardia, and miosis (pupillary constriction).

SPECIAL CONSIDERATIONS

PRECAUTIONS

• Guanabenz acetate causes sedation or drowsiness in a large fraction of patients. Use guanabenz acetate with caution in patients with severe coronary insufficiency, recent myocardial infarction, cerebrovascular disease, or severe hepatic or renal failure. Sudden cessation of therapy rarely may result in "overshoot" hypertension. Mean plasma concentrations of guanabenz acetate were higher in patients with hepatic impairment. Careful monitoring of blood pressure during guanabenz acetate dose titration is suggested in patients with coexisting hypertension and renal impairment.

PATIENT INFORMATION

• Advise patients who receive guanabenz acetate to exercise caution when operating dangerous machinery or driving motor vehicles until they determine that they do not become drowsy or dizzy from the medication. Warn patients that their tolerance for alcohol and other central nervous system depressants may be diminished. Advise patients not to discontinue therapy abruptly.

PREGNANCY AND LACTATION

• Pregnancy Category C. A teratology study in mice has indicated a possible increase in skeletal abnormalities. Fetal harm is not known. Excretion into human milk is not known.

guanadrel sulfate

(gwahn'a-drel)

Drug Class: Antiadrenergics, peripheral

Pregnancy Category: B

CLINICAL PHARMACOLOGY

Mechanism of Action: An adrenergic blocking agent that depletes norepinephrine from adrenergic nerve endings. Prevents release of norepinephrine normally produced by nerve stimulation. *Therapeutic Effect:* Reduces blood pressure (BP).

Pharmacokinetics

Rapidly and well absorbed from gastrointestinal (GI) tract. Widely distributed. Protein binding: 20%. Primarily excreted in urine. **Half-life:** 10 hrs.

AVAILABLE FORMS

- *Tablets:* 10 mg, 25 mg (Hylorel).

INDICATIONS AND DOSAGES

Hypertension

PO

Adults. Initially, 5 mg 2 times/day. Increase at 1- to 4-wk intervals. Maintenance: 20-75 mg/day in 2 divided doses. Maximum: 400 mg/day.

Elderly. Initially, 5 mg/day. May gradually increase at 1-4 wk intervals. Maintenance: 20-75 mg/day in 2 divided doses.

CONTRAINDICATIONS: Frank CHF, pheochromocytoma, hypersensitivity to guanadrel or any component of the formulation

INTERACTIONS

Drug

Tricyclic antidepressants, MAOIs, phenothiazines, sympathomimetics: May decrease antihypertensive effect.

Herbal

Licorice, yohimbine: May reduce guanadrel effectiveness.

Ma huang: May decrease hypotensive effect of guanadrel.

Food

None known.

DIAGNOSTIC TEST EFFECTS: *None known.*

SIDE EFFECTS

Frequent (42-64%)

Fatigue, headache, faintness, drowsiness, nocturia, urinary frequency, change in weight, aching limbs, shortness of breath (resting)

Occasional (21-29%)

Cough, change in vision, paresthesia, confusion, indigestion, constipation, anorexia, peripheral edema, leg cramps

Rare (<10%)

Depression, altered sleep, nausea, vomiting, dry mouth, throat, impotence, backache.

SERIOUS REACTIONS

- Overdose may produce blurred vision, severe dizziness/faintness.

SPECIAL CONSIDERATIONS

PRECAUTIONS

- Salt and water retention may occur with the use of guanadrel sulfate tablets. Use guanadrel sulfate cautiously in patients with a history of peptic ulcer. In patients with compromised renal function, decreases in renal and nonrenal clearances and an increase in the elimination half-life of guanadrel sulfate have been found. A transient increase in blood pressure has been observed in some patients.

PATIENT INFORMATION

- Advise patients about the risk of orthostatic hypotension and instruct them to sit or lie down immediately at the onset of dizziness or weakness so that they can prevent loss of consciousness. Advise patients that postural hypotension is worst in the morning and upon arising and may be exaggerated by alcohol, fever, hot weather, prolonged standing, or exercise.

PREGNANCY AND LACTATION

- Pregnancy Category B. Teratology studies performed in rats and rabbits revealed no significant harm to the fetus from guanadrel sulfate. Fetal harm is not known. Excretion into human milk is not known.

guanethidine monosulfate

(gwahn-eth'i-deen)

Drug Class: Antiadrenergics, peripheral

Pregnancy Category: C

CLINICAL PHARMACOLOGY

Mechanism of Action: An adrenergic blocker that inhibits the release of catecholamines produced by sympathetic nerve stimulation, thus suppressing peripheral sympathetic vasoconstriction. *Therapeutic Effect:* Decreases blood pressure.

Pharmacokinetics

Absorption is highly variable among patients. Protein binding: 26%. Metabolized in liver. Excreted in urine and feces. **Half-life:** 5-10 days.

AVAILABLE FORMS

- *Tablets:* 10 mg, 25 mg (Ismelin).

INDICATIONS AND DOSAGES

Hypertension

PO

Adults. Initially, 10 mg/day. May increase in 10-25 mg increments at 5-7 day intervals. Maximum: 100 mg/day. Lower initial doses are recommended for the elderly.

UNLABELED USES: Treatment of anxiety, chronic angina pectoris, hypertrophic cardiomyopathy, myocardial infarction, pheochromocytoma, syndrome of mitral valve prolapse, thyrotoxicosis, and tremors

CONTRAINDICATIONS: MAOI therapy within 1 week, overt congestive heart failure, pheochromocytoma, hypersensitivity to guanethidine or any component of the formulation

INTERACTIONS

Drug

Amphetamines, chlorpromazine, deithylpropion, epinephrine, imipramine, methylphenidate, MAOIs, prochlorperazine, tricyclic antidepressants, zotepine: May decrease antihypertensive effectiveness.

Etilefrine: May increase etilefrine effects.

Norepinephrine, phenylephrine: May cause hypertension and/or arrhythmias.

Phenylpropanolamine, pseudoephedrine: May cause a loss of blood pressure control and possible hypertensive urgency.

Herbal

Licorice, Ma huang, yohimbine: May decrease hypotensive effect of guanethidine.

Food

None known.

DIAGNOSTIC TEST EFFECTS: *None known.*

SIDE EFFECTS

Frequent

Bradycardia, dizziness, blurred vision, orthostatic hypotension, fluid retention

Occasional

Impotence, inhibition of ejaculation, nasal stuffiness

Rare

Apnea, hypertension, renal dysfunction

SERIOUS REACTIONS

- Arrhythmias, angina, and pulmonary edema have been reported.
- Overdosage may produce bradycardia, diarrhea, nausea, orthostatic hypotension, and shock.

SPECIAL CONSIDERATIONS

PRECAUTIONS

- Dosage requirements may be reduced in the presence of fever. Exercise special care when treating patients with a history of bronchial asthma. Use guanethidine monosulfate cautiously in hypertensive patients with renal disease and nitrogen retention or rising blood urea nitrogen levels. Do not give guanethidine monosulfate to patients with severe cardiac failure. Watch patients with incipient cardiac decompensation for weight gain or edema. Use guanethidine monosulfate cautiously in patients with a history of peptic ulcer or other chronic disorders that may be aggravated by a relative increase in parasympathetic tone.

PATIENT INFORMATION

• Advise the patient to take guanethidine monosulfate exactly as directed. If the patient misses a dose, instruct the patient to take only the next scheduled dose (without doubling it). Advise the patient to avoid sudden or prolonged standing or exercise and to arise slowly, especially in the morning, to reduce the orthostatic hypotensive effects of dizziness, light-headedness, or fainting. Caution the patient about ingesting alcohol because it aggravates the orthostatic hypotensive effects of guanethidine monosulfate. Advise male patients that guanethidine may interfere with ejaculation.

PREGNANCY AND LACTATION

• Pregnancy Category C. Animal reproduction studies have not been conducted with guanethidine monosulfate. Whether guanethidine monosulfate can cause fetal harm when administered to a pregnant woman or can affect reproduction capacity is not know. Guanethidine monosulfate is excreted in breast milk in very small quantity.

heparin sodium

(hep'a-rin)

Rx: Hep-Lock, Hep-Pak CVC

Drug Class: Anticoagulants

Pregnancy Category: C

Do not confuse heparin with Hespan.

CLINICAL PHARMACOLOGY

Mechanism of Action: A blood modifier that interferes with blood coagulation by blocking conversion of prothrombin to thrombin and fibrinogen to fibrin. *Therapeutic Effect:* Prevents further extension of existing thrombi or new clot formation. Has no effect on existing clots.

Pharmacokinetics

Well absorbed following subcutaneous administration. Protein binding: Very high. Metabolized in the liver. Removed from the circulation via uptake by the reticuloendothelial system. Primarily excreted in urine. Not removed by hemodialysis. **Half-life:** 1-6 hr.

AVAILABLE FORMS

• *Injection:* 10 units/ml, 100 units/ml, 1000 units/ml, 2500 units/ml, 5000 units/ml, 7500 units/ml, 10,000 units/ml, 20,000 units/ml, 25,000 units/500 ml infusion.

INDICATIONS AND DOSAGES

Line flushing

IV

Adults, Elderly, Children. 100 units q6-8h.

Infants weighing less than 10 kg. 10 units q6-8h.

Treatment of venous thrombosis, pulmonary embolism, peripheral arterial embolism, atrial fibrillation with embolism

Intermittent IV

Adults, Elderly. Initially, 10,000 units, then 50-70 units/kg (5000-10,000 units) q4-6h.

H

Children 1 yr and older. Initially, 50-100 units/kg, then 50-100 units q4h.
IV Infusion
Adults, Elderly. Loading dose: 80 units/kg, then 18 units/kg/hr, with adjustments based on aPTT. Range: 10-30 units/kg/hr.
Children 1 yr and older. Loading dose: 75 units/kg, then 20 units/kg/hr with adjustments based on aPTT.
Children younger than 1 yr. Loading dose: 75 units/kg, then 28 units/kg/hr.
Prevention of venous thrombosis, pulmonary embolism, peripheral arterial embolism, atrial fibrillation with embolism
Subcutaneous
Adult, Elderly. 5000 units q8-12h.

CONTRAINDICATIONS: Intracranial hemorrhage, severe hypotension, severe thrombocytopenia, subacute bacterial endocarditis, uncontrolled bleeding

INTERACTIONS

Drug

Antithyroid medications, cefoperazone, cefotetan, valproic acid: May cause hypoprothrombinemia.

Other anticoagulants, platelet aggregation inhibitors, thrombolytics: May increase the risk of bleeding.

Probenecid: May increase the effects of heparin.

Herbal

Feverfew, ginkgo biloba: May have additive effect.

Food

None known.

DIAGNOSTIC TEST EFFECTS: May increase free fatty acid, AST (SGOT), and ALT (SGPT) levels. May decrease serum cholesterol and triglyceride levels.

IV INCOMPATIBILITIES: Amiodarone (Cordarone), amphotericin B complex (Abelcet, AmBisome, Amphotec), ciprofloxacin (Cipro), dacarbazine (DTIC), diazepam (Valium), dobutamine (Dobutrex), doxorubicin (Adriamycin), droperidol (Inapsine), filgrastim (Neupogen), gentamicin (Garamycin), haloperidol (Haldol), idarubicin (Idamycin), labetalol (Trandate), nicardipine (Cardene), phenytoin (Dilantin), quinidine, tobramycin (Nebcin), vancomycin (Vancocin)

IV COMPATIBILITIES: Aminophylline, ampicillin/sulbactam (Unasyn), aztreonam (Azactam), calcium gluconate, cefazolin (Ancef), ceftazidime (Fortaz), ceftriaxone (Rocephin), digoxin (Lanoxin), diltiazem (Cardizem), dopamine (Intropin), enalapril (Vasotec), famotidine (Pepcid), fentanyl (Sublimaze), furosemide (Lasix), hydromorphone (Dilaudid), insulin, lidocaine, lorazepam (Ativan), magnesium sulfate, methylprednisolone (Solu-Medrol), midazolam (Versed), milrinone (Primacor), morphine, nitroglycerin, norepinephrine (Levophed), oxytocin (Pitocin), piperacillin/tazobactam (Zosyn), procainamide (Pronestyl), propofol (Diprivan)

SIDE EFFECTS

Occasional

Itching, burning (particularly on soles of feet) caused by vasospastic reaction

Rare

Pain, cyanosis of extremity 6-10 days after initial therapy lasting 4-6 hours; hypersensitivity reaction, including chills, fever, pruritus, urticaria, asthma, rhinitis, lacrimation, and headache

SERIOUS REACTIONS

• Bleeding complications ranging from local ecchymoses to major hemorrhage occur more frequently in high-dose therapy, intermittent IV infusion, and in women 60 years of age and older.

• Antidote: Protamine sulfate 1-1.5 mg, IV, for every 100 units heparin subcutaneous within 30 minutes of overdose, 0.5-0.75 mg for every 100 units heparin subcutaneous if within 30-60 minutes of overdose, 0.25-0.375 mg for every 100 units heparin subcutaneous if 2 hours have elapsed since overdose, 25-50 mg if heparin was given by IV infusion.

SPECIAL CONSIDERATIONS

PREGNANCY AND LACTATION

• Pregnancy Category C. Whether heparin sodium can cause fetal harm when administered to a pregnant woman or can affect reproduction capacity is not known. Give heparin sodium to a pregnant woman only if clearly needed. Heparin does not cross the placental barrier. Heparin is not excreted in human milk.

OCULAR CONSIDERATIONS

• Heparin can aid in ocular wound healing. Heparin in the interstitial tissue of the wound surface blocks the conversion of fibrinogen to fibrin. Adding heparin to the irrigating solution in pediatric cataract surgery decreased postoperative inflammatory and fibrinoid reactions and related complications such as synechiae, pupil irregularity, and intraocular lens decentration. (Dostalek M et al: Ligneous conjunctivitis: complication of inborn plasminogen deficiency [a case report], *Cesk Slov Oftalmol* 61[1]:38-49, 2005. Bayramlar H, Totan Y, Borazan M: Heparin in the intraocular irrigating solution in pediatric cataract surgery, *J Cataract Refract Surg* 30[10]:2163-2169, 2004.)

homatropine hydrobromide

(hoe-ma'troe-peen)

Rx: Isopto Homatropine

Drug Class: Cycloplegics; Mydriatics; Ophthalmics

Pregnancy Category: C

H

CLINICAL PHARMACOLOGY

Mechanism of Action: An ophthalmic agent that blocks response of iris sphincter muscle and the accommodative muscle of the ciliary body to cholinergic stimulation resulting in dilation and loss of accommodation. *Therapeutic Effect:* Produces cycloplegia and mydriasis for refraction.

Pharmacokinetics

Maximum mydriatic effect occurs within 10-30 min; maximum cycloplegic effect occurs within 30-90 minutes. Duration of mydriasis is 6 hrs - 4 days; duration of cycloplegia is 10-48 hrs.

AVAILABLE FORMS

• *Ophthalmic Solution:* 2%, 5% (Isopto Homatropine).

INDICATIONS AND DOSAGES

Mydriasis and cycloplegia for refraction

Ophthalmic

Adults, Elderly. Instill 1-2 drops of 2% solution or 1 drop of 5% solution before the procedure. Repeat at 5- to 10-minute intervals as needed. Maximum: 3 doses for refraction.

Children. Instill 1 drop of 2% solution immediately before the procedure. Repeat at 10-minute intervals as needed.

Uveitis

Ophthalmic

Adults, Elderly. Instill 1-2 drops of 2% or 5% 2-3 times/day up to every 3-4 hours as needed.

Children. Instill 1 drop of 2% solution 2-3 times/day.

CONTRAINDICATIONS: Narrow-angle glaucoma, acute hemorrhage, hypersensitivity to homatropine or any component of the formulation

INTERACTIONS

Drug

None known.

Herbal

None known.

Food

None known.

DIAGNOSTIC TEST EFFECTS: *None known.*

SIDE EFFECTS

Frequent

Blurred vision, photophobia

Occasional

Irritation, increased intraocular pressure, congestion

Rare

Eczematoid dermatitis, edema, exudates, follicular conjunctivitis, somnolence, vascular congestion

SERIOUS REACTIONS

• Overdosage may produce symptoms of blurred vision, urinary retention, and tachycardia. Anticholinergic toxicity is caused by strong binding of the drug to cholinergic receptors.

SPECIAL CONSIDERATIONS

PRECAUTIONS

• In infants and small children, use homatropine hydrobromide with extreme caution. Excessive use in children or in patients with a history of susceptibility to belladonna alkaloids may produce systemic symptoms of homatropine poisoning. Instruct patients to use caution when driving or when engaging in hazardous activities. Parents of children should be cautious not to get the drug into the child's mouth and to wash the child's and their hands after use of the drug. Use homatropine hydrobromide cautiously in elderly or hypertensive patients.

PREGNANCY AND LACTATION

• Pregnancy Category C. Fetal harm is not known. Very small amounts are detectable in human milk.

hydralazine hydrochloride

(hye-dral'a-zeen)

Rx: Apresoline

Drug Class: Vasodilators

Pregnancy Category: C

Do not confuse hydralazine with hydroxyzine.

CLINICAL PHARMACOLOGY

Mechanism of Action: An antihypertensive with direct vasodilating effects on arterioles. *Therapeutic Effect:* Decreases BP and systemic resistance.

Pharmacokinetics

Route	Onset	Peak	Duration
PO	20-30 min	N/A	2-4 hr
IV	5-20 min	N/A	2-6 hr

Well absorbed from the GI tract. Widely distributed. Protein binding: 85%-90%. Metabolized in the liver to active metabolite. Primarily excreted in urine. Not removed by hemodialysis. **Half-life:** 3-7 hr (increased with impaired renal function).

AVAILABLE FORMS

• *Tablets:* 10 mg, 25 mg, 50 mg, 100 mg.

• *Injection:* 20 mg/ml.

INDICATIONS AND DOSAGES

Moderate to severe hypertension

PO

Adults. Initially, 10 mg 4 times a day. May increase by 10-25 mg/dose q2-5 days. Maximum: 300 mg/day.

Children. Initially, 0.75-1 mg/kg/day in 2-4 divided doses, not to exceed 25 mg/dose. May increase over 3-4 wk. Maximum: 7.5 mg/kg/day (5 mg/kg/day in infants).

IV, IM

Adults, Elderly. Initially, 10-20 mg/dose q4-6h. May increase to 40 mg/ dose.

Children. Initially, 0.1-0.2 mg/kg/dose (maximum: 20 mg) q4-6h, as needed, up to 1.7-3.5 mg/kg/day in divided doses q4-6h.

Dosage in renal impairment

Dosage interval is based on creatinine clearance.

Creatinine Clearance	*Dosage Interval*
10-50 ml/min	q8h
less than 10 ml/min	q8-24h

UNLABELED USES: Treatment of CHF, hypertension secondary to eclampsia and preeclampsia, primary pulmonary hypertension.

CONTRAINDICATIONS: Coronary artery disease, lupus erythematosus, rheumatic heart disease

INTERACTIONS

Drug

Diuretics, other antihypertensives: May increase hypotensive effect.

Herbal

None known.

Food

None known.

DIAGNOSTIC TEST EFFECTS: May produce positive direct Coombs' test.

IV INCOMPATIBILITIES: Aminophylline, ampicillin (Polycillin), furosemide (Lasix)

IV COMPATIBILITIES: Dobutamine (Dobutrex), heparin, hydrocortisone (Solu-Cortef), nitroglycerin, potassium

SIDE EFFECTS

Frequent

Headache, palpitations, tachycardia (generally disappears in 7-10 days)

Occasional

GI disturbance (nausea, vomiting, diarrhea), paraesthesia, fluid retention, peripheral edema, dizziness, flushed face, nasal congestion

SERIOUS REACTIONS

- High dosage may produce lupus erythematosus–like reaction, including fever, facial rash, muscle and joint aches, and splenomegaly.
- Severe orthostatic hypotension, skin flushing, severe headache, myocardial ischemia, and cardiac arrhythmias may develop.
- Profound shock may occur with severe overdosage.

SPECIAL CONSIDERATIONS

PRECAUTIONS

- Hydralazine hydrochloride must be used with caution in patients with suspected coronary artery disease. Use the drug with caution in patients with cerebral vascular accidents and with advanced renal damage.

PATIENT INFORMATION

- Inform patients of possible side effects and advise them to take the medication regularly and continuously as directed.

PREGNANCY AND LACTATION

- Pregnancy Category C. Teratogenic effects observed were cleft palate and malformations of facial and cranial bones in mice. Fetal harm is not known. Hydralazine has been shown to be excreted in breast milk.

hydrochlorothiazide

(hye-droe-klor-oh-thye'a-zide)

Rx: Aquazide H, HydroDIURIL, Microzide, Oretic

Drug Class: Diuretics, thiazide and derivatives

Pregnancy Category: B

CLINICAL PHARMACOLOGY

Mechanism of Action: A sulfonamide derivative that acts as a thiazide diuretic and antihypertensive. As a diuretic blocks reabsorption of water, sodium, and potassium at the cortical diluting segment of the distal tubule. As an antihypertensive reduces plasma, extracellular fluid volume, and peripheral vascular resistance by direct effect on blood vessels. *Therapeutic Effect:* Promotes diuresis; reduces BP.

Pharmacokinetics

Route	*Onset*	*Peak*	*Duration*
PO (diuretic)	2 hr	4-6 hr	6-12 hr

Variably absorbed from the GI tract. Primarily excreted unchanged in urine. Not removed by hemodialysis. **Half-life:** 5.6-14.8 hr.

AVAILABLE FORMS

- *Capsules (Microzide):* 12.5 mg.
- *Oral Solution:* 50 mg/5 ml.
- *Tablets (Aquazide, Oretic):* 25 mg, 50 mg, 100 mg.

INDICATIONS AND DOSAGES

Edema, hypertension

PO

Adults. 12.5-100 mg/day. Maximum: 200 mg/day.

Usual pediatric dosage

PO

Children 6 mo-12 yr. 2 mg/kg/day in 2 divided doses. Maximum: 200 mg/day.

Children younger than 6 mo. 2-4 mg/kg/day in 2 divided doses. Maximum: 37.5 mg/day.

UNLABELED USES: Treatment of diabetes insipidus, prevention of calcium-containing renal calculi

CONTRAINDICATIONS: Anuria, history of hypersensitivity to sulfonamides or thiazide diuretics, renal decompensation

INTERACTIONS

Drug

Cholestyramine, colestipol: May decrease the absorption and effects of hydrochlorothiazide.

Digoxin: May increase the risk of digoxin toxicity associated with hydrochlorothiazide-induced hypokalemia.

Lithium: May increase the risk of lithium toxicity.

Herbal

None known.

Food

None known.

DIAGNOSTIC TEST EFFECTS: May increase blood glucose and serum cholesterol, LDL, bilirubin, calcium, creatinine, uric acid, and triglyceride levels. May decrease urinary calcium, and serum magnesium, potassium, and sodium levels.

SIDE EFFECTS

Expected

Increase in urinary frequency and urine volume

Frequent

Potassium depletion

Occasional

Orthostatic hypotension, headache, GI disturbances, photosensitivity

SERIOUS REACTIONS

- Vigorous diuresis may lead to profound water and electrolyte depletion, resulting in hypokalemia, hyponatremia, and dehydration.
- Acute hypotensive episodes may occur.

• Hyperglycemia may occur during prolonged therapy.
• Pancreatitis, blood dyscrasias, pulmonary edema, allergic pneumonitis, and dermatologic reactions occur rarely.
• Overdose can lead to lethargy and coma without changes in electrolytes or hydration.

SPECIAL CONSIDERATIONS

PRECAUTIONS

• Observe all patients receiving diuretic therapy for evidence of fluid or electrolyte imbalance: namely, hyponatremia, hypochloremic alkalosis, and hypokalemia. Hyperuricemia or acute gout may be precipitated in certain patients receiving thiazide diuretics. Use thiazides with caution in patients with impaired hepatic function. Calcium excretion is decreased by thiazides, and pathologic changes in parathyroid glands, with hypercalcemia and hypophosphatemia, have been observed in a few patients on prolonged thiazide therapy. In diabetic patients, dosage adjustments of insulin or oral hypoglycemic agents may be required. The antihypertensive effects of the drug may be enhanced in the postsympathectomy patient. If progressive renal impairment becomes evident, consider withholding or discontinuing diuretic therapy. Thiazides have been shown to increase the urinary excretion of magnesium; this may result in hypomagnesemia. Increases in cholesterol and triglyceride levels may be associated with thiazide diuretic therapy.

PREGNANCY AND LACTATION

• Pregnancy Category B. Studies in which hydrochlorothiazide was administered orally to pregnant mice and rats during their respective periods of major organogenesis at doses of up to 3000 and 1000 mg/kg, respectively, provided no evidence of harm to the fetus. However, no adequate and well-controlled studies in pregnant women have been done. Because animal reproduction studies are not always predictive of human response, use this drug during pregnancy only if clearly needed. Thiazides are excreted in breast milk.

OCULAR CONSIDERATIONS

• Hydrochlorothiazide can induce myopia.

H

hydrochlorothiazide; triamterene

(hye-droe-klor-oh-thye'a-zide; trye-am'ter-een)

Rx: Dyazide, Maxzide, Maxzide-25

Drug Class: Diuretics, potassium sparing; Diuretics, thiazide and derivatives

Pregnancy Category: C

CLINICAL PHARMACOLOGY

Mechanism of Action: Hydrochlorothiazide is a sulfonamide derivative that acts as a thiazide diuretic and antihypertensive. As a diuretic blocks reabsorption of water, the electrolytes sodium and potassium at cortical diluting segment of distal tubule. As an antihypertensive reduces plasma, extracellular fluid volume, decreases peripheral vascular resistance (PVR) by direct effect on blood vessels. Triamterene is a potassium-sparing diuretic that inhibits sodium, potassium, ATPase. Interferes with sodium and potassium exchange in distal tubule, cortical collecting tubule, and collecting duct. *Therapeutic Effect:* Promotes diuresis, reduces blood pressure (BP). Increases sodium and decreases potassium excretion. Also increases magnesium, decreases calcium loss.

Pharmacokinetics

Hydrochlorothiazide

Variably absorbed from the gastrointestinal (GI) tract. Primarily excreted unchanged in urine. Not removed by hemodialysis. **Half-life:** 5.6-14.8 hrs.

Triamterene

Incompletely absorbed from the gastrointestinal (GI) tract. Widely distributed. Metabolized in liver. Primarily eliminated in feces via biliary route. **Half-life:** 1.5-2.5 hrs (half-life is increased in patients with impaired renal function).

AVAILABLE FORMS

- *Capsules:* 25 mg hydrochlorothiazide and 37.5 mg triamterene (Dyazide).
- *Tablets:* 50 mg hydrochlorothiazide and 75 mg triamterene (Maxzide), 25 mg hydrochlorothiazide and 37.5 mg triamterene (Maxzide-25).

INDICATIONS AND DOSAGES

Edema, hypertension

PO

Adults. ½ to 2 tablets/capsules once daily.

CONTRAINDICATIONS: Anuria, history of hypersensitivity to sulfonamides or thiazide diuretics, renal decompensation

INTERACTIONS

Drug

Angiotensin-converting enzyme (ACE) inhibitors, such as captopril, potassium-containing medications, potassium supplements: May increase serum potassium levels.

Anticoagulants, heparin: May decrease the effects of anticoagulants and heparin.

Cholestyramine, colestipol: May decrease the absorption and effects of hydrochlorothiazide.

Lithium: May increase the risk of toxicity of lithium.

NSAIDs: May decrease the antihypertensive effect.

Herbal

None known.

Food

None known.

DIAGNOSTIC TEST EFFECTS: May increase blood glucose levels, serum cholesterol, LDL, bilirubin, calcium, creatinine, uric acid, and triglyceride levels. May decrease urinary calcium, and serum magnesium, potassium, and sodium levels.

SIDE EFFECTS

Expected

Increase in urine frequency and volume

Frequent

Hydrochlorothiazide: Potassium depletion

Triamterene: Fatigue, nausea, diarrhea, abdominal distress, leg aches, headache

Occasional

Hydrochlorothiazide: Postural hypotension, headache, gastrointestinal (GI) disturbances, photosensitivity reaction

Triamterene: Anorexia, weakness, rash, dizziness

SERIOUS REACTIONS

- Acute hypotensive episodes may occur.
- Hyperglycemia may be noted during prolonged therapy.
- GI upset, pancreatitis, dizziness, paresthesias, headache, blood dyscrasias, pulmonary edema, allergic pneumonitis, and dermatologic reactions occur rarely with hydrochlorothiazide.
- Overdosage can lead to lethargy and coma without changes in electrolytes or hydration.

• Agranulocytosis, nephrolithiasis, and thrombocytopenia occur rarely with triamterene.

SPECIAL CONSIDERATIONS

PRECAUTIONS

• Hyperkalemia is more likely to occur in patients with renal impairment and diabetes (even without evidence of renal impairment) and in the elderly or severely ill. Also avoid potassium-sparing therapy in severely ill patients in whom respiratory or metabolic acidosis may occur. Exercise caution when administering hydrochlorothiazide and triamterene to patients with diabetes because thiazides may cause hyperglycemia and glycosuria. Use thiazides with caution in patients with impaired hepatic function. Thiazides can precipitate hepatic coma in patients with severe liver disease. Electrolyte imbalance—often encountered in conditions such as heart failure, renal disease, or cirrhosis of the liver—also may be aggravated by diuretics. Dilutional hyponatremia may occur in edematous patients in hot weather. Triamterene has been found in renal stones in association with the other usual calculus components.

PREGNANCY AND LACTATION

• Pregnancy Category C. The routine use of diuretics in an otherwise healthy woman is inappropriate and exposes mother and fetus to unnecessary hazard. Fetal harm is not known. Thiazides and triamterene in combination have not been studied in nursing mothers. Triamterene appears in animal milk; this may occur in human beings. Thiazides are excreted in human breast milk.

OCULAR CONSIDERATIONS

• Adverse reactions include xanthopsia and transient blurred vision.

hydrocortisone acetate; oxytetracycline hydrochloride

(hye-droe-kor'ti-sone as'a-tate; ox-i-tet-ra-sye'kleen hye-droe-klor'ide)

Drug Class: Anti-infectives, ophthalmic; Antibiotics, tetracyclines; Corticosteroids, ophthalmic; Ophthalmics

Pregnancy Category: D

H

CLINICAL PHARMACOLOGY

Mechanism of Action: Hydrocortisone is an adrenal corticosteroid that inhibits accumulation of inflammatory cells at inflammation sites, phagocytosis, lysosomal enzyme release and synthesis or release of mediators of inflammation. Oxytetracycline is an antibiotic that binds with the 30S and 50S ribosome subunits of susceptible bacterial; cell wall synthesis is not affected. *Therapeutic Effect:* Hydrocortisone: prevents or suppresses cell-mediated immune reactions. Decreases or prevents tissue response to inflammatory process. Oxytetracycline: inhibits bacterial cell wall synthesis.

Pharmacokinetics

None reported.

AVAILABLE FORMS

• *Ophthalmic Suspension:* 10 mg/5 ml (Terra-Cortril Ophthalmic Suspension).

INDICATIONS AND DOSAGES

Superficial eye infections

Ophthalmic

Adults, Elderly. Instill 1 or 2 drops to the affected eye 3 times daily.

CONTRAINDICATIONS: Mycobacterial infection of the eye, viral disease of the cornea and conjunctiva, ocular fungal diseases, mechanical lacerations and abrasions of the eye, hypersensitivity to hydrocortisone, oxytetracycline or any component of the formulation

INTERACTIONS

Drug

None known.

Herbal

None known.

Food

None known.

DIAGNOSTIC TEST EFFECTS: *None known.*

SIDE EFFECTS

Occasional

Eye irritation, blurred vision, photophobia

SERIOUS REACTIONS

• None reported.

SPECIAL CONSIDERATIONS

PRECAUTIONS

• Renew the medication order beyond 20 ml only after slit-lamp examination. Consider the possibility of persistent fungal infections of the cornea.

hydrocortisone; neomycin sulfate; polymyxin B sulfate

(hye-droe-kor'-ti-sone; nee-oh-mye'sin sul'fate; pol-ee-mix'in bee sul'fate)

Rx: AK-Spore HC, Antibiotic-Cort Ear, Antibiotic Ear, Cortatrigen, Cortatrigen Modified, Cort-Biotic, Cortisporin Cream, Cortisporin Ophthalmic Suspension, Cortisporin Otic, Cortomycin, Cortomycin Suspension, Drotic, Ear-Eze, Oti-Sone, Pediotic, UAD Otic

Drug Class: Anti-infectives, ophthalmic; Anti-infectives, otic; Anti-infectives, topical; Antibiotics, aminoglycosides; Antibiotics, polymyxins; Corticosteroids, ophthalmic; Corticosteroids, otic; Corticosteroids, topical; Dermatologics; Ophthalmics; Otics

Pregnancy Category: C

CLINICAL PHARMACOLOGY

Mechanism of Action: Hydrocortisone is an adrenal corticosteroid that inhibits accumulation of inflammatory cells at inflammation sites, phagocytosis, lysosomal enzyme release and synthesis or release of mediators of inflammation. Polymyxin B are polypeptides that damage bacterial cytoplasmic membrane which causes leakage of intracellular components. Neomycin is an aminoglycoside antibiotic that binds to the 30s subunit of the ribosome. *Therapeutic Effect:* Inhibits bacterial cell wall synthesis. Decreases or prevents tissue response to inflammatory process.

Pharmacokinetics

Not usually absorbed through topical administration. Neomycin and hydrocortisone may be absorbed following topical administration to the eye if tissue damage is present. Neomycin, polymyxin B, and hydrocortisone may be absorbed following topical application to the ear if eardrum perforation in present.

AVAILABLE FORMS

• *Cream:* 0.5% hydrocortisone; 0.35% neomycin sulfate; 10,000 units polymyxin B sulfate (Cortisporin Cream).

• *Ophthalmic Suspension:* 1% hydrocortisone; 0.35% neomycin sulfate; 10,000 units polymyxin B sulfate (AK-Spore HC, Cortisporin Ophthalmic Suspension, Cortomycin).

• *Otic Solution:* 1% hydrocortisone, 0.35% neomycin sulfate, 10,000 units polymyxin B (Antibiotic Ear, Cort-Biotic, Cortatrigen, Cortisporin Otic, Cortomycin, Drotic, Ear-Eze, Oti-Sone).

• *Otic Suspension:* 1% hydrocortisone, 0.35% neomycin sulfate, 10,000 units polymyxin B (Antibiotic Ear, Antibiotic-Cort Ear, Cort-Biotic, Cortatrigen, Cortisporin Otic, Cortomycin, Oti-Sone, Pediotic, UAD Otic).

INDICATIONS AND DOSAGES

External auditory canal infections (swimmer's ear)

Otic

Adults, Elderly. Instill 4 drops 3-4 times/day.

Children. Instill 3 drops into affected ear 3-4 times/day.

Superficial ocular infections

Ophthalmic Ointment

Adults, Children, Elderly. Instill 1-2 drops 2-4 times/day, or more frequently as required for severe infections. For acute infections, instill 1-2 drops every 15-30 minutes gradually reducing the frequency of administration as the infection is controlled.

Skin infections

Topical

Adults, Children, Elderly. Apply a thin layer 1-4 times/day.

CONTRAINDICATIONS: Hypersensitivity to hydrocortisone, polymyxin B, neomycin, or any component of the formulation

INTERACTIONS

Drug

None known.

Herbal

None known.

Food

None known.

DIAGNOSTIC TEST EFFECTS: *None known.*

SIDE EFFECTS

Rare

Topical: Hypersensitivity reaction as evidenced by allergic contact dermatitis, burning, inflammation, and itching

Ophthalmic: Burning, itching, redness, swelling, pain

SERIOUS REACTIONS

• Severe hypersensitivity reaction, including apnea and hypotension, occurs rarely.

SPECIAL CONSIDERATIONS

PRECAUTIONS

• Renew the medication order beyond 20 ml only after slit-lamp examination. Consider the possibility of persistent fungal infections of the cornea. If the drug is used for 10 days or longer, monitor intraocular pressure. Allergic cross-reactions may occur with kanamycin, paromomycin, streptomycin, and possibly gentamicin.

PATIENT INFORMATION

• If the condition persists or gets worse or if a rash or allergic reaction develops, advise the patient to stop use and consult a physician. Give the following instructions: Do not use this product if you are allergic to any of the listed ingredients. Keep container tightly closed when not in use. Keep out of reach of children. Shake well before using.

PREGNANCY AND LACTATION

• Pregnancy Category C. This drug combination is teratogenic in rats and rabbits with topical administration. Systemically administered corticosteroids appear in human milk. Excretion of topical doses into human milk is not known.

---

hydromorphone hydrochloride

(hye-droe-mor'fone)

Rx: Dilaudid, Dilaudid-5, Dilaudid-HP, Hydrostat IR, Palladone

Drug Class: Analgesics, narcotic

Pregnancy Category: C

DEA Class: Schedule II

Do not confuse with morphine or Dilantin.

CLINICAL PHARMACOLOGY

Mechanism of Action: An opioid agonist that binds to opioid receptors in the CNS, reducing the intensity of pain stimuli from sensory nerve endings. *Therapeutic Effect:* Alters the perception of and emotional response to pain; suppresses cough reflex.

Pharmacokinetics

Route	Onset	Peak	Duration
PO	30 min	90-120 min	4 hr
IV	10-15 min	15-30 min	2-3 hr
IM	15 min	30-60 min	4-5 hr
Subcutaneous	15 min	30-90 min	4 hr
Rectal	15-30 min	N/A	N/A

Well absorbed from the GI tract after IM administration. Widely distributed. Metabolized in the liver. Excreted in urine. **Half-life:** 1-3 hr.

AVAILABLE FORMS

• *Liquid (Dilaudid):* 5 mg/5 ml.

• *Capsules (Extended-Release [Palladone]):* 12 mg, 16 mg, 24 mg, 32 mg.

• *Tablets (Dilaudid):* 2 mg, 3 mg, 4 mg, 8 mg.

• *Injection (Dilaudid):* 1 mg/ml, 2 mg/ml, 4 mg/ml.

• *Injection (Dilaudid HP):* 10 mg/ml.

• *Suppository (Dilaudid):* 3 mg.

INDICATIONS AND DOSAGES

Analgesia

PO

Adults, Elderly, Children weighing 50 kg and more. 2-4 mg q3-4h. Range: 2-8 mg/dose.

Children older than 6 mo and weighing less than 50 kg. 0.03-0.08 mg/kg/dose q3-4h.

PO (Extended-Release)

Adults, Elderly. 12-32 mg once a day.

IV

Adults, Elderly, Children weighing more than 50 kg. 0.2-0.6 mg q2-3h.

Children weighing 50 kg or less. 0.015 mg/kg/dose q3-6h as needed.

Rectal

Adults, Elderly. 3 mg q4-8h.

Patient-controlled analgesia (PCA)

IV

Adults, Elderly. 0.05-0.5 mg at 5-15 min lockout. Maximum (4-hr): 4-6 mg.

Epidural

Adults, Elderly. Bolus dose of 1-1.5 mg at rate of 0.04-0.4 mg/hr. Demand dose of 0.15 mg at 30 min lockout.

Cough

PO

Adults, Elderly, Children older than 12 yr. 1 mg q3-4h.

Children 6-12 yr. 0.5 mg q3-4h.

CONTRAINDICATIONS: None known.

INTERACTIONS

Drug

Alcohol, other CNS depressants: May increase CNS or respiratory depression and hypotension.

MAOIs: May produce a severe, sometimes fatal reaction; plan to administer one-quarter of usual hydromorphone dose.

Herbal

None known.

Food

None known.

DIAGNOSTIC TEST EFFECTS: May increase serum amylase and lipase concentrations.

IV INCOMPATIBILITIES: Amphotericin B complex (Abelcet, AmBisome, Amphotec), cefazolin (Ancef, Kefzol), diazepam (Valium), phenobarbital, phenytoin (Dilantin)

IV COMPATIBILITIES: Diltiazem (Cardizem), diphenhydramine (Benadryl), dobutamine (Dobutrex), dopamine (Intropin), fentanyl (Sublimaze), furosemide (Lasix), heparin, lorazepam (Ativan), magnesium sulfate, metoclopramide (Reglan), midazolam (Versed), milrinone (Primacor), morphine, propofol (Diprivan)

SIDE EFFECTS

Frequent

Somnolence, dizziness, hypotension (including orthostatic hypotension), decreased appetite

Occasional

Confusion, diaphoresis, facial flushing, urine retention, constipation, dry mouth, nausea, vomiting, headache, pain at injection site

Rare

Allergic reaction, depression

SERIOUS REACTIONS

- Overdose results in respiratory depression, skeletal muscle flaccidity, cold or clammy skin, cyanosis, and extreme somnolence progressing to seizures, stupor, and coma.
- The patient who uses hydromorphone repeatedly may develop a tolerance to the drug's analgesic effect as well as physical dependence.
- This drug may have a prolonged duration of action and cumulative effect in patients with hepatic or renal impairment.

SPECIAL CONSIDERATIONS

PRECAUTIONS

- Hydromorphone hydrochloride can produce drug dependence of the morphine type and therefore has the potential for being abused. Psychic dependence, physical dependence, and tolerance may develop. Respiratory depression is the chief hazard of hydromorphone hydrochloride. Use the drug with extreme caution in patients with chronic obstructive pulmonary disease or cor pulmonale and in patients having a substantially decreased respiratory reserve, hypoxia, hypercapnia, or preexisting respiratory depression. The respiratory depressant effect of hydromorphone hydrochloride with carbon dioxide retention and secondary elevation of cerebrospinal fluid pressure may be exaggerated greatly in the presence of head injury, other intracranial lesions, or preexisting increase in intracranial pressure. Hydromorphone hydrochloride may cause severe hypotension in an individual whose ability to maintain blood pressure already has been compromised by a depleted blood volume or a concurrent administration of drugs such as phenothiazines or general anesthetics. Hydromorphone hydrochloride contains sodium bisulfite, a sulfite that may cause allergic-type reactions including anaphylactic symptoms and life-threatening or less severe asthmatic episodes in certain susceptible persons. Give hydromorphone hydrochloride with caution, and reduce the initial dose in the elderly or debilitated and those with severe impairment of hepatic, pulmonary, or renal function; myxedema or hypothyroidism; adrenocortical insufficiency (e.g., Addison's disease); central nervous system depression or coma; toxic psychoses; prostatic hypertrophy or urethral stricture; gallbladder disease; acute alcoholism; delirium tremens; or kyphoscoliosis.

PATIENT INFORMATION

• Hydromorphone hydrochloride oral liquid and tablets may impair mental and/or physical ability required for the performance of potentially hazardous tasks (e.g., driving and operating machinery). Caution patients accordingly. Hydromorphone hydrochloride may produce orthostatic hypotension in ambulatory patients. The addition of other central nervous system depressants to hydromorphone hydrochloride therapy may produce additive depressant effects, and hydromorphone hydrochloride should not be taken with alcohol.

PREGNANCY AND LACTATION

• Pregnancy Category C. Fetal harm is not known. Low levels of narcotic analgesics have been detected in human milk.

OCULAR CONSIDERATIONS

• Narcotics cause miosis. Pinpoint pupils are a common sign of narcotic overdose but are not pathognomonic (e.g., pontine lesions of hemorrhagic or ischemic origin may produce similar findings), and marked mydriasis occurs when asphyxia intervenes.

---

hydroxyamphetamine hydrobromide; tropicamide

(hi-drox′-ee-am-fet-uh-meen hye-droh-bro′-mide; troe-pik′-a-mide)

Rx: Paremyd

Drug Class: Adrenergic agonists; Anticholinergics; Mydriatics; Ophthalmics

Pregnancy Category: C

CLINICAL PHARMACOLOGY

Mechanism of Action: A combination ophthalmic agent that contains an adrenergic agent (hydroxyamphetamine) and a parasympathomlytic agent (tropicamide). Hydroxyamphetamine stimulates release of norepinephrine from postganglionic adrenergic nerve terminals. Tropicamide competes with acetylcholine for receptors in the iris sphincter and ciliary muscle. *Therapeutic Effect:* Produces dilation of pupil (mydriasis); produces ciliary muscle paralysis.

Pharmacokinetics

Onset of action occurs within 15 minutes. The duration of mydriasis is about 6 to 8 hours.

AVAILABLE FORMS

• *Ophthalmic Solution:* 1% hydroxyamphetamine hydrobromide and 0.25% tropicamide (Paremyd).

INDICATIONS AND DOSAGES

Ophthalmic examinations

Ophthalmic

Adults. 1 drop in conjunctival sac.

CONTRAINDICATIONS: Angle-closure glaucoma or patients with narrow angles who are at risk of an attack of angle-closure glaucoma secondary to pupillary dilation, prior hypersensitivity to hydroxyamphetamine, tropicamide, or any component of the fixed-concentration formulation

INTERACTIONS

Drug

Cisapride: May decrease the efficacy of cisapride.

Herbal

None known.

Food

None known.

DIAGNOSTIC TEST EFFECTS: *None known.*

SIDE EFFECTS

Occasional

Blurred vision, photophobia, burning, stinging

Rare

Dry mouth, headache, nausea, vomiting

SERIOUS REACTIONS

• Cardiovascular collapse, tachycardia, myocardial infarction, ventricular fibrillation, and psychotic reactions have been reported.

SPECIAL CONSIDERATIONS

PRECAUTIONS

• Hypertension, hyperthyroidism, diabetes, or cardiac disease (i.e., arrhythmias or chronic ischemic heart disease) may occur. Monitor intraocular pressure in high-risk patients. Hydroxyamphetamine hydrobromide and tropicamide rarely may cause central nervous system disturbances that may be dangerous in infants and children. Psychotic reactions, behavioral disturbances, and vasomotor or cardiorespiratory collapse in children have been reported with the use of anticholinergic drugs.

PATIENT INFORMATION

• Advise patients to use caution when driving or engaging in other hazardous activities. Patients may experience photophobia and/or blurred vision and should protect their eyes in bright illumination while the pupils are dilated. Warn parents not to get this preparation in their child's mouth and to wash their own hands and the child's hands following administration.

PREGNANCY AND LACTATION

• Pregnancy Category C. Fetal harm is not known. Excretion into human milk is not known.

hydroxychloroquine sulfate

(hye-drox-ee-klor'oh-kwin)

Drug Class: Antiprotozoals; Disease modifying antirheumatic drugs

Pregnancy Category: C

Do not confuse hydroxychloroquine with hydrocortisone or hydroxyzine.

CLINICAL PHARMACOLOGY

Mechanism of Action: An antimalarial and antirheumatic that concentrates in parasite acid vesicles, increasing the pH of the vesicles and interfering with parasite protein synthesis. Antirheumatic action may involve suppressing formation of antigens responsible for hypersensitivity reactions. *Therapeutic Effect:* Inhibits parasite growth.

AVAILABLE FORMS

• *Tablets:* 200 mg (155 mg base).

INDICATIONS AND DOSAGES

Treatment of acute attack of malaria (dosage in mg base)

PO

Dose	Times	Adults	Children
Initial	Day 1	620 mg	10 mg/kg
Second	6 hr later	310 mg	5 mg/kg
Third	Day 2	310 mg	5 mg/kg
Fourth	Day 3	310 mg	5 mg/kg

Suppression of malaria

PO

Adults. 310 mg base weekly on same day each week, beginning 2 wk before entering an endemic area and continuing for 4-6 wk after leaving the area.

Children. 5 mg base/kg/wk, beginning 2 wk before entering an endemic area and continuing for 4-6 wk after leaving the area. If therapy is not begun before exposure, administer a loading dose of 10 mg base/kg in 2 equally divided doses 6 hr apart, followed by the ususal dosage regimen.

Rheumatoid arthritis

PO

Adults. Initially, 400-600 mg (310-465 mg base) daily for 5-10 days, gradually increased to optimum response level. Maintenance (usually within 4-12 wk): Dosage decreased by 50% and then continued at maintenance dose of 200-400 mg/day. Maximum effect may not be seen for several months.

Lupus erythematosus

PO

Adults. Initially, 400 mg once or twice a day for several weeks or months. Maintenance: 200-400 mg/day.

UNLABELED USES: Treatment of juvenile arthritis, sarcoid-associated hypercalcemia

CONTRAINDICATIONS: Long-term therapy for children, porphyria, psoriasis, retinal or visual field changes

INTERACTIONS

Drug

Penicillamine: May increase blood penicillamine concentration and the risk of hematologic, renal, or severe skin reactions.

Herbal

None known.

Food

None known.

DIAGNOSTIC TEST EFFECTS: *None known.*

SIDE EFFECTS

Frequent

Mild, transient headache; anorexia; nausea; vomiting

Occasional

Visual disturbances, nervousness, fatigue, pruritus (especially of palms, soles, and scalp), irritability, personality changes, diarrhea

Rare

Stomatitis, dermatitis, impaired hearing

SERIOUS REACTIONS

• Ocular toxicity, especially retinopathy, may occur and may progress even after drug is discontinued.

• Prolonged therapy may result in peripheral neuritis, neuromyopathy, hypotension, EKG changes, agranulocytosis, aplastic anemia, thrombocytopenia, seizures, and psychosis.

• Overdosage may result in headache, vomiting, visual disturbances, drowsiness, seizures, and hypokalemia followed by cardiovascular collapse and death.

SPECIAL CONSIDERATIONS

PRECAUTIONS

• Use antimalarial compounds with caution in patients with hepatic disease or alcoholism or along with known hepatotoxic drugs. Obtain periodic blood cell counts if patients are given prolonged therapy. If any severe blood disorder appears that is not attributable to the disease under treatment, consider discontinuation of the drug. Administer the drug with caution in patients having glucose-6-phosphate dehydrogenase deficiency. Dermatologic reactions to hydroxychloroquine sulfate may occur.

PREGNANCY AND LACTATION

• Pregnancy Category C. Radioactively tagged chloroquine administered intravenously to pregnant, pigmented CBA mice passed rapidly across the placenta. The drug accumulated selectively in the melanin structures of the fetal eyes and was retained in the ocular tissues for 5 months after the drug had been eliminated from the rest of the body.

OCULAR CONSIDERATIONS

• Irreversible retinal damage has been observed in some patients who had received long-term or high-dosage 4-aminoquinoline therapy for discoid and systemic lupus erythematosus or rheumatoid arthritis. Retinopathy has been reported to be dose related.

• When contemplating prolonged therapy with any antimalarial compound, perform initial (baseline) and periodic (every 3 months) eye examinations (including visual acuity, expert slit-lamp, funduscopic, and visual field tests).

• If there is any indication of abnormality in the visual acuity, visual field, or retinal macular areas (such as pigmentary changes, loss of foveal reflex) or any visual symptoms (such as light flashes and streaks) that are not fully explainable by difficulties of accommodation or corneal opacities, discontinue the drug immediately and observe the patient closely for possible progression. Retinal changes (and visual disturbances) may progress even after cessation of therapy.

• The methods recommended for early diagnosis of "chloroquine retinopathy" consist of (1) funduscopic examination of the macula for fine pigmentary disturbances or loss of the foveal reflex and (2) examination of the central visual field with a small red test object for pericentral or paracentral scotoma or determination of retinal thresholds to red. Regard any unexplained visual symptoms, such as light flashes or streaks, with suspicion as possible manifestations of retinopathy. If serious toxic symptoms occur from overdosage or sensitivity, it has been suggested that ammonium chloride (8 g daily in divided doses for adults) be administered orally 3 or 4 days a week for several months after therapy has been stopped because acidification of the urine increases renal excretion of the 4-aminoquinoline compounds by 20% to 90%. However, exercise caution in patients with impaired renal function and/or metabolic acidosis.

hydroxypropyl cellulose

(hye-drox-ee-proe'pil sell'yoo-lose)

Drug Class: Ocular lubricants; Ophthalmics

CLINICAL PHARMACOLOGY

Mechanism of Action: An ophthalmic agent that acts to stabilize the precorneal tear film and prolong the tear film breakup time. *Therapeutic Effect:* Lubricates and protects the eye.

Pharmacokinetics

None reported.

AVAILABLE FORMS

• *Ocular system:* 5 mg (Lacrisert).

INDICATIONS AND DOSAGES

Ocular lubricant for dry eyes

Ophthalmic

Adults, Elderly. Apply once daily into the inferior cul-de-sac beneath the base of tarsus, not in apposition to the cornea nor beneath the eyelid at the level of the tarsal plate.

CONTRAINDICATIONS: Hypersensitivity to hydroxypropyl cellulose or any component of the formulation

INTERACTIONS

Drug

None known.

Herbal

None known.

Food

None known.

DIAGNOSTIC TEST EFFECTS: *None known.*

SIDE EFFECTS

Rare

Blurred vision, ocular discomfort or irritation, matting or stickiness of eyelashes, photophobia, edema of eyelids, hyeremia

SERIOUS REACTIONS

• Hypersensitivity reactions have been reported.

SPECIAL CONSIDERATIONS

PRECAUTIONS

• If improperly placed, hydroxypropyl cellulose may result in corneal abrasion.

PATIENT INFORMATION

• Because this product may produce transient blurring of vision, instruct patients to exercise caution when operating hazardous machinery or driving a motor vehicle.

PREGNANCY AND LACTATION

• Pregnancy Category C. Feeding of hydroxypropyl cellulose to rats at levels up to 5% of their diet produced no gross or histopathologic changes or other deleterious effects.

hydroxypropyl methylcellulose

(hye-drox-ee-proe'pil meth-ill-sell'yoo-lose)

Rx: Cellugel, Gonak, Goniosoft

Drug Class: Ophthalmics

CLINICAL PHARMACOLOGY

Mechanism of Action: An ophthalmic agent that promotes corneal wetting by stabilizing and thickening the precorneal tear film and prolonging the tear film breakup time, which is usually shortened in dry eye conditions. *Therapeutic Effect:* Lubricates and protects the eye.

Pharmacokinetics

None reported.

AVAILABLE FORMS

• *Ophthalmic solution:* 2% (Cellugel), 2.5% (Gonak, Goniosoft).

INDICATIONS AND DOSAGES

Ocular lubricant for dry eyes

Ophthalmic

Adults, Elderly. Instill 1-2 drops in affected eye(s) as needed.

CONTRAINDICATIONS: Hypersensitivity to hydroxypropyl methylcellulose or any component of the formulation

INTERACTIONS

Drug

None known.

Herbal

None known.

Food

None known.

DIAGNOSTIC TEST EFFECTS: *None known.*

SIDE EFFECTS

Rare

Blurred vision, matting or stickiness of eyelashes

SERIOUS REACTIONS

• None reported.

SPECIAL CONSIDERATIONS

PRECAUTIONS

• Bion Tears: To ensure optimal effectiveness once the pouch is opened, use the containers inside the pouch within 4 days (96 hours).

• Tears Naturale Free: Make sure container is intact before use. To open, completely twist off tab. Do not pull off. To close, press tab down over container and twist. Reclosed vial may leak under pressure. Discard 12 hours after opening.

PATIENT INFORMATION

Give patients the following instructions:

• If you experience eye pain, changes in vision, or continued redness or irritation of the eye, or if the condition worsens or persists for more than 72 hours, discontinue use and consult an eye care practitioner. If solution changes color or becomes cloudy, do not use. To avoid contamination, do not touch the tip of the container to any surface. Do not reuse. Once opened, discard. Keep this and all drugs out of the reach of children.

hydroxyzine

(hye-drox'i-zeen)

Rx: Atarax, Hyzine, Vistacot, Vistaject-50, Vistaril, Vistaril IM

Drug Class: Antiemetics/antivertigo; Antihistamines, H1; Anxiolytics; Sedatives/hypnotics

Pregnancy Category: C

Do not confuse hydroxyzine with hydralazine or hydroxyurea.

H

CLINICAL PHARMACOLOGY

Mechanism of Action: A piperazine derivative that competes with histamine for receptor sites in the GI tract, blood vessels, and respiratory tract. May exert CNS depressant activity in subcortical areas. Diminishes vestibular stimulation and depresses labyrinthine function. *Therapeutic Effect:* Produces anxiolytic, anticholinergic, antihistaminic, and analgesic effects; relaxes skeletal muscle; controls nausea and vomiting.

Pharmacokinetics

Route	*Onset*	*Peak*	*Duration*
PO	15-30 min	N/A	4-6 hr

Well absorbed from the GI tract and after parenteral administration. Metabolized in the liver. Primarily excreted in urine. Not removed by hemodialysis. **Half-life:** 20-25 hr (increased in the elderly).

AVAILABLE FORMS

• *Capsules (Vistaril):* 25 mg, 50 mg, 100 mg.

• *Oral Suspension (Vistaril):* 25 mg/5 ml.

• *Syrup (Atarax):* 10 mg/5 ml.

• *Tablets (Atarax):* 10 mg, 25 mg, 50 mg, 100 mg.

• *Injection (Vistaril):*25 mg/ml, 50 mg/ml.

INDICATIONS AND DOSAGES

Anxiety

PO

Adults, Elderly. 25-100 mg 4 times a day. Maximum: 600 mg/day.

Nausea and vomiting

IM

Adults, Elderly. 25-100 mg/dose q4-6h.

Pruritus

PO

Adults, Elderly. 25 mg 3-4 times a day.

Preoperative sedation

PO

Adults, Elderly. 50-100 mg.

IM

Adults, Elderly. 25-100 mg.

Usual pediatric dosage

PO

Children. 2 mg/kg/day in divided doses q6-8h.

IM

Children. 0.5-1 mg/kg/dose q4-6h.

CONTRAINDICATIONS: None known.

INTERACTIONS

Drug

Alcohol, other CNS depressants: May increase CNS depressant effects.

MAOIs: May increase anticholinergic and CNS depressant effects.

Herbal

None known.

Food

None known.

DIAGNOSTIC TEST EFFECTS: May cause false-positive urine 17-hydroxycorticosteroid determinations.

SIDE EFFECTS

Side effects are generally mild and transient.

Frequent

Somnolence, dry mouth, marked discomfort with IM injection

Occasional

Dizziness, ataxia, asthenia, slurred speech, headache, agitation, increased anxiety

Rare

Paradoxical CNS reactions, such as hyperactivity or nervousness in children and excitement or restlessness in elderly or debilitated patients (generally noted during first 2 weeks of therapy, particularly in presence of uncontrolled pain)

SERIOUS REACTIONS

• A hypersensitivity reaction, including wheezing, dyspnea, and chest tightness, may occur.

SPECIAL CONSIDERATIONS

PRECAUTIONS

• Consider the potentiating action of hydroxyzine when using the drug along with central nervous system depressants such as narcotics, nonnarcotic analgesics, and barbiturates. Because drowsiness may occur with use of this drug, warn patients of this possibility and caution them against driving a car or operating dangerous machinery. Advise patients against the simultaneous use of other central nervous system depressant drugs, and caution them that the effect of alcohol may be increased.

PREGNANCY AND LACTATION

• Pregnancy Category C. Induced fetal abnormalities in the rat and mouse occurred at doses substantially above the human therapeutic range. Excretion into human milk is not known.

ibuprofen

(eye-byoo' pro-fen)

Rx: Advil, Advil Pediatric, Ibu, Ibu-4, Ibu-6, Ibu-8, Ibu-Tab, Motrin, Motrin Childrens, Pediacare Fever

Drug Class: Analgesics, non-narcotic; Antipyretics; Nonsteroidal anti-inflammatory drugs

Pregnancy Category: B; D, 3rd

CLINICAL PHARMACOLOGY

Mechanism of Action: An NSAID that inhibits prostaglandin synthesis. Also produces vasodilation by acting centrally on the heat-regulating center of the hypothalamus. *Therapeutic Effect:* Produces analgesic and anti-inflammatory effects and decreases fever.

Pharmacokinetics

Route	*Onset*	*Peak*	*Duration*
PO (analgesic)	0.5 hr	N/A	4-6 hr
PO (antirheumatic)	2 days	1-2 wk	N/A

Rapidly absorbed from the GI tract. Protein binding: greater than 90%. Metabolized in the liver. Primarily excreted in urine. Not removed by hemodialysis. **Half-life:** 2-4 hr.

AVAILABLE FORMS

- *Caplets (Advil, Menadol, Motrin):* 200 mg.
- *Capsules (Advil, Advil Migraine):* 200 mg.
- *Gelcaps (Advil, Motrin IB):* 200 mg.
- *Tablets (Advil, Motrin IB):* 200 mg.
- *Tablets (Motin):* 400 mg, 600 mg, 800 mg.
- *Tablets (Chewable [Children's Advil, Children's Motrin]):* 50 mg.
- *Tablets (Chewable [Junior Advil, Junior Strength Motrin]):* 100 mg.
- *Oral Suspension (Children's Advil, Children's Motrin):* 100 mg/5 ml.
- *Oral Drops (Infant Advil, Infant Motrin):* 40 mg/ml.

INDICATIONS AND DOSAGES

Acute or chronic rheumatoid arthritis, osteoarthritis, migraine pain, gouty arthritis

PO

Adults, Elderly. 400-800 mg 3-4 times a day. Maximum: 3.2 g/day.

Mild to moderate pain, primary dysmenorrhea

PO

Adults, Elderly. 200-400 mg q4-6h as needed. Maximum: 1.6 g/day.

Fever, minor aches or pain

PO

Adults, Elderly. 200-400 mg q4-6h. Maximum: 1.6 g/day.

Children. 5-10 mg/kg/dose q6-8h. Maximum: 40 mg/kg/day. OTC: 7.5 mg/kg/dose q6-8h. Maximum: 30 mg/kg/day.

Juvenile arthritis

PO

Children. 30-70 mg/kg/day in 3-4 divided doses. Maximum: 400 mg/day in children weighing less than 20 kg, 600 mg/day in children weighing 20-30 kg, 800 mg/day in children weighing greater than 30-40 kg.

UNLABELED USES: Treatment of psoriatic arthritis, vascular headaches

CONTRAINDICATIONS: Active peptic ulcer, chronic inflammation of GI tract, GI bleeding disorders or ulceration, history of hypersensitivity to aspirin or NSAIDs

INTERACTIONS

Drug

Antihypertensives, diuretics: May decrease the effects of these drugs.

Aspirin, other salicylates: May increase the risk of GI side effects such as bleeding.

Bone marrow depressants: May increase the risk of hematologic reactions.

Heparin, oral anticoagulants, thrombolytics: May increase the effects of these drugs.

Lithium: May increase the blood concentration and risk of toxicity of lithium.

Methotrexate: May increase the risk of methotrexate toxicity.

Probenecid: May increase the ibuprofen blood concentration.

Herbal

Feverfew: May decrease the effects of feverfew.

Ginkgo biloba: May increase the risk of bleeding.

Food

None known.

DIAGNOSTIC TEST EFFECTS: May prolong bleeding time. May alter blood glucose level. May increase BUN level, and serum creatinine, potassium, AST (SGOT), and ALT (SGPT) levels. May decrease blood Hgb and Hct.

SIDE EFFECTS

Occasional (9%-3%)

Nausea with or without vomiting, dyspepsia, dizziness, rash

Rare (less than 3%)

Diarrhea or constipation, flatulence, abdominal cramps or pain, pruritus

SERIOUS REACTIONS

• Acute overdose may result in metabolic acidosis.

• Rare reactions with long-term use include peptic ulcer disease, GI bleeding, gastritis, a severe hepatic reaction (cholestasis, jaundice), nephrotoxicity (dysuria, hematuria, proteinuria, nephrotic syndrome), and a severe hypersensitivity reaction (particularly in patients with systemic lupus erythematosus or other collagen diseases).

SPECIAL CONSIDERATIONS

PRECAUTIONS

• Fluid retention and edema have been reported in association with ibuprofen; therefore, use the drug with caution in patients with a history of cardiac decompensation or hypertension. Ibuprofen can inhibit platelet aggregation, but the effect is quantitatively less and of shorter duration than that seen with aspirin. Patients taking ibuprofen should report to their physicians signs or symptoms of gastrointestinal ulceration or bleeding, blurred vision or other eye symptoms, skin rash, weight gain, or edema. To avoid exacerbation of disease or adrenal insufficiency, patients who have been on prolonged corticosteroid therapy should have their therapy tapered slowly rather than discontinued abruptly when ibuprofen is added to the treatment program. The antipyretic and antiinflammatory activity of ibuprofen may reduce fever and inflammation, thus diminishing the usefulness of these as diagnostic signs in detecting complications of presumed noninfectious, noninflammatory painful conditions.

• Liver Effects: As with other nonsteroidal antiinflammatory drugs, borderline elevations of one or more liver function tests may occur in up to 15% of patients.

• Hemoglobin Levels: In cross-study comparisons with doses ranging from 1200 to 3200 mg daily for several weeks, a slight dose-response decrease in hemoglobin/hematocrit was noted.

• Aseptic Meningitis: Aseptic meningitis with fever and coma has been observed on rare occasions in patients taking ibuprofen therapy.

• Renal Effects: As with other nonsteroidal antiinflammatory drugs, long-term administration of ibuprofen to animals has resulted in renal papillary necrosis and other abnormal renal pathologic conditions.

PATIENT INFORMATION

• Ibuprofen, like other drugs of its class, is not free of side effects. The side effects of these drugs can cause discomfort, and rarely there are more serious side effects, such as gastrointestinal bleeding, which may result in hospitalization and even fatal outcomes.

• Nonsteroidal antiinflammatory drugs are often essential agents in the management of arthritis and have a major role in the treatment of pain, but they also may be used commonly for conditions that are less serious.

PREGNANCY AND LACTATION

• Pregnancy Category B; Pregnancy Category D (third trimester). Reproduction studies conducted in rats and rabbits at doses somewhat less than the maximal clinical dose did not demonstrate evidence of developmental abnormalities. However, animal reproduction studies are not always predictive of human response. Because there are no adequate and well-controlled studies in pregnant women, use this drug during pregnancy only if clearly needed. Because of the known effects of nonsteroidal antiinflammatory drugs on the fetal cardiovascular system (closure of ductus arteriosus), avoid use during late pregnancy. As with other drugs known to inhibit prostaglandin synthesis, an increased incidence of dystocia and delayed parturition occurred in rats. Administration of ibuprofen is not recommended during pregnancy. In limited studies, an assay capable of detecting 1 mg/ml did not demonstrate ibuprofen in the milk of lactating mothers.

OCULAR CONSIDERATIONS

• Blurred and diminished vision, scotomata, and changes in color vision have been reported. If a patient develops such complaints while receiving ibuprofen, discontinue the drug; the patient should have an eye examination that includes central visual fields and color vision testing.

idoxuridine

(eye-dox-yoor'i-deen)

Drug Class: Antivirals; Ophthalmics

Pregnancy Category: C

CLINICAL PHARMACOLOGY

Mechanism of Action: An analog of thymidine that produces nonselective antiviral effects. *Therapeutic Effect:* Inhibits both cellular and viral DNA synthesis.

Pharmacokinetics

Penetrates the cornea poorly. Not protein bound. Metabolized in rapidly in body tissues.

AVAILABLE FORMS

• *Ophthalmic Ointment:* 0.5% (Stoxil).

• *Ophthalmic Solution:* 0.1% (Herpes Liquifilm).

INDICATIONS AND DOSAGES

Ocular herpes simplex infections

Ophthalmic solution

Adults, Elderly. Initially, instill 1 drop into each affected eye every hour during the day and every 2 hours at night. Continue therapy for 5 to 7 days after healing is complete.

Ophthalmic ointment

Adults, Elderly. Apply a thin strip (approximately 1 cm) of ointment every 4 hours during the day.

UNLABELED USES: Treatment of nonparenchymatous sarcomas

CONTRAINDICATIONS: Hypersensitivity to idoxuridine or any component of the formulation

INTERACTIONS

Drug

Boric acid: May cause eye irritation when administered concurrently in the eye.

Herbal

None known.

Food

None known.

DIAGNOSTIC TEST EFFECTS: *None known.*

SIDE EFFECTS

Rare

Excess flow of tears, eye irritation, burning, inflammation of the eyes and lids, photophobia, allergic reactions

SERIOUS REACTIONS

• Hypersensitivity reactions have been reported.

SPECIAL CONSIDERATIONS

PRECAUTIONS

• Some strains of herpes simplex virus appear resistant to the action of idoxuridine. If there is no lessening of fluorescein staining in 14 days, undertake another form of therapy.

PREGNANCY AND LACTATION

• Pregnancy Category C. Idoxuridine has been reported to cross the placental barrier and to produce fetal malformations in rabbits when administered topically. Excretion into human milk is not known.

indocyanine green

Rx: IC-Green

Drug Class: Diagnostics, nonradioactive

Pregnancy Category: C

CLINICAL PHARMACOLOGY

Mechanism of Action: An absorbing dye that generates microbubbles by vigorous shaking during its preparation which causes the contrast effect. *Therapeutic Effect:* Causes fluorescence.

Pharmacokinetics

Rapidly bound to plasma protein after intravenous injection. Metabolized in liver. Rapidly excreted unchanged into the bile. **Half-life:** 3.28-3.5 hrs.

AVAILABLE FORMS

• *Powder for injection:* 25 mg (IC-Green).

INDICATIONS AND DOSAGES

Cardiac output

IV

Adults, Elderly. 5 mg injected using a cardiac catheter

Hepatic blood flow, hepatic function

IV

Adults, Elderly. 500 mcg/kg injected directly into arm vein rapidly.

Ophthalmic angiography

IV

Adults, Elderly. Inject directly into arm or hand vein.

CONTRAINDICATIONS: Allergy to iodide, patients at higher risk for anaphylactic reactions

INTERACTIONS

Drug

None known.

Herbal

None known.

Food

None known.

DIAGNOSTIC TEST EFFECTS: *None known.*

SIDE EFFECTS

Occasional

Urticaria

SERIOUS REACTIONS

- Anaphylaxis has been reported.

SPECIAL CONSIDERATIONS

PRECAUTIONS

- Indocyanine green is formulated with iodine and should not be used in these individuals allergic to iodine. Some persons may experience slight nausea after dye injection, but nausea usually passes quickly. Patients who are allergic to the dye can develop itching and a skin rash.

PREGNANCY AND LACTATION

- Pregnancy Category C. Animal reproduction studies have not been conducted with indocyanine green. Whether indocyanine green can cause fetal harm when administered to a pregnant woman or can affect reproduction capacity also is not known. Whether this drug is excreted in human milk is not known.

OCULAR CONSIDERATIONS

- Indocyanine green study evaluates the circulatory system of the choroid. Indocyanine green reacts to light with a longer wavelength than fluorescein. Leaking vessels in the choroid may not appear with fluorescein angiography.

indomethacin

(in-doe-meth'a-sin)

Rx: Indocin, Indocin SR

Drug Class: Analgesics, non-narcotic; Nonsteroidal anti-inflammatory drugs

Pregnancy Category: B; D, 3rd

Do not confuse Indocin with Imodium or Vicodin.

CLINICAL PHARMACOLOGY

Mechanism of Action: An NSAID that produces analgesic and anti-inflammatory effects by inhibiting prostaglandin synthesis. Also increases the sensitivity of the premature ductus to the dilating effects of prostaglandins. *Therapeutic Effect:* Reduces the inflammatory response and intensity of pain. Closure of the patent ductus arteriosus.

AVAILABLE FORMS

- *Capsules (Indocin):* 25 mg, 50 mg.
- *Capsules (Sustained-Release [Indocin SR]):* 75 mg.
- *Oral Suspension (Indocin):* 25 mg/5 ml.
- *Powder for Injection (Indocin IV):* 1 mg.
- *Suppositories:* 50 mg.

INDICATIONS AND DOSAGES

Moderate to severe rheumatoid arthritis, osteoarthritis, ankylosing spondylitis

PO

Adults, Elderly. Initially, 25 mg 2-3 times a day; increased by 25-50 mg/wk up to 150-200 mg/day. Or 75 mg/day (extended-release) up to 75 mg twice a day.

Children. 1-2 mg/kg/day. Maximum: 150-200 mg/day.

Acute gouty arthritis

PO

Adults, Elderly. Initially, 100 mg, then 50 mg 3 times a day.

Acute shoulder pain
PO
Adults, Elderly. 75-150 mg/day in 3-4 divided doses.
Usual rectal dosage
Adults, Elderly. 50 mg 4 times a day.
Children. Initially, 1.5-2.5 mg/kg/day, increased up to 4 mg/kg/day. Maximum: 150-200 mg/day.
Patent ductus arteriosus
IV
Neonates. Initially, 0.2 mg/kg. Subsequent doses are based on age, as follows:
Neonates older than 7 days. 0.25 mg/kg for second and third doses.
Neonates 2-7 days. 0.2 mg/kg for second and third doses.
Neonates less than 48 hr. 0.1 mg/kg for second and third doses.

UNLABELED USES: Treatment of fever due to malignancy, pericarditis, psoriatic arthritis, rheumatic complications associated with Paget's disease of bone, vascular headache

CONTRAINDICATIONS: Active GI bleeding or ulcerations; hypersensitivity to aspirin, indomethacin, or other NSAIDs; renal impairment, thrombocytopenia

INTERACTIONS
Drug
Aminoglycosides: May increase the blood concentration of these drugs in neonates.
Antihypertensives, diuretics: May decrease the effects of these drugs.
Aspirin, other salicylates: May increase the risk of GI side effects such as bleeding.
Bone marrow depressants: May increase the risk of hematologic reactions.
Heparin, oral anticoagulants, thrombolytics: May increase the effects of these drugs.
Lithium: May increase the blood concentration and risk of toxicity of lithium.
Methotrexate: May increase the risk of methotrexate toxicity.
Probenecid: May increase the indomethacin blood concentration.
Triamterene: May potentiate acute renal failure. Don't give concurrently.
Herbal
Feverfew: May decrease the effects of feverfew.
Ginkgo biloba: May increase the risk of bleeding.
Food
None known.

DIAGNOSTIC TEST EFFECTS: May prolong bleeding time. May alter blood glucose level. May increase BUN level, and serum creatinine, potassium, AST (SGOT), and ALT (SGPT) levels. May decrease serum sodium level and platelet count.

IV INCOMPATIBILITIES: Amino acid injection, calcium gluconate, cimetidine (Tagamet), dobutamine (Dobutrex), dopamine (Intropin), gentamicin (Garamycin), tobramycin (Nebcin)

IV COMPATIBILITIES: Insulin, potassium

SIDE EFFECTS
Frequent (11%-3%)
Headache, nausea, vomiting, dyspepsia, dizziness
Occasional (less than 3%)
Depression, tinnitus, diaphoresis, somnolence, constipation, diarrhea, bleeding disturbances in patent ductus arteriosus
Rare
Hypertension, confusion, urticaria, pruritus, rash, blurred vision

SERIOUS REACTIONS
• Paralytic ileus and ulceration of the esophagus, stomach, duodenum, or small intestine may occur.

• Patients with impaired renal function may develop hyperkalemia and worsening of renal impairment.

• Indomethacin use may aggravate epilepsy, parkinsonism, and depression or other psychiatric disturbances.

• Nephrotoxicity, including dysuria, hematuria, proteinuria, and nephrotic syndrome, occurs rarely.

• Metabolic acidosis or alkalosis, apnea, and bradycardia occur rarely in patients with patent ductus arteriosus.

SPECIAL CONSIDERATIONS

PRECAUTIONS

• Single or multiple ulcerations, including perforation and hemorrhage of the esophagus, stomach, duodenum, or small and large intestine have been reported. Serious gastrointestinal toxicity such as bleeding, ulceration, and perforation can occur. Closely monitor patients with significantly impaired renal function. Increases in serum potassium concentration, including hyperkalemia, have been reported. Indomethacin may aggravate depression or other psychiatric disturbances, epilepsy, and parkinsonism.

• Indomethacin may cause drowsiness; caution patients about engaging in activities requiring mental alertness and motor coordination, such as driving a car. Indomethacin also may cause headache and may mask the usual signs and symptoms of infection. Fluid retention and peripheral edema have been observed; therefore, use indomethacin with caution in patients with cardiac dysfunction, hypertension, or other conditions predisposing to fluid retention. Indomethacin can inhibit platelet aggregation. Use indomethacin with caution in persons with coagulation defects. Severe hepatic reactions, including jaundice and cases of fatal hepatitis, have been reported.

PATIENT INFORMATION

• Indomethacin, like other drugs of its class, is not free of side effects. The side effects of these drugs can cause discomfort, and rarely, there are more serious side effects such as gastrointestinal bleeding, which may result in hospitalization and even fatal outcomes.

• Nonsteroidal antiinflammatory drugs are often essential agents in the management of arthritis; but they also may be used commonly for conditions that are less serious.

• Eye care practitioners may wish to discuss with their patients the potential risks and likely benefits of nonsteroidal antiinflammatory drug treatment, particularly when the drugs are used for less serious conditions where treatment without nonsteroidal antiinflammatory drugs may represent an acceptable alternative to the patient and eye care practitioner.

PREGNANCY AND LACTATION

• Pregnancy category B, and category D for 3rd trimester. Indomethacin is not recommended for use in pregnant women because safety for use has not been established. The known effects of indomethacin and other drugs of this class on the human fetus during the third trimester of pregnancy include constriction of the ductus arteriosus prenatally, tricuspid incompetence, and pulmonary hypertension; nonclosure of the ductus arteriosus postnatally, which may be resistant to medical management; myocardial degenerative changes, platelet dysfunction with resultant bleeding, intracranial bleeding, renal dysfunction or failure, renal injury/dysgenesis that may result in prolonged or permanent renal failure, oligohydramnios, gastrointestinal bleeding or perforation, and increased risk of necrotizing enterocolitis. Indomethacin is excreted in the milk of lactating mothers.

OCULAR CONSIDERATIONS

• The following have an incidence less than 1%: Corneal deposits and retinal disturbances, including those of the macula, have been observed in some patients who had received prolonged therapy with indomethacin. The prescribing physician or eye care practitioner should be alert to the possible association between the changes noted and indomethacin. Discontinuation of therapy is advisable if such changes are observed. Blurred vision may be a significant symptom and warrants a thorough eye examination. Because these changes may be asymptomatic, eye examinations at periodic intervals is desirable in patients in whom therapy is prolonged.

insulin glargine

(in'su-lin glare'jeen)

Drug Class: Antidiabetic agents; Insulins

Pregnancy Category: C

CLINICAL PHARMACOLOGY

Mechanism of Action: An exogenous insulin that facilitates passage of glucose, potassium, magnesium across cellular membranes of skeletal and cardiac muscle, adipose tissue; controls storage and metabolism of carbohydrates, protein, fats. Promotes conversion of glucose to glycogen in liver. *Therapeutic Effect:* Controls glucose levels in diabetic patients.

Pharmacokinetics

Drug Form	*Onset (hrs)*	*Peak (hrs)*	*Duration (hrs)*
Insulin glargine	N/A	N/A	24

Metabolized at the carboxyl terminus of the B chain in the subcutaneous depot to form two active metabolites. Unchanged drug and degradation products are present throughout circulation.

AVAILABLE FORMS

• *Injection, solution:* 100 unit/ml, 3 ml cartridge system [package of 5] (Lantus).

INDICATIONS AND DOSAGES

Treatment of insulin-dependent type 1 diabetes mellitus, non–insulin-dependent type 2 diabetes mellitus when diet or weight control therapy has failed to maintain satisfactory blood glucose levels or in event of fever, infection, pregnancy, severe endocrine, liver or renal dysfunction, surgery, or trauma, regular insulin used in emergency treatment of ketoacidosis, to promote passage of glucose across cell membrane in hyperalimentation, to facilitate intracellular shift of potassium in hyperkalemia

Subcutaneous

Adults, Elderly, Children. 10 units once daily, preferably at bedtime, adjusted according to patient response.

CONTRAINDICATIONS: Hypersensitivity or insulin resistance may require change of type or species source of insulin

INTERACTIONS

Drug

Alcohol: May increase the effects of insulin.

Beta-adrenergic blockers: May increase the risk of hyperglycemia or hypoglycemia, mask signs of hy-

poglycemia, and prolong the period of hypoglycemia.
Glucocorticoids, thiazide diuretics: May increase blood glucose.
Herbal
Chromium, garlic, gymnema: May increase risk of hypoglycemia.
Food
None known.
DIAGNOSTIC TEST EFFECTS: May decrease serum magnesium, phosphate, and potassium concentrations.
SIDE EFFECTS
Frequent
Hypoglycemia
Occasional
Local redness, swelling, itching, caused by improper injection technique or allergy to cleansing solution or insulin
Infrequent
Systemic allergic reaction, marked by rash, angioedema, and anaphylaxis, lipodystrophy or depression at injection site due to breakdown of adipose tissue, lipohypertrophy or accumulation of subcutaneous tissue at injection site due to lack of adequate site rotation
Rare
Insulin resistance
SERIOUS REACTIONS
• Severe hypoglycemia caused by hyperinsulinism may occur in overdose of insulin, decrease or delay of food intake, excessive exercise, or those with brittle diabetes.
• Diabetic ketoacidosis may result from stress, illness, omission of insulin dose, or long-term poor insulin control.

SPECIAL CONSIDERATIONS

PRECAUTIONS
• Hypoglycemia is the most common adverse effect of insulin, including insulin glargine. As with all insulins, the timing of hypoglycemia may differ among various insulin formulations. Glucose monitoring is recommended for all patients with diabetes. Although studies have not been performed in patients with diabetes and hepatic or renal impairment, insulin glargine requirements may be diminished because of reduced insulin metabolism.
PATIENT INFORMATION
• Insulin glargine must be used only if the solution is clear and colorless with no particles visible.
• Advise patients that insulin glargine must not be diluted or mixed with any other insulin or solution. Instruct patients on self-management procedures including glucose monitoring, proper injection technique, and hypoglycemia and hyperglycemia management. Instruct patients on handling of special situations such as intercurrent conditions (illness, stress, or emotional disturbances), an inadequate or skipped insulin dose, inadvertent administration of an increased insulin dose, inadequate food intake, or skipped meals. Refer patients to the insulin glargine information in the patient circular for additional information.
• As with all patients who have diabetes, the ability to concentrate and/or react may be impaired as a result of hypoglycemia or hyperglycemia.
• Advise patients with diabetes to inform their doctor if they are pregnant or are contemplating pregnancy.
PREGNANCY AND LACTATION
• Pregnancy Category C. No well-controlled clinical studies of the use of insulin glargine in pregnant women have been performed. Whether insulin glargine is excreted in significant amounts in human

milk is not known. Many drugs, including human insulin, are excreted in human milk. For this reason, exercise caution when administering insulin glargine to a nursing woman.

OCULAR CONSIDERATIONS

- Retinopathy was evaluated in the clinical studies by means of retinal adverse events reported and fundus photography. The numbers of retinal adverse events reported for insulin glargine and NPH treatment groups were similar for patients with type 1 and type 2 diabetes. Progression of retinopathy was investigated by fundus photography using a grading protocol derived from the Early Treatment Diabetic Retinopathy Study (ETDRS). In one clinical study involving patients with type 2 diabetes, a difference in the number of subjects with progression in ETDRS scale over a 6-month period was noted by fundus photography (7.5% in insulin glargine group versus 2.7% in NPH-treated group). The overall relevance of this isolated finding cannot be determined because of the small number of patients involved, the short follow-up period, and the fact that this finding was not observed in other clinical studies.

irbesartan

(erb'ba-sar-tan)

Rx: Avapro

Drug Class: Angiotensin II receptor antagonists

Pregnancy Category: C, 1st; D, 2nd / 3rd

CLINICAL PHARMACOLOGY

Mechanism of Action: An angiotensin II receptor, type AT_1, antagonist that blocks the vasoconstrictor and aldosterone-secreting effects of angiotensin II, inhibiting the binding of angiotensin II to the AT_1 receptors. *Therapeutic Effect:* Causes vasodilation, decreases peripheral resistance, and decreases BP.

Pharmacokinetics

Rapidly and completely absorbed after PO administration. Protein binding: 90%. Undergoes hepatic metabolism to inactive metabolite. Recovered primarily in feces and, to a lesser extent, in urine. Not removed by hemodialysis. **Half-life:** 11-15 hr.

AVAILABLE FORMS

- *Tablets:* 75 mg, 150 mg, 300 mg.

INDICATIONS AND DOSAGES

Hypertension alone or in combination with other antihypertensives

PO

Adults, Elderly, Children 13 yr and older. Initially, 75-150 mg/day. May increase to 300 mg/day.

Children 6-12 yr. Initially, 75 mg/day. May increase to 150 mg/day.

Nephropathy

PO

Adults, Elderly. Target dose of 300 mg/day.

UNLABELED USES: Treatment of heart failure

CONTRAINDICATIONS: Bilateral renal artery stenosis, biliary cirrhosis or obstruction, primary hyperaldosteronism, severe hepatic insufficiency

INTERACTIONS

Drug

Hydrochlorothiazide: Further reduces BP.

Herbal

None known.

Food

None known.

DIAGNOSTIC TEST EFFECTS: May slightly increase BUN and serum creatinine levels. May decrease blood Hgb level.

SIDE EFFECTS

Occasional (9%-3%)

Upper respiratory tract infection, fatigue, diarrhea, cough

Rare (2%-1%)

Heartburn, dizziness, headache, nausea, rash

SERIOUS REACTIONS

• Overdosage may manifest as hypotension and tachycardia. Bradycardia occurs less often.

SPECIAL CONSIDERATIONS

PRECAUTIONS

• Anticipate changes in renal function in susceptible individuals. In patients with unilateral or bilateral renal artery stenosis, increases in serum creatinine or blood urea nitrogen have been reported.

PATIENT INFORMATION

• Pregnancy: Advise female patients of childbearing age about the consequences of second- and third-trimester exposure to drugs that act on the renin-angiotensin system, and inform them that these consequences do not appear to have resulted from intrauterine drug exposure that has been limited to the first trimester. Ask these patients to report pregnancies to their physicians as soon as possible.

PREGNANCY AND LACTATION

• Pregnancy Categories C (first trimester) and D (second and third trimesters). The use of drugs that act directly on the renin-angiotensin system during the second and third trimesters of pregnancy has been associated with fetal and neonatal injury, including hypotension, neonatal skull hypoplasia, anuria, reversible or irreversible renal failure, and death. Whether irbesartan is excreted in human milk is not known, but irbesartan or some metabolite of irbesartan is secreted at low concentration in the milk of lactating rats.

isosorbide

(eye-soe-sor'bide)

Drug Class: Diuretics, osmotic

Pregnancy Category: B

Do not confuse with Inderal, Isuprel, K-Dur, or Plendil.

CLINICAL PHARMACOLOGY

Mechanism of Action: A nitrate that stimulates intracellular cyclic guanosine monophosphate (GMP.)

Therapeutic Effect: Relaxes vascular smooth muscle of both arterial and venous vasculature. Decreases preload and afterload.

Pharmacokinetics

Route	*Onset*	*Peak*	*Duration*
Sublingual	2-10 min	N/A	1-2 hrs
Chewable	3 min	N/A	0.5-2 hrs
PO	45-60 min	N/A	4-6 hrs
Sustained-release	30 min	N/A	6-12 hrs

Mononitrate well absorbed after PO administration. Dinitrate poorly absorbed and metabolized in the liver to its activate metabolite isosorbide mononitrate. Excreted in urine and feces. **Half-life:** Dinitrate is 1-4 hrs and mononitrate is 4 hrs.

AVAILABLE FORMS

• *Tablets:* 5 mg (Isordil), 10 mg (Isordil, Monoket), 20 mg (Isordil, Ismo, Monoket), 30 mg (Isordil), 40 mg (Isordil).

• *Tablets (chewable):* 5 mg, 10 mg.

• *Tablets (sublingual):* 10 mg (Isordil).

• *Capsules (sustained-release):* 40 mg (Dilatrate-SR).

• *Tablets (extended-release):* 30 mg, 60 mg, 120 mg (Imdur).

INDICATIONS AND DOSAGES

Acute angina, prophylactic management in situations likely to provoke attack

Sublingual

Adults, Elderly. Initially, 2.5-5 mg. Repeat at 5- to 10-min intervals. No more than 3 doses in 15- to 30-min period.

Acute prophylactic management of angina

Sublingual

Adults, Elderly. 5-10 mg q2-3h.

Long-term prophylaxis of angina

PO

Adults, Elderly. Initially, 5-20 mg 3-4 times/day. Maintenance: 10-40 mg q6h. Consider 2-3 times/day, last dose no later than 7 pm to minimize intolerance.

PO (Mononitrate)

Adults, Elderly. 20 mg 2 times/day, 7 hrs apart. First dose upon awakening in morning.

PO (extended-release)

Adults, Elderly. Initially, 40 mg. Maintenance: 40-80 mg 2-3 times/day. Consider 1-2 times/day, last dose at 2 pm to minimize intolerance.

PO (Imdur)

Adults, Elderly. 60-120 mg/day as single dose.

Congestive heart failure

PO (Chewable)

Adults, Elderly. 5-10 mg every 2-3 hours.

UNLABELED USES: Congestive heart failure (CHF), dysphagia, pain relief, relief of esophageal spasm with gastroesophageal (GE) reflux

CONTRAINDICATIONS: Closed-angle glaucoma, gastrointestinal (GI) hypermotility or malabsorption (extended-release tablets), head trauma, hypersensitivity to nitrates, increased intracranial pressure, postural hypotension, severe anemia (extended-release tablets)

INTERACTIONS

Drug

Alcohol, antihypertensives, vasodilators: May increase risk of orthostatic hypotension.

Herbal

None known.

Food

None known.

DIAGNOSTIC TEST EFFECTS: May increase urine catecholamines, urine VMA (vanillylmandelic acid).

SIDE EFFECTS

Frequent

Burning and tingling at oral point of dissolution (sublingual), headache (may be severe) occurs mostly in early therapy, diminishes rapidly in intensity, usually disappears during continued treatment; transient flushing of face and neck, dizziness (especially if patient is standing immobile or is in a warm environment), weakness, postural hypotension, nausea, vomiting, restlessness

Occasional

GI upset, blurred vision, dry mouth

SERIOUS REACTIONS

- Blurred vision or dry mouth may occur (drug should be discontinued).
- Severe postural hypotension manifested by fainting, pulselessness, cold or clammy skin, and diaphoresis may occur.
- Tolerance may occur with repeated, prolonged therapy (minor tolerance with intermittent use of sublingual tablets). Tolerance may not occur with extended-release form.
- High dose tends to produce severe headache.

SPECIAL CONSIDERATIONS

PRECAUTIONS

- Use repetitive doses with caution, particularly in patients with diseases associated with salt retention. Ensure that patient's bladder has been emptied before surgery.

PREGNANCY AND LACTATION

• Pregnancy Category B. Reproduction studies have been preformed in rats and rabbits, and there was no evidence of impaired fertility or harm to animal fetus from isosorbide. Excretion into human milk is not known.

isotretinoin

(eye-soe-tret'i-noyn)

Rx: Accutane, Amnesteem, Claravis, Sotret

Drug Class: Retinoids

Pregnancy Category: X

Do not confuse Accutane with Accupril or Accurbron.

CLINICAL PHARMACOLOGY

Mechanism of Action: Reduces the size of sebaceous glands and inhibits their activity. *Therapeutic Effect:* Decreases sebum production; produces antikeratinizing and anti-inflammatory effects.

Pharmacokinetics

Metabolized in the liver; major metabolite active. Eliminated in urine and feces. **Half-life:** 21 hr; metabolite, 21-24 hr.

AVAILABLE FORMS

• *Capsules:* 10 mg, 20 mg, 40 mg.

INDICATIONS AND DOSAGES

Recalcitrant cystic acne that is unresponsive to conventional acne therapies

PO

Adults. Initially, 0.5-2 mg/kg/day divided into 2 doses for 15-20 wk. May repeat after at least 2 mo off therapy.

UNLABELED USES: Treatment of gram-negative folliculitis, severe keratinization disorders, severe rosacea

CONTRAINDICATIONS: Hypersensitivity to isotretinoin or parabens (component of capsules)

INTERACTIONS

Drug

Etretinate, tretinoin, vitamin A: May increase toxic effects.

Tetracycline: May increase the risk of pseudotumor cerebri.

Herbal

Dong quai, St John's wort: May cause photosensitization.

Food

None known.

DIAGNOSTIC TEST EFFECTS: May increase serum alkaline phosphatase, total cholesterol, LDH, triglyceride, ALT (SGPT), and AST (SGOT) levels; urine uric acid level; erythrocyte sedimentation rate; and fasting blood glucose level. May decrease HDL level.

SIDE EFFECTS

Frequent (90%-20%)

Cheilitis (inflammation of lips), dry skin and mucous membranes, skin fragility, pruritus, epistaxis, dry nose and mouth, conjunctivitis, hypertriglyceridemia, nausea, vomiting, abdominal pain

Occasional (16%-5%)

Musculoskeletal symptoms (including bone pain, arthralgia, generalized myalgia), photosensitivity

Rare

Decreased night vision, depression

SERIOUS REACTIONS

• Inflammatory bowel disease and pseudotumor cerebri (benign intracranial hypertension) have been associated with isotretinoin therapy.

SPECIAL CONSIDERATIONS

PATIENT INFORMATION

• Instruct females of childbearing potential that they must not be pregnant when isotretinoin therapy is initiated. Patients should not donate blood during therapy because the blood might be given to a pregnant woman whose fetus must not be exposed to isotretinoin. Inform patients that transient exacerbation (flare) of acne has been seen, generally during the initial period of therapy. Advise the patient to avoid wax epilation and skin resurfacing procedures (such as dermabrasion and laser) during isotretinoin therapy. Advise patients to avoid prolonged exposure to ultraviolet rays or sunlight. Inform patients that they may experience decreased tolerance to contact lenses during and after therapy. Inform patients that approximately 16% of patients treated with isotretinoin in a clinical trial developed musculoskeletal symptoms (including arthralgia) during treatment. In general, these symptoms were mild to moderate but occasionally required discontinuation of the drug. Transient pain in the chest has been reported less frequently. In the clinical trial, these symptoms generally cleared rapidly after discontinuation of isotretinoin, but in some cases persisted. Neutropenia and rare cases of agranulocytosis have been reported. Discontinue isotretinoin if clinically significant decreases in white cell counts occur.

PRECAUTIONS

• Hypersensitivity.

PREGNANCY AND LACTATION

• Pregnancy Category X. Avoid pregnancy. Isotretinoin must not be used by females who are pregnant or who may become pregnant while undergoing treatment. Although not every fetus exposed to isotretinoin has resulted in a deformed child, the risk is extremely high that a deformed infant can result if pregnancy occurs while the mother is taking isotretinoin in any amount even for short periods of time. Whether this drug is excreted in human milk is not known. Because of the potential for adverse effects, nursing mothers should not receive isotretinoin.

OCULAR CONSIDERATIONS

• Carefully monitor visual problems. All patients receiving isotretinoin and experiencing visual difficulties should discontinue isotretinoin treatment and have an eye examination.

• Corneal Opacities: Corneal opacities have occurred in patients receiving isotretinoin for acne and more frequently when higher drug dosages were used in patients with disorders of keratinization. The corneal opacities that have been observed in clinical trial patients treated with isotretinoin have resolved completely or were resolving at follow-up 6 to 7 weeks after discontinuation of the drug.

• Decreased Night Vision: Decreased night vision has been reported during isotretinoin therapy, and in some instances the event has persisted after therapy was discontinued. Because the onset in some patients was sudden, advise patients of this potential problem and warn them to be cautious when driving or operating any vehicle at night.

• Inform patients that they may experience decreased tolerance to contact lenses during and after therapy.

isradipine

(is-rad'i-peen)

Rx: Dynacirc, Dynacirc CR

Drug Class: Calcium channel blockers

Pregnancy Category: C

Do not confuse DynaCirc with Dynabac or Dynacin.

CLINICAL PHARMACOLOGY

Mechanism of Action: An antihypertensive that inhibits calcium movement across cardiac and vascular smooth-muscle cell membranes. Potent peripheral vasodilator that does not depress SA or AV nodes. *Therapeutic Effect:* Produces relaxation of coronary vascular smooth muscle and coronary vasodilation. Increases myocardial oxygen delivery to those with vasospastic angina.

Pharmacokinetics

Route	Onset	Peak	Duration
PO	2-3 hr	2-4 wk (with multiple doses) 8-16 hr (with single dose)	N/A
PO (Controlled-release)	2 hr	8-10 hr	N/A

Well absorbed from the GI tract. Protein binding: 95%. Metabolized in the liver (undergoes first-pass effect). Primarily excreted in urine. Not removed by hemodialysis. **Half-life:** 8 hr.

AVAILABLE FORMS

- *Capsules (Dynacirc):* 2.5 mg, 5 mg.
- *Capsules (Controlled-Release [Dynacirc-CR]):* 5 mg, 10 mg.

INDICATIONS AND DOSAGES

Hypertension

PO

Adults, Elderly. Initially 2.5 mg twice a day. May increase by 2.5 mg at 2- to 4-wk intervals. Range: 5-20 mg/day

UNLABELED USES: Treatment of chronic angina pectoris, Raynaud's phenomenon

CONTRAINDICATIONS: Cardiogenic shock, CHF, heart block, hypotension, sinus bradycardia, ventricular tachycardia

INTERACTIONS

Drug

Beta-blockers: May have additive effect.

Herbal

None known.

Food

Grapefruit, grapefruit juice: May increase the absorption of isradipine.

DIAGNOSTIC TEST EFFECTS: *None known.*

SIDE EFFECTS

Frequent (7%-4%)

Peripheral edema, palpitations (higher frequency in females)

Occasional (3%)

Facial flushing, cough

Rare (2%-1%)

Angina, tachycardia, rash, pruritus

SERIOUS REACTIONS

- Overdose produces nausea, drowsiness, confusion, and slurred speech.
- CHF occurs rarely.

SPECIAL CONSIDERATIONS

PRECAUTIONS

- Isradipine may produce hypotension. Exercise caution when using the drug in patients with congestive heart failure, particularly in combination with a beta-blocker.

PREGNANCY AND LACTATION

- Pregnancy Category C. No evidence of embryotoxicity was found at doses that were not maternotoxic, and no evidence of teratogenicity was found at any dose tested. Excretion into human milk is not known.

itraconazole

(it-ra-con'a-zol)

Rx: Sporanox

Drug Class: Antifungals

Pregnancy Category: C

Do not confuse Sporanox with Suprax.

CLINICAL PHARMACOLOGY

Mechanism of Action: A fungistatic antifungal that inhibits the synthesis of ergosterol, a vital component of fungal cell formation *Therapeutic Effect:* Damages the fungal cell membrane, altering its function.

Pharmacokinetics

Moderately absorbed from the GI tract. Absorption is increased if the drug is taken with food. Protein binding: 99%. Widely distributed, primarily in the fatty tissue, liver, and kidneys. Metabolized in the liver to active metabolite. Primarily excreted in urine. Not removed by hemodialysis. **Half-life:** 21 hr; metabolite, 12 hr.

AVAILABLE FORMS

- *Capsules:* 100 mg.
- *Oral Solution:* 10 mg/ml.
- *Injection:* 10 mg/ml (25-ml ampule).

INDICATIONS AND DOSAGES

Blastomycosis, histoplasmosis

PO

Adults, Elderly. Initially, 200 mg once a day. Maximum: 400 mg/day in 2 divided doses.

IV

Adults, Elderly. 200 mg twice a day for 4 doses, then 200 mg once a day.

Aspergillosis

PO

Adults, Elderly. 600 mg/day in 3 divided doses for 3-4 days, then 200-400 mg/day in 2 divided doses.

IV

Adults, Elderly. 200 mg twice a day for 4 doses, then 200 mg once a day.

Esophageal candidiasis

PO

Adults, Elderly. Swish 10 ml in mouth for several seconds, then swallow. Maximum: 200 mg/day.

Oropharyngeal candidiasis

PO

Adults, Elderly. Vigorously swish 10 ml in mouth for several seconds (20 ml total daily dose) once a day.

UNLABELED USES: Suppression of histoplasmosis; treatment of disseminated sporotrichosis, fungal pneumonia and septicemia, or ringworm of the hand

CONTRAINDICATIONS: Hypersensitivity to itraconazole, fluconazole, ketoconazole, or miconazole

INTERACTIONS

Drug

Antacids, didanosine, H_2 antagonists: May decrease itraconazole absorption.

Buspirone, cyclosporine, digoxin, lovastatin, simvastatin: May increase blood concentration of these drugs.

Oral anticoagulants: May increase the effect of oral anticoagulants.

Phenytoin, rifampin: May decrease itraconazole blood concentration.

Herbal

None known.

Food

Grapefruit, grapefruit juice: May alter itraconazole absorption.

DIAGNOSTIC TEST EFFECTS: May increase serum LDH serum alkaline phosphatase, serum bilirubin, AST (SGOT), and ALT (SGPT) levels. May decrease serum potassium level.

IV INCOMPATIBILITIES: Alert: Dilution compatibility of itraconazole with any solution other than 0.9% NaCl is unknown. Don't mix with D_5W or lactated Ringer's solution. Not for IV bolus administration. Don't administer any medication in same bag or through same IV line as itraconazole.

SIDE EFFECTS

Frequent (11%-9%)

Nausea, rash

Occasional (5%-3%)

Vomiting, headache, diarrhea, hypertension, peripheral edema, fatigue, fever

Rare (2% or less)

Abdominal pain, dizziness, anorexia, pruritus

SERIOUS REACTIONS

• Hepatitis (as evidenced by anorexia, abdominal pain, unusual fatigue or weakness, jaundice skin or sclera, and dark urine) occurs rarely.

SPECIAL CONSIDERATIONS

PRECAUTIONS

• Monitor hepatic enzyme test values in patients with preexisting hepatic function abnormalities or those who have experienced liver toxicity with other medications. Monitor hepatic enzyme test values periodically in all patients receiving continuous treatment for more than 1 month or at any time a patient develops signs or symptoms suggestive of liver dysfunction. Administer capsules after a full meal. The absorption of itraconazole may be decreased with the concomitant administration of antacids or gastric acid secretion suppressors.

PATIENT INFORMATION

• The topical effects of mucosal exposure may be different between the itraconazole capsules and oral solution. Only the oral solution has been demonstrated to be effective for oral and/or esophageal candidiasis. Do not use itraconazole capsules interchangeably with itraconazole oral solution. Itraconazole oral solution contains the excipient hydroxypropyl-b-cyclodextrin, which produced pancreatic adenocarcinomas in a rat carcinogenicity study. These findings were not observed in a similar mouse carcinogenicity study. The clinical relevance of these findings is unknown. Instruct patients about the signs and symptoms of congestive heart failure and that if these signs or symptoms occur during itraconazole administration, they should discontinue itraconazole and contact their health care provider immediately. Instruct patients to report any signs and symptoms that may suggest liver dysfunction so that the appropriate laboratory testing can be done. Such signs and symptoms may include unusual fatigue, anorexia, nausea and/or vomiting, jaundice, dark urine, or pale stools. Instruct patients to contact their physician before taking any concomitant medications with itraconazole to ensure there are no potential drug interactions.

• Capsules: Instruct patients to take itraconazole capsules with a full meal.

• Oral Solution: Taking itraconazole oral solution under fasted conditions improves the systemic availability of itraconazole. Instruct patients to take itraconazole oral solution without food, if possible.

PREGNANCY AND LACTATION

• Pregnancy Category C. Itraconazole was found to cause a dose-related increase in maternal toxicity, embryotoxicity, and teratogenicity in rats. No studies in pregnant women have been performed. Use itraconazole to treat systemic fungal infections in pregnancy only if the benefit outweighs the potential risk. Do not administer itraconazole capsules for the treatment of onychomycosis to pregnant patients or to women contemplating pregnancy. Do not administer itraconazole capsules to women of childbearing potential for the treatment of onychomycosis unless they are using effective measures to prevent pregnancy and they begin therapy on the second or third day following the onset of menses. Effective contraception should be continued throughout itraconazole therapy and for 2 months following the end of treatment. Itraconazole is excreted in human milk.

ketoconazole

(kee-toe-koe′na-zole)

Rx: Nizoral, Nizoral Topical

Drug Class: Antifungals; Antifungals, topical; Dermatologics

Pregnancy Category: C

Do not confuse Nizoral with Nasarel.

CLINICAL PHARMACOLOGY

Mechanism of Action: A fungistatic antifungal that inhibits the synthesis of ergosterol, a vital component of fungal cell formation. *Therapeutic Effect:* Damages the fungal cell membrane, altering its function.

AVAILABLE FORMS

- *Tablets (Nizoral):* 200 mg.
- *Cream (Nizoral):* 2%.
- *Shampoo (Nizoral AD):* 1%.

INDICATIONS AND DOSAGES

Histoplasmosis, blastomycosis, systemic candidiasis, chronic mucocutaneous candidiasis, coccidioidomycosis, paracoccidioidomycosis, chromomycosis, seborrheic dermatitis, tinea corporis, tinea capitis, tinea manus, tinea cruris, tinea pedis, tinea unguium (onychomycosis), oral thrush, candiduria

PO

Adults, Elderly. 200-400 mg/day.

Children. 3.3-6.6 mg/kg/day. Maximum: 800 mg/day in 2 divided doses.

Topical

Adults, Elderly. Apply to affected area 1-2 times a day for 2-4 wk.

Shampoo

Adults, Elderly. Use twice weekly for 4 wk, allowing at least 3 days between shampooing. Use intermittently to maintain control.

UNLABELED USES: Systemic: Treatment of fungal pneumonia, prostate cancer, septicemia

CONTRAINDICATIONS: None known.

INTERACTIONS

Drug

Alcohol, hepatotoxic medications: May increase hepatotoxicity of ketoconazole.

Antacids, anticholinergics, H_2 antagonists, omeprazole: May decrease ketoconazole absorption.

Cyclosporine, lovastatin, simvastatin: May increase blood concentration and risk of toxicity of these drugs.

Isoniazid, rifampin: May decrease blood concentration of ketoconazole.

Herbal

Echinacea: May have additive hepatotoxic effects.

Food

None known.

DIAGNOSTIC TEST EFFECTS: May increase serum alkaline phosphatase, serum bilirubin, AST (SGOT), and ALT (SGPT) levels. May decrease serum corticosteroid and testosterone concentrations.

SIDE EFFECTS

Occasional (10%-3%)

Nausea, vomiting

Rare (less than 2%)

Abdominal pain, diarrhea, headache, dizziness, photophobia, pruritus

Topical: itching, burning, irritation

SERIOUS REACTIONS

- Hematologic toxicity (as evidenced by thrombocytopenia, hemolytic anemia, and leukopenia) occurs occasionally.
- Hepatotoxicity may occur within 1 week to several months after starting therapy.
- Anaphylaxis occurs rarely.

SPECIAL CONSIDERATIONS

PRECAUTIONS

- Ketoconazole tablets have been demonstrated to lower serum testosterone. In four subjects with drug-induced achlorhydria, a marked reduction in ketoconazole absorption was observed.

PATIENT INFORMATION

- Shampoo: Ketoconazole may be irritating to mucous membranes of the eyes, and contact with this area should be avoided. Use of the shampoo has been reported to result in removal of the curl from permanently waved hair.
- Tablets: Instruct patients to report any signs and symptoms that may suggest liver dysfunction so that appropriate biochemical testing can be done. Such signs and symptoms may include unusual fatigue, anorexia, nausea and/or vomiting, jaundice, dark urine, or pale stools.

PREGNANCY AND LACTATION

- Pregnancy Category C. Ketoconazole has been shown to be teratogenic (syndactylia and oligodactylia) in the rat. Ketoconazole probably is excreted in the milk.

ketorolac tromethamine

(kee-toe'role-ak)

Rx: Acular, Acular LS, Toradol, Toradol IM, Toradol IV/IM

Drug Class: Analgesics, nonnarcotic; Nonsteroidal anti-inflammatory drugs; Ophthalmics

Pregnancy Category: C

Do not confuse Acular with Acthar or Ocular.

CLINICAL PHARMACOLOGY

Mechanism of Action: An NSAID that inhibits prostaglandin synthesis and reduces prostaglandin levels in the aqueous humor. *Therapeutic Effect:* Relieves pain stimulus and reduces intraocular inflammation.

Pharmacokinetics

Route	Onset	Peak	Duration
PO	30-60 min	1.5-4 hr	4-6 hr
IV/IM	30 min	1-2 hr	4-6 hr

Readily absorbed from the GI tract, after IM administration. Protein binding: 99%. Largely metabolized in the liver. Primarily excreted in urine. Not removed by hemodialysis. **Half-life:** 3.8-6.3 hr (increased with impaired renal function and in the elderly).

AVAILABLE FORMS

- *Tablets (Toradol):* 10 mg.
- *Injection (Toradol):* 15 mg/ml, 30 mg/ml.

K

• *Ophthalmic Solution (Acular):* 0.5%.
• *Ophthalmic Solution (Acular LS):* 0.4%.
• *Ophthalmic Solution (Acular PF):* 0.5%.

INDICATIONS AND DOSAGES

Short-term relief of mild to moderate pain (multiple doses)

PO

Adults, Elderly. 10 mg q4-6h. Maximum: 40 mg/24 hr.

IV, IM

Adults younger than 65 yr. 30 mg q6h. Maximum: 120 mg/24 hr.

Adults 65 yr and older, those with renal impairment, those weighing less than 50 kg. 15 mg q6h. Maximum: 60 mg/24 hr.

Children 2-16 yr. 0.5 mg/kg q6h.

Short-term relief of mild to moderate pain (single dose)

IV

Adults younger than 65 yr, Children 17 yr and older weighing more than 50 kg. 30 mg.

Adults 65 yr and older, with renal impairment, weighing less than 50 kg. 15 mg.

Children 2-16 yr. 0.5 mg/kg. Maximum: 15 mg.

IM

Adults younger than 65 yr, Children 17 yr and older, weighing more than 50 kg. 60 mg.

Adults 65 yr and older, with renal impairment, weighing less than 50 kg. 30 mg.

Children 2-16 yr. 1 mg/kg. Maximum: 15 kg.

Allergic conjunctivitis

Ophthalmic

Adults, Elderly, Children 3 yr and older. 1 drop 4 times a day.

Cataract extraction

Ophthalmic

Adults, Elderly. 1 drop 4 times a day. Begin 24 hr after surgery and continue for 2 wk.

Refractive surgery

Ophthalmic

Adults, Elderly. 1 drop 4 times a day for 3 days.

UNLABELED USES: Prevention or treatment of ocular inflammation- (ophthalmic form)

CONTRAINDICATIONS: Active peptic ulcer disease, chronic inflammation of GI tract, GI bleeding or ulceration, history of hypersensitivity to aspirin or NSAIDs

INTERACTIONS

Drug

Antihypertensives, diuretics: May decrease the effects of these drugs.

Aspirin, other salicylates: May increase the risk of GI side effects such as bleeding.

Bone marrow depressants: May increase the risk of hematologic reactions.

Heparin, oral anticoagulants, thrombolytics: May increase the effects of these drugs.

Lithium: May increase the blood concentration and risk of toxicity of lithium.

Methotrexate: May increase the risk of methotrexate toxicity.

Probenecid: May increase ketorolac blood concentration.

Herbal

Feverfew: May decrease the effects of feverfew.

Ginkgo biloba: May increase the risk of bleeding.

Food

None known.

DIAGNOSTIC TEST EFFECTS: May prolong bleeding time. May increase liver function test results.

IV INCOMPATIBILITIES: Promethazine (Phenergan)

IV COMPATIBILITIES: Fentanyl (Sublimaze), hydromorphone (Dilaudid), morphine, nalbuphine (Nubain)

SIDE EFFECTS

Frequent (17%-12%)

Headache, nausea, abdominal cramps or pain, dyspepsia

Occasional (9%-3%)

Diarrhea

Ophthalmic: Transient stinging and burning

Rare (3%-1%)

Constipation, vomiting, flatulence, stomatitis, dizziness

Ophthalmic: Ocular irritation, allergic reactions, superficial ocular infection, keratitis

SERIOUS REACTIONS

• Rare reactions with long-term use include peptic ulcer disease, GI bleeding, gastritis, severe hepatic reactions (cholestasis, jaundice), nephrotoxicity (glomerular nephritis, interstitial nephritis, nephrotic syndrome), and an acute hypersensitivity reaction (including fever, chills, and joint pain).

SPECIAL CONSIDERATIONS

PRECAUTIONS

• Cautious use of Acular eye solution is recommended in patients with known bleeding tendencies or who are receiving other medications that may prolong bleeding time. The potential exists for cross-sensitivity to acetylsalicylic acid, phenylacetic acid derivatives, and other nonsteroidal antiinflammatory agents.

PATIENT INFORMATION

• The patient should not administer ketorolac tromethamine while wearing contact lenses.

PREGNANCY AND LACTATION

• Pregnancy Category C. Ketorolac tromethamine administered during organogenesis was not teratogenic in rabbits or rats at oral doses. Because of the known effects of prostaglandin-inhibiting drugs on the fetal cardiovascular system (closure of the ductus arteriosus), avoid the use of Acular eye solution during late pregnancy. Exercise caution when administering Acular eye solution to a nursing woman.

OCULAR CONSIDERATIONS

• Off-label uses include for pain caused by epithelial defects or general eye pain: 1 tablet every 4 to 6 hours, 40 mg/day maximum.

---

ketotifen fumarate

(kee-toe-tye′-fen fyoo′-mah-rate)

Rx: Zaditor

Drug Class: Antihistamines, H1; Antihistamines, ophthalmic; Ophthalmics

Pregnancy Category: C

K

CLINICAL PHARMACOLOGY

Mechanism of Action: Selective histamine H_1-antagonist and mast cell stabilizer, suppresses release of mediators from cells involved in hypersensitivity reactions, and decreases chemotoxis and activation of eosinophils. *Therapeutic Effect:* Reduces symptoms of allergic conjunctivitis.

Pharmacokinetics

None reported.

AVAILABLE FORMS

• *Ophthalmic Solution:* 0.025% (Zaditor).

INDICATIONS AND DOSAGES

Allergic conjunctivitis

Ophthalmic

Adults, Elderly, Children 3 yr or older: 1 drop into affected eye q8-12h.

CONTRAINDICATIONS: Hypersensitivity to ketotifen or any component of the formulation (the preservative is benzalkonium chloride)

INTERACTIONS

Drug

None known.

Herbal

None known.

Food

None known.

DIAGNOSTIC TEST EFFECTS: *None known.*

SIDE EFFECTS

Frequent (25%-10%)

Conjunctival infection, headache, rhinitis

Occasional (5%-1%)

Allergic reaction, burning, stinging, eyelid disorder, flu-like syndrome, keratitis, mydriasis, ocular discharge/ pain, pharyngitis, photophobia, rash

SERIOUS REACTIONS

• No serious signs and symptoms have been seen after ingestion up to 20 mg.

SPECIAL CONSIDERATIONS

PATIENT INFORMATION

• Benzalkonium chloride may be absorbed by soft contact lenses. Instruct patients to wait at least 10 minutes after instilling ketotifen fumarate eye solution before they insert their contact lenses.

PREGNANCY AND LACTATION

• Pregnancy Category C. Oral doses in rats showed slight increase in postnatal mortality and slight decrease in body weight gain during the first 4 days postpartum. Oral doses in rabbits showed increased incidence of retarded ossification of the sternebrae. Fetal harm is not known with topical administration. Ketotifen fumarate has been identified in breast milk in rats following oral administration. Excretion into human milk is not known.

labetalol hydrochloride

(la-bet'a-lole)

Rx: Normodyne, Trandate

Drug Class: Antiadrenergics, beta blocking

Pregnancy Category: C

Do not confuse Trandate with tramadol or Trental.

CLINICAL PHARMACOLOGY

Mechanism of Action: An antihypertensive that blocks $alpha_1$-, $beta_1$-, and $beta_2$-(large doses) adrenergic receptor sites. Large doses increase airway resistance. *Therapeutic Effect:* Slows sinus heart rate; decreases peripheral vascular resistance, cardiac output, and BP.

Pharmacokinetics

Route	*Onset*	*Peak*	*Duration*
PO	0.5-2 hr	2-4 hr	8-12 hr
IV	2-5 min	5-15 min	2-4 hr

Completely absorbed from the GI tract. Protein binding: 50%. Undergoes first-pass metabolism. Metabolized in the liver. Primarily excreted in urine. Not removed by hemodialysis. **Half-life:** PO, 6-8 hr; IV, 5.5 hr.

AVAILABLE FORMS

• *Tablets (Normodyne, Trandate):* 100 mg, 200 mg, 300 mg.

• *Injection (Trandate):* 5 mg/ml.

INDICATIONS AND DOSAGES

Hypertension

PO

Adults. Initially, 100 mg twice a day adjusted in increments of 100 mg twice a day q2-3 days. Maintenance: 200-400 mg twice a day. Maximum: 2.4 g/day.

Elderly. Initially, 100 mg 1-2 times a day. May increase as needed.

Severe hypertension, hypertensive emergency

IV

Adults. Initially, 20 mg. Additional doses of 20-80 mg may be given at 10-min intervals, up to total dose of 300 mg.

IV Infusion

Adults. Initially, 2 mg/min up to total dose of 300 mg.

PO (after IV therapy)

Adults. Initially, 200 mg; then, 200-400 mg in 6-12 hr. Increase dose at 1-day intervals to desired level.

UNLABELED USES: Control of hypotension during surgery, treatment of chronic angina pectoris

CONTRAINDICATIONS: Bronchial asthma, cardiogenic shock, second- or third-degree heart block, severe bradycardia, uncontrolled CHF

INTERACTIONS

Drug

Diuretics, other antihypertensives: May increase hypotensive effect.

Insulin, oral hypoglycemics: May mask symptoms of hypoglycemia and prolong hypoglycemic effect of these drugs.

MAOIs: May produce hypertension.

Sympathomimetics, xanthines: May mutually inhibit effects.

Herbal

None known.

Food

None known.

DIAGNOSTIC TEST EFFECTS: May increase serum antinuclear antibody titer and BUN, serum LDH, lipoprotein, alkaline phosphatase, bilirubin, creatinine, potassium, triglyceride, uric acid, AST (SGOT), and ALT (SGPT) levels.

IV INCOMPATIBILITIES: Amphotericin B complex (Abelcet, AmBisome, Amphotec), ceftriaxone (Rocephin), furosemide (Lasix), heparin, nafcillin (Nafcil), thiopental

IV COMPATIBILITIES: Aminophylline, amiodarone (Cordarone), calcium gluconate, diltiazem (Cardizem), dobutamine (Dobutrex), dopamine (Intropin), enalapril (Vasotec), fentanyl (Sublimaze), hydromorphone (Dilaudid), lidocaine, lorazepam (Ativan), magnesium sulfate, midazolam (Versed), milrinone (Primacor), morphine, nitroglycerin, norepinephrine (Levophed), potassium chloride, potassium phosphate, propofol (Diprivan)

SIDE EFFECTS

Frequent

Drowsiness, difficulty sleeping, unusual fatigue or weakness, diminished sexual ability, transient scalp tingling

Occasional

Dizziness, dyspnea, peripheral edema, depression, anxiety, constipation, diarrhea, nasal congestion, nausea, vomiting, abdominal discomfort

Rare

Altered taste, dry eyes, increased urination, paresthesia

SERIOUS REACTIONS

- Labetolol administration may precipitate or aggravate CHF beacause of decreased myocardial stimulation.
- Abrupt withdrawal may precipitate ischemic heart disease, producing sweating, palpitations, headache, and tremor.
- May mask signs and symptoms of acute hypoglycemia (tachycardia, BP changes) in patients with diabetes.

SPECIAL CONSIDERATIONS

PRECAUTIONS

• Use labetalol hydrochloride with caution in patients with impaired hepatic function because metabolism of the drug may be diminished.

PATIENT INFORMATION

• As with all drugs with beta-blocking activity, certain advice to patients being treated with labetalol hydrochloride is warranted. This information is intended to aid in the safe and effective use of this medication. Such advice is not a disclosure of all possible adverse or intended effects. Although no incident of the abrupt withdrawal phenomenon (exacerbation of angina pectoris) has been reported with labetalol hydrochloride, dosing with labetalol hydrochloride tablets should not be interrupted or discontinued without a physician's advice. Patients being treated with labetalol hydrochloride tablets should consult a physician at any signs or symptoms of impending cardiac failure or hepatic dysfunction. Also, transient scalp tingling may occur, usually when treatment with labetalol hydrochloride tablets is initiated.

PREGNANCY AND LACTATION

• Pregnancy Category C. Hypotension, bradycardia, hypoglycemia, and respiratory depression have been reported in infants of mothers who were treated with labetalol hydrochloride for hypertension during pregnancy. Oral administration of labetalol to rats caused a decrease in neonatal survival. Small amounts of labetalol (approximately 0.004% of the maternal dose) are excreted in human milk.

lansoprazole

(lan-soe-pray'-zole)

Rx: Prevacid, Prevacid SoluTab

Drug Class: Gastrointestinals; Proton pump inhibitors

Pregnancy Category: B

Do not confuse Prevacid with Pepcid, Pravachol, or Prevpac.

CLINICAL PHARMACOLOGY

Mechanism of Action: A proton pump inhibitor that selectively inhibits the parietal cell membrane enzyme system (hydrogen-potassium adenosine triphosphatase) or proton pump. *Therapeutic Effect:* Suppresses gastric acid secretion.

Pharmacokinetics

Route	Onset	Peak	Duration
PO (15 mg)	2-3 hr	N/A	24 hr
PO (30 mg)	1-2 hr	N/A	longer than 24 hr

Rapid and complete absorption (food may decrease absorption) once drug has left stomach. Protein binding: 97%. Distributed primarily to gastric parietal cells and converted to two active metabolites. Extensively metabolized in the liver. Eliminated in bile and urine. Not removed by hemodialysis. **Half-life:** 1.5 hr (increased in the elderly and in those with hepatic impairment).

AVAILABLE FORMS

• *Capsules (Delayed-Release [Prevacid]):* 15 mg, 30 mg.

• *Granules for Oral Suspension (Prevacid):* 15 mg/pack; 30 mg/pack.

• *Injection Powder for Reconstitution (Prevacid IV):* 30 mg.

• *Oral-disintegrating Tablets (Prevacid Solu-Tab):* 15 mg, 30 mg.

INDICATIONS AND DOSAGES

Duodenal ulcer

PO

Adults, Elderly. 15 mg/day, before eating, preferably in the morning, for up to 4 wks.

Erosive esophagitis

PO

Adults, Elderly. 30 mg/day, before eating, for up to 8 wks. If healing does not occur within 8 wk (in 5%-10% of cases), may give for additional 8 wk. Maintenance: 15 mg/day.

IV

Adults, Elderly. 30 mg once a day for up to 7 days. Switch to oral lansoprazole therapy as soon as patient can tolerate oral route.

Gastric ulcer

PO

Adults. 30 mg/day for up to 8 wk.

NSAID gastric ulcer

PO

Adults, Elderly. (Healing): 30 mg/day for up to 8 wk. (Prevention): 15 mg/day for up to 12 wk.

Healed duodenal ulcer, gastroesophageal reflux disease

PO

Adults. 15 mg/day.

Usual pediatric dosage

Children 3 mo-14 yr, weighing more than 20 kg. 30 mg once daily.

Children 3 mo-14 yr, weighing 10-20 kg. 15 mg once daily.

Children 3 mo-14 yr, weighing less than 10 kg. 7.5 mg once daily.

Helicobacter pylori *infection*

PO

Adults. 30 mg twice a day for 10 days (with amoxicillin and clarithromycin).

Pathologic hypersecretory conditions (including Zollinger-Ellison syndrome)

PO

Adults, Elderly. 60 mg/day. Individualize dosage according to patient needs and for as long as clinically indicated. Administer up to 120 mg/day in divided doses.

CONTRAINDICATIONS: None known.

INTERACTIONS

Drug

Ampicillin, digoxin, iron salts, ketoconazole: May interfere with the absorption of ampicillin, digoxin, iron salts, and ketoconazole.

Sucralfate: May delay the absorption of lansoprazole.

Herbal

None known.

Food

None known.

DIAGNOSTIC TEST EFFECTS: May increase LDH, serum alkaline phosphatase, bilirubin, cholesterol, creatinine, AST (SGOT), ALT (SGPT), triglyceride, and uric acid levels. May produce abnormal albumin/globulin ratio, electrolyte balance, and platelet, RBC, and WBC counts. May increase Hgb and Hct.

SIDE EFFECTS

Occasional (3%-2%)

Diarrhea, abdominal pain, rash, pruritus, altered appetite

Rare (1%)

Nausea, headache

SERIOUS REACTIONS

• Bilirubinemia, eosinophilia, and hyperlipemia occur rarely.

SPECIAL CONSIDERATIONS

PRECAUTIONS

• Serious and occasionally fatal hypersensitivity (anaphylactic) reactions have been reported in patients taking penicillin therapy. Pseudomembranous colitis has been reported with nearly all antibacterial agents and may range in severity from mild to life threatening. Symptomatic response to therapy with lansoprazole does not preclude the presence of gastric malignancy.

PATIENT INFORMATION

• Instruct patients to take lansoprazole delayed-release capsules before eating.

PREGNANCY AND LACTATION

• Lansoprazole, Pregnancy Category B; clarithromycin, Pregnancy Category C. Teratology studies performed in pregnant rats and rabbits have revealed no evidence of impaired fertility or harm to the fetus from lansoprazole. Do not use clarithromycin in pregnant women except in clinical circumstances where no alternative therapy is appropriate. If pregnancy occurs while the patient is taking clarithromycin, apprise the patient of the potential hazard to the fetus. Lansoprazole or its metabolites are excreted in the milk of rats. Excretion into human milk is not known.

latanoprost

(la-ta′-noe-prost)

Rx: Xalatan

Drug Class: Ophthalmics; Prostaglandins

Pregnancy Category: C

Do not confuse with Xanax.

CLINICAL PHARMACOLOGY

Mechanism of Action: An ophthalmic agent that is a prostanoid selective FP receptor agonist. *Therapeutic Effect:* Reduces intraocular pressure (IOP) by reducing aqueous humor production.

Pharmacokinetics

Absorbed through the cornea where the isopropyl ester prodrug is hydrolyzed to acid form to become biologically active. Highly lipophilic. The acid of latanoprost can be measured in the aqueous humor during the first 4 hours and in the plasma only during the first hour after local administration. Cornea, latanoprost, is hydrolyzed to the biologically active acid. Metabolized in liver if it reaches systemic circulation. Metabolized to 1,2-dinor metabolite and 1,2,3,4-tetranor metabolite. Primarily eliminated by the kidneys. **Half-life:** 17 min.

AVAILABLE FORMS

• *Ophthalmic Solution:* 0.005% (Xalatan).

INDICATIONS AND DOSAGES

Glaucoma, ocular hypertension

Ophthalmic

Adults, Elderly. 1 drop (1.5 mcg) in affected eye(s) once daily, in the evening.

CONTRAINDICATIONS: Hypersensitivity to latanoprost or benzalkonium chloride, or any other component of the formulation

INTERACTIONS

Drug

Pilocarpine: May decrease latanoprost efficacy.

Thimerosal: May cause precipitation in the eye.

Herbal

None known.

Food

None known.

DIAGNOSTIC TEST EFFECTS: *None known.*

SIDE EFFECTS

Frequent

Blurred vision

Occasional

Eyelash changes, eyelid skin darkening, iris pigmentation

Rare

Macular edema

SERIOUS REACTIONS

• Pigmentation is expected to increase as long as latanoprost is administered but after discontinuation, pigmentation of the iris is likely to be permanent while pigmentation of the periorbital tissue and eyelash changes has been reported as reversible.

- Inflammation (iritis/uveitis) and macular edema, including cystoid macular edema have been reported.

SPECIAL CONSIDERATIONS

PRECAUTIONS

- Patients may develop increased brown pigmentation of the iris. Use latanoprost with caution in patients with iritis and uveitis. Macular edema may occur in aphakic patients and pseudophakic patients. Use latanoprost with caution in patients with renal or hepatic impairment. Do not administer latanoprost while the patient is wearing contact lenses.

PATIENT INFORMATION

- The possibility exists of iris color change caused by an increase of the brown pigment. The possibility exists of eyelash changes in the treated eye, which may result in a disparity between eyes in lash length, thickness, pigmentation, and/or number. The possibility of eyelid skin darkening exists. Changes may be permanent. If any ocular reactions, particularly conjunctivitis and lid reactions, should develop, instruct the patient to seek an eye care practitioner's advice. Latanoprost contains benzalkonium chloride, which may be absorbed by contact lenses. Contact lenses may be reinserted 15 minutes following administration.

PREGNANCY AND LACTATION

- Pregnancy Category C. Twenty-five percent of rabbit dams had no viable fetuses with oral doses. Fetal harm is not known with topical administration. Excretion into human milk is not known.

levobetaxolol hydrochloride

(le-vo-bay-tax'oh-lol)

Rx: Betaxon

Drug Class: Antiadrenergics, beta blocking; Ophthalmics

Pregnancy Category: C

Do not confuse with levobunolol.

CLINICAL PHARMACOLOGY

Mechanism of Action: An antiglaucoma agent that blocks $beta_1$-adrenergic receptors. Reduces aqueous humor production. *Therapeutic Effect:* Reduces intraocular pressure (IOP).

Pharmacokinetics

Route	*Onset*	*Peak*	*Duration*
Eye drops	30 min	2 hrs	12 hrs

May be systemically absorbed.

AVAILABLE FORMS

- *Ophthalmic Solution:* 0.5% (Betaxon).

INDICATIONS AND DOSAGES

Glaucoma, ocular hypertension

Ophthalmic

Adults, Elderly. Instill 1 drop 2 times/day.

CONTRAINDICATIONS: Sinus bradycardia, second- or third-degree atrioventricular (AV) block, cardiogenic shock, overt heart failure, hypersensitivity to betaxolol, levobetaxolol, or any component of levobetaxolol formulations

INTERACTIONS

Drug

Fenoldopam: May exaggerate hypotensive response.

Herbal

Dong quai: May decrease blood pressure.

L

Licorice, Ma huang, St. John's wort, yohimbine: May decrease effectiveness of levobetaxolol.

Food

None known.

DIAGNOSTIC TEST EFFECTS: *None known.*

SIDE EFFECTS

Frequent

Ocular discomfort

Occasional

Blurred vision

Rare

Anxiety, dizziness, vertigo, headache

SERIOUS REACTIONS

• Diabetes, hypothyroidism, bradycardia, tachycardia, hypertension, hypotension, heart block, alopecia, dermatitis, psoriasis, arthritis, tendonitis, dyspnea and other respiratory symptoms (e.g., bronchitis, pneumonia, rhinitis, sinusitits, pharyngitis) occur rarely.

• Ophthalmic overdosage may produce bradycardia, hypotension, bronchospasm, and acute cardiac failure.

SPECIAL CONSIDERATIONS

PRECAUTIONS

• Diabetes Mellitus: Administer levobetaxolol with caution in patients subject to spontaneous hypoglycemia or to diabetic patients.

• Thyrotoxicosis: Levobetaxolol may mask certain clinical signs (e.g., tachycardia) of hyperthyroidism.

• Muscle Weakness: Levobetaxolol potentiates muscle weakness consistent with certain myasthenic symptoms (e.g., diplopia, ptosis, and generalized weakness).

• Major Surgery: Initiate gradual withdrawal before general anesthesia because of the reduced ability of the heart to respond to beta-adrenergically mediated sympathetic reflex stimuli.

• Pulmonary: Exercise caution in the treatment of patients with glaucoma who have excessive restriction of pulmonary function. Reports have been made of asthmatic attacks and pulmonary distress during betaxolol treatment.

PATIENT INFORMATION

• Patients with a history of atopy or a history of severe anaphylactic reaction may be unresponsive to the usual doses of epinephrine used to treat anaphylactic reactions.

PREGNANCY AND LACTATION

• Pregnancy Category C. Postimplantation loss occurred in rabbits with oral doses. Fetal harm is not known with topical administration. Excretion into human milk is not known.

---

levobunolol hydrochloride

(lee-vo-byoo'no-lol)

Rx: AK-Beta, Betagan

Drug Class: Antiadrenergics, beta blocking; Ophthalmics

Pregnancy Category: C

Do not confuse with levobetaxolol.

CLINICAL PHARMACOLOGY

Mechanism of Action: A nonselective beta-blocker that blocks $beta_1$- and $beta_2$-adrenergenic receptors. *Therapeutic Effect:* Reduces intraocular pressure. Decreases production of aqueous humor.

Pharmacokinetics

Well absorbed after administration. Metabolized in liver. Primarily excreted in urine. **Half-life:** 6.1 hrs.

AVAILABLE FORMS

• *Ophthalmic Solution:* 0.25%, 0.5% (AK-Beta, Betagan).

INDICATIONS AND DOSAGES

Glaucoma, ocular hypertension

Ophthalmic

Adults, Elderly. Instill 1-2 drops in affected eye(s) once daily.

UNLABELED USES: Bronchial asthma, chronic obstructive pulmonary disease (COPD), cardiogenic shock, overt cardiac failure, second- or third-degree AV block, severe sinus bradycardia, hypersensitivity to levobunolol or any component of the formulation

CONTRAINDICATIONS: Cardiogenic shock, overt cardiac failure, second- or third-degree heart block, sinus bradycardia, hypersensitivity to levobunolol or any component of the formulation

INTERACTIONS

Drug

Amiodarone: May increase risk of hypotension, bradycardia, and cardiac arrest.

Diuretics, fentanyl, other hypotensives: May increase hypotensive effect.

NSAIDs: May decrease antihypertensive effect.

Sympathomimetics, xanthines: May mutually inhibit hypotensive effects and may mask symptoms of hypoglycemia.

Herbal

Dong quai: May increase hypotensive effect.

Licorice, Ma huang, St. John's wort, yohimbine: May decrease effectiveness of levobunolol.

Food

None known.

DIAGNOSTIC TEST EFFECTS: *None known.*

SIDE EFFECTS

Frequent

Burning/stinging, eye irritation, visual disturbances

Occasional

Increased light sensitivity, watering of eye

Rare

Dry eye, conjunctivitis, eye pain, diarrhea, dyspepsia

SERIOUS REACTIONS

- Abrupt withdrawal may result in sweating, headache, and fatigue.
- Ophthalmic overdosage may produce bradycardia, hypotension, bronchospasm, and acute cardiac failure.

SPECIAL CONSIDERATIONS

PRECAUTIONS

- Exercise caution in patients with diminished pulmonary function. Additive effects occur with orally administered beta-adrenergic blocking agents. Use levobunolol hydrochloride cautiously in patients with cerebrovascular insufficiency. If levobunolol hydrochloride is used to reduce elevated intraocular pressure in angle-closure glaucoma, follow it with a miotic and not alone.
- Muscle Weakness: Levobunolol hydrochloride may potentiate muscle weakness consistent with certain myasthenic symptoms (e.g., diplopia, ptosis, and generalized weakness).

PATIENT INFORMATION

- Instruct patients not to wear soft contact lenses while they are using this medicine. This medicine contains a preservative that can be absorbed by soft contact lenses and cause eye irritation.

PREGNANCY AND LACTATION

- Pregnancy Category C. Fetotoxicity has been observed in rabbits with oral doses. Teratogenic studies in rats showed no evidence of fetal malformations. Fetal harm is not known with topical administration. Systemically effective beta-blockers and topical timolol maleate are known to be excreted in human milk. Excretion into human milk is not known.

levocabastine

(levo-cab'a-steen)

Rx: Livostin

Drug Class: Antihistamines, H1; Antihistamines, ophthalmic; Ophthalmics

Pregnancy Category: C

CLINICAL PHARMACOLOGY

Mechanism of Action: An antiallergic agent that selectively antagonizes H_1 receptor. *Therapeutic Effect:* Blocks histamine-associated symptoms of seasonal allergic conjunctivitis.

Pharmacokinetics

Duration of action is about 2 hours. Minimal systemic absorbtion.

AVAILABLE FORMS

- *Ophthalmic Suspension:* 0.05% (Livostin).

INDICATIONS AND DOSAGES

Allergic conjunctivitis

Ophthalmic

Adults, Elderly, Children 12 yr or older. 1 drop 4 times/day, for up to 2 wks.

CONTRAINDICATIONS: Wearing of soft contact lenses (product contains benzalkonium chloride), hypersensitivity to levocabastine or any component of the formulation

INTERACTIONS

Drug

None known.

Herbal

None known.

Food

None known.

DIAGNOSTIC TEST EFFECTS: *None known.*

SIDE EFFECTS

Frequent

Transient stinging, burning, discomfort, headache

Occasional

Dry mouth, fatigue, eye dryness, lacrimation/discharge, eyelid edema

Rare

Rash, erythema, nausea, dyspnea

SERIOUS REACTIONS

- None reported.

SPECIAL CONSIDERATIONS

PATIENT INFORMATION

- Instruct patients to shake the container well before using.

PREGNANCY AND LACTATION

- Pregnancy Category C. Teratogenicity (polydactyly, hydrocephaly, brachygnathia), embryotoxicity, and maternal toxicity were observed in rats. About 0.5 mg excreted into breast milk daily after ocular administration in one nursing woman.

levofloxacin

(levo-flox'a-sin)

Rx: IQUIX, Levaquin, Levaquin Leva-Pak, Quixin

Drug Class: Anti-infectives, ophthalmic; Antibiotics, quinolones; Ophthalmics

Pregnancy Category: C

CLINICAL PHARMACOLOGY

Mechanism of Action: A fluoroquinolone that inhibits the enzyme DNA enzyme gyrase in susceptible microorganisms, interfering with bacterial cell replication and repair. *Therapeutic Effect:* Bactericidal.

Pharmacokinetics

Well absorbed after both PO and IV administration. Protein binding: 24%-8%. Penetrates rapidly and extensively into leukocytes, epithelial cells, and macrophages. Lung concentrations are 2-5 times higher than those of plasma. Eliminated unchanged in the urine. Partially removed by hemodialysis. **Half-life:** 8 hr.

AVAILABLE FORMS

- *Oral Solution:* 25 mg/ml.
- *Tablets (Levaquin):* 250 mg, 500 mg, 750 mg.
- *Injection (Levaquin):* 500-mg/20-ml vials.
- *Premixed Solution (Levaquin):* 250 mg/50 ml, 500 mg/100 ml, 750 mg/150 ml.
- *Ophthalmic Solution (Quixin):* 1.5%
- *Ophthalmic Solution (Iquix):* 0.5%.

INDICATIONS AND DOSAGES

Bronchitis

PO, IV

Adults, Elderly. 500 mg q24h for 7 days.

Community-acquired pneumonia

PO

Adults, Elderly. 750 mg/day for 5 days.

Pneumonia

PO, IV

Adults, Elderly. 500 mg q24h for 7-14 days.

Acute maxillary sinusitis

PO, IV

Adults, Elderly. 500 mg q24h for 10-14 days.

Skin and skin-structure infections

PO, IV

Adults, Elderly. 500 mg q24h for 7-10 days.

UTIs, acute pyelonephritis

PO, IV

Adults, Elderly. 250 mg q24h for 10 days.

Bacterial conjunctivitis

Ophthalmic

Adults, Elderly, Children 1 yr and older. 1-2 drops q2h for 2 days (up to 8 times a day), then 1-2 drops q4h for 5 days.

Corneal ulcer

Ophthalmic

Adults, Elderly, Children older than 5 yr. Days 1-3: Instill 1-2 drops q30min to 2 hours while awake and 4-6 hours after retiring. Days 4 through completion: 1-2 drops q1-4h while awake.

Dosage in renal impairment

For bronchitis, pneumonia, sinusitis, and skin and skin-structure infections, dosage and frequency are modified based on creatinine clearance.

Creatinine Clearance	*Dosage*
50-80 ml/min	No change
20-49 ml/min	500 mg initially, then 250 mg q24h
10-19 ml/min	500 mg initially, then 250 mg q48h

Dialysis 500 mg initially, then 250 mg q48h

For UTIs and pyelonephritis, dosage and frequency are modified based on creatinine clearance.

Creatinine Clearance	*Dosage*
20 ml/min	No change
10-19 ml/min	250 mg initially, then 250 mg q48h

CONTRAINDICATIONS: Hypersensitivity to levofloaxcin, other fluoroquinolones, or nalidixic acid

INTERACTIONS

Drug

Antacids, iron preparations, sucralfate, zinc: Decrease levofloxacin absorption.

NSAIDs: May increase the risk of CNS stimulation or seizures.

Herbal

None known.

Food

None known.

DIAGNOSTIC TEST EFFECTS: May alter blood glucose levels.

IV INCOMPATIBILITIES: Furosemide (Lasix), heparin, insulin, nitroglycerin, propofol (Diprivan)

IV COMPATIBILITIES: Aminophylline, dobutamine (Dobutrex), dopamine (Intron), fentanyl (Sublimaze), lidocaine, lorazepam (Ativan), morphine

SIDE EFFECTS

Occasional (3%-1%)

Diarrhea, nausea, abdominal pain, dizziness, drowsiness, headache, light-headedness

Ophthalmic: Local burning or discomfort, margin crusting, crystals or scales, foreign body sensation, ocular itching, altered taste

Rare (less than 1%)

Flatulence; altered taste; pain; inflammation or swelling in calves, hands, or shoulder; chest pain; difficulty breathing; palpitations; edema; tendon pain

Ophthalmic: Corneal staining, keratitis, allergic reaction, eyelid swelling, tearing, reduced visual acuity

SERIOUS REACTIONS

• Antibiotic-associated colitis and other superinfections may occur from altered bacterial balance. Hypersensitivity reactions, including photosensitivity (as evidenced by rash, pruritus, blisters, edema, and burning skin), have occurred in patients receiving fluoroquinolones.

SPECIAL CONSIDERATIONS

PRECAUTIONS

• Do not inject levofloxacin eye solution subconjunctivally, and do not introduce it directly into the anterior chamber of the eye. In patients receiving systemically effective quinolones, serious and occasionally fatal hypersensitivity (anaphylactic) reactions have been reported, some following the first dose. Some reactions were accompanied by cardiovascular collapse, loss of consciousness, angioedema (including laryngeal, pharyngeal, or facial edema), airway obstruction, dyspnea, urticaria, and itching. If an allergic reaction to levofloxacin occurs, discontinue the drug. Serious acute hypersensitivity reactions may require immediate emergency treatment. Administer oxygen and airway management as clinically indicated.

• As with other antiinfective drugs, prolonged use may result in overgrowth of nonsusceptible organisms, including fungi. If superinfection occurs, discontinue use and institute alternative therapy. Whenever clinical judgment dictates, examine the patient with the aid of magnification, such as slit-lamp biomicroscopy, and where appropriate, fluorescein staining. Advise patients not to wear contact lenses if they have signs and symptoms of bacterial conjunctivitis.

PATIENT INFORMATION

• Instruct patients to avoid contaminating the applicator tip with material from the eye, fingers, or other source. Systemically effective quinolones have been associated with hypersensitivity reactions, even following a single dose. Instruct patients to discontinue use immediately and to contact their physician at the first sign of a rash or allergic reaction.

PREGNANCY AND LACTATION

• Pregnancy Category C. Fetal harm is not known. Levofloxacin has not been measured in human milk. Based on data from ofloxacin, it can be presumed that levofloxacin is excreted in human milk. Exercise caution when administering levofloxacin to a nursing mother.

OCULAR CONSIDERATIONS

• Ocular Indications and Usage: Levofloxacin eye solution is indicated for the treatment of bacterial conjunctivitis caused by susceptible strains of the following organisms: aerobic gram-positive microorganisms—*Corynebacterium* species, *Staphylococcus aureus* (methicillin-susceptible strains only), *Staphylococcus epidermidis* (methicillin-susceptible strains only), *Streptococcus pneumoniae, Streptococcus* (groups C and F), *Streptococcus* (group G), and viridans group streptococci; aerobic gram-negative microorganisms—*Acinetobacter lwoffi, Haemophilus influenzae,* and *Serratia marcescens.*

OCULAR DOSAGE AND ADMINISTRATION

• Gram-positive or gram-negative bacterial conjunctivitis: Days 1 and 2, instill 1 to 2 drops in the affected eye(s) every 2 hours while awake, up to 8 times per day. Days 3 to 7, instill 1 to 2 drops in the affected eye(s) every 4 hours while awake, up to 4 times per day.

levothyroxine

(lee-voe-thye-rox'een)

Rx: Eltroxin, Levothroid, Synthroid

Drug Class: Hormones/hormone modifiers; Thyroid agents

Pregnancy Category: A

Do not confuse levothyroxine with liothyronine.

CLINICAL PHARMACOLOGY

Mechanism of Action: A synthetic isomer of thyroxine involved in normal metabolism, growth, and development, especially of the CNS in infants. Possesses catabolic and anabolic effects. *Therapeutic Effect:* Increases basal metabolic rate, enhances gluconeogenesis and stimulates protein synthesis.

Pharmacokinetics

Variable, incomplete absorption from the GI tract. Protein binding: greater than 99%. Widely distributed. Deiodinated in peripheral tissues, minimal metabolism in the liver. Eliminated by biliary excretion. **Half-life:** 6-7 days.

AVAILABLE FORMS

• *Tablets (Levo-T, Levothroid, Levoxyl, Synthroid, Unithroid):* 0.025 mg, 0.05 mg, 0.075 mg, 0.088 mg, 0.1 mg, 0.112 mg, 0.125 mg, 0.137 mg, 0.15 mg, 0.175 mg, 0.2 mg, 0.3 mg.

• *Injection (Synthroid):* 200 mcg, 500 mcg.

INDICATIONS AND DOSAGES

Hypothyroidism

PO

Adults, Elderly. Initially, 12.5-50 mcg. May increase by 25-50 mcg/day q2-4wk. Maintenance: 100-200 mcg/day.

Children 13 yr and older. 150 mcg/day.

Children 6-12 yr. 100-125 mcg/day.

Children 1-5 yr. 75-100 mcg/day.

Children 7-11 mo. 50-75 mcg/day.

Children older than 3-6 mo. 25-50 mcg/day.

Children 3 mo and younger. 10-15 mcg/day.

Thyroid suppression therapy

PO

Adults, Elderly. 2-6 mcg/kg/day for 7-10 days.

Thyroid stimulating hormone suppression in thyroid cancer, nodules, euthyroid goiters

PO

Adults, Elderly. 2-6 mcg/kg/day for 7-10 days.

IV

Adults, Elderly, Children. Initial dosage approximately half the previously established oral dosage.

CONTRAINDICATIONS: Hypersensitivity to tablet components, such as tartrazine; allergy to aspirin; lactose intolerance; MI and thyrotoxicosis uncomplicated by hypothyroidism; treatment of obesity

INTERACTIONS

Drug

Cholestyramine, colestipol: May decrease the absorption of levothyroxine.

Oral anticoagulants: May alter the effects of oral anticoagulants

Sympathomimetics: May increase the risk of coronary insufficiency and the effects of levothyroxine.

Herbal

None known.

Food

None known.

DIAGNOSTIC TEST EFFECTS: *None known.*

IV INCOMPATIBILITIES: Do not use or mix with other IV solutions.

SIDE EFFECTS

Occasional

Reversible hair loss at the start of therapy (in children)

Rare

Dry skin, GI intolerance, rash, hives, pseudotumor cerebri or severe headache in children

SERIOUS REACTIONS

- Excessive dosage produces signs and symptoms of hyperthyroidism, including weight loss, palpitations, increased appetite, tremors, nervousness, tachycardia, hypertension, headache, insomnia, and menstrual irregularities.
- Cardiac arrhythmias occur rarely.

SPECIAL CONSIDERATIONS

PRECAUTIONS

- Use levothyroxine sodium with caution in patients with cardiovascular disorders, including angina, coronary artery disease, and hypertension, and in the elderly who have a greater likelihood of occult cardiac disease. Concomitant administration with sympathomimetic agents to patients with coronary artery disease may increase the risk of coronary insufficiency. Use in patients with concomitant diabetes mellitus, diabetes insipidus, or adrenal cortical insufficiency may aggravate the intensity of their symptoms. Treatment of myxedema coma may require simultaneous administration of glucocorticoids.
- Closely monitor prothrombin time in patients taking levothyroxine and oral anticoagulants. Lithium blocks the thyroid-stimulating hormone–mediated release of thyroxin and triiodothyronine.

PATIENT INFORMATION

Give patients the following instructions:

- Levothyroxine sodium is intended to replace a hormone that normally is produced by your thyroid gland. It generally is taken for life, except in cases of temporary hypothyroidism associated with an inflammation of the thyroid gland.
- Before or at any time while using levothyroxine sodium, you should tell your doctor if you are allergic to any foods or medicines, are pregnant or intend to become pregnant, are breast-feeding, are taking or start taking any other prescription or nonprescription (over-the-counter) medications, or have any other medical problems (especially hardening of the arteries, heart dis-

ease, high blood pressure, or history of thyroid, adrenal, or pituitary gland problems).

• Use levothyroxine sodium only as prescribed by your doctor. Do not discontinue levothyroxine sodium or change the amount you take or how often you take it, except as directed by your doctor.

• Levothyroxine sodium, like all medicines obtained from your doctor, must be used only by you and for the condition determined appropriate by your doctor.

• It may take a few weeks for levothyroxine sodium to begin working. Until it begins working, you may not notice any change in your symptoms.

• You should notify your doctor if you experience any of the following symptoms or if you experience any other unusual medical event: chest pain, shortness of breath, hives or skin rash, rapid or irregular heartbeat, headache, irritability, nervousness, sleeplessness, diarrhea, excessive sweating, heat intolerance, changes in appetite, vomiting, weight gain or loss, changes in menstrual periods, fever, hand tremors, or leg cramps.

• You should inform your doctor or dentist that you are taking levothyroxine sodium before having any kind of surgery.

• You should notify your doctor if you become pregnant while taking levothyroxine sodium. Your dose of this medicine likely will have to be increased while you are pregnant.

• If you have diabetes, your dose of insulin or oral antidiabetic agent may need to be changed after starting levothyroxine sodium. You should monitor your blood or urinary glucose levels as directed by your doctor and report any changes to your doctor immediately.

• If you are taking an oral anticoagulant drug such as warfarin, your dose may need to be changed after starting levothyroxine sodium. You should have your coagulation status checked often to determine whether a change in dose is required.

• Partial hair loss may occur rarely during the first few months of levothyroxine sodium therapy, but it is usually temporary.

• Synthroid is the trade name for tablets containing the thyroid hormone levothyroxine, manufactured by Knoll Pharmaceutical Company. Other manufacturers also make tablets containing levothyroxine. You should not change to another manufacturer's product without discussing that change with your doctor first. Repeat blood tests and a change in the amount of levothyroxine sodium you take may be required.

• Keep levothyroxine sodium out of the reach of children. Store away from heat and moisture.

PREGNANCY AND LACTATION

• Pregnancy Category A. Studies in pregnant women have not shown that levothyroxine sodium increases the risk of fetal abnormalities if administered during pregnancy. Minimal amounts of thyroid hormones are excreted in human milk.

lidocaine

(lye'doe-kane)

Rx: Anestacon, Ela-Max, Ela-Max Plus, Laryng-O-Jet Spray, Lida Mantle, Lidoderm, LidoSite, LMX 4, LMX 4 with Tegaderm, LMX 5, Xylocaine 10% Oral, Xylocaine Jelly, Xylocaine Topical, Xylocaine Viscous

Drug Class: Anesthetics, topical; Dermatologics

Pregnancy Category: B

CLINICAL PHARMACOLOGY

Mechanism of Action: An amide anesthetic that inhibits conduction of nerve impulses. *Therapeutic Effect:* Causes temporary loss of feeling and sensation. Also an antiarrhythmic that decreases depolarization, automaticity, excitability of the ventricle during diastole by direct action. *Therapeutic Effect:* Inhibits ventricular arrhythmias.

Pharmacokinetics

Route	Onset	Peak	Duration
IV	30-90 sec	N/A	10-20 min
Local anesthetic	2.5 min	N/A	30-60 min

Completely absorbed after IM administration. Protein binding: 60% to 80%. Widely distributed. Metabolized in the liver. Primarily excreted in urine. Minimally removed by hemodialysis. **Half-life:** 1-2 hr.

AVAILABLE FORMS

- *IM Injection:* 300 mg/3 ml.
- *Direct IV Injection:* 10 mg/ml, 20 mg/ml.
- *IV Admixture Injection:* 40 mg/ml, 100 mg/ml, 200 mg/ml.
- *IV Infusion:* 2 mg/ml, 4 mg/ml, 8 mg/ml.
- *Injection (anesthesia):* 0.5%, 1%, 1.5%, 2%, 4%.
- *Liquid:* 2.5%, 5%.
- *Ointment:* 2.5%, 5%.
- *Cream:* 0.5%.
- *Gel:* 0.5%, 2.5%.
- *Topical Spray:* 0.5%.
- *Topical Solution:* 2%, 4%.
- *Topical Jelly:* 2%.
- *Dermal Patch:* 5%.

INDICATIONS AND DOSAGES

Rapid control of acute ventricular arrhythmias after an MI, cardiac catheterization, cardiac surgery, or digitalis-induced ventricular arrhythmias

IM

Adults, Elderly. 300 mg (or 4.3 mg/kg). May repeat in 60-90 min.

IV

Adults, Elderly. Initially, 50-100 mg (1 mg/kg) IV bolus at rate of 25-50 mg/min. May repeat in 5 min. Give no more than 200-300 mg in 1 hr. Maintenance: 20-50 mcg/kg/min (1-4 mg/min) as IV infusion.

Children, Infants. Initially, 0.5-1 mg/kg IV bolus; may repeat but total dose not to exceed 3-5 mg/kg. Maintenance: 10-50 mcg/kg/min as IV infusion.

Dental or surgical procedures, childbirth

Infiltration or nerve block

Adults. Local anesthetic dosage varies with procedure, degree of anesthesia, vascularity, duration. Maximum dose: 4.5 mg/kg. Do not repeat within 2 hrs.

Local skin disorders (minor burns, insect bites, prickly heat, skin manifestations of chickenpox, abrasions), and mucous membrane disorders (local anesthesia of oral, nasal, and laryngeal mucous membranes; local anesthesia of respiratory, urinary tract; relief of discomfort of pruritus ani, hemorrhoids, pruritus vulvae)

Topical

Adults, Elderly. Apply to affected areas as needed.

Treatment of shingles-related skin pain

Topical (Dermal patch)

Adults, Elderly. Apply to intact skin over most painful area (up to 3 applications once for up to 12 hrs in a 24-hr period).

CONTRAINDICATIONS: Adams-Stokes syndrome, hypersensitivity to amide-type local anesthetics, septicemia (spinal anesthesia), supraventricular arrhythmias, Wolff-Parkinson-White syndrome

INTERACTIONS

Drug

Anticonvulsants: May increase cardiac depressant effects.

Beta-adrenergic blockers: May increase risk of toxicity.

Other antiarrhythmics: May increase cardiac effects.

Herbal

None known.

Food

None known.

DIAGNOSTIC TEST EFFECTS: IM lidocaine may increase creatine kinase level (used to diagnose acute MI). Therapeutic blood level is 1.5 to 6 mcg/ml; toxic blood level is greater than 6 mcg/ml.

IV INCOMPATIBILITIES: Amphotericin B complex (Abelcet, AmBisome, Amphotec), thiopental

IV COMPATIBILITIES: Aminophylline, amiodarone (Cordarone), calcium gluconate, digoxin (Lanoxin), diltiazem (Cardizem), dobutamine (Dobutrex), dopamine (Intropin), enalapril (Vasotec), furosemide (Lasix), heparin, insulin, nitroglycerin, potassium chloride

SIDE EFFECTS

CNS effects are generally dose-related and of short duration.

Occasional

IM: Pain at injection site

Topical: Burning, stinging, tenderness at application site

Rare

Generally with high dose: Drowsiness; dizziness; disorientation; light-headedness; tremors; apprehension; euphoria; sensation of heat, cold, or numbness; blurred or double vision; ringing or roaring in ears (tinnitus); nausea

SERIOUS REACTIONS

- Although serious adverse reactions to lidocaine are uncommon, high dosage by any route may produce cardiovascular depression, bradycardia, hypotension, arrhythmias, heart block, cardiovascular collapse, and cardiac arrest.
- Potential for malignant hyperthermia.
- CNS toxicity may occur, especially with regional anesthesia use, progressing rapidly from mild side effects to tremors, somnolence, seizures, vomiting, and respiratory depression.
- Methemoglobinemia (evidenced by cyanosis) has occurred following topical application of lidocaine for teething discomfort and laryngeal anesthetic spray.

SPECIAL CONSIDERATIONS

OCULAR CONSIDERATIONS

- Topical anesthesia with preservative-free 2% lidocaine drops has been used successfully in clear corneal phacoemulsification with intraocular lens implantation. (Chuang LH et al: Efficacy and safety of phacoemulsification with intraocular lens implantation under topical anesthesia, *Chang Gung Med J* 27[8]:609-613, 2004.)

lisinopril

(ly-sin'oh-pril)

Rx: Prinivil, Zestril

Drug Class: Angiotensin converting enzyme inhibitors

Pregnancy Category: C, 1st; D, 2nd / 3rd

Do not confuse lisinopril with fosinopril; Prinivil with Desyrel, Plendil, Proventil, or Restoril; Fibsol with Lioresal; or Zestril with Zostrix. Do not confuse lisinopril's combination form Zestoretic with Prilosec.

CLINICAL PHARMACOLOGY

Mechanism of Action: This angiotensin-converting enzyme (ACE) inhibitor suppresses the renin-angiotensin-aldosterone system and prevents conversion of angiotensin I to angiotensin II, a potent vasoconstrictor; may also inhibit angiotensin II at local vascular and renal sites. Decreases plasma angiotensin II, increases plasma renin activity, and decreases aldosterone secretion. *Therapeutic Effect:* Reduces peripheral arterial resistance, BP, afterload, pulmonary capillary wedge pressure (preload), and pulmonary vascular resistance. In those with heart failure, also decreases heart size, increases cardiac output, and exercise tolerance time.

Pharmacokinetics

Route	*Onset*	*Peak*	*Duration*
PO	1 hr	6 hr	24 hr

Incompletely absorbed from the GI tract. Protein binding: 25%. Primarily excreted unchanged in urine. Removed by hemodialysis. **Half-life:** 12 hr (half-life is prolonged in those with impaired renal function).

AVAILABLE FORMS

- *Tablets (Prinivil, Zestril):* 2.5 mg, 5 mg, 10 mg, 20 mg, 30 mg, 40 mg.

INDICATIONS AND DOSAGES

Hypertension (used alone)

PO

Adults. Initially, 10 mg/day. May increase by 5-10 mcg/day at 1-2 wk intervals. Maximum: 40 mg/day.

Elderly. Initially, 2.5-5 mg/day. May increase by 2.5-5 mg/day at 1- to 2-wk intervals. Maximum: 40 mg/day.

Hypertension (used in combination with other antihypertensives)

PO

Adults. Initially, 2.5-5 mg/day titrated to patient's needs.

Adjunctive therapy for management of heart failure

PO

Adults, Elderly. Initially, 2.5-5 mg/day. May increase by no more than 10 mg/day at intervals of at least 2 wk. Maintenance: 5-40 mg/day.

Improve survival in patients after a myocardial infarction (MI)

PO

Adults, Elderly. Initially, 5 mg, then 5 mg after 24 hr, 10 mg after 48 hr, then 10 mg/day for 6 wk. For patients with low systolic BP, give 2.5 mg/day for 3 days, then 2.5-5 mg/day.

Dosage in renal impairment

Titrate to patient's needs after giving the following initial dose:

Creatinine Clearance	*% Normal Dose*
10-50 ml/min	50-75
less than 10 ml/min	25-50

UNLABELED USES: Treatment of hypertension or renal crises with scleroderma

CONTRAINDICATIONS: History of angioedema from previous treatment with ACE inhibitors

INTERACTIONS

Drug

Alcohol, diuretics, hypotensive agents: May increase the effects of lisinopril.
Lithium: May increase lithium blood concentration and risk of toxicity.
NSAIDs: May decrease the effects of lisinopril.
Potassium-sparing diuretics, potassium supplements: May cause hyperkalemia.

Herbal

None known.

Food

None known.

DIAGNOSTIC TEST EFFECTS: May increase BUN, serum alkaline phosphatase, serum bilirubin, serum creatinine, serum potassium, AST (SGOT), and ALT (SGPT) levels. May decrease serum sodium levels. May cause positive ANA titer.

SIDE EFFECTS

Frequent (12%-5%)
Headache, dizziness, postural hypotension
Occasional (4%-2%)
Chest discomfort, fatigue, rash, abdominal pain, nausea, diarrhea, upper respiratory infection
Rare (1% or less)
Palpitations, tachycardia, peripheral edema, insomnia, paresthesia, confusion, constipation, dry mouth, muscle cramps

SERIOUS REACTIONS

• Excessive hypotension ("first-dose syncope") may occur in patients with CHF and severe salt and volume depletion.

• Angioedema (swelling of face and lips) and hyperkalemia occurs rarely.

• Agranulocytosis and neutropenia may be noted in patients with collagen vascular disease, including scleroderma and systemic lupus erythematosus, and impaired renal function.

• Nephrotic syndrome may be noted in patients with history of renal disease.

SPECIAL CONSIDERATIONS

PRECAUTIONS

• Anticipate changes in renal function in susceptible individuals. Elevated serum potassium was observed in hypertensive patients in clinical trials. Cough has been reported with all angiotensin-converting enzyme (ACE) inhibitors. In patients undergoing major surgery or during anesthesia with agents that produce hypotension, enalapril may block angiotensin II formation following compensatory renin release.

PATIENT INFORMATION

• Angioedema: Angioedema, including laryngeal edema, may occur at any time during treatment with ACE inhibitors, including lisinopril. Advise patients to report immediately any signs or symptoms suggesting angioedema (swelling of face, extremities, eyes, lips, or tongue and difficulty in swallowing or breathing) and to take no more drug until they have consulted with the prescribing physician.

• Symptomatic Hypotension: Caution patients to report light-headedness especially during the first few days of therapy. If actual syncope occurs, instruct patients to discontinue the drug until they have consulted with the prescribing physician.

• Caution all patients that excessive perspiration and dehydration may lead to an excessive fall in blood pressure because of reduction in fluid volume. Other causes of volume depletion such as vomiting or diarrhea also may lead to a fall in blood pressure; advise patients to consult with their physician.

• Hyperkalemia: Instruct patients not to use salt substitutes containing potassium without consulting their physician.

• Leukopenia/Neutropenia: Instruct patients to report promptly any indication of infection (e.g., sore throat or fever), which may be a sign of leukopenia/neutropenia.

• Pregnancy: Advise female patients of childbearing age about the consequences of second- and third-trimester exposure to ACE inhibitors, and advise them that these consequences do not appear to have resulted from intrauterine ACE inhibitor exposure that has been limited to the first trimester. Ask these patients to report pregnancies to their physicians as soon as possible.

• NOTE: As with many other drugs, certain advice to patients being treated with lisinopril is warranted. This information is intended to aid in the safe and effective use of this medication. Such advice is not a disclosure of all possible adverse or intended effects.

PREGNANCY AND LACTATION

• Pregnancy Categories C (first trimester) and D (second and third trimesters). The use of angiotensin-converting enzyme inhibitors during the second and third trimesters of pregnancy has been associated with fetal and neonatal injury, including hypotension, neonatal skull hypoplasia, anuria, reversible or irreversible renal failure, and death. Excretion into human milk is not known.

lithium carbonate/lithium citrate

(lith'-ee-um)

Rx: Eskalith, Eskalith-CR, Lithobid

Drug Class: Antipsychotics

Pregnancy Category: D

Do not confuse Lithobid with Levbid, Lithostat, or Lithotabs.

CLINICAL PHARMACOLOGY

Mechanism of Action: A psychotherapeutic agent that affects the storage, release, and reuptake of neurotransmitters. Antimanic effect may result from increased norepinephrine reuptake and serotonin receptor sensitivity. *Therapeutic Effect:* Produces antimanic and antidepressant effects.

Pharmacokinetics

Rapidly and completely absorbed from the GI tract. Primarily excreted unchanged in urine. Removed by hemodialysis. **Half-life:** 18-24 hr (increased in elderly).

AVAILABLE FORMS

• *Capsules:* 150 mg, 300 mg, 600 mg.

• *Syrup:* 300 mg/ml.

• *Tablets:* 300 mg.

• *Tablets (Controlled-Release):* 450 mg.

• *Tablets (Slow-Release):* 300 mg.

INDICATIONS AND DOSAGES:

Alert During acute phase, a therapeutic serum lithium concentration of 1-1.4 mEq/L is required. For long-term control, the desired level is 0.5-1.3 mEq/L. Monitor serum drug concentration and clinical response to determine proper dosage.

Prevention or treatment of acute mania, manic phase of bipolar disorder (manic-depressive illness)

PO

Adults. 300 mg 3-4 times a day or 450-900 mg slow-release form twice a day. Maximum: 2.4 g/day.

Elderly. 300 mg twice a day. May increase by 300 mg/day q1wk. Maintenance: 900-1200 mg/day.

Children 12 yr and older. 600-1800 mg/day in 3-4 divided doses (2 doses/day for slow-release).

Children younger than 12 yr. 15-60 mg/kg/day in 3-4 divided doses.

UNLABELED USES: Prevention of vascular headache; treatment of depression, neutropenia

CONTRAINDICATIONS: Debilitated patients, severe cardiovascular disease, severe dehydration, severe renal disease, severe sodium depletion

INTERACTIONS

Drug

Antithyroid medications, iodinated glycerol, potassium iodide: May increase the effects of these drugs.

Diuretics, NSAIDs: May increase lithium serum concentration and risk of toxicity.

Haloperidol: May increase extrapyramidal symptoms and the risk of neurologic toxicity.

Molindone: May increase the risk of neurotoxicity.

Phenothiazines: May decrease the absorption of phenothiazines, increase the intracellular concentration and renal excretion of lithium, and increase delirium and extrapyramidal symptoms. Antiemetic effect of some phenothiazines may mask early signs of lithium toxicity.

Herbal

None known.

Food

None known.

DIAGNOSTIC TEST EFFECTS: May increase blood glucose, immunoreactive parathyroid hormone, and serum calcium levels. Therapeutic serum level is 0.6-1.2 mEq/L; toxic serum level is greater than 1.5 mEq/L.

SIDE EFFECTS

AlertSide effects are dose related and seldom occur at lithium serum levels less than 1.5 mEq/L.

Occasional

Fine hand tremor, polydipsia, polyuria, mild nausea

Rare

Weight gain, bradycardia or tachycardia, acne, rash, muscle twitching, cold and cyanotic extremities, pseudotumor cerebri (eye pain, headache, tinnitus, vision disturbances)

SERIOUS REACTIONS

- A lithium serum concentration of 1.5-2.0 mEq/L may produce vomiting, diarrhea, drowsiness, confusion, incoordination, coarse hand tremor, muscle twitching, and T-wave depression on EKG.
- A lithium serum concentration of 2.0-2.5 mEq/L may result in ataxia, giddiness, tinnitus, blurred vision, clonic movements, and severe hypotension.
- Acute toxicity may be characterized by seizures, oliguria, circulatory failure, coma, and death.

SPECIAL CONSIDERATIONS

PRECAUTIONS

- Cases of pseudotumor cerebri (increased intracranial pressure and papilledema) have been reported with lithium use. If undetected, this condition may result in enlargement of the blind spot, constriction of visual fields, and eventual blindness caused by optic atrophy.

• Exophthalmos has been reported as a side effect.

• Acetazolamide can lower serum lithium concentrations by increasing urinary lithium excretion.

Iodoxamide

(Ioe-dox'a-mide)

Rx: Alomide

Drug Class: Mast cell stabilizers; Ophthalmics

Pregnancy Category: B

CLINICAL PHARMACOLOGY

Mechanism of Action: A mast cell stabilizer that prevents increase in cutaneous vascular permeability, antigen-stimulated histamine release and may prevent calcium influx into mast cells. *Therapeutic Effect:* Inhibits sensitivity reaction.

Pharmacokinetics

Nondetectable absorption. **Half-life:** 8.5 hrs.

AVAILABLE FORMS

• *Ophthalmic Solution:* 0.1% (Alomide).

INDICATIONS AND DOSAGES

Treatment of vernal keratoconjunctivitis, conjunctivitis, and keratitis

Ophthalmic

Adults, Elderly, Children 2 yr or older. 1-2 drops 4 times/day, for up to 3 mos.

CONTRAINDICATIONS: Wearing soft contact lenses (product contains benzalkonium chloride), hypersensitivity to Iodoxamide tromethamine or any component of the formulation

INTERACTIONS

Drug

None known.

Herbal

None known.

Food

None known.

DIAGNOSTIC TEST EFFECTS: *None known.*

SIDE EFFECTS

Frequent

Transient stinging, burning, instillation discomfort

Occasional

Ocular itching, blurred vision, dry eye, tearing/discharge/foreign body sensation, headache

Rare

Scales on lid/lash, ocular swelling, sticky sensation, dizziness, somnolence, nausea, sneezing, dry nose, rash

SERIOUS REACTIONS

• None reported.

SPECIAL CONSIDERATIONS

PRECAUTIONS

• Transient burning or stinging may occur.

PREGNANCY AND LACTATION

• Pregnancy Category B. Animal studies produced no evidence of developmental toxicity with oral doses. However, no adequate and well-controlled studies have been performed in pregnant women. Excretion into human milk is not known.

OCULAR CONSIDERATIONS

• Off-label uses include seasonal allergic conjunctivitis.

loratadine

(loer-at'ah-deen)

Drug Class: Antihistamines, H1

Pregnancy Category: B

CLINICAL PHARMACOLOGY

Mechanism of Action: A long-acting antihistamine that competes with histamine for H_1 receptor sites on effector cells. *Therapeutic Effect:*

Prevents allergic responses mediated by histamine, such as rhinitis, urticaria, and pruritus.

Pharmacokinetics

Route	*Onset*	*Peak*	*Duration*
PO	1-3 hr	8-12 hr	longer than 24 hr

Rapidly and almost completely absorbed from the GI tract. Protein binding: 97%; metabolite, 73%-77%. Distributed mainly to the liver, lungs, GI tract, and bile. Metabolized in the liver to active metabolite; undergoes extensive first-pass metabolism. Eliminated in urine and feces. Not removed by hemodialysis. **Half-life:** 8.4 hr; metabolite, 28 hr (increased in elderly and hepatic impairment).

AVAILABLE FORMS

- *Syrup (Claritin):* 10 mg/10 ml.
- *Tablets (Alavert, Claritin, Tavist ND):* 10 mg.
- *Tablets (Rapid-Disintegrating [Alavert, Claritin RediTab]):* 10 mg.

INDICATIONS AND DOSAGES

Allergic rhinitis, urticaria

PO

Adults, Elderly, Children 6 yr and older. 10 mg once a day.

Children 2-5 yr. 5 mg once a day.

Dosage in hepatic impairment

For adults, elderly, and children 6 years and older dosage is reduced to 10 mg every other day.

UNLABELED USES: Adjunct treatment of bronchial asthma

CONTRAINDICATIONS: Hypersensitivity to loratadine or its ingredients

INTERACTIONS

Drug

Clarithromycin, erythromycin, fluconazole, ketoconazole: May increase the loratadine blood concentration.

Herbal

None known.

Food

All foods: Delay the absorption of loratadine.

DIAGNOSTIC TEST EFFECTS: May suppress wheal and flare reactions to antigen skin testing unless the drug is discontinued 4 days before testing.

SIDE EFFECTS

Frequent (12%-8%)

Headache, fatigue, somnolence

Occasional (3%)

Dry mouth, nose, or throat

Rare

Photosensitivity

SERIOUS REACTIONS

- None known.

L

SPECIAL CONSIDERATIONS

PRECAUTIONS

- Give patients with liver impairment or renal insufficiency (glomerular filtration rate less than 30 ml/min) a lower initial dose (10 mg every other day).

PREGNANCY AND LACTATION

- Pregnancy Category B. No evidence of animal teratogenicity was found in studies performed in rats and rabbits at oral doses. Loratadine and its metabolite, descarboethoxyloratadine, pass easily into breast milk and achieve concentrations.

OCULAR CONSIDERATIONS

Loratadine has been shown to increase corneal and conjunctival staining and decrease tear flow and volume.

lorazepam

(lor-a′ze-pam)

Rx: Ativan

Drug Class: Anxiolytics; Benzodiazepines

Pregnancy Category: D

DEA Class: Schedule IV

Do not confuse lorazepam with Alprazolam.

CLINICAL PHARMACOLOGY

Mechanism of Action: A benzodiazepine that enhances the action of the inhibitory neurotransmitter gamma-aminobutyric acid in the CNS, affecting memory, as well as motor, sensory, and cognitive function. *Therapeutic Effect:* Produces anxiolytic, anticonvulsant, sedative, muscle relaxant, and antiemetic effects.

Pharmacokinetics

Route	*Onset*	*Peak*	*Duration*
PO	60 min	N/A	8-12 hr
IV	15-30 min	N/A	8-12 hr
IM	30-60 min	N/A	8-12 hr

Well absorbed after PO and IM administration. Protein binding: 85%. Widely distributed. Metabolized in the liver. Primarily excreted in urine. Not removed by hemodialysis. **Half-life:** 10-20 hr.

AVAILABLE FORMS

- *Tablets (Ativan):* 0.5 mg, 1 mg, 2 mg.
- *Injection (Ativan):* 2 mg/ml, 4 mg/ml.
- *Oral solution (Lorazepam Intensol):* 2 mg/ml.

INDICATIONS AND DOSAGES

Anxiety

PO

Adults. 1-10 mg/day in 2-3 divided doses. Average: 2-6 mg/day.

Elderly. Initially, 0.5-1 mg/day. May increase gradually. Range: 0.5-4 mg.

IV

Adults, Elderly. 0.02-0.06 mg/kg q2-6h.

IV Infusion

*Adults, Elderly.*0.01-0.1 mg/kg/h.

PO, IV

Children. 0.05 mg/kg/dose q4-8h. Range: 0.02-0.1 mg/kg. Maximum: 2 mg/dose.

Insomnia due to anxiety

PO

Adults. 2-4 mg at bedtime.

Elderly. 0.5-1 mg at bedtime.

Preoperative sedation

IV

Adults, Elderly. 0.044 mg/kg 15-20 min before surgery. Maximum total dose: 2 mg.

IM

Adults, Elderly. 0.05 mg/kg 2 hr before procedure. Maximum total dose: 4 mg.

Status epilepticus

IV

Adults, Elderly. 4 mg over 2-5 min. May repeat in 10-15 min. Maximum: 8 mg in 12-hr period.

Children. 0.1 mg/kg over 2-5 min. May give second dose of 0.05 mg/kg in 15-20 min. Maximum: 4 mg.

Neonates. 0.05 mg/kg. May repeat in 10-15 min.

UNLABELED USES: Treatment of alcohol withdrawal, panic disorders, skeletal muscle spasms, chemotherapy-induced nausea or vomiting, tension headache, tremors; adjunctive treatment before endoscopic procedures (diminishes patient recall)

CONTRAINDICATIONS: Angle-closure glaucoma; preexisting CNS depression; severe hypotension; severe uncontrolled pain

INTERACTIONS
Drug
Alcohol, other CNS depressants: May increase CNS depression.
Herbal
Kava kava, valerian: May increase CNS depression.
Food
None known.

DIAGNOSTIC TEST EFFECTS: *None known.* Therapeutic serum drug level is 50-240 ng/ml; toxic serum drug level is unknown.

IV INCOMPATIBILITIES: Aldesleukin (Proleukin), aztreonam (Azactam), idarubicin (Idamycin), ondansetron (Zofran), sufentanil (Sufenta)

IV COMPATIBILITIES: Bumetanide (Bumex), cefepime (Maxipime), diltiazem (Cardizem), dobutamine (Dobutrex), dopamine (Intropin), heparin, labetalol (Normodyne, Trandate), milrinone (Primacor), norepinephrine (Levophed), piperacillin and tazobactam (Zosyn), potassium, propofol (Diprivan)

SIDE EFFECTS
Frequent
Somnolence (initially in the morning), ataxia, confusion
Occasional
Blurred vision, slurred speech, hypotension, headache
Rare
Paradoxical CNS restlessness or excitement in elderly or debilitated

SERIOUS REACTIONS

- Abrupt or too-rapid withdrawal may result in pronounced restlessness, irritability, insomnia, hand tremor, abdominal or muscle cramps, diaphoresis, vomiting, and seizures.
- Overdose results in somnolence, confusion, diminished reflexes, and coma.

SPECIAL CONSIDERATIONS

PRECAUTIONS

- Lorazepam is not recommended for use in patients with a primary depressive disorder or psychosis. In patients with depression accompanying anxiety, bear in mind a possibility for suicide. Abrupt withdrawal of any antianxiety agent may result in symptoms similar to those for which patients are being treated: anxiety, agitation, irritability, tension, insomnia, and occasional convulsions. Observe the usual precautions for treating patients with impaired renal or hepatic function.

PATIENT INFORMATION

- To ensure the safe and effective use of lorazepam, inform patients that because benzodiazepines may produce psychological and physical dependence, it is advisable that they consult with their physician before increasing the dose or abruptly discontinuing this drug. As appropriate, inform the patient of the pharmacologic effects of the drug, such as sedation, relief of anxiety, and lack of recall, and the duration of these effects (about 8 hours) so that they adequately may perceive the risks as and the benefits to be derived from its use. Caution patients who receive lorazepam injection as a premedicant to delay driving an automobile or operating hazardous machinery or engaging in a hazardous sport for 24 to 48 hours following the injection. Sedatives, tranquilizers, and narcotic analgesics may produce a more prolonged and profound effect when administered along with injectable lorazepam. This effect may take the form of excessive sleepiness or drowsiness and on rare occasions may interfere with recall and recognition of events of the day of surgery and the day after. Getting out of bed unassisted may result in falling and injury if undertaken within 8 hours of receiving lorazepam injection. Instruct patients not to consume alcoholic beverages for at least 24 to 48 hours after receiving lorazepam injectable because of the additive effects on central nervous system depression seen with benzodiazepines in general. Advise elderly patients that lorazepam injection may make them sleepy for a period longer than 6 to 8 hours following surgery.

PREGNANCY AND LACTATION

• Pregnancy Category D. Occasional anomalies (reduction of tarsals, tibia, metatarsals, malrotated limbs, gastroschisis, malformed skull, and microphthalmia) were seen in drug-treated rabbits without relationship to dosage. Do not administer injectable lorazepam to nursing mothers because as with other benzodiazepines, the possibility exists that lorazepam may be excreted in human milk and may sedate the infant. Whether oral lorazepam is excreted in human milk like the other benzodiazepine tranquilizers is not known.

losartan

(lo-sar'tan)

Rx: Cozaar

Drug Class: Angiotensin II receptor antagonists

Pregnancy Category: C; D, 2nd / 3rd

Do not confuse Cozaar with Zocor.

CLINICAL PHARMACOLOGY

Mechanism of Action: An angiotensin II receptor, type AT_1, antagonist that blocks vasoconstrictor and aldosterone-secreting effects of angiotensin II, inhibiting the binding of angiotensin II to the AT_1 receptors. *Therapeutic Effect:* Causes vasodilation, decreases peripheral resistance, and decreases BP.

Pharmacokinetics

Route	*Onset*	*Peak*	*Duration*
PO	N/A	6 hr	24 hr

Well absorbed after PO administration. Protein binding: 98%. Undergoes first-pass metabolism in the liver to active metabolites. Excreted in urine and via the biliary system. Not removed by hemodialysis. **Half-life:** 2 hr, metabolite: 6-9 hr.

AVAILABLE FORMS

• *Tablets:* 25 mg, 50 mg, 100 mg.

INDICATIONS AND DOSAGES

Hypertension

PO

Adults, Elderly. Initially, 50 mg once a day. Maximum: May be given once or twice a day, with total daily doses ranging from 25-100 mg.

Nephropathy

PO

Adults, Elderly. Initially, 50 mg/day. May increase to 100 mg/day based on BP response.

Stroke reduction

PO

Adults, Elderly. 50 mg/day. Maximum: 100 mg/day.

Hypertension in patients with impaired hepatic function

PO

Adults, Elderly. Initially, 25 mg/day.

CONTRAINDICATIONS: None known.

INTERACTIONS

Drug

Cimetidine: May increase the effects of losartan.

Ketoconazole, troleandomycin: May inhibit the effects of these drugs.

Lithium: May increase lithium blood concentration and risk of lithium toxicity.
Phenobarbital, rifampin: May decrease the effects of losartan.
Herbal
None known.
Food
Grapefruit, grapefruit juice: May alter the absorption of losartan.
DIAGNOSTIC TEST EFFECTS: May increase BUN, serum alkaline phosphatase, serum bilirubin, serum creatinine, AST (SGOT), and ALT (SGPT) levels. May decrease blood Hgb and Hct levels.
SIDE EFFECTS
Frequent (8%)
Upper respiratory tract infection
Occasional (4%-2%)
Dizziness, diarrhea, cough
Rare (1% or less)
Insomnia, dyspepsia, heartburn, back and leg pain, muscle cramps, myalgia, nasal congestion, sinusitis
SERIOUS REACTIONS
• Overdosage may manifest as hypotension and tachycardia. Bradycardia occurs less often.

SPECIAL CONSIDERATIONS

PRECAUTIONS
• Anaphylactic reactions have been reported. Consider a lower dose for patients with impaired liver function. Changes in renal function have been reported in susceptible individuals. Patients with unilateral or bilateral renal artery stenosis and increases in serum creatinine or blood urea nitrogen have been reported.
PATIENT INFORMATION
• Pregnancy: Advise female patients of childbearing age about the consequences of second- and third-trimester exposure to drugs that act on the renin-angiotensin system, and advise them that these consequences do not appear to have resulted from intrauterine drug exposure that has been limited to the first trimester. Ask these patients to report pregnancies to their physicians as soon as possible.
• Potassium Supplements: Instruct a patient receiving losartan potassium not to use potassium supplements or salt substitutes containing potassium without consulting the prescribing physician.
PREGNANCY AND LACTATION
• Pregnancy Categories C (first trimester) and D (second and third trimesters). The use of drugs that act directly on the renin-angiotensin system during the second and third trimesters of pregnancy has been associated with fetal and neonatal injury, including hypotension, neonatal skull hypoplasia, anuria, reversible or irreversible renal failure, and death. Whether losartan is excreted in human milk is not known, but significant levels of losartan and its active metabolite were shown to be present in rat milk.

loteprednol

(loh-teh-pred′nol)
Rx: Alrex, Lotemax
Drug Class: Corticosteroids, ophthalmic; Ophthalmics
Pregnancy Category: C

CLINICAL PHARMACOLOGY
Mechanism of Action: A glucocorticoid that inhibits accumulation of inflammatory cells at inflammation sites, phagocytosis, lysosomal enzyme release and synthesis and/or release of mediators of inflammation. *Therapeutic Effect:* Prevents and suppresses cell and tissue immune reactions, inflammatory process.

Pharmacokinetics
Metabolized by enzymes in the eye, minimizing systemic adverse effects.

AVAILABLE FORMS

• *Ophthalmic Suspension:* 0.2% (Alrex), 0.5% (Lotemax).

INDICATIONS AND DOSAGES

Treatment of seasonal allergic conjunctivitis, giant papillary conjunctivitis, ureitis
Ophthalmic
Adults, Elderly. Instill 1 drop 4 times/day for 4-6 weeks.

CONTRAINDICATIONS: Acute epithelial herpes simplex keratitis, fungal diseases of ocular structures, vaccinia, varicella, ocular tuberculosis, hypersensitivity, after removal of corneal foreign body, mycobacterial eye infection, acute, purulent, untreated eye infection

INTERACTIONS

Drug
None known.

Herbal
None known.

Food
None known.

DIAGNOSTIC TEST EFFECTS: *None known.*

SIDE EFFECTS

Frequent
Blurred vision

Occasional
Decreased vision, watering of eyes, eye pain, nausea, vomiting, burning, stinging, redness of eyes

SERIOUS REACTIONS

• Glaucoma with optic nerve damage, cataract formation, and secondary ocular infection occur rarely.

SPECIAL CONSIDERATIONS

PRECAUTIONS

• Renew the medication order beyond 14 days after slit-lamp examination. If no improvement occurs after 2 days, reevaluate the patient. If loteprednol etabonate is used for 10 days or longer, monitor intraocular pressure. Fungal infections of the cornea are particularly prone to develop coincidentally with long-term local steroid application.

PATIENT INFORMATION

• Advise patients not to wear a contact lens if their eye is red. Benzalkonium chloride may be absorbed by soft contact lenses. Instruct patients to wait at least 10 minutes before they insert their contact lenses.

PREGNANCY AND LACTATION

• Pregnancy Category C. Loteprednol etabonate has been shown to be embryotoxic (delayed ossification) and teratogenic (increased incidence of meningocele, abnormal left common carotid artery, and limb flexures) when administered orally to rabbits. Systemic steroids appear in human milk and could suppress growth, interfere with endogenous corticosteroid production, or cause other untoward effects.

loteprednol etabonate; tobramycin

(loe-te-pred'nol; toe-bra-mye'sin)

Rx: Zylet

Drug Class: Anti-infectives, ophthalmic; Antibiotics, aminoglycosides; Corticosteroids, ophthalmic

Pregnancy Category: C

CLINICAL PHARMACOLOGY

Mechanism of Action: A combination ophthalmic product of an aminoglycoside and a glucocorticoid. Loteprednol is a glucocorticoid that inhibits accumulation of inflammatory cells at inflammation sites, phagocytosis, lysosomal enzyme release and synthesis and/or release of mediators of inflammation Tobramycin is an antibiotic that irreversibly binds to protein on bacterial ribosomes. *Therapeutic Effect:* Prevents and suppresses cell and tissue immune reactions and inflammatory process. Interferes in protein synthesis of susceptible microorganisms.

Pharmacokinetics

Limited systemic absorption.

AVAILABLE FORMS

• *Ophthalmic Solution:* 0.5% loteprednol etabonate and 0.3% tobramycin (Zylet).

INDICATIONS AND DOSAGES

Steroid-responsive inflammatory ocular conditions for which a corticosteroid is indicated and where superficial bacterial ocular infection or a risk of bacterial ocular infection exists

Ophthalmic

Adults, Elderly. Apply 1 or 2 drops into the affected eye(s) q4-6h. During the initial 24 to 48 hours, the dosing may be increased to every 1 to 2 hours. Gradually decrease by improvement in clinical signs.

CONTRAINDICATIONS: Viral diseases of the cornea and conjunctiva including epithelial herpes simplex keratitis (dendritic keratitis), vaccinia, varicella, and mycobacterial infection of the eye and fungal diseases of ocular structures, hypersensitivity to any of loteprednol, tobramycin or any component of the formulation and to other corticosteroids

INTERACTIONS

Drug

None known.

Herbal

None known.

Food

None known.

DIAGNOSTIC TEST EFFECTS: *None known.*

SIDE EFFECTS

Frequent

Blurred vision

Occasional

Tearing, burning, itching, redness, swelling of eyelid, decreased vision, eye pain

Rare

Nausea, vomiting

SERIOUS REACTIONS

• Glaucoma with optic nerve damage, cataract formation, and secondary ocular infection occurs rarely.
• Secondary infection, especially fungal infections of the cornea, may occur after use of this medication. These infections are more frequent with long-term applications.

lovastatin

(lo′va-sta-tin)

Rx: Altocor, Mevacor

Drug Class: Antihyperlipidemics; HMG CoA reductase inhibitors

Pregnancy Category: X

Do not confuse lovastatin with Leustatin or Livostin, or Mevacor with Mivacron.

CLINICAL PHARMACOLOGY

Mechanism of Action: An antihyperlipidemic that inhibits HMG-CoA reductase, the enzyme that catalyzes the early step in cholesterol synthesis. *Therapeutic Effect:* Decreases LDL cholesterol, VLDL cholesterol, plasma triglycerides; increases HDL cholesterol.

Pharmacokinetics

Route	*Onset*	*Peak*	*Duration*
PO	3 days	4-6 wk	N/A

Incompletely absorbed from the GI tract (increased on empty stomach). Protein binding: 95%. Hydrolyzed in the liver to active metabolite. Primarily eliminated in feces. Not removed by hemodialysis. **Half-life:** 1.1-1.7 hr.

AVAILABLE FORMS

- *Tablets (Mevacor):* 10 mg, 20 mg, 40 mg.
- *Tablets (Extended-Release [Altoprev]):* 20 mg, 40 mg, 60 mg.

INDICATIONS AND DOSAGES

Hyperlipoproteinemia, primary prevention of coronary artery disease

PO

Adults, Elderly. Initially, 20-40 mg/day with evening meal. Increase at 4-wk intervals up to maximum of 80 mg/day. Maintenance: 20-80 mg/day in single or divided doses.

PO (Extended-Release)

Adults, Elderly. Initially, 20 mg/day. May increase at 4-wk intervals up to 60 mg/day.

Children 10-17 yr. 10-40 mg/day with evening meal.

Heterozygous familial hypercholesterolemia

PO

Children 10-17 yr. Initially, 10 mg/day. May increase to 20 mg/day after 8 wk and 40 mg/day after 16 wk if needed.

CONTRAINDICATIONS: Active liver disease, pregnancy, unexplained elevated liver function tests

INTERACTIONS

Drug

Cyclosporine, erythromycin, gemfibrozil, immunosuppressants, niacin: Increases the risk of acute renal failure and rhabdomyolysis.

Erythromycin, itraconazole, ketoconazole: May increase lovastatin blood concentration causing severe muscle inflammation, myalgia, and weakness.

Herbal

None known.

Food

Grapefruit juice: Large amounts of grapefruit juice may increase risk of side effects, such as myalgia and weakness.

DIAGNOSTIC TEST EFFECTS: May increase serum creatine kinase and serum transaminase concentrations.

SIDE EFFECTS

Generally well tolerated. Side effects usually mild and transient.

Frequent (9%-5%)

Headache, flatulence, diarrhea, abdominal pain or cramps, rash and pruritus

Occasional (4%-3%)

Nausea, vomiting, constipation, dyspepsia

Rare (2%-1%)

Dizziness, heartburn, myalgia, blurred vision, eye irritation

SERIOUS REACTIONS

- There is a potential for cataract development.

SPECIAL CONSIDERATIONS

PRECAUTIONS

- Lovastatin may elevate creatine phosphokinase and transaminase levels. 3-Hydroxy-3-methylglutaryl–coenzyme A reductase inhibitors interfere with cholesterol synthesis and might theoretically blunt adrenal and/or gonadal steroid production.

PATIENT INFORMATION

- Advise patients to report promptly unexplained muscle pain, tenderness, or weakness.

PREGNANCY AND LACTATION

- Pregnancy Category X. Administer lovastatin to women of childbearing age only when such patients are highly unlikely to conceive. If the patient becomes pregnant while taking this drug, discontinue lovastatin immediately and apprise the patient of the potential hazard to the fetus. Excretion into human milk is not known.

OCULAR CONSIDERATIONS

- A high prevalence of baseline lenticular opacities occurred in the patient population included in the early clinical trials with lovastatin. During these trials, the appearance of new opacities was noted in the lovastatin and placebo groups. No clinically significant change in visual acuity was reported in the patients who had new opacities, and no patient, including those with opacities noted at baseline, discontinued therapy because of a decrease in visual acuity. Cataracts were seen in dogs treated for 11 and 28 weeks at 180 mg/kg per day and 1 year at 60 mg/kg per day.
- A 3-year, double-blind, placebo-controlled study in hypercholesterolemic patients to assess the effect of lovastatin on the human lens demonstrated that there were no clinically or statistically significant differences between the lovastatin and placebo groups in the incidence, type, or progression of lenticular opacities. No controlled clinical data assessing the lens are available for treatment beyond 3 years.
- Lovastatin produced optic nerve degeneration (wallerian degeneration of retinogeniculate fibers) in clinically normal dogs in a dose-dependent fashion starting at 60 mg/kg per day, a dose that produced mean plasma drug levels about 30 times higher than the mean drug level in human beings taking the highest recommended dose (as measured by total enzyme inhibitory activity). Vestibulocochlear wallerian-like degeneration and retinal ganglion cell chromatolysis also were seen in dogs treated for 14 weeks at 180 mg/kg per day, a dose that resulted in a mean plasma drug level (maximum concentration) similar to that seen with the 60 mg/kg per day dose.

mannitol

(man′i-tall)

Rx: Osmitrol, Resectisol

Drug Class: Diuretics, osmotic

Pregnancy Category: C

CLINICAL PHARMACOLOGY

Mechanism of Action: An osmotic diuretic, antiglaucoma, and antihemolytic agent that elevates osmotic pressure of the glomerular filtrate, inhibiting tubular reabsorption of water and electrolytes, resulting in increased flow of water into interstitial fluid and plasma. *Therapeutic Effect:* Produces diuresis; reduces IOP; reduces ICP and cerebral edema.

Pharmacokinetics

Route	Onset	Peak	Duration
IV (diuresis)	15-30 min	N/A	2-8 hr
IV (Reduced ICP)	15-30 min	N/A	3-8 hr
IV (Reduced IOP)	N/A	30-60 min	4-8 hr

Remains in extracellular fluid. Primarily excreted in urine. Removed by hemodialysis. **Half-life:** 100 min.

AVAILABLE FORMS

- *Injection:* 5%, 10%, 15%, 20%, 25%.

INDICATIONS AND DOSAGES

Prevention and treatment of oliguric phase of acute renal failure; to promote urinary excretion of toxic substances (such as aspirin, barbiturates, bromides, and imipramine); to reduce increased ICP due to cerebral edema or edema of injured spinal cord; to reduce increased IOP due to acute glaucoma

IV

Adults, Elderly, Children. Initially, 0.5-1 g/kg, then 0.25-0.5 g/kg q4-6h.

CONTRAINDICATIONS: Dehydration, intracranial bleeding, severe pulmonary edema and congestion, severe renal disease

INTERACTIONS

Drug

Digoxin: May increase the risk of digoxin toxicity associated with mannitol-induced hypokalemia.

Herbal

None known.

Food

None known.

DIAGNOSTIC TEST EFFECTS: May decrease serum phosphate, potassium, and sodium levels.

IV INCOMPATIBILITIES: Cefepime (Maxipime), doxorubicin liposomal (Doxil), filgrastim (Neupogen)

IV COMPATIBILITIES: Cisplatin (Platinol), ondansetron (Zofran), propofol (Diprivan)

SIDE EFFECTS

Frequent

Dry mouth, thirst

Occasional

Blurred vision, increased urinary frequency and urine volume, headache, arm pain, backache, nausea, vomiting, urticaria, dizziness, hypotension or hypertension, tachycardia, fever, angina-like chest pain

SERIOUS REACTIONS

- Fluid and electrolyte imbalance may occur from rapid administration of large doses or inadequate urine output resulting in overexpansion of extracellular fluid.
- Circulatory overload may produce pulmonary edema and CHF.
- Excessive diuresis may produce hypokalemia and hyponatremia.
- Fluid loss in excess of electrolyte excretion may produce hypernatremia and hyperkalemia.

SPECIAL CONSIDERATIONS

PRECAUTIONS

- Clinical evaluation and periodic laboratory determinations are necessary to monitor changes in fluid balance, electrolyte concentrations, and acid-base balance during parenteral therapy with mannitol solutions. Use these solutions with care in patients with hypervolemia, renal insufficiency, urinary tract obstruction, or impending or frank cardiac decompensation. Mannitol administration may obscure and intensify inadequate hydration or hypovolemia by sustaining diuresis.

PREGNANCY AND LACTATION

- Pregnancy Category C. Whether mannitol injections USP can cause fetal harm when administered to a pregnant woman or can affect reproduction capacity is not known. Excretion into human milk is not known.

OCULAR CONSIDERATIONS

Mannitol can be used to dehydrate the vitreous and overcome malignant glaucoma and refractory intraocular pressure elevation.

mecamylamine

(mek-a-mil-'a-meen hye-droe-klor-ide)

Rx: Inversine

Drug Class: Antiadrenergics, peripheral

Pregnancy Category: C

CLINICAL PHARMACOLOGY

Mechanism of Action: A ganglionic blocker that inhibits acetylcholine at the autonomic ganglia. Blocks central nicotinic cholinergic receptors, which inhibits effects of nicotine. *Therapeutic Effect:* Reduces blood pressure; decreases desire to smoke.

Pharmacokinetics

Completely absorbed following PO administration. Widely distributed. Excreted in urine. **Half-life:** 24 hrs.

AVAILABLE FORMS

- *Tablets:* 2.5 mg (Inversine).

INDICATIONS AND DOSAGES

Hypertension

PO

Adults. Initially, 2.5 mg q12h for 2 days, then increase by 2.5 mg increments at more than 2-day intervals until desired blood pressure is achieved. The average daily dose is 25 mg in 3 divided doses.

Smoking cessation

PO

Adults. Initially, 2.5 mg q12h for 2 days, then increase by 2.5 mg increments during the first week of therapy. Range: 10-20 mg in divided doses.

UNLABELED USES: Tourette's syndrome, hyperreflexia

CONTRAINDICATIONS: Coronary insufficiency, pyloric stenosis, glaucoma, uremia, recent myocardial infarction, unreliable patients

INTERACTIONS

Drug

Sulfonamides, antibiotics: May increase the effect of mecamylamine.

Herbal

None known.

Food

None known.

DIAGNOSTIC TEST EFFECTS: *None known.*

IV INCOMPATIBILITIES: None known.

IV COMPATIBILITIES: None known.

SIDE EFFECTS

Occasional

Nausea, diarrhea, orthostatic hypotension, tachycardia, drowsiness, urinary retention, blurred vision, dilated pupils, confusion, mental depression, decreased sexual ability, loss of appetite

Rare

Pulmonary edema, pulmonary fibrosis, paresthesias

SERIOUS REACTIONS

- Overdosage includes symptoms such as hypotension, nausea, vomiting, urinary retention and constipation.

SPECIAL CONSIDERATIONS

PRECAUTIONS

- Use of mecamylamine hydrochloride in patients with marked cerebral and coronary arteriosclerosis or after a recent cerebral accident requires caution. Mecamylamine hydrochloride may be potentiated by excessive heat, fever, infection, hemorrhage, pregnancy, anesthesia, surgery, vigorous exercise, other antihypertensive drugs, alcohol, and salt depletion as a result of diminished intake or increased excretion. Caution is required in patients with prostatic hypertrophy, bladder neck obstruction, and urethral stricture. Frequent loose bowel movements with abdominal distention and decreased borborygmi may be the first signs of paralytic ileus.

PATIENT INFORMATION

• Mecamylamine hydrochloride may cause dizziness, light-headedness, or fainting, especially when one is rising from a lying or sitting position. This effect may be increased by alcoholic beverages and exercise or during hot weather. Getting up slowly may help alleviate such a reaction.

PREGNANCY AND LACTATION

• Pregnancy Category C. Animal reproduction studies have not been conducted with mecamylamine hydrochloride. Fetal harm is not known. Because of the potential for serious adverse reactions in nursing infants from mecamylamine hydrochloride, decide whether to discontinue nursing or to discontinue the drug, taking into account the importance of the drug to the mother. Excretion into human milk is not known.

OCULAR CONSIDERATIONS

• Mecamylamine hydrochloride is contraindicated in patients with glaucoma.

meclizine

(mek'li-zeen)

Rx: Antivert, Meclicot, Meni-D

Drug Class: Antiemetics/antivertigo; Antihistamines, H1

Pregnancy Category: B

Do not confuse Antivert with Axert.

CLINICAL PHARMACOLOGY

Mechanism of Action: An anticholinergic that reduces labyrinthine excitability and diminishes vestibular stimulation of the labyrinth, affecting the chemoreceptor trigger zone. *Therapeutic Effect:* Reduces nausea, vomiting, and vertigo.

Pharmacokinetics

Route	*Onset*	*Peak*	*Duration*
PO	30-60 min	N/A	12-24 hr

Well absorbed from the GI tract. Widely distributed. Metabolized in the liver. Primarily excreted in urine. **Half-life:** 6 hr.

AVAILABLE FORMS

• *Tablets (Antivert):* 12.5 mg, 25 mg, 50 mg.

• *Tablets (Chewable [Bonine]):*25 mg.

INDICATIONS AND DOSAGES

Motion sickness

PO

Adults, Elderly, Children 12 yr and older. 12.5-25 mg 1 hr before travel. May repeat q12-24h. May require a dose of 50 mg.

Vertigo

PO

Adults, Elderly, Children 12 yr and older. 25-100 mg/day in divided doses, as needed.

CONTRAINDICATIONS: None known.

INTERACTIONS

Drug

Alcohol, CNS depression-producing medications: May increase CNS depressant effect.

Herbal

None known.

Food

None known.

DIAGNOSTIC TEST EFFECTS: May produce false-negative results in antigen skin testing unless meclizine is discontinued 4 days before testing.

SIDE EFFECTS

Frequent

Drowsiness

Occasional
Blurred vision; dry mouth, nose, or throat

SERIOUS REACTIONS

• A hypersensitivity reaction, marked by eczema, pruritus, rash, cardiac disturbances, and photosensitivity, may occur.
• Overdose may produce CNS depression (manifested as sedation, apnea, cardiovascular collapse, or death) or severe paradoxical reactions (such as hallucinations, tremor, and seizures).
• Children may experience paradoxical reactions, including restlessness, insomnia, euphoria, nervousness, and tremors.
• Overdose in children may result in hallucinations, seizures, and death.

SPECIAL CONSIDERATIONS

PATIENT INFORMATION

• Because drowsiness may occur occasionally with use of this drug, warn patients of this possibility and caution them against driving a car or operating dangerous machinery. Patients should avoid alcoholic beverages while taking this drug. Because of the potential anticholinergic action of meclizine hydrochloride, use this drug with caution in patients with asthma, glaucoma, or enlargement of the prostate gland.

PREGNANCY AND LACTATION

• Pregnancy Category B. Reproduction studies in rats have shown cleft palates at 25 to 50 times the human dose. Epidemiologic studies in pregnant women, however, do not indicate that meclizine increases the risk of abnormalities when administered during pregnancy. Despite the animal findings, it would appear that the possibility of fetal harm is remote. Nevertheless, meclizine, or any other medication, should be used during pregnancy only if clearly necessary.

medrysone

(me'dri-sone)

Rx: HMS

Drug Class: Corticosteroids, ophthalmic; Ophthalmics

Pregnancy Category: C

CLINICAL PHARMACOLOGY

Mechanism of Action: A topical synthetic corticosteroid that inhibits accumulation of inflammatory cells at inflammation sites. *Therapeutic Effect:* Inhibits inflammatory process.

Pharmacokinetics

Absorbed through aqueous humor. Metabolized in liver if absorbed. Excreted in urine and feces.

AVAILABLE FORMS

• *Ophthalmic suspension:* 1% (HMS Liquifilm).

INDICATIONS AND DOSAGES

Ophthalmic disorders

Ophthalmic

Adults, Elderly, Children 3 yrs and older. Instill 1 drop up to every 4 hours.

CONTRAINDICATIONS: Active superficial herpes simplex, conjunctival or corneal viral disease, fungal diseases of the eye, ocular tuberculosis, hypersensitivity to medrysone or any component of the formulation

INTERACTIONS

Drug

None known.

Herbal

None known.

Food

None known.

DIAGNOSTIC TEST EFFECTS: *None known.*

SIDE EFFECTS

Frequent

Blurred vision

Occasional

Decreased vision, watering of eyes, eye pain, burning, stinging, redness of eyes, nausea, vomiting

SERIOUS REACTIONS

• Systemic absorption may occur with topical application.

• Cataracts, corneal thinning, corneal ulcers, delayed wound healing, optic nerve damage, and glaucoma have been reported.

SPECIAL CONSIDERATIONS

PRECAUTIONS

• Determine intraocular pressure and examine the lens periodically. In persistent corneal ulceration, suspect fungal infection.

PREGNANCY AND LACTATION

• Pregnancy Category C. Medrysone is embryocidal and causes early resorptions in rabbits. Excretion into human milk is not known.

---

memantine hydrochloride

(meh-man′-teen)

Rx: Namenda

Drug Class: NMDA receptor antagonists

Pregnancy Category: B

CLINICAL PHARMACOLOGY

Mechanism of Action: A neurotransmitter inhibitor that decreases the effects of glutamate, the principle excitatory neurotransmitter in the brain. Persistent CNS excitation by glutamate is thought to cause the symptoms of Alzheimer's disease. *Therapeutic Effect:* May reduce clinical deterioration in moderate to severe Alzheimer's disease.

Pharmacokinetics

Rapidly and completely absorbed after PO administration. Protein binding: 45%. Undergoes little metabolism; most of the dose is excreted unchanged in urine. **Half-life:** 60-80 hr.

AVAILABLE FORMS

• *Tablets:* 5 mg, 10 mg.

INDICATIONS AND DOSAGES

Alzheimer's disease

PO

Adults, Elderly. Initially, 5 mg once a day. May increase dosage at intervals of at least 1 wk in 5-mg increments to 10 mg/day (5 mg twice a day), then 15 mg/day (5 mg and 10 mg as separate doses), and finally 20 mg/day (10 mg twice a day). Target dose: 20 mg/day.

CONTRAINDICATIONS: Severe renal impairment

INTERACTIONS

Drug

Carbonic anhydrase inhibitors, sodium bicarbonate: May decrease the renal elimination of memantine.

Herbal

None known.

Food

None known.

DIAGNOSTIC TEST EFFECTS: *None known.*

SIDE EFFECTS

Occasional (7%-4%)

Dizziness, headache, confusion, constipation, hypertension, cough

Rare (3%-2%)
Back pain, nausea, fatigue, anxiety, peripheral edema, arthralgia, insomnia

SERIOUS REACTIONS
• None known.

SPECIAL CONSIDERATIONS

OCULAR CONSIDERATIONS
• Memantine (Namenda) is in Food and Drug Administration clinical trials for the treatment of glaucoma. Memantine seems to possess neuroprotective properties and may help to prevent retinal ganglion cell loss. Memantine binds to the glutamate receptor molecules on the cell surface and prevents the attachment of glutamate to the nerve cells. Calcium is unable to enter the nerve cells. The nerve cells are protected from excess calcium and cell toxicity. (Bonner H: Ocular drug preview: spotlight on emerging pharmaceuticals, *Rev Optometry* vol 141, issue 12, 2004. http://www.revoptom.com/index.asp?page=2_1309.htm.)

meperidine hydrochloride

(me-per'i-deen)
Rx: Demerol HCl
Drug Class: Analgesics, narcotic; Preanesthetics
Pregnancy Category: C
DEA Class: Schedule II
Do not confuse with Demulen or Dymelor.

CLINICAL PHARMACOLOGY
Mechanism of Action: An opioid agonist that binds to opioid receptors in the CNS. *Therapeutic Effect:* Alters the perception of and emotional response to pain.

Pharmacokinetics

Route	Onset	Peak	Duration
PO	15 min	60 min	2-4 hr
IV	less than 5 min	5-7 min	2-3 hr
IM	10-15 min	30-50 min	2-4 hr
Subcutaneous	10-15 min	30-50 min	2-4 hr

Variably absorbed from the GI tract; well absorbed after IM administration. Protein binding: 60%-80%. Widely distributed. Metabolized in the liver to active metabolite. Primarily excreted in urine. Not removed by hemodialysis. **Half-life:** 2.4-4 hr; metabolite 8-16 hr (increased in hepatic impairment and disease).

AVAILABLE FORMS
• *Syrup:* 50 mg/5 ml.
• *Tablets:* 50 mg, 100 mg.
• *Injection:* 25 mg/ml, 50 mg/ml, 75 mg/ml, 100 mg/ml.

INDICATIONS AND DOSAGES
Analgesia
PO, IM, Subcutaneous
Adults, Elderly. 50-150 mg q3-4h.
Children. 1.1-1.5 mg/kg q3-4h. Don't exceed single dose of 100 mg.

Patient-controlled analgesia (PCA)
IV
Adults. Loading dose: 50-100 mg. Intermittent bolus: 5-30 mg. Lockout interval: 10-20 min. Continuous infusion: 5-40 mg/hr. Maximum (4-hr): 200-300 mg.

Dosage in renal impairment
Dosage is based on creatinine clearance.

Creatinine Clearance	Dosage
10-50 ml/min	75% of usual dose
less than 10 ml/min	50% of usual dose

CONTRAINDICATIONS: Delivery of premature infant, diarrhea due to poisoning, use within 14 days of MAOIs

INTERACTIONS

Drug

Alcohol, other CNS depressants: May increase CNS or respiratory depression and hypotension.

MAOIs: May produce a severe, sometimes fatal reaction. Meperidine use is contraindicated.

Herbal

Valerian: May increase CNS depression.

Food

None known.

DIAGNOSTIC TEST EFFECTS: May increase serum amylase and lipase levels. Therapeutic serum level is 100-550 ng/ml; toxic serum level is greater than 1000 ng/ml.

IV INCOMPATIBILITIES: Allopurinol (Aloprim), amphotericin B complex (Abelcet, AmBisome, Amphotec), cefepime (Maxipime), cefoperazone (Cefobid), doxorubicin liposomal (Doxil), furosemide (Lasix), idarubicin (Idamycin), nafcillin (Nafcil)

IV COMPATIBILITIES: Atropine, bumetanide (Bumex), diltiazem (Cardizem), diphenhydramine (Benadryl), dobutamine (Dobutrex), dopamine (Intropin), glycopyrrolate (Robinul), heparin, hydroxyzine (Vistaril), insulin, lidocaine, magnesium, midazolam (Versed), oxytocin (Pitocin), potassium

SIDE EFFECTS

Frequent

Sedation, hypotension (including orthostatic hypotension), diaphoresis, facial flushing, dizziness, nausea, vomiting, constipation

Occasional

Confusion, arrhythmias, tremors, urine retention, abdominal pain, dry mouth, headache, irritation at injection site, euphoria, dysphoria

Rare

Allergic reaction (rash, pruritus), insomnia

SERIOUS REACTIONS

• Overdose results in respiratory depression, skeletal muscle flaccidity, cold or clammy skin, cyanosis, and extreme somnolence progressing to seizures, stupor, and coma. The antidote is 0.4 mg naloxone.

• The patient who uses meperidine repeatedly may develop a tolerance to the drug's analgesic effect and physical dependence.

SPECIAL CONSIDERATIONS

PRECAUTIONS

• Use meperidine hydrochloride with extreme caution in patients having an acute asthmatic attack, patients with chronic obstructive pulmonary disease or cor pulmonale, patients having a substantially decreased respiratory reserve, and patients with preexisting respiratory depression, hypoxia, or hypercapnia. Drug administration may result in severe hypotension in the postoperative patient or any individual whose ability to maintain blood pressure has been compromised by a depleted blood volume or the administration of drugs such as the phenothiazines or certain anesthetics. Meperidine hydrochloride may produce orthostatic hypotension in ambulatory patients. Use meperidine hydrochloride with caution in patients with atrial flutter and other supraventricular tachycardias because of a possible vagolytic action that may produce a significant increase in the ventricular response rate. Meperidine hydrochloride may aggravate preexisting convulsions in patients with convulsive disorders. If dosage is escalated substantially above recommended levels because of tolerance development, convulsions may occur in individuals without a history of convulsive disorders. Meperidine hydrochloride may obscure the diagnosis of clinical course in patients with acute abdominal conditions. Give meperidine hydrochloride with caution and reduce the initial dose in certain patients such as the elderly or debilitated and in those with severe impairment of hepatic or renal function, hypothyroidism, Addison's disease, and prostatic hypertrophy or urethral stricture.

PATIENT INFORMATION

- Meperidine may impair the mental and/or physical abilities required for the performance of potentially hazardous tasks such as driving a car or operating machinery. Caution the patient accordingly.

PREGNANCY AND LACTATION

- Pregnancy Category B. Do not use meperidine hydrochloride in pregnant women before the labor period. When used as an obstetric analgesic, meperidine crosses the placental barrier and can produce depression of respiration and psychophysiologic functions in the newborn. Meperidine appears in the milk of nursing mothers receiving the drug.

metformin hydrochloride

(met-for'min)

Rx: Glucophage, Glucophage XR, Riomet

Drug Class: Antidiabetic agents; Biguanides

Pregnancy Category: C

CLINICAL PHARMACOLOGY

Mechanism of Action: An antihyperglycemic that decreases hepatic production of glucose. Decreases absorption of glucose and improves insulin sensitivity. *Therapeutic Effect:* Improves glycemic control, stabilizes or decreases body weight, and improves lipid profile.

Pharmacokinetics

Slowly, incompletely absorbed after oral administration. Food delays or decreases the extent of absorption. Protein binding: Negligible. Primarily distributed to intestinal mucosa and salivary glands. Primarily excreted unchanged in urine. Removed by hemodialysis. **Half-life:** 3-6 hr.

AVAILABLE FORMS

- *Oral Solution (Riomet):* 100 mg/ml.
- *Tablets (Glucophage):* 500 mg, 850 mg, 1000 mg.
- *Tablets (Extended-Release [Glucophage XL]):* 500 mg, 750 mg.
- *Tablets (Extended-Release [Fortamet]):* 500 mg, 1000 mg.

INDICATIONS AND DOSAGES

Diabetes mellitus

PO (500-mg, 1000-mg tablet)

Adults, Elderly. Initially, 500 mg twice a day, with morning and evening meals. May increase in 500-mg increments every week, in divided doses. May give twice a day up to 2000 mg/day (for example, 1000 mg twice a day [with morning

M

and evening meals]). If 2,500 mg/day is required, give 3 times a day with meals. Maximum: 2,500 mg/day.

Children 10-16 yr. Initially, 500 mg twice a day. May increase by 500 mg/day at weekly intervals. Maximum: 2,000 mg/day.

PO (850-mg tablet)

Adults, Elderly. Initially, 850-mg/day, with morning meal. May increase dosage in 850-mg increments every other week, in divided doses. Maintenance: 850 mg twice a day, with morning and evening meals. Maximum: 2550 mg/day (850 mg 3 times a day).

PO (Extended-Release tablets)

Adults, Elderly. Initially, 500 mg once a day. May increase by 500 mg/day at weekly intervals. Maximum: 2000 mg once a day.

Adjunct to insulin therapy

PO

Adults, Elderly. Initially, 500 mg/day. May increase by 500 mg at 7-day intervals. Maximum: 2500 mg/day (2000 mg/day for extended-release form).

UNLABELED USES: Treatment of metabolic complications of AIDS, prediabetes, weight reduction

CONTRAINDICATIONS: Acute CHF, MI, cardiovascular collapse, renal disease or dysfunction, respiratory failure, septicemia

INTERACTIONS

Drug

Alcohol, amiloride, cimetidine, digoxin, furosemide, morphine, nifedipine, procainamide, quinidine, quinine, ranitidine, triamterene, trimethoprim, vancomycin: Increase metformin blood concentration.

Furosemide, hypoglycemia-causing medications: May require a decrease in metformin dosage.

Iodinated contrast studies: May cause acute renal failure and increased risk of lactic acidosis.

Herbal

None known.

Food

None known.

DIAGNOSTIC TEST EFFECTS: *None known.*

SIDE EFFECTS

Occasional (greater than 3%)

GI disturbances (including diarrhea, nausea, vomiting, abdominal bloating, flatulence, and anorexia) that are transient and resolve spontaneously during therapy.

Rare (3%-1%)

Unpleasant or metallic taste that resolves spontaneously during therapy

SERIOUS REACTIONS

• Lactic acidosis occurs rarely but is a fatal complication in 50% of cases. Lactic acidosis is characterized by an increase in blood lactate levels (greater than 5 mmol/L), a decrease in blood pH, and electrolyte disturbances. Signs and symptoms of lactic acidosis include unexplained hyperventilation, myalgia, malaise, and somnolence, which may advance to cardiovascular collapse (shock), acute CHF, acute MI, and prerenal azotemia.

SPECIAL CONSIDERATIONS

PRECAUTIONS

• Metformin is known to be substantially excreted by the kidney, and the risk of metformin accumulation and lactic acidosis increases with the degree of impairment of renal function. Thus patients with serum creatinine levels above the upper limit of normal for their age should not receive metformin hydrochloride. Cardiovascular collapse (shock) from whatever cause, acute congestive heart failure, acute myocardial infarction, and other conditions characterized by hypoxemia have been associated with lactic acidosis and also may cause prerenal azotemia. Temporarily suspend metformin hydrochloride therapy for any surgical procedure. Alcohol is known to potentiate the effect of metformin on lactate metabolism. Hypoglycemia does not occur in patients receiving metformin hydrochloride alone under usual circumstances of use but could occur when caloric intake is deficient, when strenuous exercise is not compensated by caloric supplementation, or during concomitant use with other glucose-lowering agents (such as sulfonylureas and insulin) or ethanol. Elderly, debilitated, or malnourished patients and those with adrenal or pituitary insufficiency or alcohol intoxication are particularly susceptible to hypoglycemic effects. Hypoglycemia may be difficult to recognize in the elderly and in persons who are taking beta-adrenergic blocking drugs. When a patient stabilized on any diabetic regimen is exposed to stress such as fever, trauma, infection, or surgery, a temporary loss of glycemic control may occur. At such times, it may be necessary to withhold metformin hydrochloride and temporarily administer insulin.

PATIENT INFORMATION

- Inform patients of the potential risks and benefits of metformin hydrochloride and of alternative modes of therapy. Also inform patients about the importance of adherence to dietary instructions, of a regular exercise program, and of regular testing of blood glucose, glycosylated hemoglobin, renal function, and hematologic parameters.
- Explain the risks of lactic acidosis, its symptoms, and conditions that predispose to its development. Advise patients to discontinue metformin hydrochloride immediately and promptly to notify their health care practitioner if unexplained hyperventilation, myalgia, malaise, unusual somnolence, or other nonspecific symptoms occur. Once a patient is stabilized on any dose level of metformin hydrochloride, gastrointestinal symptoms, which are common during initiation of metformin therapy, are unlikely to be drug related. Later occurrence of gastrointestinal symptoms could be due to lactic acidosis or other serious disease.
- Counsel patients against excessive alcohol intake, acute or chronic, while receiving metformin hydrochloride.
- Metformin hydrochloride alone usually does not cause hypoglycemia, although hypoglycemia may occur when metformin hydrochloride is used along with orally administered sulfonylureas and insulin. When initiating combination therapy, explain the risks of hypoglycemia, its symptoms and treatment, and conditions that predispose to its development to patients and responsible family members.

PREGNANCY AND LACTATION

- Pregnancy Category B. No adequate and well-controlled studies have been performed in pregnant women with metformin hydrochloride. Metformin was not teratogenic in rats and rabbits at doses up to 600 mg/kg per day. Studies in lactating rats show that metformin is excreted into milk and reaches levels comparable to those in plasma. Excretion into human milk is not known.

methadone hydrochloride

(meth'a-done)

Rx: Dolophine

Drug Class: Analgesics, narcotic

Pregnancy Category: B

DEA Class: Schedule II

CLINICAL PHARMACOLOGY

Mechanism of Action: An opioid agonist that binds with opioid receptors in the CNS. *Therapeutic Effect:* Alters the perception of and emotional response to pain; reduces withdrawal symptoms from other opioid drugs.

Pharmacokinetics

Route	*Onset*	*Peak*	*Duration*
Oral	0.5-1 hr	1.5-2 hr	6-8 hr
IM	10-20 min	1-2 hr	4-5 hr
IV	N/A	15-30 min	3-4 hr

Well absorbed after IM injection. Protein binding: 80%-85%. Metabolized in the liver. Primarily excreted in urine. Not removed by hemodialysis. **Half-life:** 15-25 hr.

AVAILABLE FORMS

- *Oral Concentrate (Methadone Intensol, Methadose):* 10 mg/ml.
- *Oral Solution:* 5 mg/5 ml, 10 mg/5 ml.
- *Tablets (Dolophine, Methadose):* 5 mg, 10 mg.
- *Tablets (Dispersible [Methadose]):* 40 mg.
- *Injection (Dolophine):* 10 mg/ml.

INDICATIONS AND DOSAGES

Analgesia

PO, IV, IM, Subcutaneous

Adults. 2.5-10 mg q3-8h as needed up to 5-20 mg q6-8h.

Elderly. 2.5 mg q8-12h.

Children. Initially, 0.1 mg/kg/dose q4h for 2-3 doses, then q6-12h. Maximum: 10 mg/dose.

Detoxification

PO

Adults, Elderly. 15-40 mg/day.

Temporary maintenance treatment of narcotic abstinence syndrome

PO

Adults, Elderly. 20-120 mg/day.

CONTRAINDICATIONS: Delivery of premature infant, diarrhea due to poisoning, hypersensitivity to narcotics, labor

INTERACTIONS

Drug

Alcohol, other CNS depressants: May increase CNS or respiratory depression and hypotension.

MAOIs: May produce a severe, sometimes fatal reaction; plan to administer one quarter of usual methadone dose.

Herbal

Valerian: May increase CNS depression.

Food

None known.

DIAGNOSTIC TEST EFFECTS: May increase serum amylase and lipase levels.

SIDE EFFECTS

Frequent

Sedation, decreased BP (including orthostatic hypotension), diaphoresis, facial flushing, constipation, dizziness, nausea, vomiting

Occasional

Confusion, urine retention, palpitations, abdominal cramps, visual changes, dry mouth, headache, decreased appetite, anxiety, insomnia

Rare

Allergic reaction (rash, pruritus)

SERIOUS REACTIONS

- Overdose results in respiratory depression, skeletal muscle flaccidity, cold or clammy skin, cyanosis, and extreme somnolence progressing to seizures, stupor, and coma. The antidote is 0.4 mg naloxone.

• The patient who uses methadone long-term may develop a tolerance to the drug's analgesic effect and physical dependence.

SPECIAL CONSIDERATIONS

PRECAUTIONS

• Use methadone hydrochloride with caution and in reduced dosage in patients who are concurrently receiving other narcotic analgesics, general anesthetics, phenothiazines, other tranquilizers, sedative-hypnotics, tricyclic antidepressants, and other central nervous system depressants (including alcohol). Respiratory depression, hypotension, and profound sedation or coma may result. The respiratory depressant effects of methadone and its capacity to elevate cerebrospinal fluid pressure may be exaggerated greatly in the presence of increased intracranial pressure. Use methadone hydrochloride with caution in patients having an acute asthmatic attack, in those with chronic obstructive pulmonary disease or cor pulmonale, and in individuals with a substantially decreased respiratory reserve, preexisting respiratory depression, hypoxia, or hypercapnia. Drug administration may result in severe hypotension in individuals whose ability to maintain their blood pressure already has been compromised by a depleted blood volume or concurrent administration of drugs such as the phenothiazines or certain anesthetics. Methadone hydrochloride may obscure the diagnosis or clinical course in patients with acute abdominal conditions. Give methadone hydrochloride with caution in the elderly or debilitated and those with severe impairment of hepatic or renal function, hypothyroidism, Addison's disease, prostatic hypertrophy, or urethral stricture.

PATIENT INFORMATION

• Methadone hydrochloride may impair the mental and/or physical abilities required for the performance of potentially hazardous tasks such as driving a car or operating machinery. Caution the patient accordingly.

PREGNANCY AND LACTATION

• Pregnancy Category C. Fetal harm is not known. Excretion into human milk is not known.

---

methazolamide

(meth-ah-zole'ah-mide)

Rx: Glauctabs, Neptazane

Drug Class: Carbonic anhydrase inhibitors

Pregnancy Category: C

Do not confuse with nefazodone.

M

CLINICAL PHARMACOLOGY

Mechanism of Action: A noncompetitive inhibitor of carbonic anhydrase that inhibits the enzyme at the luminal border of cells of the proximal tubule. Increases urine volume and changes to an alkaline pH with subsequent decreases in the excretion of titratable acid and ammonia. *Therapeutic Effect:* Produces a diuretic and antiglaucoma effect.

Pharmacokinetics

PO route onset 2-4 hrs, peak 6-8 hrs, duration10-18 hrs. Well absorbed slowly from the GI tract. Protein binding: 55%. Distributed into the tissues (including CSF). Metabolized slowly from the gastrointestinal (GI) tract. Partially excreted in urine. Not removed by hemodialysis. **Half-life:** 14 hrs.

AVAILABLE FORMS

• *Tablets:* 25 mg, 50 mg.

INDICATIONS AND DOSAGES

Glaucoma

PO

Adults, Elderly. 50-100 mg/day 2-3 times/day.

UNLABELED USES: Motion sickness, essential tremor

CONTRAINDICATIONS: Kidney or liver dysfunction, severe pulmonary obstruction, hypersensitivity to methazolamide or any component of the formulation

INTERACTIONS

Drug

Amphetamines, quinidine, procainamide, methenamine, phenobarbital, salicylates: May increase the excretion of these drugs.

Aspirin: May increase the risk for anorexia, tachypnea, lethargy, coma and death have been reported when receiving high-dose aspirin and methazolamide concomitantly.

Diuretics: May increase the risk of hypokalemia.

Lithium: May increase the excretion of lithium.

Memantine: May decrease the clearance of memantine.

Steroids: May increase the risk of hypokalemia.

Topiramate: May increase the risk of nephrolithiasis.

Herbal

None known.

Food

None known.

DIAGNOSTIC TEST EFFECTS: *None known.*

SIDE EFFECTS

Occasional

Paresthesias, hearing dysfunction or tinnitus, fatigue, malaise, loss of appetite, taste alteration, nausea, vomiting, diarrhea, polyuria, drowsiness, confusion, hypokalemia

Rare

Metabolic acidosis, electrolyte imbalance, transient myopia, urticaria, melena, hematuria, glycosuria, hepatic insufficiency, flaccid paralysis, photosensitivity, convulsions, and rarely, crystalluria, renal calculi

SERIOUS REACTIONS

• Malaise and complaints of tiredness and myalgia are signs of excessive dosing and acidosis in the elderly.

• Stevens-Johnson syndrome, toxic epidermal necrolysis, fulminant hepatic necrosis, agranulocytosis, aplastic anemia, and other blood dyscrasias have been reported and have caused fatalities.

SPECIAL CONSIDERATIONS

PRECAUTIONS

• Potassium excretion is increased initially upon administration of methazolamide, and in patients with cirrhosis or hepatic insufficiency, potassium excretion could precipitate a hepatic coma.

• In patients with pulmonary obstruction or emphysema, where alveolar ventilation may be impaired, use methazolamide with caution because it may precipitate or aggravate acidosis.

PATIENT INFORMATION

• Adverse reactions common to all sulfonamide derivatives may occur: anaphylaxis, fever, rash (including erythema multiforme, Stevens-Johnson syndrome, and toxic epidermal necrolysis), crystalluria, renal calculus, bone marrow depression, thrombocytopenic purpura, hemolytic anemia, leukopenia, pancytopenia, and agranulocytosis. Precaution is advised for early detection of such reactions and the drug should be discontinued and appropriate therapy instituted.

• Caution is advised for patients receiving high-dose aspirin and methazolamide concomitantly.

PREGNANCY AND LACTATION

• Pregnancy Category C. Methazolamide has been shown to be teratogenic (skeletal anomalies) in rats when given in doses approximately 40 times the human dose. Excretion into human milk is not known.

methotrexate sodium

(meth-oh-trex'ate)

Rx: Rheumatrex Dose Pack, Trexall

Drug Class: Antineoplastics, antimetabolites; Disease modifying antirheumatic drugs

Pregnancy Category: X

Do not confuse Trexall with Trexan.

CLINICAL PHARMACOLOGY

Mechanism of Action: An antimetabolite that competes with enzymes necessary to reduce folic acid to tetrahydrofolic acid, a component essential to DNA, RNA, and protein synthesis. This action inhibits DNA, RNA, and protein synthesis. *Therapeutic Effect:* Causes death of cancer cells.

Pharmacokinetics

Variably absorbed from the GI tract. Completely absorbed after IM administration. Protein binding: 50%-60%. Widely distributed. Metabolized intracellularly in the liver. Primarily excreted in urine. Removed by hemodialysis but not by peritoneal dialysis. **Half-life:** 8-12 hr (large doses, 8-15 hr).

AVAILABLE FORMS

• *Tablets (Rheumatrex):* 2.5 mg.

• *Tablets (Trexall):* 5 mg, 7.5 mg, 10 mg, 15 mg.

• *Injection Solution:* 25 mg/ml.

• *Injection Powder for Reconstitution:* 20 mg, 1 g.

INDICATIONS AND DOSAGES

Trophoblastic neoplasms

PO, IM

Adults, Elderly. 15-30 mg/day for 5 days; repeat in 7 days for 3-5 courses.

Head and neck cancer

PO, IV, IM

Adults, Elderly. 25-50 mg/m^2 once weekly.

Choriocarcinoma, chorioadenoma destruens, hydatidiform mole

PO, IM

Adults, Elderly. 15-30 mg/day for 5 days; repeat 3-5 times with 1-2 wk between courses.

Breast cancer

IV

Adults, Elderly. 30-60 mg/m^2 days 1 and 8 q3-4wk.

Acute lymphocytic leukemia

PO, IV, IM

Adults, Elderly. Induction: 3.3 mg/m^2/day in combination with other chemotherapeutic agents.

Maintenance: 30 mg/m^2/wk PO or IM in divided doses or 2.5 mg/kg IV every 14 days.

Burkitt's lymphoma

PO

Adults. 10-25 mg/day for 4-8 days; repeat with 7- to 10-day rest between courses.

Lymphosarcoma

PO

Adults, Elderly. 0.625-2.5 mg/kg/day.

Mycosis fungoides

PO

Adults, Elderly. 2.5-10 mg/day.

IM

Adults, Elderly. 50 mg/wk or 25 mg twice a week.

Rheumatoid arthritis
PO
Adults, Elderly. 7.5 mg once weekly or 2.5 mg q12h for 3 doses once weekly. Maximum: 20 mg/wk.
Juvenile rheumatoid arthritis
PO, IM, Subcutaneous
Children. 5-15 mg/m^2/wk as a single dose or in 3 divided doses given q12h.
Psoriasis
PO
Adults, Elderly. 10-25 mg once weekly or 2.5-5 mg q12h for 3 doses once weekly.
IM
Adults, Elderly. 10-25 mg once weekly.
Antineoplastic dosage for children
PO, IM
Children. 7.5-30 mg/m^2/wk or q2wk.
IV
Children. 10-33,000 mg/m^2 bolus or continuous infusion over 6-42 hr.
Dosage in renal impairment
Creatinine clearance 61-80 ml/min. Reduce dose by 25%.
Creatinine clearance 51-60 ml/min. Reduce dose by 33%.
Creatinine clearance 10-50 ml/min. Reduce dose by 50%-70%.

UNLABELED USES: Treatment of acute myelocytic leukemia; bladder, cervical, ovarian, prostatic, renal, and testicular carcinomas; psoriatic arthritis; systemic dermatomyositis

CONTRAINDICATIONS: Preexisting myelosuppression, severe hepatic or renal impairment

INTERACTIONS
Drug
Acyclovir (parenteral): May increase the risk of neurotoxicity.
Alcohol, hepatotoxic medications: May increase the risk of hepatotoxicity.
Asparaginase: May decrease the effects of methotrexate.
Bone marrow depressants: May increase myelosuppression.
Live-virus vaccines: May potentiate virus replication, increase vaccine side effects, and decrease the patient's antibody response to the vaccine.
NSAIDs: May increase the risk of methotrexate toxicity.
Probenecid, salicylates: May increase blood methotrexate concentration and risk of toxicity.
Herbal
None known.
Food
None known.

DIAGNOSTIC TEST EFFECTS: May increase serum uric acid and AST (SGOT) levels.

IV INCOMPATIBILITIES: Chlorpromazine (Thorazine), droperidol (Inapsine), gemcitabine (Gemzar), idarubicin (Idamycin), midazolam (Versed), nalbuphine (Nubain)

IV COMPATIBILITIES: Cisplatin (Platinol AQ), cyclophosphamide (Cytoxan), daunorubicin (DaunoXome), doxorubicin (Adriamycin), etoposide (VePesed), 5-fluorouracil, granisetron (Kytril), leucovorin, mitomycin (Mutamycin), ondansetron (Zofran), paclitaxel (Taxol), vinblastine (Velban), vincristine (Oncovin), vinorelbine (Navelbine)

SIDE EFFECTS
Frequent (10%-3%)
Nausea, vomiting, stomatitis; burning and erythema at psoriatic site (in patients with psoriasis)
Occasional (3%-1%)
Diarrhea, rash, dermatitis, pruritus, alopecia, dizziness, anorexia, malaise, headache, drowsiness, blurred vision

SERIOUS REACTIONS
• GI toxicity may produce gingivitis, glossitis, pharyngitis, stomatitis, enteritis, and hematemesis.

• Hepatotoxicity is more likely to occur with frequent small doses than with large intermittent doses.

• Pulmonary toxicity may be characterized by interstitial pneumonitis.

• Hematologic toxicity, which may develop rapidly from marked myelosuppression, may be manifested as leukopenia, thrombocytopenia, anemia, and hemorrhage.

• Dermatologic toxicity may produce a rash, pruritus, urticaria, pigmentation, photosensitivity, petechiae, ecchymosis, and pustules.

• Severe nephrotoxicity may produce azotemia, hematuria, and renal failure.

SPECIAL CONSIDERATIONS

PRECAUTIONS

• Methotrexate has the potential for serious toxicity. Toxic effects may be related in frequency and severity to dose or frequency of administration but have been seen at all doses. Because toxic effects can occur at any time during therapy, it is necessary to follow patients closely who are taking methotrexate. If vomiting, diarrhea, or stomatitis occur, which may result in dehydration, discontinue methotrexate until recovery occurs. Use methotrexate with extreme caution in the presence of peptic ulcer disease or ulcerative colitis. Methotrexate can suppress hematopoiesis and cause anemia, leukopenia, and/or thrombocytopenia. In patients with psoriasis and rheumatoid arthritis, stop methotrexate immediately if there is a significant drop in blood counts. Methotrexate has the potential for acute (elevated transaminases) and chronic (fibrosis and cirrhosis) hepatotoxicity. In patients with rheumatoid arthritis, age at first use of methotrexate and duration of therapy have been reported as risk factors for hepatotoxicity; other risk factors, similar to those observed in patients with psoriasis, may be present in patients with rheumatoid arthritis but have not been confirmed to date.

• Use methotrexate with extreme caution in the presence of active infection; it usually is contraindicated in patients with overt or laboratory evidence of immunodeficiency syndromes. Hypogammaglobulinemia has been reported rarely. Leukoencephalopathy following intravenous administration of methotrexate to patients who have had craniospinal irradiation has been reported. A transient acute neurologic syndrome has been observed in patients treated with high-dosage regimens. Pulmonary symptoms (especially a dry, nonproductive cough) or a nonspecific pneumonitis occurring during methotrexate therapy may be indicative of a potentially dangerous lesion and require interruption of treatment and careful investigation. High doses of methotrexate used to treat osteosarcoma may cause renal damage leading to acute renal failure. Severe, occasionally fatal, dermatologic reactions, including toxic epidermal necrolysis, Stevens-Johnson syndrome, exfoliative dermatitis, skin necrosis, and erythema multiforme, have been reported in children and adults, within days of oral, intramuscular, intravenous, or intrathecal methotrexate administration. Use methotrexate with extreme caution in the presence of debility. Lesions of psoriasis may be aggravated by concomitant exposure to ultraviolet radiation. Radiation dermatitis and sunburn may be "recalled" by the use of methotrexate.

PATIENT INFORMATION

• Inform patients of the early signs and symptoms of toxicity, of the need to see their physician promptly if these signs occur, and of the need for close follow-up, including periodic laboratory tests to monitor toxicity.

• The physician and pharmacist should emphasize to the patient that the recommended dose is taken weekly for rheumatoid arthritis and psoriasis and that mistaken daily use of the recommended dose has led to fatal toxicity. Encourage patients to read the patient instructions sheet within the dose pack. Do not write or refill prescriptions on an as-needed basis.

• Inform patients of the potential benefit and risk in the use of methotrexate. Discuss the risk of effects on reproduction with male and female patients taking methotrexate.

PREGNANCY AND LACTATION

• Pregnancy Category D. Psoriasis and rheumatoid arthritis: Methotrexate is in Pregnancy Category X. Because of the potential for serious adverse reactions from methotrexate in breast-fed infants, its use is contraindicated in nursing mothers.

methoxsalen

(meth-ox'a-len)

Rx: 8-Mop, Oxsoralen, Uvadex

Drug Class: Photosensitizers; Psoralens

Pregnancy Category: C

Do not confuse with methsuximide or methotrexate.

CLINICAL PHARMACOLOGY

Mechanism of Action: A member of the family of psoralens that induces an augmented sunburn reaction followed by hyperpigmentation in the presence of long-wave ultraviolet radiation. Bonds covalently to pyrimidine bases in DNA, inhibits the synthesis of DNA, and suppresses cell division. The augmented sunburn reaction involves excitation of the methoxsalen molecule by radiation in the long-wave ultraviolet light (UVA), resulting in transference of energy to the methoxsalen molecule producing an excited state or "triplet electronic state." The molecule, in this "triplet state," then reacts with cutaneous DNA. *Therapeutic Effect:* Results in symptomatic control of severe, recalcitrant disabling psoriasis, repigmentation of idiopathic vitiligo, palliative treatment of skin manifestations of cutaneous T-cell lymphoma (CTCL), repigmentation of idiopathic vitiligo, and palliative treatment of skin manifestations of CTCL.

Pharmacokinetics

Absorption varies. Food increases peak serum levels. Reversibly bound to albumin. Metabolized in the liver. Excreted in the urine. **Half-life:** 2 hrs.

AVAILABLE FORMS

• *Capsule:* 10 mg (8-MOP).

• *Gelcap:* 10 mg (Oxsoralen-Ultra).

• *Lotion:* 1% (Oxsoralen).

• *Solution:* 20 mcg/ml (Uvadex).

INDICATIONS AND DOSAGES

Psoriasis

PO

Adults, Elderly. 10-70 mg 1.5 -2 hrs before exposure to UVA light, repeated 2-3 times/week. Give at least 48 hours apart. Dosage is based upon patient's body weight and skin type:

Less than 30 kg: 10 mg, *30-50 kg:* 20 mg, *51-65 kg:* 30 mg, *66-80 kg:* 40 mg, *81-90 kg:* 50 mg, *91-115 kg:* 60 mg, *more than 115 kg:* 70 mg.

Vitiligo

PO

Adults, Elderly, Children older than 12 yr. 20 mg 2-4 hrs before exposure to UVA light. Give at least 48 hours apart.

Topical

Adults, Elderly, Children older than 12 yr. Apply 1-2 hrs before exposure to UVA light, no more than once weekly.

CTCL

Extracorporeal

Adults, Elderly. Inject 200 mcg into the photoactivation bag during collection cycle using the UVAR photopheresis system, 2 consecutive days every 4 weeks for a minimum of 7 treatment cycles.

UNLABELED USES: Dermographism, eczema, hypereosinophilic syndrome, hypopigmented sarcoidosis, ichthyosis linearis circumflexa, lymphomatoid papulosis, mycosis fungoides, palmoplantar pustulosis, pruritus, scleromyxedema, systemic sclerosis

CONTRAINDICATIONS: Cataract, invasive squamous cell cancer, aphakia, melanoma, pregnancy (Uvadex), diseases associated with photosensitivity, hypersensitivity to methoxsalen (psoralens) or any component of the formulation

INTERACTIONS

Drug

Caffeine: May inhibit caffeine metabolism.

Phenytoin, fosphenytoin: May decrease the effectiveness of methoxsalen.

Herbal

None known.

Food

None known.

SIDE EFFECTS

Occasional

Nausea, pruritus, edema, hypotension, nervousness, vertigo, depression, dizziness, headache, malaise, painful blistering, burning, rash, urticaria, loss of muscle coordination, leg cramps

SERIOUS REACTIONS

- Hypersensitivity reaction, such as nausea and severe burns, may occur.

SPECIAL CONSIDERATIONS

PRECAUTIONS

- Patients must not sunbathe during the 24 hours before methoxsalen ingestion and UV exposure.

PREGNANCY AND LACTATION

- Pregnancy Category C. Fetal harm is not known. Excretion into human milk is not known.

OCULAR CONSIDERATIONS

- Cataractogenicity
- Animal Studies: Exposure to large doses of UVA causes cataracts in animals, and this effect is enhanced by the administration of methoxsalen.
- Human Studies: The concentration of methoxsalen in the lens has been found to be proportional to the serum level. If the lens is exposed to UVA during the time methoxsalen is present in the lens, photochemical action may lead to irreversible binding of methoxsalen to proteins and the DNA components of the lens. However, if the lens is shielded from UVA, the methoxsalen will diffuse out of the lens in a 24-hour period. Advise patients emphatically to wear UVA absorbing, wrap-around sunglasses for the 24-hour period following ingestion of methoxsalen whether exposed to direct or indirect sunlight in the open or through window glass.

• Among patients using proper eye protection, there is no evidence for a significantly increased risk of cataracts in association with psoralen plus UVA therapy. Thirty-five of 1380 patients have developed cataracts in the 5 years since their first psoralen plus UVA treatment. This incidence is comparable to that expected in a population of this size and age distribution. No relationship between psoralen plus UVA dose and cataract risk in this group has been noted.

---

methyldopa

(meth-ill-doe′pa)

Rx: Aldomet, Methyldopate

Drug Class: Antiadrenergics, central

Pregnancy Category: B

Do not confuse Aldomet with Anzemet.

CLINICAL PHARMACOLOGY

Mechanism of Action: An antihypertensive agent that stimulates central inhibitory alpha-adrenergic receptors, lowers arterial pressure, and reduces plasma renin activity. *Therapeutic Effect:* Reduces BP.

AVAILABLE FORMS

- *Tablets:* 250 mg, 500 mg.
- *Injection:* 50 mg/ml.

INDICATIONS AND DOSAGES

Moderate to severe hypertension

PO

Adults. Initially, 250 mg 2-3 times a day for 2 days. Adjust dosage at intervals of 2 days (minimum).

Elderly. Initially, 125 mg 1-2 times a day. May increase by 125 mg q2-3 days. Maintenance: 500 mg to 2 g/day in 2-4 divided doses.

Children. Initially, 10 mg/kg/day in 2-4 divided doses. Adjust dosage at intervals of 2 days (minimum). Maximum: 65 mg/kg/day or 3 g/day, whichever is less.

IV

Adults. 250-1000 mg q6-8h. Maximum: 4 g/day.

Children. Initially, 2-4 mg/kg/dose. May increase to 5-10 mg/kg/dose in 4-6h if no response. Maximum: 65 mg/kg/day or 3 g/day, whichever is less.

CONTRAINDICATIONS: Hepatic disease, pheochromocytoma

INTERACTIONS

Drug

Hypotensive-producing medications, such as antihypertensives and diuretics: May increase the effects of methyldopa.

Lithium: May increase the risk of lithium toxicity.

MAOIs: May cause hyperexcitability.

NSAIDs, tricyclic antidepressants: May decrease the effects of methyldopa.

Other sympathomimetics: May decrease the effects of sympathomimetics.

Herbal

None known.

Food

None known.

DIAGNOSTIC TEST EFFECTS: May increase BUN and serum prolactin, alkaline phosphatase, bilirubin, creatinine, potassium, sodium, uric acid, AST (SGOT), and ALT (SGPT) levels. May produce false-positive Coombs' test and prolong prothrombin time.

SIDE EFFECTS

Frequent

Peripheral edema, somnolence, headache, dry mouth

Occasional

Mental changes (such as anxiety, depression), decreased sexual function or libido, diarrhea, swelling of breasts, nausea, vomiting, lightheadedness, paraesthesia, rhinitis

SERIOUS REACTIONS

• Hepatotoxicity (abnormal liver function test results, jaundice, hepatitis), hemolytic anemia, unexplained fever and flu-like symptoms may occur. If these conditions appear, discontinue the medication and contact the physician.

SPECIAL CONSIDERATIONS

PRECAUTIONS

• Use methyldopa with caution in patients with a history of previous liver disease or dysfunction. Some patients taking methyldopa experience clinical edema or weight gain that may be controlled by use of a diuretic. Hypertension has recurred occasionally after dialysis in patients.

PREGNANCY AND LACTATION

• Tablets: Pregnancy Category B; injection: Pregnancy Category C. Published reports of the use of methyldopa tablets during all trimesters indicate that if this drug is used during pregnancy, the possibility of fetal harm appears remote. Whether methyldopate hydrochloride injection can effect reproduction capacity or can cause fetal harm when given to a pregnant woman is not known. Methyldopa crosses the placental barrier, appears in cord blood, and appears in breast milk.

methylphenidate hydrochloride

(meth-ill-fen'i-date)

Rx: Concerta, Metadate CD, Metadate ER, Methylin, Methylin ER, Ritalin, Ritalin LA, Ritalin-SR

Drug Class: Stimulants, central nervous system

Pregnancy Category: C

DEA Class: Schedule II

Do not confuse Ritalin with Rifadin.

CLINICAL PHARMACOLOGY

Mechanism of Action: A CNS stimulant that blocks the reuptake of norepinephrine and dopamine into presynaptic neurons. *Therapeutic Effect:* Decreases motor restlessness and fatigue; increases motor activity, attention span, and mental alertness; produces mild euphoria.

Pharmacokinetics

Onset	*Peak*	*Duration*
Immediate-release	2 hr	3-5 hr
Sustained-release	4-7 hr	3-8 hr
Extended-release	N/A	8-12 hr

Slowly and incompletely absorbed from the GI tract. Protein binding: 15%. Metabolized in the liver. Eliminated in urine and in feces by biliary system. Unknown if removed by hemodialysis. **Half-life:** 2-4 hr.

AVAILABLE FORMS

• *Capsules (Extended-Release [Metadate CD]):* 10 mg, 20 mg, 30 mg.

• *Capsules (Extended-Release [Ritalin LA]):* 20 mg, 30 mg, 40 mg.

• *Tablets (Ritalin):* 5 mg, 10 mg, 20 mg.

M

• *Tablets (Extended-Release [Mentadate ER, Mehtylin ER]):* 10 mg, 20 mg.
• *Tablets (Extended-Release [Concerta]):* 18 mg, 27 mg, 36 mg, 54 mg, 72 mg.
• *Tablets (Sustained-Release [Ritalin SR]):* 20 mg.
• *Tablets (Chewable [Methylin]):* 2.5 mg, 5 mg, 10 mg.
• *Oral Solution (Methylin):* 5 mg/5 ml, 10 mg/5 ml.

INDICATIONS AND DOSAGES

Attention deficit hyperactivity disorder (ADHD)

PO

Children 6 yr and older. Immediate release: Initially, 2.5-5 mg before breakfast and lunch. May increase by 5-10 mg/day at weekly intervals. Maximum: 60 mg/day.

PO (Concerta)

Children 6 yr and older. Initially, 18 mg once a day; may increase by 18 mg/day at weekly intervals. Maximum: 72 mg/day.

PO (Metadate CD)

Children 6 yr and older. Initially, 20 mg/day. May increase by 20 mg/day at weekly intervals. Maximum: 60 mg/day.

PO (Ritalin LA)

Children 6 yr and older. Initially, 20 mg/day. May increase by 10 mg/day at weekly intervals. Maximum: 60 mg/day.

Narcolepsy

PO

Adults, Elderly. 10 mg 2-3 times a day. Range: 10-60 mg/day.

UNLABELED USES: Treatment of secondary mental depression

CONTRAINDICATIONS: Use within 14 days of MAOIs

INTERACTIONS

Drug

MAOIs: May increase the effects of methylphenidate.

Other CNS stimulants: May have an additive effect.

Herbal

None known.

Food

None known.

DIAGNOSTIC TEST EFFECTS: *None known.*

SIDE EFFECTS

Frequent

Anxiety, insomnia, anorexia

Occasional

Dizziness, drowsiness, headache, nausea, abdominal pain, fever, rash, arthralgia, vomiting

Rare

Blurred vision, Tourette syndrome (marked by uncontrolled vocal outbursts, repetitive body movements, and tics), palpitations

SERIOUS REACTIONS

• Prolonged administration to children with ADHD may delay growth.
• Overdose may produce tachycardia, palpitations, arrhythmias,chest pain, psychotic episode, seizures, and coma.
• Hypersensitivity reactions and blood dyscrasias occur rarely.

SPECIAL CONSIDERATIONS

PRECAUTIONS

• Periodic complete blood count, differential, and platelet count are advised during prolonged therapy.

PATIENT INFORMATION

• Inform patients that Concerta should be swallowed whole with the aid of liquids. Instruct patients not to chew, divide, or crush tablets. The medication is contained within a nonabsorbable shell designed to release the drug at a controlled rate. The tablet shell, along with insoluble core components, is eliminated from the body; patients should not be concerned if they occasionally notice in their stool something that looks like a tablet. To ensure safe and effective use of Concerta, discuss with patients the information and instructions provided in the patient information.

PREGNANCY AND LACTATION

• Pregnancy Category C. Methylphenidate has been shown to have teratogenic effects in rabbits. Adequate animal reproduction studies to establish safe use of Ritalin during pregnancy have not been conducted. Whether methylphenidate is excreted in human milk is not known.

OCULAR CONSIDERATIONS

• Methylphenidate hydrochloride can cause mydriasis and reduction of intraocular pressure. Symptoms of visual disturbances have been encountered in rare cases. Difficulties with accommodation and blurring of vision have been reported.

methylprednisolone acetate

(meth-ill-pred'nis-oh-lone ass'eh-tate)

Drug Class: Corticosteroids

Pregnancy Category: B

Do not confuse with Mebaral or medroxyprogesterone.

CLINICAL PHARMACOLOGY

Mechanism of Action: An adrenal corticosteroid that suppresses migration of polymorphonuclear leukocytes, reverses increased capillary permeability. *Therapeutic Effect:* Decreases inflammation.

Pharmacokinetics

Route	*Onset*	*Peak*	*Duration*
IM	N/A	4- 8 days	1- 4 wks

Well absorbed from the gastrointestinal (GI) tract after IM administration. Widely distributed. Metabolized in liver. Excreted in urine. Removed by hemodialysis. **Half-life:** longer than 3. 5 hrs.

AVAILABLE FORMS

• *Injection:* 20 mg/ml, 40 mg/ml, 80 mg/ml (Depo-Medrol).

INDICATIONS AND DOSAGES

Substitution therapy of deficiency states: acute or chronic adrenal insufficiency, adrenal insufficiency secondary to pituitary insufficiency, congenital adrenal hyperplasia, and nonendocrine disorders, such as allergic, collagen, intestinal tract, liver, ocular, renal, and skin diseases, arthritis, bronchial asthma, cerebral edema, malignancies, and rheumatic carditis

IM (Methylprednisolone Acetate)

Adults, Elderly. 10-80 mg/day.

CONTRAINDICATIONS: Administration of live-virus vaccines, systemic fungal infection, hypersensitivity to methylprednisolone or any component of the formulation

INTERACTIONS

Drug

Amphotericin: May increase hypokalemia.

Digoxin: May increase the risk of toxicity of this drug caused by hypokalemia.

Diuretics, insulin, oral hypoglycemics, potassium supplements: May decrease the effects of diuretics, insulin, oral hypoglycemics, and potassium supplements.

Liver enzyme inducers: May decrease the effects of methylprednisolone.

Live-virus vaccines: May decrease the patient's antibody response to vaccine, increase vaccine side effects, and potentiate virus replication.

Herbal

None known.

Food

None known.

DIAGNOSTIC TEST EFFECTS: May decrease serum calcium, potassium, and thyroxine levels. May increase blood glucose levels, serum lipids, amylase, and sodium levels. May interfere with skin tests.

SIDE EFFECTS

Frequent

Insomnia, heartburn, nervousness, abdominal distention, diaphoresis, acne, mood swings, increased appetite, facial flushing, GI distress, delayed wound healing, increased susceptibility to infection, diarrhea or constipation

Occasional

Headache, edema, tachycardia, change in skin color, frequent urination, depression

Rare

Psychosis, increased blood coagulability, hallucinations

SERIOUS REACTIONS

• The serious reactions of long-term therapy are hypocalcemia, hypokalemia, muscle wasting, especially in arms and legs, osteoporosis, spontaneous fractures, amenorrhea, cataracts, glaucoma, peptic ulcer disease, and congestive heart failure (CHF).

• Abruptly withdrawing the drug after long-term therapy may cause anorexia, nausea, fever, headache, sudden severe joint pain, rebound inflammation, fatigue, weakness, lethargy, dizziness, and orthostatic hypotension.

methylprednisolone sodium succinate

(meth-il-pred-nis'oh-lone)

Drug Class: Corticosteroids

Pregnancy Category: C

Do not confuse with Mebaral or medroxyprogesterone.

CLINICAL PHARMACOLOGY

Mechanism of Action: An adrenal corticosteroid that suppresses migration of polymorphonuclear leukocytes, reverses increased capillary permeability. *Therapeutic Effect:* Decreases inflammation.

Pharmacokinetics

Well absorbed from the gastrointestinal (GI) tract after IM administration. Widely distributed. Metabolized in liver. Excreted in urine. Removed by hemodialysis. **Half-life:** longer than 3.5 hrs

AVAILABLE FORMS

• *Powder for Injection:* 40 mg, 125 mg, 500 mg, 1 g, 2 g (A-Methapred, Solu-Medrol).

INDICATIONS AND DOSAGES

Substitution therapy of deficiency states: acute or chronic adrenal insufficiency, adrenal insufficiency secondary to pituitary insufficiency, congenital adrenal hyperplasia, and nonendocrine disorders, such as allergic, collagen, intestinal tract, liver, ocular, renal, and skin diseases, arthritis, bronchial asthma, cerebral edema, malignancies, and rheumatic carditis

IV

Adults, Elderly. 40-250 mg q4-6h. High dose: 30 mg/kg over at least 30 min. Repeat q4-6h for 48-72 hrs.

Intra-articular, intralesional

Adults, Elderly. 4-40 mg, up to 80 mg q1-5wks.

CONTRAINDICATIONS: Administration of live virus vaccines, systemic fungal infection, hypersensitivity to methylprednisolone sodium succinate or any component of the formulation

INTERACTIONS

Drug

Amphotericin: May increase hypokalemia.

Digoxin: May increase the risk of toxicity of this drug caused by hypokalemia.

Diuretics, insulin, oral hypoglycemics, potassium supplements: May decrease the effects of diuretics, insulin, oral hypoglycemics, and potassium supplements.

Liver enzyme inducers: May decrease the effects of methylprednisolone.

Live-virus vaccines: May decrease the patient's antibody response to vaccine, increase vaccine side effects, and potentiate virus replication.

Herbal

None known.

Food

None known.

DIAGNOSTIC TEST EFFECTS: May decrease serum calcium, potassium, and thyroxine levels. May increase blood glucose levels, serum lipids, amylase, and sodium levels. May interfere with skin tests.

IV INCOMPATIBILITIES: Ciprofloxacin (Cipro), diltiazem (Cardizem), docetaxel (Taxotere), etoposide (VePesid), filgrastim (Neupogen), gemcitabine (Gemzar), paclitaxel (Taxol), potassium chloride, propofol (Diprivan), vinorelbine (Navelbine)

IV COMPATIBILITIES: Dopamine (Intropin), heparin, midazolam (Versed), theophylline

SIDE EFFECTS

Frequent

Insomnia, heartburn, nervousness, abdominal distention, diaphoresis, acne, mood swings, increased appetite, facial flushing, GI distress, delayed wound healing, increased susceptibility to infection, diarrhea or constipation

Occasional

Headache, edema, tachycardia, change in skin color, frequent urination, depression

Rare

Psychosis, increased blood coagulability, hallucinations

SERIOUS REACTIONS

- The serious reactions of long-term therapy are hypocalcemia, hypokalemia, muscle wasting, especially in arms and legs, osteoporosis, spontaneous fractures, amenorrhea, cataracts, glaucoma, peptic ulcer disease, and congestive heart failure (CHF).
- Abruptly withdrawing the drug after long-term therapy may cause anorexia, nausea, fever, headache, sudden severe joint pain, rebound inflammation, fatigue, weakness, lethargy, dizziness, and orthostatic hypotension.

SPECIAL CONSIDERATIONS

PRECAUTIONS

- Average and large doses of cortisone or hydrocortisone can cause elevation of blood pressure, salt and water retention, and increased excretion of potassium. All corticosteroids increase calcium excretion.
- Administration of live or live attenuated vaccines is contraindicated in patients receiving immunosuppressive doses of corticosteroids.
- The use of methylprednisolone acetate in patients with active tuberculosis should be restricted to those cases of fulminating or dissemi-

nated tuberculosis in which the corticosteroid is used for the management of the disease along with an appropriate antituberculous regimen.

• If corticosteroids are indicated in patients with latent tuberculosis or tuberculin reactivity, close observation is necessary because reactivation of the disease may occur. During prolonged corticosteroid therapy, these patients should receive chemoprophylaxis.

• Because rare instances of anaphylactoid reactions have occurred in patients receiving parenteral corticosteroid therapy, take appropriate precautionary measures before administration, especially when the patient has a history of allergy to any drug.

• Persons who are taking drugs that suppress the immune system are more susceptible to infections than healthy individuals. Chickenpox and measles, for example, can have a more serious or even fatal course in nonimmune children or adults taking corticosteroids. In such children or adults who have not had these diseases, advise them to take particular care to avoid exposure.

• Similarly, use corticosteroids with great care in patients with known or suspected *Strongyloides* (threadworm) infestation.

• Minimize drug-induced secondary adrenocortical insufficiency by gradual reduction of dosage. This type of relative insufficiency may persist for months after discontinuation of therapy; therefore in any situation of stress occurring during that period, reinstate hormone therapy. Because mineralocorticoid secretion may be impaired, administer salt and/or a mineralocorticoid concurrently. An enhanced effect of corticosteroids occurs in patients with hypothyroidism and in those with cirrhosis.

• Psychic derangements may appear when corticosteroids are used, ranging from euphoria, insomnia, mood swings, personality changes, and severe depression to frank psychotic manifestations. Also, corticosteroids may aggravate existing emotional instability or psychotic tendencies.

• Use steroids with caution in patients with nonspecific ulcerative colitis, if there is a probability of impending perforation, abscess, or other pyogenic infection. Use caution also in patients with diverticulitis, fresh intestinal anastomoses, active or latent peptic ulcer, renal insufficiency, hypertension, osteoporosis, and myasthenia gravis when steroids are used as direct or adjunctive therapy.

• Carefully follow the growth and development of infants and children on prolonged corticosteroid therapy.

• Kaposi sarcoma has been reported to occur in patients receiving corticosteroid therapy.

PREGNANCY AND LACTATION

• Pregnancy Category B. Because adequate human reproduction studies have not been done with corticosteroids, the use of these drugs in pregnancy, nursing mothers, or women of childbearing potential requires that the possible benefits of the drug be weighed against the potential hazards to the mother and embryo or fetus. Carefully observe infants born of mothers who have received substantial doses of corticosteroids during pregnancy for signs of hypoadrenalism.

PATIENT INFORMATION

• Warn patients who are taking immunosuppressant doses of corticosteroids to avoid exposure to chickenpox or measles. Advise patients that if they are exposed, they should seek medical advice without delay.

OCULAR CONSIDERATIONS

• **PRECAUTION:** Use corticosteroids cautiously in patients with ocular herpes simplex for fear of corneal perforation.

• Ocular Indications and Usage: Anterior uveitis, chorioretinitis, diffuse posterior uveitis and choroiditis, pars planitis, optic neuritis, sympathetic ophthalmia, acute retinal necrosis, and anterior segment inflammation

• Ocular Contraindications: Prolonged use of corticosteroids may produce posterior subcapsular cataracts and glaucoma with possible damage to the optic nerves and may enhance the establishment of secondary ocular infections caused by fungi or viruses.

• Ocular Adverse Reactions: Posterior subcapsular cataracts, increased intraocular pressure, glaucoma, and exophthalmos

• Ocular Injection: Temporary or permanent visual impairment including blindness; increased intraocular pressure; ocular and periocular inflammation including allergic reactions, infection, residue, or slough at injection site

OCULAR DOSAGE AND ADMINISTRATION

• Anterior Uveitis: Periocular repository steroids 40 to 80 mg subtenons if uveitis is severe and is not responding well to topical steroids at full strength for 6 weeks

• Optic Neuritis: Vision 20/50 or worse, methylprednisolone 250 mg IV given over 30 minutes q6h for 12 doses, followed by prednisone 1 mg/kg per day PO for 11 days, then 20 mg for 1 day, and then 15 mg every other day for doses.

• Pars Planitis: Methylprednisolone 40 mg subtenons repeated every 1 to 2 months until vision and cystoid macular edema are no longer improving, and then slowly taper frequency of injections

• Acute Retinal Necrosis: Some administer methylprednisolone 250 mg IV qid for 3 days followed by prednisone 60 mg PO bid for 1 to 2 weeks. Others wait 1 to 2 weeks until retinitis clears, and administer prednisone 60 to 80 mg/day for 1 to 2 weeks followed by taper over 2 to 6 weeks.

• For an intraocular foreign body and traumatic optic neuropathy in the presence of sinus wall fracture or penetrating orbital injury, consider methylprednisolone 250 mg IV q6h for 12 doses plus ranitidine 150 mg orally bid (treatment is controversial).

M

metipranolol hydrochloride

(met-ee-pran'oh-lol)

Rx: OptiPranolol

Drug Class: Antiadrenergics, beta blocking; Ophthalmics

Pregnancy Category: C

Do not confuse with metoprolol or propranolol.

CLINICAL PHARMACOLOGY

Mechanism of Action: An antiglaucoma agent that nonselectively blocks beta-adrenergic receptors. Reduces aqueous humor production. *Therapeutic Effect:* Reduces intraocular pressure (IOP).

Pharmacokinetics

Route	Onset	Peak	Duration
Eye drops	0.5-3 hrs	2-7 hrs	24 hrs or more

Systemic absorption may occur.

AVAILABLE FORMS

- *Ophthalmic Solution:* 0.3% (OptiPranolol).

INDICATIONS AND DOSAGES

Glaucoma, ocular hypertension

Ophthalmic

Adults, Elderly. Instill 1 drop 2 times/day.

CONTRAINDICATIONS: Bronchial asthma or chronic obstructive pulmonary disease, cardiogenic shock, overt cardiac failure, second or third degree heart AV block, severe sinus bradycardia, hypersensitivity to metipranolol or any component of the formulation.

INTERACTIONS

Drug

None known.

Herbal

None known.

Food

None known.

DIAGNOSTIC TEST EFFECTS: *None known.*

SIDE EFFECTS

Frequent

Eye burning/stinging, hyperemia, blurred vision, headache, fatigue

Occasional

Sensitivity to light, dizziness, hypotension

Rare

Dry eye, conjunctivitis, eye pain, rash, muscle pain

SERIOUS REACTIONS

- Ophthalmic overdosage may produce bradycardia, hypotension, bronchospasm, and acute cardiac failure.
- Arrhythmias and myocardial infarction have been reported.
- Ocular Adverse Reactions: Transient local discomfort, conjunctivitis, eyelid dermatitis, blepharitis, blurred vision, tearing, browache, abnormal vision, photophobia, and edema may occur.

SPECIAL CONSIDERATIONS

PRECAUTIONS

- Use metipranolol hydrochloride with caution in patients with cerebrovascular insufficiency. Gradual withdrawal of beta-adrenergic receptor blocking agents in patients undergoing elective surgery is recommended. Use caution in patients with diabetes (especially labile diabetes) because of possible masking of signs and symptoms of acute hypoglycemia. Metipranolol hydrochloride may mask certain signs and symptoms of hyperthyroidism. Metipranolol hydrochloride is reported to potentiate muscle weakness consistent with certain myasthenic symptoms (e.g., diplopia, ptosis, and generalized weakness). Patients with a history of severe anaphylactic reaction may be unresponsive to the usual doses of epinephrine used to treat allergic reaction.
- Ocular: With angle-closure glaucoma, use metipranolol hydrochloride only with concomitant administration of a miotic agent.

PREGNANCY AND LACTATION

- Pregnancy Category C. Metipranolol hydrochloride is shown to increase fetal resorption, fetal death, and delayed development when administered orally to rabbits. Fetal harm is not known with topical administration. Excretion into human milk is not known.

metoprolol tartrate

(me-toe'pro-lole)

Rx: Lopressor, Toprol XL

Drug Class: Antiadrenergics, beta blocking

Pregnancy Category: C

Do not confuse metoprolol with metaproterenol or metolazone.

CLINICAL PHARMACOLOGY

Mechanism of Action: An antianginal, antihypertensive, and MI adjunct that selectively blocks $beta_1$-adrenergic receptors; high dosages may block $beta_2$-adrenergic receptors. Decreases oxygen requirements. Large doses increase airway resistance. *Therapeutic Effect:* Slows sinus node heart rate, decreases cardiac output, and reduces BP. Also decreases myocardial ischemia severity.

Pharmacokinetics

Route	Onset	Peak	Duration
PO	10-15 min	N/A	6 hr
PO (extended release)	N/A	6-12 hr	24 hr
IV	Immediate	20 min	5-8 hr

Well absorbed from the GI tract. Protein binding: 12%. Widely distributed. Metabolized in the liver (undergoes significant first-pass metabolism). Primarily excreted in urine. Removed by hemodialysis. **Half-life:** 3-7 hr.

AVAILABLE FORMS

- *Tablets (Lopressor):* 25 mg, 50 mg, 100 mg.
- *Tablets (Extended-Release [Toprol XL]):* 25 mg, 50 mg, 100 mg, 200 mg.
- *Injection (Lopressor):* 1 mg/ml.

INDICATIONS AND DOSAGES

Mild to moderate hypertension

PO

Adults. Initially, 100 mg/day as single or divided dose. Increase at weekly (or longer) intervals. Maintenance: 100-450 mg/day.

Elderly. Initially, 25 mg/day. Range: 25-300 mg/day.

PO (Extended-Release)

Adults. 50-100 mg/day as single dose. May increase at least at weekly intervals until optimum BP attained. Maximum: 200 mg/day.

Chronic, stable angina pectoris

PO

Adults. Initially, 100 mg/day as single or divided dose. Increase at weekly (or longer) intervals. Maintenance: 100-450 mg/day.

PO (Extended-Release)

Adults. Initially, 100 mg/day as single dose. May increase at least at weekly intervals until optimum clinical response achieved. Maximum: 200 mg/day.

Congestive heart failure

PO (Extended-Release)

Adults. Initially, 25 mg/day. May double dose q2wk. Maximum: 200 mg/day.

Early treatment of MI

IV

Adults. 5 mg q2min for 3 doses, followed by 50 mg orally q6h for 48 hr. Begin oral dose 15 min after last IV dose. Or, in patients who do not tolerate full IV dose, give 25-50 mg orally q6h, 15 min after last IV dose.

Late treatment and maintenance after an MI

PO

Adults. 100 mg twice a day for at least 3 mo.

UNLABELED USES: To increase survival rate in diabetic patients with coronary artery disease (CAD); treatment or prevention of anxiety; cardiac arrhythmias; hypertrophic cardiomyopathy; mitral valve prolapse syndrome; pheochromocytoma; tremors; thyrotoxicosis; vascular headache

CONTRAINDICATIONS: Cardiogenic shock, MI with a heart rate less than 45 beats/minute or systolic BP less than 100 mm Hg, overt heart failure, second- or third-degree heart block, sinus bradycardia

INTERACTIONS

Drug

Cimetidine: May increase metoprolol blood concentration.

Diuretics, other antihypertensives: May increase hypotensive effect.

Insulin, oral hypoglycemics: May mask symptoms of hypoglycemia and prolong hypoglycemic effect of these drugs.

NSAIDs: May decrease antihypertensive effect.

Sympathomimetics, xanthines: May mutually inhibit effects.

Herbal

None known.

Food

None known.

DIAGNOSTIC TEST EFFECTS: May increase serum antinuclear antibody titer and BUN, serum lipoprotein, serum LDH, serum alkaline phosphatase, serum bilirubin, serum creatinine, serum potassium, serum uric acid, AST (SGOT), ALT (SGPT), and serum triglyceride levels.

IV INCOMPATIBILITIES: Amphotericin B complex (Abelcet, AmBisome, Amphotec)

IV COMPATIBILITIES: Alteplase (Activase)

SIDE EFFECTS

Metoprolol is generally well tolerated, with transient and mild side effects.

Frequent

Diminished sexual function, drowsiness, insomnia, unusual fatigue or weakness

Occasional

Anxiety, nervousness, diarrhea, constipation, nausea, vomiting, nasal congestion, abdominal discomfort, dizziness, difficulty breathing, cold hands or feet

Rare

Altered taste, dry eyes, nightmares, paraesthesia, allergic reaction (rash, pruritus)

SERIOUS REACTIONS

- Overdose may produce profound bradycardia, hypotension, and bronchospasm.
- Abrupt withdrawal of metoprolol may result in diaphoresis, palpitations, headache, tremulousness, exacerbation of angina, MI, and ventricular arrhythmias.
- Metoprolol administration may precipitate CHF and MI in patients with heart disease; thyroid storm in those with thyrotoxicosis; and peripheral ischemia in those with existing peripheral vascular disease.
- Hypoglycemia may occur in patients with previously controlled diabetes.

SPECIAL CONSIDERATIONS

PRECAUTIONS

- Use metoprolol with caution in patients with impaired hepatic function. use metoprolol with caution in diabetic patients if a beta-blocking agent is required. Patients with bronchospastic diseases should not receive beta-blockers. Metoprolol produces a decrease in sinus heart rate in most patients. Beta-adrenergic blockade may mask certain clinical signs (e.g., tachycardia) of hyperthyroidism. Sympathetic stimulation is a vital component supporting circulatory function in congestive heart failure, and beta-blockade carries the potential hazard of further depressing myocardial contractility and precipitating more severe failure.

PATIENT INFORMATION

- Advise patients to take metoprolol regularly and continuously as directed with or immediately following meals. If the patient misses a dose, instruct the patient to take only the next scheduled dose (without doubling it). Patients should not discontinue metoprolol without consulting the physician.
- Advise patients (1) to avoid operating automobiles and machinery or engaging in other tasks requiring alertness until their response to therapy with metoprolol has been determined; (2) to contact the physician if any difficulty in breathing occurs; (3) to inform the physician or dentist before any type of surgery that they are taking metoprolol.

PREGNANCY AND LACTATION

- Pregnancy Category C. Metoprolol has been shown to increase postimplantation loss and decrease neonatal survival in rats. Metoprolol is excreted in breast milk in very small quantity.

miglitol

(mig-lee'tall)

Rx: Glyset

Drug Class: Alpha glucosidase inhibitors; Antidiabetic agents

Pregnancy Category: B

CLINICAL PHARMACOLOGY

Mechanism of Action: An alpha-glucosidase inhibitor that delays the digestion of ingested carbohydrates into simple sugars such as glucose. *Therapeutic Effect:* Produces smaller rise in blood glucose concentration after meals.

AVAILABLE FORMS

- *Tablets:* 25 mg, 50 mg, 100 mg.

INDICATIONS AND DOSAGES

Diabetes mellitus

PO

Adults, Elderly. Initially, 25 mg 3 times a day with first bite of each main meal. Maintenance: 50 mg 3 times a day. Maximum: 100 mg 3 times a day.

CONTRAINDICATIONS: Colonic ulceration, diabetic ketoacidosis, hypersensitivity to miglitol, inflammatory bowel disease, partial intestinal obstruction

INTERACTIONS

Drug

Digoxin, propranolol, ranitidine: May decrease the blood concentrations and effects of these drugs.

Herbal

None known.

Food

None known.

DIAGNOSTIC TEST EFFECTS: *None known.*

SIDE EFFECTS

Frequent (40%-10%)

Flatulence, loose stools, diarrhea, abdominal pain

Occasional (5%)

Rash

SPECIAL CONSIDERATIONS

PRECAUTIONS

- Miglitol should not cause hypoglycemia in the fasted or postprandial state. When diabetic patients are exposed to stress such as fever, trauma, infection, or surgery, a temporary loss of control of blood glucose may occur. At such times, temporary insulin therapy may be necessary. Plasma concentrations of miglitol in renally impaired volunteers were increased proportionally relative to the degree of renal dysfunction.

PATIENT INFORMATION

• Miglitol should be taken orally 3 times a day at the start (with the first bite) of each main meal. It is important to continue to adhere to dietary instructions, a regular exercise program, and regular testing of urine and/or blood glucose. Miglitol itself does not cause hypoglycemia even when administered to patients in the fasted state. Sulfonylurea drugs and insulin, however, can lower blood sugar levels enough to cause symptoms or sometimes life-threatening hypoglycemia. Because miglitol given in combination with a sulfonylurea or insulin will cause a further lowering of blood sugar, it may increase the hypoglycemic potential of these agents. Ensure that patients and family members understand well the risk of hypoglycemia, its symptoms and treatment, and conditions that predispose to its development. Because miglitol prevents the breakdown of table sugar, a source of glucose (dextrose, D-glucose) should be readily available to treat symptoms of low blood sugar when taking miglitol in combination with a sulfonylurea or insulin. If side effects occur with miglitol, they usually develop during the first few weeks of therapy. Side effects are most commonly mild to moderate dose-related gastrointestinal effects, such as flatulence, soft stools, diarrhea, or abdominal discomfort, and they generally diminish in frequency and intensity with time. Discontinuation of drug usually results in rapid resolution of the gastrointestinal symptoms.

PREGNANCY AND LACTATION

• Pregnancy Category B. The safety of miglitol in pregnant women has not been established. Miglitol has been shown to be excreted in human milk to a very small degree.

minocycline hydrochloride

(mi-noe-sye'kleen)

Rx: Arestin, Dynacin, Minocin, Vectrin

Drug Class: Antibiotics, tetracyclines

Pregnancy Category: D

Do not confuse Dynacin with Dynabac or Minocin with Mithracin or niacin.

CLINICAL PHARMACOLOGY

Mechanism of Action: A tetracycline antibiotic that inhibits bacterial protein synthesis by binding to ribosomes. *Therapeutic Effect:* Bacteriostatic.

AVAILABLE FORMS

• *Capsules (Dynacin, Minocin):* 50 mg, 75 mg, 100 mg.

• *Capsules (Pellet-filled [Minocin]):* 50 mg, 100 mg.

• *Tablets (Minocin, Myrac):* 50 mg, 75 mg, 100 mg.

• *Powder for Injection (Minocin, Myrac):* 100 mg.

INDICATIONS AND DOSAGES

Mild, moderate, or severe prostate, urinary tract, and CNS infections (excluding meningitis); uncomplicated gonorrhea; inflammatory acne; brucellosis; skin granulomas; cholera; trachoma; nocardiasis; yaws; and syphilis when penicillins are contraindicated

PO

Adults, Elderly. Initially, 100-200 mg, then 100 mg q12h or 50 mg q6h.

IV

Adults, Elderly. Initially, 200 mg, then 100 mg q12h up to 400 mg/day.

PO, IV

Children older than 8 yr. Initially, 4 mg/kg, then 2 mg/kg q12h.

UNLABELED USES: Treatment of atypical mycobacterial infections, rheumatoid arthritis, scleroderma

CONTRAINDICATIONS: Children younger than 8 years, hypersensitivity to tetracyclines, last half of pregnancy

INTERACTIONS

Drug

Carbamazepine, phenytoin: May decrease minocycline blood concentration.

Cholestyramine, colestipol: May decrease minocycline absorption.

Oral contraceptives: May decrease the effects of oral contraceptives.

Herbal

St. John's wort: May increase the risk of photosensitivity.

Food

None known.

DIAGNOSTIC TEST EFFECTS: May increase serum alkaline phosphatase, amylase, bilirubin, AST (SGOT), and ALT (SGPT) levels.

IV INCOMPATIBILITIES: Piperacillin and tazobactam (Zosyn)

IV COMPATIBILITIES: Heparin, magnesium, potassium

SIDE EFFECTS

Frequent

Dizziness, light-headedness, diarrhea, nausea, vomiting, abdominal cramps, possibly severe photosensitivity, drowsiness, vertigo

Occasional

Altered pigmentation of skin or mucous membranes, rectal or genital pruritus, stomatitis

SERIOUS REACTIONS

- Superinfection (especially fungal), anaphylaxis, and benign intracranial hypertension may occur.
- Bulging fontanelles occur rarely in infants.

SPECIAL CONSIDERATIONS

PRECAUTIONS

- As with other antibiotic preparations, use of this drug may result in overgrowth of nonsusceptible organisms, including fungi. Pseudotumor cerebri (benign intracranial hypertension) in adults has been associated with the use of tetracyclines. The usual clinical manifestations are headache and blurred vision. Bulging fontanels have been associated with the use of tetracyclines in infants. Perform incision and drainage or other surgical procedures along with antibiotic therapy when indicated.

PATIENT INFORMATION

- Photosensitivity manifested by an exaggerated sunburn reaction has been observed in some individuals taking tetracyclines. Advise patients apt to be exposed to direct sunlight or ultraviolet light that this reaction can occur with tetracycline drugs and to discontinue treatment at the first evidence of skin erythema. This reaction has been reported rarely with use of minocycline. Caution patients who experience central nervous system symptoms about driving vehicles or using hazardous machinery while taking minocycline therapy. Concurrent use of tetracycline may render oral contraceptives less effective.

PREGNANCY AND LACTATION

- Pregnancy Category D. Results of animal studies indicate that tetracyclines cross the placenta, are found in fetal tissues, and can have toxic effects on the developing fetus (often related to retardation of skeletal development). Tetracyclines are present in the milk of lactating women.

OCULAR CONSIDERATIONS

For lid disease, minocycline for 2 weeks at 50 mg/day, then monthly at 100 mg/day. Taper minocycline for long-term management. Minocycline can be taken bid, has fewest side effects, and induces minimal photosensitization.

• Minocycline hydrochloride can cause papilledema and blue-gray or brownish sclera.

minoxidil

(min-nox'i-dill)

Rx: Loniten

Drug Class: Vasodilators

Pregnancy Category: C

Do not confuse Loniten with Lotensin.

CLINICAL PHARMACOLOGY

Mechanism of Action: An antihypertensive and hair growth stimulant that has direct action on vascular smooth muscle, producing vasodilation of arterioles. *Therapeutic Effect:* Decreases peripheral vascular resistance and BP; increases cutaneous blood flow; stimulates hair follicle epithelium and hair follicle growth.

Pharmacokinetics

Route	Onset	Peak	Duration
PO	0.5 hr	2-8 hr	2-5 days

Well absorbed from the GI tract; minimal absorption after topical application. Protein binding: None. Widely distributed. Metabolized in the liver to active metabolite. Primarily excreted in urine. Removed by hemodialysis. **Half-life:** 4.2 hr.

AVAILABLE FORMS

• *Tablets (Loniten):* 2.5 mg, 10 mg.
• *Topical Solution (Rogaine):* 2% (20 mg/ml).
• *Topical Solution (Rogaine Extra Strength):* 5% (50 mg/ml).

INDICATIONS AND DOSAGES

Severe symptomatic hypertension, hypertension associated with organ damage, hypertension that has failed to respond to maximal therapeutic dosages of a diuretic or two other antihypertensives

PO

Adults. Initially, 5 mg/day. Increase with at least 3-day intervals to 10 mg, then 20 mg, then up to 40 mg/day in 1-2 doses.

Elderly. Initially, 2.5 mg/day. May increase gradually. Maintenance: 10-40 mg/day. Maximum: 100 mg/day.

Children. Initially, 0.1-0.2 mg/kg (5 mg maximum) daily. Gradually increase at a minimum of 3-day intervals. Maintenance: 0.25-1 mg/kg/day in 1-2 doses. Maximum: 50 mg/day.

Hair regrowth

Topical

Adults. 1 ml to affected areas of scalp 2 times a day. Total daily dose not to exceed 2 ml.

CONTRAINDICATIONS: Pheochromocytoma

INTERACTIONS

Drug

NSAIDs: May decrease the hypotensive effects of minoxidil.

Parenteral antihypertensives: May increase hypotensive effect.

Herbal

None known.

Food

None known.

DIAGNOSTIC TEST EFFECTS: May increase plasma renin activity and BUN, serum alkaline phosphatase, serum creatinine, and serum sodium levels. May decrease blood Hgb and Hct levels and erythrocyte count.

SIDE EFFECTS

Frequent

PO: Edema with concurrent weight gain, hypertrichosis (elongation, thickening, increased pigmentation of fine body hair; develops in 80% of patients within 3-6 weeks after beginning therapy)

Occasional

PO: T-wave changes (usually revert to pretreatment state with continued therapy or drug withdrawal)

Topical: Pruritus, rash, dry or flaking skin, erythema

Rare

PO: Breast tenderness, headache, photosensitivity reaction

Topical: Allergic reaction, alopecia, burning sensation at scalp, soreness at hair root, headache, visual disturbances

SERIOUS REACTIONS

- Tachycardia and angina pectoris may occur because of increased oxygen demands associated with increased heart rate and cardiac output.
- Fluid and electrolyte imbalance and CHF may occur, especially if a diuretic is not given concurrently with minoxidil.
- Too-rapid reduction in BP may result in syncope, CVA, MI, and ocular or vestibular ischemia.
- Pericardial effusion and tamponade may be seen in patients with impaired renal function who are not on dialysis.

SPECIAL CONSIDERATIONS

PRECAUTIONS

- Monitor fluid and electrolyte balance and body weight. Minoxidil tablets have not been used in patients who have had a myocardial infarction within the preceding month. Possible hypersensitivity can manifest as a skin rash. Patients with renal failure or dialysis patients may require smaller doses.

PATIENT INFORMATION

- The patient should be fully aware of the importance of continuing all of the antihypertensive medications and of the nature of symptoms that would suggest fluid overload. A patient brochure has been prepared and is included with each minoxidil package.

PREGNANCY AND LACTATION

- Pregnancy Category C. Oral administration of minoxidil has been associated with evidence of increased fetal resorption in rabbits. Fetal harm is not known. One report indicates minoxidil excretion in the breast milk of a woman treated with 5 mg oral minoxidil twice daily for hypertension.

mitomycin

(my-toe-my'-sin)

Rx: Mutamycin

Drug Class: Antineoplastics, antibiotics

Pregnancy Category: C

CLINICAL PHARMACOLOGY

Mechanism of Action: An antibiotic that acts similar to an alkylating agent, cross-linking with strands of DNA. *Therapeutic Effect:* Inhibits DNA and RNA synthesis.

Pharmacokinetics

Widely distributed. Does not cross the blood-brain barrier. Primarily metabolized in the liver and excreted in urine. **Half-life:** 50 min.

AVAILABLE FORMS

- *Powder for Injection:* 5 mg, 20 mg, 40 mg.

INDICATIONS AND DOSAGES

Disseminated adenocarcinoma of pancreas and stomach

IV

Adults, Elderly, Children. Initially, 10-20 mg/m^2 as single dose. Repeat q6-8wk. Give additional courses only after platelet and WBC counts are within acceptable levels, as shown below.

Leukocytes/ mm^3	*Platelets/ mm^3*	*% of Prior Dose to Give*
4000	more than 100,000	100%
3000-3999	75,000-99,000	100%
2000-2999	25,000-74,999	70%
1999 or less	less than 25,000	50%

Dosage in renal impairment

Patients with creatinine clearance less than 10 ml/min should receive 75% of normal dose.

UNLABELED USES: Treatment of biliary, bladder, breast, cervical, colorectal, head and neck, and lung carcinomas; chronic myelocytic leukemia

CONTRAINDICATIONS: Coagulation disorders and bleeding tendencies, platelet count less than 75,000/mm^3, serious infection, serum creatinine level greater than 1.7 mg/dl, WBC count less than 3000/mm^3

INTERACTIONS

Drug

Bone marrow depressants: May increase myelosuppression.

Live-virus vaccines: May potentiate virus replication, increase vaccine side effects, and decrease the patient's antibody response to the vaccine.

Herbal

None known.

Food

None known.

DIAGNOSTIC TEST EFFECTS: May increase BUN and serum creatinine levels.

IV INCOMPATIBILITIES: Aztreonam (Azactam), bleomycin (Blenoxane), cefepime (Maxipime), filgrastim (Neupogen), heparin, piperacillin/tazobactam (Zosyn), sargramostin (Leukine), vinorelbine (Navelbine)

IV COMPATIBILITIES: Cisplatin (Platinol AQ), cyclophosphamide (Cytoxan), doxorubicin (Adriamycin), 5-fluorouracil, granisetron (Kytril), leucovorin, methotrexate, ondansetron (Zofran), vinblastine (Velban), vincristine (Oncovin)

SIDE EFFECTS

Frequent (greater than 10%)

Fever, anorexia, nausea, vomiting

Occasional (10%-2%)

Stomatitis, paraesthesia, purple color bands on nails, rash, alopecia, unusual fatigue

Rare (less than 1%)

Thrombophlebitis, cellulitis, extravasation

SERIOUS REACTIONS

• Marked myelosuppression may result in hematologic toxicity (manifested as leukopenia, thrombocytopenia and to a lesser extent, anemia), usually within 2 to 4 weeks after the start of therapy.

• Renal toxicity (manifested as increased BUN and serum creatinine levels) and pulmonary toxicity (manifested as dyspnea, cough, hemoptysis, and pneumonia) may occur.

• Long-term therapy may produce hemolytic uremic syndrome, characterized by hemolytic anemia, thrombocytopenia, renal failure, and hypertension.

SPECIAL CONSIDERATIONS

OCULAR CONSIDERATIONS

• Topical mitomycin has been used for primary and recurrent pterygia after surgical excision. A dose of 1.0 mg/ml caused conjunctival irritation, excessive lacrimation, and mild superficial punctate keratitis, whereas 0.4 mg/ml minimized side effects. (Singh G, Wilson MR, Foster CS: Mitomycin eye drops as treatment for pterygium, *Ophthalmology* 95[6]:813-821, 1988.)

• Intraoperatively administered mitomycin C has been used during deep sclerectomy and has a significant effect on the postoperative intraocular pressure and increases the probability of achieving target intraocular pressures. (Anand N, Atherley C: Deep sclerectomy augmented with mitomycin C, *Eye* 19[4]:442-450, 2005.)

moexipril hydrochloride

(moe-ex'a-prile)

Rx: Univasc

Drug Class: Angiotensin converting enzyme inhibitors

Pregnancy Category: C, 1st; D, 2nd / 3rd

CLINICAL PHARMACOLOGY

Mechanism of Action: An ACE inhibitor that suppresses the renin-angiotensin-aldosterone system and prevents conversion of angiotensin I to angiotensin II, a potent vasoconstrictor; may also inhibit angiotensin II at local vascular and renal sites. *Therapeutic Effect:* Reduces peripheral arterial resistance and lowers BP.

Pharmacokinetics

Route	*Onset*	*Peak*	*Duration*
PO	1 hr	3-6 hr	24 hr

Incompletely absorbed from the GI tract. Food decreases drug absorption. Rapidly converted to active metabolite. Protein binding: 50%. Primarily recovered in feces, partially excreted in urine. Unknown if removed by dialysis. **Half-life:** 1 hr, metabolite 2-9 hr.

AVAILABLE FORMS

• *Tablets:* 7.5 mg, 15 mg.

INDICATIONS AND DOSAGES

Hypertension

PO

Adults, Elderly. For patients not receiving diuretics, initial dose is 7.5 mg once a day 1 hr before meals. Adjust according to BP effect. Maintenance: 7.5-30 mg a day in 1-2 divided doses 1 hr before meals.

Hypertension in patients with impaired renal function

PO

Adults, Elderly. 3.75 mg once a day in patients with creatinine clearance of 40 ml/min. Maximum: May titrate up to 15 mg/day.

CONTRAINDICATIONS: History of angioedema from previous treatment with ACE inhibitors

INTERACTIONS

Drug

Alcohol, antihypertensives, diuretics: May increase the effects of moexipril.

Lithium: May increase lithium blood concentration and risk of lithium toxicity.

NSAIDs: May decrease the effects of moexipril.

Potassium-sparing diuretics, potassium supplements: May cause hyperkalemia.

Herbal

None known.

Food

None known.

DIAGNOSTIC TEST EFFECTS: May increase BUN, serum alkaline phosphatase, serum bilirubin, serum creatinine, serum potassium, AST (SGOT), and ALT (SGPT) levels. May decrease serum sodium levels. May cause positive serum antinuclear antibody titer.

SIDE EFFECTS

Occasional

Cough, headache (6%); dizziness (4%); fatigue (3%)

Rare

Flushing, rash, myalgia, nausea, vomiting

SERIOUS REACTIONS

- Excessive hypotension ("first-dose syncope") may occur in patients with CHF and in those who are severely salt or volume depleted.
- Angioedema (swelling of face and lips) and hyperkalemia occur rarely.
- Agranulocytosis and neutropenia may be noted in those with collagen vascular disease, including scleroderma and systemic lupus erythematosus, and impaired renal function.
- Nephrotic syndrome may be noted in those with history of renal disease.

SPECIAL CONSIDERATIONS

PRECAUTIONS

- Anticipate changes in renal function in susceptible individuals. Hypertensive patients with congestive heart failure may be associated with oliguria and/or progressive azotemia and, rarely, acute renal failure or death. Elevated serum potassium was observed in hypertensive patients in clinical trials. Cough has been reported with all angiotensin-converting enzyme (ACE) inhibitors. In patients undergoing major surgery or during anesthesia with agents that produce hypotension, enalapril may block angiotensin II formation following compensatory renin release.

PATIENT INFORMATION

- Food: Advise patients to take moexipril 1 hour before meals.
- Angioedema: Angioedema, including laryngeal edema, may occur with treatment with ACE inhibitors, usually occurring early in therapy (within the first month). Advise patients to report immediately any signs or symptoms suggesting angioedema (swelling of the face, extremities, eyes, lips, and tongue and difficulty in breathing) and to take no more moexipril hydrochloride until they have consulted with the prescribing physician.
- Symptomatic Hypotension: Caution patients that light-headedness can occur with moexipril hydrochloride, especially during the first few days of therapy. If fainting occurs, the patient should stop taking moexipril hydrochloride and consult the prescribing physician.
- Caution all patients that excessive perspiration and dehydration may lead to an excessive fall in blood pressure because of reduction in fluid volume. Other causes of volume depletion such as vomiting or diarrhea also may lead to a fall in blood pressure; advise patients to consult their physician if they develop these conditions.
- Hyperkalemia: Instruct patients not to use potassium supplements or salt substitutes containing potassium without consulting their physician.
- Neutropenia: Instruct patients to report promptly any indication of infection (e.g., sore throat or fever) that could be a sign of neutropenia.

• Pregnancy: Advise female patients of childbearing age about the consequences of second- and third-trimester exposure to ACE inhibitors, and advise them that these consequences do not appear to have resulted from intrauterine ACE inhibitor exposure that has been limited to the first trimester. Ask patients to report pregnancies to their physicians as soon as possible.

PREGNANCY AND LACTATION

• Pregnancy Categories C (first trimester) and D (second and third trimesters). The use of ACE inhibitors during the second and third trimesters of pregnancy has been associated with fetal and neonatal injury, including hypotension, neonatal skull hypoplasia, anuria, reversible or irreversible renal failure, and death. Excretion into human milk is not known.

mometasone furoate monohydrate

(mo-met'a-sone)

Rx: Elocon, Nasonex

Drug Class: Corticosteroids, inhalation; Corticosteroids, topical; Dermatologics

Pregnancy Category: C

CLINICAL PHARMACOLOGY

Mechanism of Action: An adrenocorticosteroid that inhibits the release of inlammatory cells into nasal tissue, preventing early activation of the allergic reaction. *Therapeutic Effect:* Decreases response to seasonal and perennial rhinitis.

Pharmacokinetics

Undetectable in plasma. Protein binding: 98%-99%. The swallowed portion undergoes extensive metabolism. Excreted primarily through bile and, to a lesser extent, urine.

AVAILABLE FORMS

• *Nasal Spray:* 50 mg/spray.

INDICATIONS AND DOSAGES

Allergic rhinitis

Nasal Spray

Adults, Elderly, Children 12 yr and older. 2 sprays in each nostril once a day.

Children 2-11 yr. 1 spray in each nostril once a day.

CONTRAINDICATIONS: Hypersensitivity to any corticosteroid, persistently positive sputum cultures for *Candida albicans*, systemic fungal infections, untreated localized infection involving nasal mucosa.

INTERACTIONS

Drug

None known.

Herbal

None known.

Food

None known.

DIAGNOSTIC TEST EFFECTS: *None known.*

SIDE EFFECTS

Occasional

Nasal irritation, stinging

Rare

Nasal or pharyngeal candidiasis

SERIOUS REACTIONS

• An acute hypersensitivity reaction, including urticaria, angioedema, and severe bronchospasm, occurs rarely.

• Transfer from systemic to local steroid therapy may unmask previously suppressed bronchial asthma condition.

SPECIAL CONSIDERATIONS

PRECAUTIONS

• Mometasone furoate may cause a reduction in growth velocity when administered to pediatric patients.

Use nasally administered corticosteroids with caution in patients with active or quiescent tuberculous infection tract or in untreated fungal, bacterial, systemic viral infections or ocular herpes simplex. When nasal corticosteroids are used at excessive doses, systemic corticosteroid effects such as hypercorticism and adrenal suppression may appear.

PATIENT INFORMATION

• Give patients being treated with mometasone furoate nasal spray, 50 mg, the following information and instructions. This information is intended to aid in the safe and effective use of this medication. Such advice is not a disclosure of all intended or possible adverse effects. Patients should use mometasone furoate nasal spray, 50 mg, at regular intervals (once daily) because its effectiveness depends on regular use. Improvement in nasal symptoms of allergic rhinitis has been shown to occur within 11 hours after the first dose based on one single-dose, parallel-group study of patients in an outdoor "park" setting (park study) and one environmental exposure unit study and within 2 days after the first dose in two randomized, double blind, placebo-controlled, parallel-group seasonal allergic rhinitis studies. Maximum benefit usually is achieved within 1 to 2 weeks after initiation of dosing. Patients should take the medication as directed and should not increase the prescribed dosage by using it more than once a day in an attempt to increase its effectiveness. Patients should contact their physician if symptoms do not improve or if the condition worsens. To ensure proper use of this nasal spray and to attain maximum benefit, patients should read and follow the accompanying patient's instructions for use carefully. Caution patients not to spray mometasone furoate nasal spray, 50 mg, into the eyes or directly onto the nasal septum. Warn persons who are taking immunosuppressant doses of corticosteroids to avoid exposure to chickenpox or measles, and advise patients that if they are exposed, they should seek medical advice without delay.

PREGNANCY AND LACTATION

• Pregnancy Category C. Mometasone furoate caused cleft palate in mice. Fetal harm is not known. Excretion into human milk is not known.

OCULAR CONSIDERATIONS

• Glaucoma and cataract formation was evaluated in one controlled study of 12 weeks' duration and one uncontrolled study of 12 months' duration in patients treated with mometasone furoate nasal spray, 50 mg, at 200 mg/day, using intraocular pressure measurements and slit-lamp examination. No significant change from baseline was noted in the mean intraocular pressure measurements for the 141 patients treated with mometasone furoate in the 12-week study, as compared with 141 placebo-treated patients. No individual patient treated with mometasone furoate was noted to have developed a significant elevation in intraocular pressure or cataracts in this 12-week study. Likewise, no significant change from baseline was noted in the mean intraocular pressure measurements for the 139 patients treated with mometasone furoate in the 12-month study, and again no cataracts were detected in these patients. Nonetheless, nasal and inhaled corticosteroids have been associated with the development of glaucoma and/or cataracts. Therefore, close follow-up is warranted in patients with a change in vision and with a history of glaucoma and/or cataracts.

• Rare instances of nasal septum perforation and increased intraocular pressure also have been reported following the intranasal application of aerosolized corticosteroids. As with any long-term topical treatment of the nasal cavity, patients using mometasone furoate nasal spray, 50 mg, over several months or longer should be examined periodically for possible changes in the nasal mucosa.

montelukast

(mon-te'loo-kast)

Rx: Singulair

Drug Class: Leucotriene antagonists/inhibitors

Pregnancy Category: B

CLINICAL PHARMACOLOGY

Mechanism of Action: An antiasthmatic that binds to cysteinyl leukotriene receptors, inhibiting the effects of leukotrienes on bronchial smooth muscle. *Therapeutic Effect:* Decreases bronchoconstriction, vascular permeability, mucosal edema, and mucus production.

Pharmacokinetics

Route	*Onset*	*Peak*	*Duration*
PO	N/A	N/A	24 hr
PO (chewable)	N/A	N/A	24 hr

Rapidly absorbed from the GI tract. Protein binding: 99%. Extensively metabolized in the liver. Excreted almost exclusively in feces. **Half-life:** 2.7-5.5 hr (slightly longer in the elderly).

AVAILABLE FORMS

- *Oral Granules:* 4 mg.
- *Tablets:* 10 mg.
- *Tablets (Chewable):* 4 mg, 5 mg.

INDICATIONS AND DOSAGES

Bronchial asthma

PO

Adults, Elderly, Adolescents older than 14 yr. One 10-mg tablet a day, taken in the evening.

Children 6-14 yr. One 5-mg chewable tablet a day, taken in the evening.

Children 1-5 yr. One 4-mg chewable tablet a day, taken in the evening.

CONTRAINDICATIONS: None known.

INTERACTIONS

Drug

Phenobarbital, rifampin: May decrease montelukasts's duration of action.

Herbal

None known.

Food

None known.

DIAGNOSTIC TEST EFFECTS: May increase AST (SGOT) and ALT (SGPT) levels.

SIDE EFFECTS

Adults, Adolescents 15 years and older

Frequent (18%)

Headache

Occasional (4%)

Influenza

Rare (3%-2%)

Abdominal pain, cough, dyspepsia, dizziness, fatigue, dental pain

Children 6-14 years

Rare (less than 2%)

Diarrhea, laryngitis, pharyngitis, nausea, otitis media, sinusitis, viral infection

SERIOUS REACTIONS

• None known.

SPECIAL CONSIDERATIONS

PRECAUTIONS

• Montelukast sodium should not be substituted abruptly for inhaled or oral corticosteroids. Montelukast sodium should not be used as monotherapy for exercise-induced bronchospasm. Patients with known aspirin sensitivity should continue avoidance of aspirin or nonsteroidal antiinflammatory agents while taking montelukast.

PATIENT INFORMATION

• Advise patients to take montelukast daily as prescribed, even when they are asymptomatic, as well as during periods of worsening asthma, and to contact their physicians if their asthma is not well controlled. Advise patients that oral tablets of montelukast are not for the treatment of acute asthma attacks. Patients should have appropriate short-acting inhaled beta-agonist medication available to treat asthma exacerbations. Advise patients that while using montelukast, they should seek medical attention if short-acting inhaled bronchodilators are needed more often than usual or if more than the maximum number of inhalations of short-acting bronchodilator treatment prescribed for 24-hour period are needed. Instruct patients receiving montelukast not to decrease the dose or stop taking any other antiasthma medications unless instructed by a physician. Instruct patients who have exacerbations of asthma after exercise to continue to use their usual regimen of inhaled beta-agonists as prophylaxis unless otherwise instructed by their physician. All patients should have available for rescue a short-acting inhaled beta-agonist. Advise patients with known aspirin sensitivity to continue avoidance of aspirin or nonsteroidal antiinflammatory agents while taking montelukast. Inform phenylketonuric patients that the 4- and 5-mg chewable tablets contain phenylalanine.

PREGNANCY AND LACTATION

• Pregnancy Category B. No teratogenicity was observed in rats or rabbits. Montelukast crosses the placenta following oral dosing in rats and rabbits. Fetal harm is not known. Studies in rats have shown that montelukast is excreted in milk. Whether montelukast is excreted in human milk is not known.

---

morphine sulfate

(mor'feen)

Rx: Astramorph PF, Avinza, DepoDur, Duramorph PF, Infumorph, Kadian, MS/S, MS Contin, MSIR, Oramorph SR, Rapi-Ject, RMS, Roxanol, Roxanol-T

Drug Class: Analgesics, narcotic

Pregnancy Category: C

DEA Class: Schedule II

Do not confuse morphine with hydromorphone, or Roxanol with Roxicet.

CLINICAL PHARMACOLOGY

Mechanism of Action: An opioid agonist that binds with opioid receptors in the CNS. *Therapeutic Effect:* Alters the perception of and emotional response to pain; produces generalized CNS depression.

Pharmacokinetics

Route	Onset	Peak	Duration
Oral Solution	N/A	1 hr	3-5 hr
Tablets	N/A	1 hr	3-5 hr
Tablets (ER)	N/A	3-4 hr	8-12 hr
IV	Rapid	0.3 hr	3-5 hr
IM	5-30 min	0.5-1 hr	3-5 hr
Epidural	N/A	1 hr	12-20 hr
Subcutaneous	N/A	1.1-5 hr	3-5 hr
Rectal	N/A	0.5-1 hr	3-7 hr

Variably absorbed from the GI tract. Readily absorbed after IM or subcutaneous administration. Protein binding: 20%-35%. Widely distributed. Metabolized in the liver. Primarily excreted in urine. Removed by hemodialysis. **Half-life:** 2-3 hr. (increased in patients with hepatic disease)

AVAILABLE FORMS

- *Capsules (Extended-Release [Kadian]):* 20 mg, 30 mg, 50 mg, 60 mg, 100 mg.
- *Capsules (Extended-Release [Avinza]):* 30 mg, 60 mg, 90 mg, 120 mg.
- *Capsules (MSIR):* 15 mg, 30 mg.
- *Solution for Injection:* 2 mg/ml, 4 mg/ml, 5 mg/ml, 8 mg/ml, 10 mg/ml, 15 mg/ml, 25 mg/ml.
- *Solution for Injection (Preservative-Free):* 10 mg/ml, 15 mg/ml, 25 mg/ml, 50 mg/ml.
- *Epidural and Intrathecal via Infusion Device (Infumorph):* 10 mg/ml, 25 mg/ml.
- *Epidural, Intrathecal, IV Infusion (Astramorph, Duramorph):* 0.5 mg/ml, 1 mg/ml.
- *Oral Solution (MSIR):* 10 mg/ml, 20 mg/ml.
- *Oral Solution (Roxanol):* 20 mg/ml, 100 mg/ml.
- *Suppositories (RMS):* 5 mg, 10 mg, 20 mg, 30 mg.
- *Tablets (MSIR):* 15 mg, 30 mg.
- *Tablets (Extended-Release [MS Contin]):* 15 mg, 30 mg, 60 mg, 100 mg, 200 mg.
- *Tablets (Extended-Release [Oramorph SR]):* 15 mg, 30 mg, 60 mg, 100 mg.
- *Liposomal Injection (DepoDur):* 10 mg/ml, 15 mg/1.5 ml, 20 mg/2 ml.

INDICATIONS AND DOSAGES: Alert Dosage should be titrated to desired effect.

Analgesia

PO (Prompt-release)

Adults, Elderly. 10-30 mg q3-4h as needed.

Children. 0.2-0.5 mg/kg q3-4h as needed.

Alert: For the Avinza dosage below, be aware that this drug is to be administered once a day only.

Alert: For the Kadian dosage information below, be aware that this drug is to be administered q12h or once a day only.

Alert: Be aware that pediatric dosages of extended-release preparations Kadian and Avinza have not been established.

Alert: For the MSContin and Oramorph SR dosage information below, be aware that the daily dosage is divided and given q8h or q12h.

PO (Extended-Release [Avinza])

Adults, Elderly. Dosage requirement should be established using prompt-release formulations and is based on total daily dose. Avinza is given once a day only.

PO (Extended-Release [Kadian])

Adults, Elderly. Dosage requirement should be established using prompt-release formulations and is based on total daily dose. Dose is given once a day or divided and given q12h.

PO (Extended-Release [MSContin, Oramorph SR])

Adults, Elderly. Dosage requirement should be established using prompt-release formulations and is based on total daily dose. Daily dose is divided and given q8h or q12h.

Children. 0.3-0.6 mg/kg/dose q12h.

IV

Adults, Elderly. 2.5-5 mg q3-4h as needed. Note: Repeated doses (e.g. 1-2 mg) may be given more frequently (e.g. every hour) if needed.

Children. 0.05-0.1 mg/kg q3-4h as needed.

IV Continuous Infusion

Adults, Elderly. 0.8-10 mg/hr. Range: Up to 80 mg/hr.

Children. 10-30 mcg/kg/hr.

IM

Adults, Elderly. 5-10 mg q3-4h as needed.

Children. 0.1 mg/kg q3-4h as needed.

Epidural

Adults, Elderly. Initially, 1-6 mg bolus, infusion rate: 0.1-1 mg/hr. Maximum: 10 mg/24 hr.

Intrathecal

Adults, Elderly. One-tenth of the epidural dose: 0.2-1 mg/dose.

PCA

IV

Adults, Elderly. Loading dose: 5-10 mg. Intermittent bolus: 0.5-3 mg. Lockout interval: 5-12 min. Continuous infusion: 1-10 mg/hr. 4-hr limit: 20-30 mg.

CONTRAINDICATIONS: Acute or severe asthma, GI obstruction, severe hepatic or renal impairment, severe respiratory depression, asthma, severe liver or renal impairment

INTERACTIONS

Drug

Alcohol, other CNS depressants: May increase CNS or respiratory depression and hypotension.

MAOIs: May produce a severe, sometimes fatal reaction; expect to administer one-quarter of usual morphine dose.

Herbal

None known.

Food

None known.

DIAGNOSTIC TEST EFFECTS: May increase serum amylase and lipase levels.

IV INCOMPATIBILITIES: Amphotericin B complex (Abelcet, AmBisome, Amphotec), cefepime (Maxipime), doxorubicin liposomal (Doxil), thiopental

IV COMPATIBILITIES: Amiodarone (Cordarone), atropine, bumetanide (Bumex), bupivacaine (Marcaine, Sensorcaine), diltiazem (Cardizem), diphenhydramine (Benadryl), dobutamine (Dobutrex), dopamine (Intropin), glycopyrrolate (Robinul), heparin, hydroxyzine (Vistaril), lidocaine, lorazepam (Ativan), magnesium, midazolam (Versed), milrinone (Primacor), nitroglycerin, potassium, propofol (Diprivan)

SIDE EFFECTS

Frequent

Sedation, decreased BP (including orthostatic hypotension), diaphoresis, facial flushing, constipation, dizziness, somnolence, nausea, vomiting

Occasional

Allergic reaction (rash, pruritus), dyspnea, confusion, palpitations, tremors, urine retention, abdominal cramps, vision changes, dry mouth, headache, decreased appetite, pain or burning at injection site

Rare

Paralytic ileus

SERIOUS REACTIONS

• Overdose results in respiratory depression, skeletal muscle flaccidity, cold or clammy skin, cyanosis, and extreme somnolence progressing to seizures, stupor, and coma.

• The patient who uses morphine repeatedly may develop a tolerance to the drug's analgesic effect and physical dependence.

• The drug may have a prolonged duration of action and cumulative effect in those with hepatic and renal impairment.

SPECIAL CONSIDERATIONS

PRECAUTIONS

• Respiratory depression is the chief hazard of all morphine preparations. Morphine sulfate should be used with extreme caution in patients with chronic obstructive pulmonary disease or cor pulmonale and in patients having a substantially decreased respiratory reserve (e.g., severe kyphoscoliosis), hypoxia, hypercapnia, or preexisting respiratory depression. The respiratory depressant effects of morphine with carbon dioxide retention and secondary elevation of cerebrospinal fluid pressure may be exaggerated greatly in the presence of head injury, other intracranial lesions, or preexisting increase in intracranial pressure. Morphine sulfate may cause severe hypotension in an individual whose ability to maintain blood pressure already has been compromised by a depleted blood volume or a concurrent administration of drugs such as phenothiazines or general anesthetics. Administer morphine with caution to patients in circulatory shock. Do not give morphine sulfate to patients with gastrointestinal obstruction, particularly paralytic ileus. Use morphine sulfate with caution and in reduced dosages in elderly or debilitated patients, patients with severe renal or hepatic insufficiency, and patients with Addison's disease, myxedema, hypothyroidism, prostatic hypertrophy, or urethral stricture. Exercise caution in the administration of morphine sulfate to patients with central nervous system depression, toxic psychosis, acute alcoholism and delirium tremens, and convulsive disorders. Morphine sulfate may aggravate preexisting convulsions in patients with convulsive disorders.

PATIENT INFORMATION

If clinically advisable, the eye care practitioner should give patients receiving morphine sulfate controlled-release capsules the following instructions:

• Although psychological dependence (addiction) to morphine used in the treatment of pain is rare, morphine is one of a class of drugs known to be abused and should be handled accordingly.

• The dose of the drug should not be adjusted without consulting a physician.

• Morphine may impair mental and/or physical ability required for the performance of potentially hazardous tasks (e.g., driving or operating machinery). Patients started on morphine sulfate extended-release tablets or whose dose has been changed should refrain from dangerous activity until it is established that they are not adversely affected.

• Morphine should not be taken with alcohol or other central nervous system depressants (sleep aids, tranquilizers) because additive effects including central nervous system depression may occur. The patient should consult a physician if other prescription medications are being used currently or are prescribed for future use.

• For women of childbearing potential who become or are planning to become pregnant, they should consult a physician regarding analgesics and other drug use.

• Upon completion of therapy, it may be appropriate to taper morphine dose, rather than abruptly discontinue it.

• The morphine sulfate controlled-release 200-mg tablet is for use only in opioid-tolerant patients requiring daily morphine equivalent dosages of 400 mg or more. Patients must take special care to avoid accidental ingestion or the use by individuals (including children) other than the patient for whom the morphine sulfate originally was prescribed, because such unsupervised use may have severe, even fatal, consequences.

• Morphine sulfate controlled-release capsules should not be opened, chewed, crushed, or dissolved. The pellets in the controlled-release capsules should not be chewed or dissolved.

• As with other opioids, advise patients taking morphine sulfate that severe constipation could occur, and initiate appropriate laxatives, stool softeners, and other appropriate treatments from the beginning of opioid therapy.

PREGNANCY AND LACTATION

• Pregnancy Category C. Teratogenic effects of morphine have been reported in the animal literature. Low levels of morphine have been detected in human milk.

moxifloxacin hydrochloride

(moks-i-floks'a-sin)

Rx: Avelox, Avelox I.V., Vigamox

Drug Class: Anti-infectives, ophthalmic; Antibiotics, quinolones; Ophthalmics

Pregnancy Category: C

Do not confuse Avelox with Avonex.

CLINICAL PHARMACOLOGY

Mechanism of Action: A fluoroquinolone that inhibits two enzymes, topoisomerase II and IV, in susceptible microorganisms. *Therapeutic Effect:* Interferes with bacterial DNA replication. Prevents or delays emergence of resistant organisms. Bactericidal.

Pharmacokinetics

Well absorbed from the GI tract after PO administration. Protein binding: 50%. Widely distributed throughout body with tissue concentration often exceeding plasma concentration. Metabolized in liver. Primarily excreted in urine with a lesser amount in feces. **Half-life:** 10.7-13.3 hr.

AVAILABLE FORMS

• *Tablets (Avelox):* 400 mg.

• *Injection (Avelox IV):* 400 mg.

• *Ophthalmic Solution (Vigamox):* 0.5%.

INDICATIONS AND DOSAGES

Acute bacterial sinusitis, community-acquired pneumonia

PO, IV

Adults, Elderly. 400 mg q24h for 10 days.

Acute bacterial exacerbation of chronic bronchitis

PO, IV

Adults, Elderly. 400 mg q24h for 5 days.

Skin and skin-structure infection
PO, IV
Adults, Elderly. 400 mg once a day for 7 days.
Topical treatment of bacterial conjunctivitis due to susceptible strains of bacteria
Ophthalmic
Adults, Elderly, Children older than 1 yr. 1 drop 3 times/day for 7 days.

CONTRAINDICATIONS: Hypersensitivity to quinolones

INTERACTIONS

Drug
Antacids, didanosine chewable, buffered tablets or pediatric powder for oral solution, iron preparations, sucralfate: May decrease moxifloxacin absorption.

Herbal
None known.

Food
None known.

DIAGNOSTIC TEST EFFECTS: *None known.*

IV INCOMPATIBILITIES: Do not add or infuse other drugs simultaneously through the same IV line. Flush line before and after use if same IV line is used with other medications.

SIDE EFFECTS

Frequent (8%-6%)
Nausea, diarrhea
Occasional (3%-2%)
Dizziness, headache, abdominal pain, vomiting
Ophthalmic (6%-1%): conjunctival irritation, reduced visual acuity, dry eye, keratitis, eye pain, ocular itching, swelling of tissue around cornea, eye discharge, fever, cough, pharyngitis, rash, rhinitis
Rare (1%)
Change in sense of taste, dyspepsia (heartburn, indigestion), photosensitivity

SERIOUS REACTIONS

- Pseudomembranous colitis as evidenced by fever, severe abdominal cramps or pain, and severe watery diarrhea may occur.
- Superinfection manifested as anal or genital pruritus, moderate to severe diarrhea, and stomatitis may occur.

nadolol

(nay-doe'lole)
Rx: Corgard
Drug Class: Antiadrenergics, beta blocking
Pregnancy Category: C

CLINICAL PHARMACOLOGY

Mechanism of Action: A nonselective beta-blocker that blocks $beta_1$- and $beta_2$-adrenergenic receptors. Large doses increase airway resistance. *Therapeutic Effect:* Slows sinus heart rate, decreases cardiac output and BP. Decreases myocardial ischemia severity by decreasing oxygen requirements.

AVAILABLE FORMS

- *Tablets:* 20 mg, 40 mg, 80 mg, 120 mg, 160 mg.

INDICATIONS AND DOSAGES

Mild to moderate hypertension, angina
PO
Adults. Initially, 40 mg/day. May increase by 40-80 mg at 3-7 day intervals. Maximum: 240-360 mg/day.
Elderly. Initially, 20 mg/day. May increase gradually. Range: 20-240 mg/day.

Dosage in renal impairment
Dosage is modified based on creatinine clearance.

Creatinine Clearance	*% Usual Dosage*
10-50 ml/min	50
less than 10 ml/min	25

UNLABELED USES: Treatment of arrhythmias, hypertrophic cardiomyopathy, MI, mitral valve prolapse syndrome, neuroleptic-induced akathisia, pheochromocytoma, tremors, thyrotoxicosis, vascular headaches

CONTRAINDICATIONS: Bronchial asthma, cardiogenic shock, CHF secondary to tachyarrhythmias, COPD, patients receiving MAOI therapy, second- or third-degree heart block, sinus bradycardia, uncontrolled cardiac failure

INTERACTIONS

Drug

Cimetidine: May increase nadolol blood concentration.

Diuretics, other antihypertensives: May increase hypotensive effect.

Insulin, oral hypoglycemics: May mask symptoms of hypoglycemia and prolong the hypoglycemic effect of insulin and oral hypoglycemics.

NSAIDs: May decrease antihypertensive effect.

Sympathomimetics, xanthines: May mutually inhibit effects.

Herbal

None known.

Food

None known.

DIAGNOSTIC TEST EFFECTS: May increase serum antinuclear antibody titer and BUN, serum LDH, serum lipoprotein, serum alkaline phosphatase, serum bilirubin, serum creatinine, serum potassium, serum uric acid, AST (SGOT), ALT (SGPT), and serum triglyceride levels.

SIDE EFFECTS

Nadolol is generally well tolerated, with transient and mild side effects.

Frequent

Diminished sexual ability, drowsiness, unusual fatigue or weakness

Occasional

Bradycardia, difficulty breathing, depression, cold hands or feet, diarrhea, constipation, anxiety, nasal congestion, nausea, vomiting

Rare

Altered taste, dry eyes, itching

SERIOUS REACTIONS

- Overdose may produce profound bradycardia and hypotension.
- Abrupt withdrawal of nadolol may result in diaphoresis, palpitations, headache, tremors, exacerbation of angina, MI, and ventricular arrhythmias.
- Nadolol administration may precipitate CHF and MI in patients with cardiac disease; thyroid storm in those with thyrotoxicosis; and peripheral ischemia in those with existing peripheral vascular disease.
- Hypoglycemia may occur in patients with previously controlled diabetes.

SPECIAL CONSIDERATIONS

PRECAUTIONS

- Use nadolol with caution in patients with impaired renal function. Sympathetic stimulation may be a vital component supporting circulatory function in patients with congestive heart failure, and its inhibition by beta-blockade may precipitate more severe failure. Patients with bronchospastic diseases in general should not receive beta-blockers. Beta-adrenergic blockade may prevent the appearance of premonitory signs and symptoms (e.g., tachycardia and blood pressure changes) of acute hypoglycemia. Beta-adrenergic blockade may mask certain clinical signs (e.g., tachycardia) of hyperthyroidism. Patients with a history of severe anaphylactic reactions to a variety of allergens may be more reactive to repeated challenge. Such patients may be unresponsive to the usual doses of epinephrine used to treat allergic reactions.

PATIENT INFORMATION

- Warn patients, especially those with evidence of coronary artery insufficiency, against interruption or discontinuation of nadolol therapy without the physician's advice. Although cardiac failure rarely occurs in properly selected patients, advise patients being treated with beta-adrenergic blocking agents to consult the physician at the first sign or symptom of impending failure. Also advise the patient of a proper course in the event of an inadvertently missed dose.

PREGNANCY AND LACTATION

- Pregnancy Category C. In animal reproduction studies with nadolol, evidence of embryotoxicity and fetotoxicity was found in rabbits, but not in rats or hamsters, at doses 5 to 10 times greater than the maximum indicated human dose. Nadolol is excreted in human milk.

nafcillin

(naph-sil-'in)

Rx: Nallpen, Unipen

Drug Class: Antibiotics, penicillins

Pregnancy Category: B

CLINICAL PHARMACOLOGY

Mechanism of Action: A penicillin that acts as a bactericidal in susceptible microorganisms. *Therapeutic Effect:* Inhibits bacterial cell wall synthesis. Bactericidal.

Pharmacokinetics

Poorly absorbed from gastrointestinal (GI) tract. Protein binding: 87%-90%. Metabolized in liver. Primarily excreted in urine. Not removed by hemodialysis. **Half-life:** 10.5-1 hr (half-life increased with imparied renal function, neonates).

AVAILABLE FORMS

- *Tablets:* 500 mg (Unipen).
- *Capsules:* 250 mg (Unipen).
- *Powder for Injection:* 1 g, 2 g, 10 g (Nafcil, Nallpen, Unipen).

INDICATIONS AND DOSAGES

Staphylococcal infections

IV

Adults, Elderly. 3-6 g/24 hrs in divided doses.

Children. 25 mg/kg 2 times/day.

Neonates 7 days and older. 75 mg/kg/day in 4 divided doses.

Neonates less than 7 days old. 50 mg/kg/day in 2-3 divided doses.

IM

Adults, Elderly. 500 mg q4-6h.

Children. 25 mg/kg 2 times/day.

Neonates 7 days and older. 75 mg/kg/day in 4 divided doses.

Neonates less than 7 days old. 50 mg/kg/day in 2-3 divided doses.

PO

Adults, Elderly. 250 mg to 1 g q4-6h.

Children. 25-50 mg/kg/day in 4 divided doses.

UNLABELED USES: Surgical prophylaxis

CONTRAINDICATIONS: Hypersensitivity to any penicillin

INTERACTIONS

Drug

Probenecid: May increase nafcillin blood concentration and risk for nafcillin toxicity.

Herbal

None known.

Food

None known.

DIAGNOSTIC TEST EFFECTS: May cause positive Coombs' test.

IV INCOMPATIBILITIES: Diltiazem (Cardizem), droperidol (Inapsine), fentanyl, insulin, labetalol (Normodyne, Trandate), midazolam (Versed), nalbuphine (Nubain), vancomycin (Vancocin), verapamil (Isoptin)

IV COMPATIBILITIES: None known.

SIDE EFFECTS

Frequent

Mild hypersensitivity reaction (fever, rash, pruritus), GI effects (nausea, vomiting, diarrhea) more frequent with oral administration

Occasional

Hypokalemia with high IV doses, phlebitis, thrombophlebitis (more common in elderly)

Rare

Extravasation with IV administration

SERIOUS REACTIONS

• Superinfections, potentially fatal antibiotic-associated colitis may result from altered bacterial balance.

• Hematologic effects (especially involving platelets, WBCs), severe hypersensitivity reactions, and anaphylaxis occur rarely.

SPECIAL CONSIDERATIONS

PRECAUTIONS

• Nafcillin sodium generally should not be administered to patients with a history of sensitivity to any penicillin. The use of antibiotics may result in overgrowth of nonsusceptible organisms. Exercise caution when treating patients with concomitant hepatic insufficiency and renal dysfunction with nafcillin.

PREGNANCY AND LACTATION

• Pregnancy Category B. Reproduction studies have been performed in the mouse with oral doses up to 20 times the human dose and orally in the rat at doses up to 40 times the human dose and have revealed no evidence of impaired fertility or harm to the rodent fetus from nafcillin sodium. Penicillins are excreted in human milk.

naphazoline

(naf-az'oh-leen)

Rx: AK-Con, Albalon, Allersol, Nafazair, Ocu-Zoline

Drug Class: Decongestants, nasal; Decongestants, ophthalmic; Ophthalmics

CLINICAL PHARMACOLOGY

Mechanism of Action: A sympathomimetic that directly acts on alpha-adrenergic receptors in conjunctival arterioles and nasal blood vessels. *Therapeutic Effect:* Causes vasoconstriction, resulting in decreased congestion.

AVAILABLE FORMS

• *Ophthalmic Solution:* 0.012%, 0.1%.

• *Nasal Drops:* 0.05%.

• *Nasal Spray:* 0.05%.

INDICATIONS AND DOSAGES

Nasal congestion due to acute or chronic rhinitis, common cold, hay fever, or other allergies

Intranasal

Adults, Elderly, Children older than 12 yr. 1-2 drops or sprays in each nostril q3-6h.

Children 6-12 yr. 1 spray or drop in each nostril q6h as needed.

Control of hyperemia in patients with superficial corneal vascularity; relief of congestion and inflammation; for use during ocular diagnostic procedures

Ophthalmic

Adults, Elderly, Children older than 6 yr. 1-2 drops in affected eye q3-4h for 3-4 days.

CONTRAINDICATIONS: Angle-closure glaucoma, before peripheral iridectomy, patients with a narrow angle who do not have glaucoma

INTERACTIONS

Drug

Maprotiline, tricyclic antidepressants: May increase the effects of naphazoline.

Herbal

None known.

Food

None known.

DIAGNOSTIC TEST EFFECTS: *None known.*

SIDE EFFECTS

Occasional

Nasal: Burning, stinging, or drying of nasal mucosa; sneezing; rebound congestion

Ophthalmic: Blurred vision, dilated pupils, increased eye irritation

SERIOUS REACTIONS

• If naphazoline is systemically absorbed, the patient may experience tachycardia, palpitations, headache, insomnia, light-headedness, nausea, nervousness, and tremor.

• Large doses may produce tachycardia, palpitations, light-headedness, nausea, and vomiting.

• Overdose in patients older than 60 years may produce hallucinations, CNS depression, and seizures.

SPECIAL CONSIDERATIONS

PRECAUTIONS

• Use caution in the presence of hypertension, cardiovascular abnormalities, hyperglycemia, hyperthyroidism, and other medications.

naproxen

(na-prox′en)

Rx: Aflaxen, Anaprox, Anaprox-DS, EC Naprosyn, Naprelan ′375′, Naprelan ′500′, Naprosyn

Drug Class: Analgesics, non-narcotic; Nonsteroidal anti-inflammatory drugs

Pregnancy Category: B

Do not confuse Aleve with Allese or Anaprox with Anaspaz.

CLINICAL PHARMACOLOGY

Mechanism of Action: An NSAID that produces analgesic and anti-inflammatory effects by inhibiting prostaglandin synthesis. *Therapeutic Effect:* Reduces the inflammatory response and intensity of pain.

Pharmacokinetics

Route	*Onset*	*Peak*	*Duration*
PO (analgesic)	less than 1 hr	N/A	7 hr or less
PO (antirheumatic)	less than 14 days	2-4 wk	N/A

Completely absorbed from the GI tract. Protein binding: 99%. Metabolized in the liver. Primarily excreted in urine. Not removed by hemodialysis. **Half-life:** 13 hr.

AVAILABLE FORMS

• *Gelcaps (Aleve):* 220 mg naproxen sodium (equivalent to 200 mg naproxen).

• *Oral Suspension (Naprosyn):* 125 mg/5 ml naproxen.

• *Tablets (Aleve):* 220 mg naproxen.

• *Tablets (Anaprox):* 275 mg naproxen sodium (equivalent to 250 mg naproxen).

- *Tablets (Anaprox DS):* 550 mg naproxen sodium (equivalent to 500 mg naproxen).
- *Tablets (Controlled-Release [EC-Naprosyn]):* 375 mg naproxen, 500 mg naproxen.
- *Tablets (Controlled-Release [Naprelan]):* 421 mg naproxen, 550 mg naproxen sodium (equivalent to 500 mg naproxen).

INDICATIONS AND DOSAGES

Rheumatoid arthritis, osteoarthritis, ankylosing spondylitis

PO

Adults, Elderly. 250-500 mg naproxen (275-550 mg naproxen sodium) twice a day or 250 mg naproxen (275 mg naproxen sodium) in morning and 500 mg naproxen (550 mg naproxen sodium) in evening. Naprelan: 750-1000 mg once a day.

Acute gouty arthritis

PO

Adults, Elderly. Initially, 750 mg naproxen (825 mg naproxen sodium), then 250 mg naproxen (275 mg naproxen sodium) q8h until attack subsides. Naprelan: Initially, 1000-1500 mg, then 1000 mg once a day until attack subsides.

Mild to moderate pain, dysmenorrhea, bursitis, tendinitis

PO

Adults, Elderly. Initially, 500 mg naproxen (550 mg naproxen sodium), then 250 mg naparoxen (275 mg naproxen sodium) q6-8h as needed. Maximum: 1.25 g/day naproxen (1.375 g/day naproxen sodium). Naprelan: 1000 mg once a day.

Juvenile rheumatoid arthritis

PO (naproxen only)

Children. 10-15 mg/kg/day in 2 divided doses. Maximum: 1000 mg/day.

UNLABELED USES: Treatment of vascular headaches

CONTRAINDICATIONS: Hypersensitivity to aspirin, naproxen, or other NSAIDs

INTERACTIONS

Drug

Antihypertensives, diuretics: May decrease the effects of these drugs.

Aspirin, other salicylates: May increase the risk of GI side effects such as bleeding.

Bone marrow depressants: May increase the risk of hematologic reactions.

Heparin, oral anticoagulants, thrombolytics: May increase the effects of these drugs.

Lithium: May increase the blood concentration and risk of toxicity of lithium.

Methotrexate: May increase the risk of methotrexate toxicity.

Probenecid: May increase the naproxen blood concentration.

Herbal

Feverfew: May decrease the effects of feverfew.

Ginkgo biloba: May increase the risk of bleeding.

Food

None known.

DIAGNOSTIC TEST EFFECTS: May prolong bleeding time and alter blood glucose level. May increase serum hepatic function test results. May decrease serum sodium and uric acid levels.

SIDE EFFECTS

Frequent (9%-4%)

Nausea, constipation, abdominal cramps or pain, heartburn, dizziness, headache, somnolence

Occasional (3%-1%)

Stomatitis, diarrhea, indigestion

Rare (less than 1%)

Vomiting, confusion

SERIOUS REACTIONS

- Rare reactions with long-term use include peptic ulcer disease, GI bleeding, gastritis, severe hepatic reactions (cholestasis, jaundice), nephrotoxicity (dysuria, hematuria, proteinuria, nephrotic syndrome), and a severe hypersensitivity reaction (fever, chills, bronchospasm).

naproxen sodium

(na-prox'-en soe'-dee-um)
Drug Class: Analgesics, non-narcotic; Nonsteroidal anti-inflammatory drugs
Pregnancy Category: B

CLINICAL PHARMACOLOGY

Mechanism of Action: A nonsteroidal anti-inflammatory that produces analgesic and anti-inflammatory effect by inhibiting prostaglandin synthesis. *Therapeutic Effect:* Reduces inflammatory response and intensity of pain stimulus reaching sensory nerve endings.

Pharmacokinetics

Route	Onset	Peak	Duration
PO (analgesic)	less than 1 hr	N/A	7 hrs or less
PO (antirheumatic)	14 days or less	2-4 wks	N/A

Completely absorbed from the gastrointestinal (GI) tract. Protein binding: 99%. Metabolized in liver. Primarily excreted in urine. Not removed by hemodialysis. **Half-life:** 13 hrs.

AVAILABLE FORMS

- *Tablets:* 275 mg (Anaprox), 550 mg (Anaprox DS, Aflaxen).
- *Tablets (extended-release):* 412.5 mg (Naprelan '375'), 550 mg (Napralen '500').
- *Powder for Compounding:* 100%.

INDICATIONS AND DOSAGES

Rheumatoid arthritis, osteoarthritis, ankylosing spondylitis

PO

Adults, Elderly. 250-500 mg (275-550 mg) 2 times/day or 250 mg (275 mg) in morning and 500 mg (550 mg) in evening.

Acute gouty arthritis

PO

Adults, Elderly. Initially, 750 (825) mg, then 250 (275) mg q8h until attack subsides. Mild to moderate pain, dysmenorrhea, bursitis, tendinitis

PO

Adults, Elderly. Initially, 500 (550) mg, then 250 (275) mg q6-8h as needed. Total daily dose not to exceed 1. 25 (1.375) g.

UNLABELED USES: Treatment of vascular headaches

CONTRAINDICATIONS: Hypersensitivity to aspirin, naproxen, or other NSAIDs

INTERACTIONS

Drug

Antihypertensives, diuretics: May decrease the effects of antihypertensives and diuretics.

Aspirin, salicylates: May increase the risk of GI bleeding and side effects.

Bone marrow depressants: May increase risk of hematologic reactions.

Heparin, oral anticoagulants, thrombolytics: May increase the effects of heparin, oral anticoagulants, and thrombolytics.

Lithium: May increase the blood concentration and risk of toxicity of lithium.

Methotrexate: May increase the risk of toxicity of methotrexate.

Probenecid: May increase naproxen blood concentration.

Herbal

Feverfew: May decrease the effects of feverfew.

Ginkgo biloba: May increase the risk of bleeding.

Food

None known.

DIAGNOSTIC TEST EFFECTS: May prolong bleeding time, alter blood glucose levels. May increase liver function tests. May decrease serum sodium and uric acid levels.

SIDE EFFECTS

Frequent (9%-4%)

Nausea, constipation, abdominal cramps/pain, heartburn, dizziness, headache, drowsiness

Occasional (3%-1%)

Stomatitis, diarrhea, indigestion-

Rare (less than 1%)

Vomiting, confusion

SERIOUS REACTIONS

• Peptic ulcer disease, GI bleeding, gastritis, and severe hepatic reaction, such as cholestasis and jaundice, occur rarely.

• Nephrotoxicity, including dysuria, hematuria, proteinuria, and nephrotic syndrome, and severe hypersensitivity reaction, marked by fever, chills, and bronchospasm, occur rarely.

SPECIAL CONSIDERATIONS

PRECAUTIONS

• Naproxen sodium should not be used concomitantly with the related drug naproxen because they circulate in plasma as the naproxen anion. In human beings, there have been reports of acute interstitial nephritis with hematuria, proteinuria, and occasionally nephrotic syndrome. In patients with prerenal conditions, administration of a nonsteroidal antiinflammatory drug may cause a dose-dependent reduction in prostaglandin formation and may precipitate overt renal decompensation. Naproxen sodium and its metabolites are eliminated primarily by the kidneys; therefore, use the drug with great caution in patients with significantly impaired renal function. Chronic alcoholic liver disease and probably other forms of cirrhosis reduce the total plasma concentration of naproxen, but the plasma concentration of unbound naproxen is increased. As with other nonsteroidal antiinflammatory drugs, borderline elevations of one or more liver function tests may occur in up to 15% of patients. If steroid dosage is reduced or eliminated during therapy, reduce the steroid dosage slowly and closely observe the patients for any evidence of adverse effects, including adrenal insufficiency and exacerbation of symptoms of arthritis. Patients with initial hemoglobin values of 10 g or less who are to receive long-term therapy should have hemoglobin values determined periodically. Peripheral edema has been observed in some patients. The antipyretic and antiinflammatory activities of the drug may reduce fever and inflammation, thus diminishing their usefulness as diagnostic signs in detecting complications of presumed noninfectious, noninflammatory, painful conditions.

PATIENT INFORMATION

• Naproxen sodium, like other drugs of its class, is not free of side effects. The side effects of these drugs can cause discomfort, and rarely there are more serious side effects, such as gastrointestinal bleeding, which may result in hospitalization and even fatal outcomes. Nonsteroidal antiinflammatory drugs are often essential agents in the management of arthritis and have a major role in the treatment of pain, but they also may be used commonly for conditions that are less serious. Eye care practitioners may wish to discuss with their patients the potential risks and likely benefits of nonsteroidal antiinflammatory drug treatment, particularly when the drugs are used for less serious conditions where treatment without nonsteroidal antiinflammtory drugs may represent an acceptable alternative to the patient and eye care practitioner. Patients whose activities require alertness should exercise caution if they experience drowsiness, dizziness, vertigo, or depression during therapy with the drug.

PREGNANCY AND LACTATION

- Pregnancy Category B. Reproduction studies have been performed in rats, rabbits, and mice at doses up to 6 times the human dose and have revealed no evidence of impaired fertility or harm to the fetus from the drug. The naproxen anion has been found in the milk of lactating women at a concentration of approximately 1% of that found in the plasma.

OCULAR CONSIDERATIONS

PRECAUTION:

- Because of adverse eye findings in animal studies with drugs of this class, it is recommended that an eye examination be performed if any change or disturbance in vision occurs.

natamycin

(na-ta-mye'-sin)

Rx: Natacyn

Drug Class: Antifungals, ophthalmic; Ophthalmics

Pregnancy Category: C

Do not confuse with naproxen.

CLINICAL PHARMACOLOGY

Mechanism of Action: A polyene antifungal agent that increases cell membrane permeability in susceptible fungi. *Therapeutic Effect:* Fungicidal.

Pharmacokinetics

Minimal systemic absorption. Adheres to cornea and retained in conjunctival fornices.

AVAILABLE FORMS

- *Ophthalmic Suspension:* 5% (Natacyn).

INDICATIONS AND DOSAGES

Fungal keratitis, ophthalmic fungal infections

Ophthalmic

Adults, Elderly. Instill 1 drop in conjunctival sac every 1-2 hours. After 3-4 days, reduce to 1 drop 6-8 times daily. Usual course of therapy is 2-3 weeks.

UNLABELED USES: Oral and vaginal candidiasis, onychomycosis, pulmonary aspergillosis

CONTRAINDICATIONS: Hypersensitivity to natamycin or any component of the formulation

INTERACTIONS

Drug

Topical corticosteroids: May increase risk of toxicity. Concomitant use is contraindicated.

Herbal

None known.

Food

None known.

DIAGNOSTIC TEST EFFECTS: *None known.*

IV INCOMPATIBILITIES: None known.

IV COMPATIBILITIES: None known.

SIDE EFFECTS

Occasional (10%-3%)

Blurred vision, eye irritation, eye pain, photophobia

SERIOUS REACTIONS

• Vomiting and diarrhea have occurred with large doses in the treatment of systemic mycoses.

SPECIAL CONSIDERATIONS

PRECAUTIONS

• Failure of improvement of keratitis following 7 to 10 days of administration of the drug suggests that the infection may be caused by a microorganism not susceptible to natamycin. Adherence of the suspension to areas of epithelial ulceration or retention of the suspension in the fornices occurs regularly.

PREGNANCY AND LACTATION

• Pregnancy Category C. Fetal harm is not known with topical administration. Excretion into human milk is not known.

nateglinide

(na-teg'lin-ide)

Rx: Starlix

Drug Class: Antidiabetic agents; Meglitinides

Pregnancy Category: C

CLINICAL PHARMACOLOGY

Mechanism of Action: An antihyperglycemic that stimulates release of insulin from beta cells of the pancreas by depolarizing beta cells, leading to an opening of calcium channels. Resulting calcium influx induces insulin secretion. *Therapeutic Effect:* Lowers blood glucose concentration.

AVAILABLE FORMS

• *Tablets:* 60 mg, 120 mg.

INDICATIONS AND DOSAGES

Diabetes mellitus

PO

Adult, Elderly. 120 mg 3 times a day before meals. Initially, 60 mg may be given.

CONTRAINDICATIONS: Diabetic ketoacidosis, type 1 diabetes mellitus

INTERACTIONS

Drug

Beta-blockers, MAOIs, NSAIDs, salicylates: May increase hypoglycemic effect of nateglinide.

Corticosteroids, thiazide diuretics, thyroid medication, sympathomimetics: May decrease hypoglycemic effect of nateglinide.

Herbal

None known.

Food

Liquid meal: Peak plasma levels may be significantly reduced if administered 10 minutes before a liquid meal.

DIAGNOSTIC TEST EFFECTS: *None known.*

SIDE EFFECTS

Frequent (10%)

Upper respiratory tract infection

Occasional (4%-3%)

Back pain, flu symptoms, dizziness, arthropathy, diarrhea

Rare (3% or less)

Bronchitis, cough

SERIOUS REACTIONS

• Hypoglycemia occurs in less than 2% of patients.

SPECIAL CONSIDERATIONS

PRECAUTIONS

• All oral blood glucose–lowering drugs that are absorbed systemically are capable of producing hypoglycemia. Geriatric patients, malnourished patients, and those with adrenal or pituitary insufficiency are more susceptible to the glucose-lowering effect of these treatments. Use nateglinide with caution in patients with moderate to severe liver disease. Transient loss of glycemic control may occur with fever, infection, trauma, or surgery.

PATIENT INFORMATION

• Inform patients of the potential risks and benefits of nateglinide and of alternative modes of therapy. Explain the risks and management of hypoglycemia. Instruct patients to take nateglinide 1 to 30 minutes before ingesting a meal but to skip their scheduled dose if they skip the meal to reduce the risk of hypoglycemia. Discuss drug interactions with patients. Inform patients of potential drug-drug interactions with nateglinide.

PREGNANCY AND LACTATION

• Pregnancy Category C. In the rabbit, embryonic development was affected adversely with oral doses. Studies in lactating rats showed that nateglinide is excreted in the milk. Excretion into human milk is not known.

nedocromil sodium

(ned-oh-crow'mil)

Rx: Alocril

Drug Class: Mast cell stabilizers

Pregnancy Category: B

CLINICAL PHARMACOLOGY

Mechanism of Action: A mast cell stabilizer that prevents the activation and release of inflammatory mediators, such as histamine, leukotrienes, mast cells, eosinophils, and monocytes. *Therapeutic Effect:* Prevents both early and late asthmatic responses.

AVAILABLE FORMS

• *Aerosol for Inhalation (Tilade):* 1.75 mg/activation.

• *Ophthalmic Solution (Alocril):* 2%.

INDICATIONS AND DOSAGES

Mild to moderate asthma

Oral Inhalation

Adults, Elderly, Children 6 yr and older. 2 inhalations 4 times a day. May decrease to 3 times a day then twice a day as asthma becomes controlled.

Allergic conjunctivitis

Ophthalmic

Adults, Elderly, Children 3 yr and older. 1-2 drops in each eye twice a day.

UNLABELED USES: Prevention of bronchospasm in patients with reversible obstructive airway disease

CONTRAINDICATIONS: None known.

INTERACTIONS

Drug

None known.

Herbal

None known.

Food

None known.

DIAGNOSTIC TEST EFFECTS: *None known.*

SIDE EFFECTS

Frequent (10%-6%)

Cough, pharyngitis, bronchospasm, headache, altered taste

Occasional (5%-1%)

Rhinitis, upper respiratory tract infection, abdominal pain, fatigue

Rare (less than 1%)

Diarrhea, dizziness

SERIOUS REACTIONS

• None known.

neomycin sulfate; polymyxin B sulfate

(nee-oh-mye'sin sul'fate; pol-ee-mix'in bee sul'fate)

Drug Class: Anti-infectives, ophthalmic; Antibiotics, aminoglycosides; Antibiotics, polymyxins; Irrigants, genitourinary; Ophthalmics

Pregnancy Category: D

CLINICAL PHARMACOLOGY

Mechanism of Action: Polymyxin B damages bacterial cytoplasmic membrane which causes leakage of intracellular components. Neomycin is an aminoglycoside antibiotic that binds to the 30s subunit of the ribosome. *Therapeutic Effect:* Inhibits bacterial cell wall synthesis.

Pharmacokinetics

Neomycin and polymyxin B are absorbed in clinically insignificant quantities after prophylactic irrigation.

AVAILABLE FORMS

- *Cream:* 3.5 mg neomycin and 10,000 units of polymyxin B per gram (Neosporin Cream).
- *Solution, irrigant:* 40 mg neomycin and 200,000 units polymyxin B sulfate per ml (Neosporin G.U. Irrigant).

INDICATIONS AND DOSAGES

Short term as a continuous irrigant or rinse in the urinary bladder to prevent bacteriuria and gram-negative rod septicemia associated with the use of indwelling catheters

Bladder irrigation

Adults, Elderly. Add 1 ml irrigant to 1 L isotonic saline solution and connect container to the inflow of lumen of 3-way catheter. Continuous irrigant or rinse in the urinary bladder for up to a maximum of 10 days with administration rate adjusted to patient's urine output. Usually no more than 1 L of irrigant is used per day.

Minor bacterial skin infections

Topical

Adults, Elderly. Apply to affected area 1-3 times/day.

CONTRAINDICATIONS: History of hypersensitivity or serious toxic reaction to an aminoglycoside, hypersensitivity to polymyxin B, neomycin, or any component of the formulation

INTERACTIONS

Drug

None known.

Herbal

None known.

Food

None known.

DIAGNOSTIC TEST EFFECTS: *None known.*

SIDE EFFECTS

Occasional

Topical: skin sensitization

Bladder irrigation: irritation of the urinary bladder mucosa

SERIOUS REACTIONS

- Otoxicity, nephrotoxicity, and neuromuscular blockade may occur if systemically absorbed.

SPECIAL CONSIDERATIONS

PRECAUTIONS

- Renew the medication order beyond 20 ml or 8 g after slit-lamp examination with fluorescein staining.

PREGNANCY AND LACTATION

- Pregnancy Category D. Aminoglycosides, when absorbed, can cause fetal harm when administered to a pregnant woman. Aminoglycoside antibiotics cross the placenta, and there have been several reports of total, irreversible, bilateral, congenital deafness in children whose mothers received streptomycin during pregnancy. Excretion into human milk is not known.

neomycin sulfate; polymyxin B sulfate; prednisolone acetate

(nee-oh-mye'-sin; pol-i-mix'-in bee; pred-niss'-oh-lone as'-i-tate)

Rx: Poly Pred

Drug Class: Anti-infectives, ophthalmic; Antibiotics, aminoglycosides; Antibiotics, polymyxins; Corticosteroids, ophthalmic; Ophthalmics

Pregnancy Category: C

CLINICAL PHARMACOLOGY

Mechanism of Action: Polymyxin B damages bacterial cytoplasmic membrane which causes leakage of intracellular components. Neomycin is an aminoglycoside antibiotic that binds to the 30s subunit of the ribosome. Prednisolone is an adrenal corticosteroid that inhibits accumulation of inflammatory cells at inflammation sites, phagocytosis, lysosomal enzyme release and synthesis, and release of mediators of inflammation. *Therapeutic Effect:* Inhibits bacterial cell wall synthesis. Prevents or suppresses cell-mediated immune reactions. Decreases or prevents tissue response to inflammatory process.

Pharmacokinetics

None reported.

AVAILABLE FORMS

• *Ophthalmic suspension:* 0.35% neomycin sulfate, 10,000 units polymyxin B sulfate, and 0.5% prednisolone acetate per ml (Poly-Pred).

INDICATIONS AND DOSAGES

Steroid-responsive inflammatory ocular condition in which bacterial infection or a risk of bacterial ocular infection exists

Ophthalmic

Adults, Elderly. Instill 1-2 drops every 3-4 hours. Acute infections may require every 30 minute instillations initially with frequency of administration reduced as the infection is brought under control.

CONTRAINDICATIONS: Epithelial herpes simplex keratitis, vaccinia, varicella, and other viral diseases of the cornea and conjunctiva, mycobacterial infection of the eye, fungal disease of the eye, and hypersensitivity to polymyxin B, neomycin, prednisolone or any component of the formulation

INTERACTIONS

Drug

None known.

Herbal

None known.

Food

None known.

DIAGNOSTIC TEST EFFECTS: *None known.*

SIDE EFFECTS

Rare

Stinging or burning, elevated intraocular pressure, posterior cataract formation

SERIOUS REACTIONS

• Optic nerve damage and delayed wound healing have been reported.

• Secondary infections occur rarely.

SPECIAL CONSIDERATIONS

PRECAUTIONS

• Renew the medication order beyond 20 ml after slit-lamp examination with fluorescein staining. Consider the possibility of fungal infections of the cornea after prolonged steroid dosing. Exercise great caution in treatment of patients with herpes simplex.

niacin, nicotinic acid

(nye'a-sin)

Rx: Niaspan ER

Drug Class: Antihyperlipidemics; Nicotinic acid derivatives; Vitamins/minerals

Pregnancy Category: C

Do not confuse niacin, Niacor, or Niaspan with minocin or Nitro-Bid.

OTC

CLINICAL PHARMACOLOGY

Mechanism of Action: An antihyperlipidemic, water-soluble vitamin that is a component of two coenzymes needed for tissue respiration, lipid metabolism, and glycogenolysis. Inhibits synthesis of VLDLs. *Therapeutic Effect:* Reduces total, LDL, and VLDL cholesterol levels and triglyceride levels; increases HDL cholesterol concentration.

Pharmacokinetics

Readily absorbed from the GI tract. Widely distributed. Metabolized in the liver. Primarily excreted in urine. **Half-life:** 45 min.

AVAILABLE FORMS

- *Capsules (Timed-Release):* 125 mg, 250 mg, 400 mg, 500 mg.
- *Tablets (Niacor):* 50 mg, 100 mg, 250 mg, 500 mg.
- *Tablets (Timed-Release [Slo-Niacin]):* 250 mg, 500 mg, 750 mg.
- *Tablets (Timed-Release [Niaspan]):* 500 mg, 750 mg, 1000 mg.
- *Elixir (Nicotinex):* 50 mg/5 ml.

INDICATIONS AND DOSAGES

Hyperlipidemia

PO (Immediate-Release)

Adults, Elderly. Initially, 50-100 mg twice a day for 7 days. Increase gradually by doubling dose qwk up to 1-1.5 g/day in 2-3 doses. Maximum: 3 g/day.

Children. Initially, 100-250 mg/day (maximum: 10 mg/kg/day) in 3 divided doses. May increase by 100 mg/wk or 250 mg q2-3wks. Maximum: 2250 mg/day.

PO (Timed-Release)

Adults, Elderly. Initially, 500 mg/day in 2 divided doses for 1 wk; then increase to 500 mg twice a day. Maintenance: 2 g/day.

Nutritional supplement

PO

Adults, Elderly. 10-20 mg/day. Maximum: 100 mg/day.

Pellegra

PO

Adults, Elderly. 50-100 mg 3-4 times a day. Maximum: 500 mg/day.

Children. 50-100 mg 3 times a day.

CONTRAINDICATIONS: Active peptic ulcer disease, arterial hemorrhaging, hepatic dysfunction, hypersensitivity to niacin or tartrazine (frequently seen in patients sensitive to aspirin), severe hypotension

INTERACTIONS

Drug

Alcohol: May increase risk of niacin side effects, such as flushing.

Lovastatin, pravastatin, simvastatin: May increase the risk of acute renal failure and rhabdomyolysis.

Herbal

None known.

Food

None known.

DIAGNOSTIC TEST EFFECTS: May increase serum uric acid level.

SIDE EFFECTS

Frequent

Flushing (especially of the face and neck) occurring within 20 minutes of drug administration and lasting for 30-60 minutes, GI upset, pruritus

Occasional

Dizziness, hypotension, headache, blurred vision, burning or tingling of skin, flatulence, nausea, vomiting, diarrhea

Rare

Hyperglycemia, glycosuria, rash, hyperpigmentation, dry skin

SERIOUS REACTIONS

• Arrhythmias occur rarely.

SPECIAL CONSIDERATIONS

PRECAUTIONS

• Use with caution in patients who consume substantial quantities of alcohol and/or have a history of liver disease. Active liver diseases or unexplained transaminase elevations are contraindication to the use of nicotinic acid. Frequently monitor liver function tests and blood glucose to ascertain that the drug is producing no adverse effects on these organ systems. Diabetic patients may experience a dose-related rise in glucose intolerance, the clinical significance of which is unclear. Also use caution when nicotinic acid is used in patients with unstable angina or in the acute phase of myocardial infarction. Use niacin with caution in patients predisposed to gout. This product contains FD&C yellow No. 5 (tartrazine), which may cause allergic-type reactions (including bronchial asthma) in certain susceptible persons.

PREGNANCY AND LACTATION

• Pregnancy Category C. Animal reproduction studies have not been conducted with nicotinic acid. Whether nicotinic acid at doses typically used for lipid disorders can cause fetal harm when administered to pregnant women or whether it can affect reproductive capacity is not known. Excretion into human milk is not known.

OCULAR CONSIDERATIONS

• Adverse reactions include toxic amblyopia and cystoid macular edema.

• Niacin has been associated with the discoloration of the eyelids, decreased vision, dry eyes, cystoid macular edema, loss of eyebrows and eyelashes, proptosis, eyelid edema, and superficial punctuate keratitis. (Fraunfelder FW: Ocular side effects from herbal medicines and nutritional supplements, *Am J Ophthalmol* 138[4]:639-647, 2004.)

nicardipine hydrochloride

(nye-card'i-peen)

Rx: Cardene, Cardene IV, Cardene SR

Drug Class: Calcium channel blockers

Pregnancy Category: C

Do not confuse nicardipine with nifedipine, Cardene with codeine, or Cardene SR with Cardizem SR or codeine.

CLINICAL PHARMACOLOGY

Mechanism of Action: An antianginal and antihypertensive agent that inhibits calcium ion movement across cell membranes, depressing contraction of cardiac and vascular smooth muscle. *Therapeutic Effect:* Increases heart rate and cardiac output. Decreases systemic vascular resistance and BP.

Pharmacokinetics

Route	Onset	Peak	Duration
PO	N/A	1-2 hr	8 hr

Rapidly, completely absorbed from the GI tract. Protein binding: 95%. Undergoes first-pass metabolism in the liver. Primarily excreted in urine. Not removed by hemodialysis. **Half-life:** 2-4 hr.

AVAILABLE FORMS

- *Capsules (Cardene):* 20 mg, 30 mg.
- *Capsules, (Sustained-Release [Cardene SR]):* 30 mg, 45 mg, 60 mg.
- *Injection (Cardene IV):* 2.5 mg/ml.

INDICATIONS AND DOSAGES

Chronic stable (effort-associated) angina

PO

Adults, Elderly. Initially, 20 mg 3 times a day. Range: 20-40 mg 3 times a day.

Essential hypertension

PO

Adults, Elderly. Initially, 20 mg 3 times a day. Range: 20-40 mg 3 times a day.

PO (Sustained-Release)

Adults, Elderly. Initially, 30 mg twice a day. Range: 30-60 mg twice a day.

Short-term treatment of hypertension when oral therapy is not feasible or desirable (substitute for oral nicardipine)

IV

Adults, Elderly. 0.5 mg/hr (for patient receiving 20 mg PO q8h); 1.2 mg/hr (for patient receiving 30 mg PO q8h); 2.2 mg/hr (for patient receiving 40 mg PO q8h).

Patients not already receiving nicardipine

IV

Adults, Elderly (gradual BP decrease). Initially, 5 mg/hr. May increase by 2.5 mg/hr q15min. After BP goal is achieved, decrease rate to 3 mg/hr.

Adults, Elderly (rapid BP decrease). Initially, 5 mg/hr. May increase by 2.5 mg/hr q5min. Maximum: 15 mg/hr until desired BP attained. After BP goal achieved, decrease rate to 3 mg/hr.

Changing from IV to oral antihypertensive therapy

Adults, Elderly. Begin antihypertensives other than nicardipine when IV has been discontinued; for nicardipine, give first dose 1 hr before discontinuing IV.

Dosage in hepatic impairment

For adults and elderly patients, initially give 20 mg twice a day; then titrate.

Dosage in renal impairment

For adults and elderly patients, initially give 20 mg q8h (30 mg twice a day [sustained-release capsules]); then titrate.

UNLABELED USES: Treatment of associated neurologic deficits, Raynaud's phenomenon, subarachnoid hemorrhage, vasospastic angina

CONTRAINDICATIONS: Atrial fibrillation or flutter associated with accessory conduction pathways, cardiogenic shock, CHF, second- or third-degree heart block, severe hypotension, sinus bradycardia, ventricular tachycardia, within several hours of IV beta-blocker therapy

INTERACTIONS

Drug

Beta-blockers: May have additive effect.

Digoxin: May increase nicardipine blood concentration.

Hypokalemia-producing agents (such as furosemide and certain other diuretics): May increase risk of arrhythmias.

Procainamide, quinidine: May increase risk of QT-interval prolongation.

Herbal

None known.

Food

Grapefruit, grapefruit juice: May alter absorption of nicardipine.

DIAGNOSTIC TEST EFFECTS: *None known.*

IV INCOMPATIBILITIES: Furosemide (Lasix), heparin, thiopental (Pentothal)

IV COMPATIBILITIES: Diltiazem (Cardizem), dobutamine (Dobutrex), dopamine (Intropin), epinephrine, hydromorphone (Dilaudid), labetalol (Trandate), lorazepam (Ativan), midazolam (Versed), milrinone (Primacor), morphine, nitroglycerin, norepinephrine (Levophed)

SIDE EFFECTS

Frequent (10%-7%)

Headache, facial flushing, peripheral edema, light-headedness, dizziness

Occasional (6%-3%)

Asthenia (loss of strength, energy), palpitations, angina, tachycardia

Rare (less than 2%)

Nausea, abdominal cramps, dyspepsia, dry mouth, rash

SERIOUS REACTIONS

• Overdose produces confusion, slurred speech, somnolence, marked hypotension, and bradycardia.

SPECIAL CONSIDERATIONS

PRECAUTIONS

• Increased angina has been reported. Exercise caution when using the drug in patients with congestive heart failure, particularly in combination with a beta-blocker. Nicardipine hydrochloride may produce hypotension. Use the drug with caution in patients having impaired liver function or reduced hepatic blood flow.

PREGNANCY AND LACTATION

• Pregnancy Category C. Nicardipine was embryocidal when administered orally to pregnant rabbits during organogenesis. Fetal harm is not known. Studies in rats have shown significant concentrations of nicardipine hydrochloride in maternal milk following oral administration. For this reason, it is recommended that women who wish to breast-feed should not take this drug.

OCULAR CONSIDERATIONS

• Concomitant administration of nicardipine and cyclosporine increases cyclosporine levels. Therefore, closely monitor plasma concentrations of cyclosporine and reduce its dosage accordingly in patients treated with nicardipine.

nifedipine

(nye-fed'i-peen)

Rx: Adalat CC, Procardia, Procardia XL

Drug Class: Calcium channel blockers

Pregnancy Category: C

Do not confuse nifedipine with nicardipine or nimodipine.

CLINICAL PHARMACOLOGY

Mechanism of Action: An antianginal and antihypertensive agent that inhibits calcium ion movement across cell membranes, depressing contraction of cardiac and vascular smooth muscle. *Therapeutic Effect:* Increases heart rate and cardiac output. Decreases systemic vascular resistance and BP.

Pharmacokinetics

Route	Onset	Peak	Duration
Sublingual	1-5 min	N/A	N/A
PO	20-30 min	N/A	4-8 hr
PO (extended release)	2 hr	N/A	24 hr

Rapidly, completely absorbed from the GI tract. Protein binding: 92%-98%. Undergoes first-pass metabolism in the liver. Primarily excreted in urine. Not removed by hemodialysis. **Half-life:** 2-5 hr.

AVAILABLE FORMS

- *Capsules (Procardia):* 10 mg.
- *Tablets (Extended-Release [Adalat CC, Procardia XL]):* 30 mg, 60 mg, 90 mg.
- *Tablets (Extended-Release [Nifedical XL}):* 30 mg, 60 mg.

INDICATIONS AND DOSAGES

Prinzmetal's variant angina, chronic stable (effort-associated) angina

PO

Adults, Elderly. Initially, 10 mg 3 times a day. Increase at 7- to 14-day intervals. Maintenance: 10 mg 3 times a day up to 30 mg 4 times a day.

PO (Extended-Release)

Adults, Elderly. Initially, 30-60 mg/day. Maintenance: Up to 120 mg/day.

Essential hypertension

PO (Extended-Release)

Adults, Elderly. Initially, 30-60 mg/day. Maintenance: Up to 120 mg/day.

UNLABELED USES: Treatment of Raynaud's phenomenon

CONTRAINDICATIONS: Advanced aortic stenosis, severe hypotension

INTERACTIONS

Drug

Beta-blockers: May have additive effect.

Digoxin: May increase digoxin blood concentration.

Hypokalemia-producing agents (such as furosemide and certain other diuretics): May increase risk of arrhythmias.

Herbal

None known.

Food

Grapefruit, grapefruit juice: May increase nifedipine plasma concentration.

DIAGNOSTIC TEST EFFECTS: May cause positive ANA and direct Coombs' test.

SIDE EFFECTS

Frequent (30%-11%)

Peripheral edema, headache, flushed skin, dizziness

Occasional (12%-6%)

Nausea, shakiness, muscle cramps and pain, somnolence, palpitations, nasal congestion, cough, dyspnea, wheezing

Rare (5%-3%)

Hypotension, rash, pruritus, urticaria, constipation, abdominal discomfort, flatulence, sexual difficulties

SERIOUS REACTIONS

- Nifedipine may precipitate CHF and MI in patients with cardiac disease and peripheral ischemia.
- Overdose produces nausea, somnolence, confusion, and slurred speech.

SPECIAL CONSIDERATIONS

PRECAUTIONS

- Patients recently withdrawn from beta-blockers may develop a withdrawal syndrome with increased angina, probably related to increased sensitivity to catecholamines. Because nifedipine decreases peripheral vascular resistance, careful monitoring of blood pressure during the initial administration and titration of nifedipine is suggested. Mild to moderate peripheral edema may be associated with use.

PATIENT INFORMATION

Give patients the following instructions:

- Extended-Release Tablets: Nifedipine extended-release tablets should be swallowed whole. Do not chew, divide, or crush tablets. Do not be concerned if you occasionally notice in your stool something that looks like a tablet. In nifedipine the medication is contained within a nonabsorbable shell that has been specially designed to release the drug slowly for your body to absorb. When this process is completed, the empty tablet is eliminated from your body. Adalat CC should be taken on an empty stomach. It should not be administered with food.

PREGNANCY AND LACTATION

- Pregnancy Category C. Nifedipine administration was associated with a variety of embryotoxic, placentotoxic, and fetotoxic effects. Fetal harm is not known. Excretion into human milk is not known.

nisoldipine

(nye-soul-dih-peen)

Rx: Sular

Drug Class: Calcium channel blockers

Pregnancy Category: C

Do not confuse with nicardipine.

CLINICAL PHARMACOLOGY

Mechanism of Action: A calcium channel blocker that inhibits calcium ion movement across cell membrane, depressing contraction of cardiac and vascular smooth muscle. *Therapeutic Effect:* Increases heart rate and cardiac output. Decreases systemic vascular resistance and blood pressure (BP).

Pharmacokinetics

Poor absorption from the gastrointestinal (GI) tract. Food increases bioavailability. Protein binding: more than 99%. Metabolism occurs in the gut wall. Primarily excreted in urine. Not removed by hemodialysis. **Half-life:** 7-12 hrs.

AVAILABLE FORMS

- *Tablets (extended-release):* 10 mg, 20 mg, 30 mg, 40 mg (Sular).

INDICATIONS AND DOSAGES

Hypertension

PO

Adults. Initially, 20 mg once daily, then increase by 10 mg per week, or longer intervals until therapeutic BP response is attained.

Elderly. Initially, 10 mg once daily. Increase by 10 mg per week to therapeutic response. Maintenance: 20-40 mg once daily. Maximum: 60 mg once daily.

UNLABELED USES: Stable angina pectoris, CHF

CONTRAINDICATIONS: Sick-sinus syndrome/second- or third-degree AV block (except in presence of pacemaker), hypersensitivity to nisoldipine or any component of the formulation

INTERACTIONS

Drug

Amiodarone: May increase risk of bradycardia, atrioventricular block and/or sinus arrest.

Beta-blockers: May have additive effect.

Delavirdine, ketoconazole, voriconazole: May increase serum nisoldipine concentrations.

Digoxin: May increase digoxin blood concentration.

Epirubicin: May increase risk of heart failure.

Fentanyl: May increase risk of severe hypotension.
Phenytoin, fosphenytoin: May decrease nisoldipine concentrations.
NSAIDs, oral anticoagulants: May increase risk of gastrointestinal hemorrhage and/or antagonism of hypotensive effect.
Quinidine: May increase risk of quinidine toxicity.
Quinupristin/dalfopristin, saquinavir: May increase risk of nisoldipine toxicity.
Rifampin: May decrease nisoldipine efficacy.

Herbal

Licorice, Ma huang, peppermint oil, yohimbine: May decrease effectiveness of nisoldipine.
St. John's wort: May decrease bioavailability of nisoldipine.

Food

Grapefruit and grapefruit juice: May increase nisoldipine plasma concentration.

DIAGNOSTIC TEST EFFECTS: *None known.*

IV INCOMPATIBILITIES: None known.

IV COMPATIBILITIES: None known.

SIDE EFFECTS

Frequent

Giddiness, dizziness, lightheadedness, peripheral edema, headache, flushing, weakness, nausea

Occasional

Transient hypotension, heartburn, muscle cramps, nasal congestion, cough, wheezing, sore throat, palpitations, nervousness, mood changes

Rare

Increase in frequency, intensity, duration of anginal attack during initial therapy

SERIOUS REACTIONS

- May precipitate congestive heart failure (CHF) and myocardial infarction (MI) in patients with cardiac disease and peripheral ischemia.
- Overdose produces nausea, drowsiness, confusion, and slurred speech.

SPECIAL CONSIDERATIONS

PRECAUTIONS

- Because nisoldipine, like other vasodilators, decreases peripheral vascular resistance, careful monitoring of blood pressure during the initial administration and titration of nisoldipine is recommended. Therefore, exercise caution when using nisoldipine in patients with heart failure or compromised ventricular function, particularly in combination with a beta-blocker. Administer nisoldipine cautiously in patients with severe hepatic dysfunction.

PREGNANCY AND LACTATION

- Pregnancy Category C. Nisoldipine was fetotoxic but not teratogenic in rats and rabbits.
- Fetal harm is not known. Excretion into human milk is not known.

norfloxacin

(nor-flox'a-sin)

Rx: Chibroxin, Noroxin

Drug Class: Anti-infectives, ophthalmic; Antibiotics, quinolones; Ophthalmics

Pregnancy Category: C

CLINICAL PHARMACOLOGY

Mechanism of Action: A quinolone that inhibits DNA gyrase in susceptible microorganisms, interfering with bacterial cell replication and repair. *Therapeutic Effect:* Bactericidal.

AVAILABLE FORMS

- *Tablets:* 400 mg.
- *Ophthalmic Solution (Chibroxin):* 0.3%.

INDICATIONS AND DOSAGES

Bacterial conjunctivitis

The recommended dose in adults and pediatric patients (1 year and older) is 1 or 2 drops 4 times/day for up to 7 days. First day of therapy may be 1 or 2 drops every 2 hours during the waking hours.

Urinary tract infections (UTIs)

PO

Adults, Elderly. 400 mg twice a day for 7-21 days.

Prostatitis

PO

Adults. 400 mg twice a day for 28 days.

Uncomplicated gonococcal infections

PO

Adults. 800 mg as a single dose.

Dosage in renal impairment

Dosage and frequency are modified based on creatinine clearance.

Creatinine Clearance	*Dosage*
30 ml/min or higher	400 mg twice a day
less than 30 ml/min	400 mg once a day

CONTRAINDICATIONS: Children younger than 18 years because of risk arthropathy; hypersensitivity to norfloxacin, other quinolones, or their components

INTERACTIONS

Drug

Antacids, sucralfate: May decrease norfloxacin absorption.

Oral anticoagulants: May increase effects of oral anticoagulants.

Theophylline: Decreases clearance and may increase blood concentration and risk of toxicity of theophylline.

Herbal

None known.

Food

None known.

DIAGNOSTIC TEST EFFECTS: May increase BUN level and serum alkaline phosphatase, bilirubin, creatinine, LDH, AST (SGOT), and ALT (SGPT) levels.

SIDE EFFECTS

Burning or discomfort. Other reactions were conjunctival hyperemia, chemosis, corneal deposits, photophobia, and a bitter taste following installation.

Frequent

Nausea, headache, dizziness

Rare

Vomiting, diarrhea, dry mouth, bitter taste, nervousness, drowsiness, insomnia, photosensitivity, tinnitus, crystalluria, rash, fever, seizures

SERIOUS REACTIONS

• Superinfection, anaphylaxis, Stevens-Johnson syndrome, and arthropathy occur rarely.

• Hypersensitivity reactions, including photosensitivity (as evidenced by rash, pruritus, blisters, edema, and burning skin), have occurred in patients receiving fluoroquinolones.

SPECIAL CONSIDERATIONS

PRECAUTIONS

• Prolonged use may result in overgrowth of fungi. If superinfection occurs, initiate appropriate measures.

PATIENT INFORMATION

• Administration of norfloxacin may be associated with hypersensitivity reactions. Advise patients not to wear contact lenses if they have signs and symptoms of bacterial conjunctivitis.

PREGNANCY AND LACTATION

• Pregnancy Category C. Norfloxacin produced embryonic loss in monkeys with oral doses. Fetal harm is not known with topical administration. Excretion into human milk is not known.

nystatin

(nye-stat'in)

Rx: Bio-Statin, Mycostatin, Mycostatin Pastilles, Mycostatin Topical, Nystat-Rx, Nystex, Nystop, Pedi-Dri

Drug Class: Antifungals; Antifungals, topical; Dermatologics

Pregnancy Category: C

Do not confuse nystatin or Mycostatin with Nitrostat.

CLINICAL PHARMACOLOGY

Mechanism of Action: A fungistatic antifungal that binds to sterols in the fungal cell membrane. *Therapeutic Effect:* Increases fungal cell-membrane permeability, allowing loss of potassium and other cellular components.

Pharmacokinetics

PO: Poorly absorbed from the GI tract. Eliminated unchanged in feces. Topical: Not absorbed systemically from intact skin.

AVAILABLE FORMS

- *Oral Suspension (Mycostatin):* 100,000 units/ml.
- *Tablets (Mycostatin):* 500,000 units.
- *Vaginal Tablets:* 100,000 units.
- *Cream (Mycostatin):* 100,000 units/g.
- *Ointment:* 100,000 units/g.
- *Topical Powder (Mycostatin, Nystop):* 100,000 units/g.

INDICATIONS AND DOSAGES

Intestinal infections

PO

Adults, Elderly. 500,000-1,000,000 units q8h.

Oral candidiasis

PO

Adults, Elderly, Children. 400,000-600,000 units 4 times/day.

Infants. 200,000 units 4 times/day.

Vaginal infections

Vaginal

Adults, Elderly, Adolescents. 1 tablet/day at bedtime for 14 days.

Cutaneous candidal infections

Topical

Adults, Elderly, Children. Apply 2-4 times/day.

UNLABELED USES: Prophylaxis and treatment of oropharyngeal candidiasis, tinea barbae, tinea capitis

CONTRAINDICATIONS: None known.

INTERACTIONS

Drug

None known.

Herbal

None known.

Food

None known.

DIAGNOSTIC TEST EFFECTS: *None known.*

SIDE EFFECTS

Occasional

PO: None known

Topical: Skin irritation

Vaginal: Vaginal irritation

SERIOUS REACTIONS

- High dosages of oral form may produce nausea, vomiting, diarrhea, and GI distress.

SPECIAL CONSIDERATIONS

OCULAR CONSIDERATIONS

- Nystatin has been used for fungal conjunctivitis. Systemic administration may be necessary for resistant fungal ulcers. Topical fortified antifungal drops have been dosed initially every hour during the day and every 2 hours overnight. (Manzouri B, Vafidis GC, Wyse RK: Pharmacotherapy of fungal eye infections, *Expert Opin Pharmacother* 2[11]:1849-1857, 2001. Alexandrakis G: Keratitis: fungal, e-Medicine.com. Retrieved May 18, 2004, from http://www.emedicine.com/oph/topic99.htm.)

ofloxacin

(o-flox'a-sin)

Rx: Floxin, Floxin Otic, Ocuflox

Drug Class: Anti-infectives, ophthalmic; Antibiotics, quinolones; Ophthalmics

Pregnancy Category: C

Do not confuse Floxin with Flexeril or Flexon, or Ocuflox with Ocufen.

CLINICAL PHARMACOLOGY

Mechanism of Action: A fluoroquinolone antibiotic that inhibits DNA gyrase in susceptible microorganisms, interfering with bacterial cell replication and repair. *Therapeutic Effect:* Bactericidal.

Pharmacokinetics

Rapidly and well absorbed from the GI tract. Protein binding: 20%-25%. Widely distributed (including to CSF). Metabolized in the liver. Primarily excreted in urine. Removed by hemodialysis. **Half-life:** 4.7-7 hr (increased in impaired renal function, cirrhosis, and the elderly).

AVAILABLE FORMS

- *Tablets (Floxin):* 200 mg, 300 mg, 400 mg.
- *Injection Solution (Floxin):* 40 mg/ml.
- *Premixed Infusion Solution (Floxin):* 200 mg/50 ml, 400 mg/100 ml.
- *Ophthalmic Solution (Ocuflox):* 0.3%.
- *Otic Solution (Floxin):* 0.3%.

INDICATIONS AND DOSAGES

UTIs

PO, IV

Adults. 200 mg q12h.

Pelvic inflammatory disease (PID)

PO

Adults. 400 mg q12h for 10-14 days.

Lower respiratory tract, skin and skin-structure infections

PO, IV

Adults. 400 mg q12h for 10 days.

Prostatitis, sexually transmitted diseases (cervicitis, urethritis)

PO

Adults. 300 mg q12h.

Prostatitis

IV

Adults. 300 mg q12h.

Sexually transmitted diseases

IV

Adults. 400 mg as a single dose.

Acute, uncomplicated gonorrhea

PO

Adults. 400 mg 1 time.

Usual elderly dosage

PO

Elderly. 200-400 mg q12-24h for 7 days up to 6 wk.

Bacterial conjunctivitis

Ophthalmic

Adults, Elderly. 1-2 drops q2-4h for 2 days, then 4 times a day for 5 days.

Corneal ulcers

Ophthalmic

Adults. 1-2 drops q30min while awake for 2 days, then q60min while awake for 5-7 days, then 4 times a day.

Acute otitis media

Otic

Children 1-12 yr. 5 drops into the affected ear 2 times/day for 10 days.

Otitis externa

Otic

Adults, Elderly, Children 12 yr and older. 10 drops into the affected ear once a day for 7 days.

Children 6 mo-11 yr. 5 drops into the affected ear once a day for 7 days.

Dosage in renal impairment

After a normal initial dose, dosage and frequency are based on creatinine clearance.

Creatinine Clearance	*Adjusted Dose*	*Dosage Interval*
greater than 50 ml/min	None	q12h
10-50 ml/min	None	q24h
less than 10 ml/min	½	q24h

CONTRAINDICATIONS: Children younger than 18 years, hypersensitivity to any quinolones

INTERACTIONS

Drug

Antacids, sucralfate: May decrease absorption and effects of ofloxacin.

Caffeine: May increase the effects of caffeine.

Theophylline: May increase theophylline blood concentration and risk of toxicity.

Herbal

None known.

Food

None known.

DIAGNOSTIC TEST EFFECTS: *None known.*

IV INCOMPATIBILITIES: Amphotericin B complex (Abelcet, AmBisome, Amphotec), cefepime (Maxipime), doxorubicin liposomal (Doxil)

IV COMPATIBILITIES: Propofol (Diprivan)

SIDE EFFECTS

Frequent (10%-7%)

Nausea, headache, insomnia

Occasional (5%-3%)

Abdominal pain, diarrhea, vomiting, dry mouth, flatulence, dizziness, fatigue, drowsiness, rash, pruritus, fever

Rare (less than 1%)

Constipation, paraesthesia

SERIOUS REACTIONS

- Antibiotic-associated colitis and other superinfections may occur from altered bacterial balance.
- Hypersensitivity reactions, including photosensitivity (as evidenced by rash, pruritus, blisters, edema, and burning skin), have occurred in patients receiving fluoroquinolones.
- Arthropathy (swelling, pain, and clubbing of fingers and toes, degeneration of stress-bearing portion of a joint) may occur if the drug is given to children.

SPECIAL CONSIDERATIONS

PRECAUTIONS

- Superinfection may occur with prolonged use.

PATIENT INFORMATION

- Hypersensitivity

PREGNANCY AND LACTATION

- Pregnancy Category C. Oral doses resulted in decreased fetal body weight and increased fetal mortality in rats and rabbits. Fetal harm is not known with topical administration. In lactating females, a single 200-mg oral dose of ofloxacin resulted in concentrations of ofloxacin in milk. Excretion of topical doses into human milk is not known.

olanzapine

(oh-lan′za-peen)

Rx: Zyprexa, Zyprexa Zydis

Drug Class: Antipsychotics

Pregnancy Category: C

Do not confuse olanzapine with olsalazine, or Zyprexa with Zyrtec.

CLINICAL PHARMACOLOGY

Mechanism of Action: A dibenzepin derivative that antagonizes alpha$_1$-adrenergic, dopamine, histamine, muscarinic, and serotonin receptors. Produces anticholinergic, histaminic, and CNS depressant effects. *Therapeutic Effect:* Diminishes manifestations of psychotic symptoms.

Pharmacokinetics

Well absorbed after PO administration. Protein binding: 93%. Extensively distributed throughout the body. Undergoes extensive first-pass metabolism in the liver. Excreted primarily in urine and, to a lesser extent, in feces. Not removed by dialysis. **Half-life:** 21-54 hr.

AVAILABLE FORMS

- *Tablets (Zyprexa):* 2.5 mg, 5 mg, 7.5 mg, 10 mg, 15 mg, 20 mg).
- *Tablets (Orally-Disintegrating [Zyprexa Zydis]):* 5 mg, 10 mg, 15 mg, 20 mg.
- *Injection (Zyprexa Intramuscular):* 10 mg.

INDICATIONS AND DOSAGES

Schizophrenia

PO

Adults. Initially, 5-10 mg once daily. May increase by 10 mg/day at 5-7 day intervals. If further adjustments are indicated, may increase by 5-10 mg/day at 7-day intervals. Range: 10-30 mg/day.

Elderly. Initially, 2.5 mg/day. May increase as indicated. Range: 2.5-10 mg/day.

Children. Initially, 2.5 mg/day. Titrate as necessary up to 20 mg/day.

Bipolar mania

PO

Adults. Initially, 10-15 mg/day. May increase by 5 mg/day at intervals of at least 24 hr. Maximum: 20 mg/day.

Children. Initially, 2.5 mg/day. Titrate as necessary up to 20 mg/day.

Dosage for elderly or debilitated patients and those predisposed to hypotensive reactions

The initial dosage for these patients is 5 mg/day.

Control agitation in schizophrenic or bipolar patients

IM

Adults, Elderly. 2.5-10 mg. May repeat 2 hr after first dose and 4 hr after 2nd dose. Maximum: 30 mg/day.

UNLABELED USES: Treatment of anorexia, maintenance of long-term treatment response in schizophrenic patients, nausea, vomiting

CONTRAINDICATIONS: None known.

INTERACTIONS

Drug

Alcohol, other CNS depressants: May increase CNS depressant effects.

Antihypertensives: May increase the hypotensive effects of these drugs.

Carbamazepine: Increases olanzapine clearance.

Ciprofloxacin, fluvoxamine: May increase the olanzapine blood concentration.

Dopamine agonists, levodopa: May antagonize the effects of these drugs.

Imipramine, theophylline: May inhibit the metabolism of these drugs.

Herbal

None known.

Food

None known.

DIAGNOSTIC TEST EFFECTS: May significantly increase serum GGT, prolactin, AST (SGOT), and ALT (SGPT) levels.

SIDE EFFECTS

Frequent

Somnolence (26%), agitation (23%), insomnia (20%), headache (17%), nervousness (16%), hostility (15%), dizziness (11%), rhinitis (10%)

O

Occasional
Anxiety, constipation (9%); nonaggressive atypical behavior (8%); dry mouth (7%); weight gain (6%); orthostatic hypotension, fever, arthralgia, restlessness, cough, pharyngitis, visual changes (dim vision) (5%)
Rare
Tachycardia; back, chest, abdominal, or extremity pain; tremor

SERIOUS REACTIONS

• Rare reactions include seizures and neuroleptic malignant syndrome, a potentially fatal syndrome-characterized by hyperpyrexia, muscle rigidity, irregular pulse or BP, tachycardia, diaphoresis, and cardiac arrhythmias.

• Extrapyramidal symptoms and dysphagia may also occur.

• Overdose (300 mg) produces drowsiness and slurred speech.

SPECIAL CONSIDERATIONS

PRECAUTIONS

• Neuroleptic malignant syndrome has been reported in association with administration of antipsychotic drugs, including olanzapine. Clinical manifestations of neuroleptic malignant syndrome are hyperpyrexia, muscle rigidity, altered mental status, and evidence of autonomic instability (irregular pulse or blood pressure, tachycardia, diaphoresis and cardiac dysrhythmia). Possible risk exists of tardive dyskinesia, orthostatic hypotension, seizures, suicidal tendencies, and hyperprolactinemia. Exercise caution in patients with signs and symptoms of hepatic impairment. Somnolence was a commonly reported adverse event associated with olanzapine treatment. Appropriate care is advised when prescribing olanzapine for patients who will be experiencing conditions that may contribute to an elevation in core body temperature, such as exercising strenuously, exposure to extreme heat, receiving concomitant medication with anticholinergic activity, or being subject to dehydration. Esophageal dysmotility and aspiration have been associated with antipsychotic drug use.

PATIENT INFORMATION

• Physicians are advised to discuss the following issues with patients for whom they prescribe olanzapine.

• Orthostatic Hypotension: Advise patients of the risk of orthostatic hypotension, especially during the period of initial dose titration and in association with the concomitant use of drugs that may potentiate the orthostatic effect of olanzapine, such as diazepam or alcohol.

• Interference with Cognitive and Motor Performance: Because olanzapine has the potential to impair judgment, thinking, or motor skills, caution patients about operating hazardous machinery, including automobiles, until they are reasonably certain that olanzapine therapy does not affect them adversely.

• Pregnancy: Advise patients to notify their physician if they become pregnant or intend to become pregnant during therapy with olanzapine.

• Nursing: Advise patients not to breast-feed an infant if they are taking olanzapine.

• Concomitant Medication: Advise patients to inform their physicians if they are taking, or plan to take, any prescription or over-the-counter drugs, because a potential for interactions exists.

• Alcohol: Advise patients to avoid alcohol while taking olanzapine and to avoid overheating and dehydration.

• Phenylketonurics (Orally Disintegrating Tablets Only): Olanzapine orally disintegrating tablets contain phenylalanine (0.34 and 0.45 mg per 5- and 10-mg tablet, respectively).

PREGNANCY AND LACTATION

• Pregnancy Category C. Fetal harm is not known. Olanzapine was excreted in milk of treated rats during lactation. Whether olanzapine is excreted in human milk is not known. Recommend that women receiving olanzapine not breast-feed.

OCULAR CONSIDERATIONS

• Adverse reactions include conjunctivitis (frequent); abnormality of accommodation, blepharitis, cataract, corneal lesion, deafness, diplopia, dry eyes, ear pain, eye hemorrhage, eye inflammation, eye pain, ocular muscle abnormality, taste perversion, and tinnitus (infrequent); and glaucoma, keratoconjunctivitis, macular hypopigmentation, miosis, mydriasis, and pigment deposits lens (rare).

olopatadine

(oh-loe-pa-ta'deen)

Rx: Patanol

Drug Class: Antihistamines, H1; Ophthalmics

Pregnancy Category: C

CLINICAL PHARMACOLOGY

Mechanism of Action: An antihistamine that inhibits histamine release from the mast cell. *Therapeutic Effect:* Inhibits symptoms associated with allergic conjunctivitis.

Pharmacokinetics

The time to peak concentration is less than 2 hours and duration of action is 8 hours. Minimal absorption after topical administration. Metabolized to inactive metabolites. Primarily excreted in urine. **Half-life:** 3 hrs.

AVAILABLE FORMS

• *Ophthalmic Solution:* 0.1% (Patanol).

INDICATIONS AND DOSAGES

Allergic conjunctivitis

Ophthalmic

Adults, Elderly, Children 3 yr and older. 0.1% 1-2 drops in affected eye(s) twice daily q6-8h. 0.2% once daily 1-2 drops in affected eye(s).

CONTRAINDICATIONS: Hypersensitivity to olopatadine hydrochloride or any other component of the formulation

INTERACTIONS

Drug

None known.

Herbal

None known.

Food

None known.

DIAGNOSTIC TEST EFFECTS: *None known.*

SIDE EFFECTS

Occasional

Headache, weakness, cold syndrome, taste perversion, burning, stinging, dry eyes, foreign body sensation, hyperemia, keratitis, eyelid edema, itching, pharyngitis, rhinitis, sinusitis

SERIOUS REACTIONS

• None reported.

SPECIAL CONSIDERATIONS

PATIENT INFORMATION

• Advise patients not to wear contact lenses if their eye is red. Olopatadine hydrochloride eye solution 0.1% should not be used to treat contact lens irritation. The preservative in Patanol, benzalkonium chloride, may be absorbed by soft contact lenses. Instruct patients who wear soft contact lenses and whose eyes are not red to wait at least 10 minutes after drug instillation before they insert their contact lenses.

PREGNANCY AND LACTATION

• Pregnancy Category C. Rats and rabbits showed a decrease in live fetuses. Fetal harm is not known with topical administration. Olopatadine has been identified in the milk of nursing rats following oral administration. Excretion of topical doses into human milk is not known.

omeprazole

(oh-mep′-rah-zole)

Rx: Prilosec, Zegerid

Drug Class: Gastrointestinals; Proton pump inhibitors

Pregnancy Category: C

Do not confuse Prilosec with prilocaine, Prinivil, or Prozac.

CLINICAL PHARMACOLOGY

Mechanism of Action: A benzimidazole that is converted to active metabolites that irreversibly bind to and inhibit hydrogen-potassium adenosine triphosphatase, an enzyme on the surface of gastric parietal cells. Inhibits hydrogen ion transport into gastric lumen. *Therapeutic Effect:* Increases gastric pH, reduces gastric acid production.

Pharmacokinetics

Route	Onset	Peak	Duration
PO	1 hr	2 hr	72 hr

Rapidly absorbed from the GI tract. Protein binding: 99%. Primarily distributed into gastric parietal cells. Metabolized extensively in the liver. Primarily excreted in urine. Unknown if removed by hemodialysis. **Half-life:** 0.5-1 hr (increased in patients with hepatic impairment).

AVAILABLE FORMS

• *Capsules (Delayed-Release [Prilosec]):* 10 mg, 20 mg, 40 mg.

• *Oral Suspension (Zegerid):*20 mg.

INDICATIONS AND DOSAGES

Erosive esophagitis, poorly responsive gastroesophageal reflux disease, active duodenal ulcer, prevention and treatment of NSAID-induced ulcers

PO

Adults, Elderly. 20 mg/day.

To maintain healing of erosive esophagitis

PO

Adults, Elderly. 20 mg/day.

Pathologic hypersecretory conditions

PO

Adults, Elderly. Initially, 60 mg/day up to 120 mg 3 times a day.

***Duodenal ulcer caused by* Helibacter pylori**

PO

Adults, Elderly. 20 mg twice a day for 10 days.

Active benign gastric ulcer

PO

Adults, Elderly. 40 mg/day for 4-8 wk.

Usual pediatric dosage

Children older than 2 yr, weighing 20 kg or more. 20 mg/day.

Children older than 2 yr, weighing less than 20 kg. 10 mg/day.

UNLABELED USES: *H. pylori*–associated duodenal ulcer (with amoxicillin and clarithromycin), prevention and treatment of NSAID-induced ulcers, treatment of active benign gastric ulcers

CONTRAINDICATIONS: None known.

INTERACTIONS

Drug

Diazepam, oral anticoagulants, phenytoin: May increase the blood concentration of diazepam, oral anticoagulants, and phenytoin.

Herbal

None known.

Food

None known.

DIAGNOSTIC TEST EFFECTS: May increase serum alkaline phosphatase, AST (SGOT), and ALT (SGPT) levels.

SIDE EFFECTS

Frequent (7%)

Headache

Occasional (3%-2%)

Diarrhea, abdominal pain, nausea

Rare (2%)

Dizziness, asthenia or loss of strength, vomiting, constipation, upper respiratory tract infection, back pain, rash, cough

SERIOUS REACTIONS

• None known.

SPECIAL CONSIDERATIONS

PRECAUTIONS

• Serious and occasionally fatal hypersensitivity (anaphylactic) reactions have been reported in patients taking penicillin therapy. Pseudomembranous colitis has been reported with nearly all antibacterial agents and may range in severity from mild to life threatening. Symptomatic response to therapy with omeprazole does not preclude the presence of gastric malignancy. Atrophic gastritis has been noted occasionally in gastric corpus biopsies from patients treated long term with omeprazole.

PATIENT INFORMATION

• Instruct patients to take omeprazole delayed-release capsules before eating. Caution patients that the omeprazole delayed-release capsule should not be opened, chewed, or crushed and should be swallowed whole.

PREGNANCY AND LACTATION

• Pregnancy Category C. In rabbits, omeprazole produced dose-related increases in embryolethality, fetal resorptions, and pregnancy disruptions. Do not use clarithromycin in pregnant women except in clinical circumstances where no alternative therapy is appropriate. If pregnancy occurs while the patient is taking clarithromycin, apprise the patient of the potential hazard to the fetus. Fetal harm is not known. In rats, omeprazole administration during late gestation and lactation resulted in decreased weight gain in pups. Excretion into human milk is not known.

oxycodone

(ox-ee-koe'done)

Rx: M-Oxy, OxyContin, Oxydose, Oxyfast, OxyIR, Percolone, Roxicodone

Drug Class: Analgesics, narcotic

DEA Class: Schedule II

Do not confuse oxycodone with oxybutynin.

CLINICAL PHARMACOLOGY

Mechanism of Action: An opioid analgesic that binds with opioid receptors in the CNS. *Therapeutic Effect:* Alters the perception of and emotional response to pain.

Pharmacokinetics

Route	Onset	Peak	Duration
PO, Immediate-release	N/A	N/A	4-5 hr
PO, Controlled-release	N/A	N/A	12 hr

Moderately absorbed from the GI tract. Protein binding: 38%-45%. Widely distributed. Metabolized in the liver. Excreted in urine. Unknown if removed by hemodialysis. **Half-life:** 2-3 hr (3.2 hr controlled-release).

AVAILABLE FORMS

- *Capsules (Immediate-Release [OxyIR]):* 5 mg.
- *Oral Concentrate (Oxydose, OxyFast, Roxicodone Intensol):* 20 mg/ml.
- *Oral Solution (Roxicodone):* 5 mg/5 ml.
- *Tablets (Roxicodone):* 5 mg, 15 mg, 30 mg.
- *Tablets (Extended-Release [OxyContin]):* 10 mg, 20 mg, 40 mg, 80 mg, 160 mg.

INDICATIONS AND DOSAGES

Analgesia

PO (Controlled-Release)

Adults, Elderly. Initially, 10 mg q12h. May increase every 1-2 days by 25%-50%. Usual: 40 mg/day (100 mg/day for cancer pain).

PO (Immediate-Release)

Adults, Elderly. Initially, 5 mg q6h as needed. May increase up to 30 mg q4h. Usual: 10-30 mg q4h as needed.

Children. 0.05-0.15 mg/kg/dose q4-6h.

CONTRAINDICATIONS: None known.

INTERACTIONS

Drug

Alcohol, other CNS depressants: May increase CNS or respiratory depression and hypotension.

MAOIs: May produce a severe, sometimes fatal reaction; expect to administer one-quarter of usual oxycodone dose.

Herbal

None known.

Food

None known.

DIAGNOSTIC TEST EFFECTS: May increase serum amylase and lipase levels.

SIDE EFFECTS

Frequent

Somnolence, dizziness, hypotension (including orthostatic hypotension), anorexia

Occasional

Confusion, diaphoresis, facial flushing, urine retention, constipation, dry mouth, nausea, vomiting, headache

Rare

Allergic reaction, depression, paradoxical CNS hyperactivity or nervousness in children, paradoxical excitement and restlessness in elderly or debilitated patients

SERIOUS REACTIONS

- Overdose results in respiratory depression, skeletal muscle flaccidity, cold or clammy skin, cyanosis, and extreme somnolence progressing to seizures, stupor, and coma.
- Hepatotoxicity may occur with overdose of the acetaminophen

component of fixed-combination products.

• The patient who uses oxycodone repeatedly may develop a tolerance to the drug's analgesic effect and physical dependence.

SPECIAL CONSIDERATIONS

PRECAUTIONS

• Respiratory depression is the chief hazard from oxycodone. Use oxycodone with extreme caution in patients with significant chronic obstructive pulmonary disease or cor pulmonale and in patients having a substantially decreased respiratory reserve, hypoxia, hypercapnia, or preexisting respiratory depression. The respiratory depressant effects of opioids include carbon dioxide retention and secondary elevation of cerebrospinal fluid pressure and may be exaggerated greatly in the presence of head injury, intracranial lesions, or other sources of preexisting increased intracranial pressure. Oxycodone may cause severe hypotension. Oxycodone may be expected to have additive effects when used along with alcohol, other opioids, or illicit drugs that cause central nervous system depression.

• Reserve oxycodone for cases where the benefits of opioid analgesia outweigh the known risks of respiratory depression, altered mental state, and postural hypotension. Use oxycodone only with caution in the following conditions: acute alcoholism; adrenocortical insufficiency (e.g., Addison's disease); central nervous system depression or coma; delirium tremens; debilitated patients; kyphoscoliosis associated with respiratory depression; myxedema or hypothyroidism; prostatic hypertrophy or urethral stricture; severe impairment of hepatic, pulmonary, or renal function; and toxic psychosis. Oxycodone may obscure the diagnosis or clinical course in patients with acute abdominal conditions. Oxycodone may aggravate convulsions in patients with convulsive disorders.

PATIENT INFORMATION

• Patients should be aware that OxyContin tablets contain oxycodone, which is a morphinelike substance.

• Advise patients that OxyContin tablets were designed to work properly only if swallowed whole. OxyContin tablets will release all their contents at once if broken, chewed, or crushed, resulting in a risk of fatal overdose.

• Advise patients to report episodes of breakthrough pain and adverse experiences occurring during therapy. Individualization of dosage is essential to make optimal use of this medication.

• Advise patients not to adjust the dose of OxyContin without consulting the prescribing professional.

• Advise patients that OxyContin may impair mental and/or physical ability required for the performance of potentially hazardous tasks (e.g., driving or operating heavy machinery).

• Patients should not combine OxyContin with alcohol or other central nervous system depressants (sleep aids, tranquilizers) except by the orders of the prescribing physician, because dangerous additive effects may occur, resulting in serious injury or death.

• Advise women of childbearing potential who become, or are planning to become, pregnant to consult their physician regarding the effects of analgesics and other drug use during pregnancy on themselves and their unborn child.

- Advise patients that OxyContin is a potential drug of abuse. Patients should protect the drug from theft, and it should never be given to anyone other than the individual for whom it was prescribed.
- Advise patients that they may pass empty matrix "ghosts" (tablets) via colostomy or in the stool and that this is of no concern because the active medication already has been absorbed.
- Advise patients that if they have been receiving treatment with OxyContin for more than a few weeks and cessation of therapy is indicated, it may be appropriate to taper the OxyContin dose, rather than abruptly discontinue it, because of the risk of precipitating withdrawal symptoms. Their physician can provide a dose schedule to accomplish a gradual discontinuation of the medication.
- Instruct patients to keep OxyContin in a secure place out of the reach of children. When OxyContin is no longer needed, the unused tablets should be destroyed by flushing down the toilet.

PREGNANCY AND LACTATION

- Pregnancy Category C. Reproduction studies performed in rats and rabbits by oral doses did not reveal evidence of harm to the fetus. Low concentrations of oxycodone have been detected in breast milk.

oxytetracycline hydrochloride; polymyxin B sulfate

(ox-i-tet-ra-sye'kleen hye-droe-klor'ide; pol-ee-mix'in bee sul'fate)

Rx: Terak, Terramycin with Polymyxin B Sulfate

Drug Class: Anti-infectives, ophthalmic; Antibiotics, polymyxins; Antibiotics, tetracyclines; Ophthalmics

Pregnancy Category: D

CLINICAL PHARMACOLOGY

Mechanism of Action: Oxytetracycline is an antibiotic that binds with the 30S and 50S ribosome subunits of susceptible bacterial; cell wall synthesis is not affected. Polymyxin B damages bacterial cytoplasmic membrane which causes leakage of intracellular components. *Therapeutic Effect:* Inhibits bacterial cell wall synthesis.

Pharmacokinetics

None reported.

AVAILABLE FORMS

- *Ophthalmic ointment:* 5 mg oxytetracycline hydrochloride and 10,000 units of polymyxin B per gram (Terak, Terramycin w/Polymyxin B Ophthalmic).

INDICATIONS AND DOSAGES

Superficial eye infections involving the conjunctiva and/or cornea

Ophthalmic

Adults, Elderly. Apply ½ inch of ointment onto the lower lid of affected eye 2-4 times/day.

CONTRAINDICATIONS: Hypersensitivity to oxytetracycline, polymyxin B or any component of the formulation

INTERACTIONS

Drug

None known.

Herbal

None known.

Food

None known.

DIAGNOSTIC TEST EFFECTS: *None known.*

SIDE EFFECTS

Rare

Allergic or inflammatory reactions

SERIOUS REACTIONS

• Superinfection may occur.

SPECIAL CONSIDERATIONS

PRECAUTIONS

• Administration of oxytetracycline hydrochloride and polymyxin B sulfate may result in overgrowth of fungi. If superinfection occurs, discontinue the antibiotic and institute appropriate specific therapy.

pamidronate disodium

(pam-id'drow-nate)

Rx: Aredia, Pamidronate Disodium Novaplus

Drug Class: Bisphosphonates

Pregnancy Category: C

Do not confuse Aredia with Adriamcyin.

CLINICAL PHARMACOLOGY

Mechanism of Action: A bisphosphate that binds to bone and inhibits osteoclast-mediated calcium resorption. *Therapeutic Effect:* Lowers serum calcium concentrations.

Pharmacokinetics

Route	*Onset*	*Peak*	*Duration*
IV	24-48 hr	5-7 days	N/A

After IV administration, rapidly absorbed by bone. Slowly excreted unchanged in urine. Unknown if removed by hemodialysis. **Half-life:** bone, 300 days; unmetabolized, 2.5 hr.

AVAILABLE FORMS

• *Powder for Injection:* 30 mg, 90 mg.

• *Injection Solution:*3 mg/ml, 6 mg/ml, 9 mg/ml.

INDICATIONS AND DOSAGES

Hypercalcemia

IV Infusion

Adults, Elderly. Moderate hypercalcemia (corrected serum calcium level12-13.5 mg/dl): 60-90 mg. Severe hypercalcemia (corrected serum calcium level greater than 13.5 mg/dl): 90 mg.

Paget's disease

IV Infusion

Adults, Elderly. 30 mg/day for 3 days.

Osteolytic bone lesion

IV Infusion

Adults, Elderly. 90 mg over 2-4 hr once a month.

CONTRAINDICATIONS: Hypersensitivity to other bisphosphonates, such as etidronate, tiludronate, risedronate, and alendronate

INTERACTIONS

Drug

Calcium-containing medications, vitamin D: May antagonize effects of pamidronate in treatment of hypercalcemia.

Herbal

None known.

Food

None known.

DIAGNOSTIC TEST EFFECTS: May decrease serum phosphate, magnesium, calcium, and potassium levels.

IV INCOMPATIBILITIES: Calcium-containing IV fluids

SIDE EFFECTS

Frequent (greater than 10%)

Temperature elevation (at least 1 °C) 24-48 hr after administration (27%); redness, swelling, induration, pain at catheter site with in patients receiving 90 mg (18%); anorexia, nausea, fatigue

Occasional (10%-1%)

Constipation, rhinitis

SERIOUS REACTIONS

- Hypophosphatemia, hypokalemia, hypomagnesemia, and hypocalcemia occur more frequently with higher dosages.
- Anemia, hypertension, tachycardia, atrial fibrillation, and somnolence occur more frequently with 90-mg doses.
- GI hemorrhage occurs rarely.

SPECIAL CONSIDERATIONS

PRECAUTIONS

- Rare cases of uveitis, iritis, scleritis, and episcleritis have been reported, including one case of scleritis and one case of uveitis on separate rechallenges.

paroxetine hydrochloride

(par-ox'e-teen)

Rx: Paxil, Paxil CR, Pexeva

Drug Class: Antidepressants, serotonin specific reuptake inhibitors

Pregnancy Category: C

Do not confuse paroxetine with pyridoxine, or Paxil with Doxil or Taxol.

CLINICAL PHARMACOLOGY

Mechanism of Action: An antidepressant, anxiolytic, and antiobsessional agent that selectively blocks uptake of the neurotransmitter serotonin at neuronal presynaptic membranes, thereby increasing its availability at postsynaptic receptor sites. *Therapeutic Effect:* Relieves depression, reduces obsessive-compulsive behavior, decreases anxiety.

Pharmacokinetics

Well absorbed from the GI tract. Protein binding: 95%. Widely distributed. Metabolized in the liver. Excreted in urine. Not removed by hemodialysis. **Half-life:** 24 hr.

AVAILABLE FORMS

- *Oral Suspension (Paxil):* 10 mg/5 ml.
- *Tablets (Paxil, Pexeva):* 10 mg, 20 mg, 30 mg, 40 mg.
- *Tablets (Controlled-Release [Paxil CR]):* 12.5 mg, 25 mg, 37.5 mg.

INDICATIONS AND DOSAGES

Depression

PO

Adults. Initially, 20 mg/day. May increase by 10 mg/day at intervals of more than 1 wk. Maximum: 50 mg/day.

PO (Controlled-Release)

Adults. Initially, 25 mg/day. May increase by 12.5 mg/day at intervals of more than 1 wk. Maximum: 62.5 mg/day.

Generalized anxiety disorder

PO

Adults. Initially, 20 mg/day. May increase by 10 mg/day at intervals of more than 1 wk. Range: 20-50 mg/day.

Obsessive compulsive disorder

PO

Adults. Initially, 20 mg/day. May increase by 10 mg/day at intervals of more than 1 wk. Range: 20-60 mg/day.

Panic disorder

PO

Adults. Initially, 10-20 mg/day. May increase by 10 mg/day at intervals of more than 1 wk. Range: 10-60 mg/day.

Social anxiety disorder

PO

Adults. Initially 20 mg/day. Range: 20-60 mg/day.

Post traumatic stress disorder

PO

Adults. Initially, 20 mg/day. May increase by 10 mg/day at intervals of more than 1 wk. Range: 20-50 mg/day.

Premenstrual dysphoric disorder

PO (Paxil CR)

Adults. Initially, 12.5 mg/day. May increase by 12.5 mg at weekly intervals to a maximum of 25 mg/day.

Usual elderly dosage

PO: Initially, 10 mg/day. May increase by 10 mg/day at intervals of more than 1 wk. Maximum: 40 mg/day.

PO (Controlled-Release): Initially, 12.5 mg/day. May increase by 12.5 mg/day at intervals of more than 1 wk. Maximum: 50 mg/day.

CONTRAINDICATIONS: Use within 14 days of MAOIs

INTERACTIONS

Drug

Cimetidine: May increase paroxetine blood concentration.

MAOIs: May cause serotonin syndrome, marked by excitement, diaphoresis, rigidity, hyperthermia, autonomic hyperactivity, and coma, and neuroleptic malignant syndrome.

Phenytoin: May decrease paroxetine blood concentration.

Risperidone: May increase risperidone blood concentration and cause extrapyramidal symptoms.

Herbal

St. John's wort: May increase paroxetine's pharmacologic effects and risk of toxicity.

Food

None known.

DIAGNOSTIC TEST EFFECTS: May increase serum hepatic enzyme levels. May decrease blood Hgb level, Hct, and WBC count.

SIDE EFFECTS

Frequent

Nausea (26%); somnolence (23%); headache, dry mouth (18%); asthenia (15%); constipation (15%); dizziness, insomnia (13%); diarrhea (12%); diaphoresis (11%); tremor (8%)

Occasional

Decreased appetite, respiratory disturbance (such as increased cough) (6%); anxiety, nervousness (5%); flatulence, paresthesia, yawning (4%); decreased libido, sexual dysfunction, abdominal discomfort (3%)

Rare

Palpitations, vomiting, blurred vision, altered taste, confusion

SERIOUS REACTIONS

• None known.

SPECIAL CONSIDERATIONS

PRECAUTIONS

• Use paroxetine hydrochloride cautiously in patients with a history of mania; it can activate mania/hypomania. Use the drug cautiously in patients with a history of seizures. The possibility of a suicide attempt is inherent in depression and may persist until significant remission occurs. Several cases of hyponatremia have been reported. Several reports of abnormal bleeding (mostly ecchymosis and purpura) associated with paroxetine treatment have been made. Caution is advisable in using Paxil in patients with diseases or conditions that could affect metabolism or hemodynamic responses. Increased plasma concentrations of paroxetine occur in patients with severe renal impairment.

PATIENT INFORMATION

• Instruct the patient not to chew or crush Paxil and to swallow it whole.

• Interference with Cognitive and Motor Performance: Any psychoactive drug may impair judgment, thinking, or motor skills. Although in controlled studies immediate-release paroxetine hydrochloride has not been shown to impair psychomotor performance, caution patients about operating hazardous machinery, including automobiles, until they are reasonably certain that Paxil therapy does not affect their ability to engage in such activities.

• Completing Course of Therapy: Although patients may notice improvement with Paxil therapy in 1 to 4 weeks, advise them to continue therapy as directed.

• Concomitant Medication: Advise patients to inform their physician if they are taking, or plan to take, any prescription or over-the-counter drugs because there is a potential for interactions.

• Alcohol: Although immediate-release paroxetine hydrochloride has not been shown to increase the impairment of mental and motor skills caused by alcohol, advise patients to avoid alcohol while taking Paxil.

• Pregnancy: Advise patients to notify their physician if they become pregnant or intend to become pregnant during therapy.

• Nursing: Advise patients to notify their physician if they are breast-feeding an infant.

PREGNANCY AND LACTATION

• Pregnancy Category C. In rats an increase in pup deaths occurred during the first 4 days of lactation when dosing occurred during the last trimester of gestation and continued throughout lactation. Fetal harm is not known. Like many other drugs, paroxetine is secreted in human milk; exercise caution when administering Paxil to a nursing woman.

OCULAR CONSIDERATIONS

• Adverse Reactions: Conjunctivitis (frequent); abnormality of accommodation, eye appendage disorder, eye disorder, eye hemorrhage, keratoconjunctivitis, mydriasis, as well as amblyopia, anisocoria, blepharitis, blurred vision, cataract, conjunctival edema, conjunctivitis, corneal ulcer, deafness, exophthalmos, eye pain, glaucoma, night blindness, photophobia, ptosis, retinal hemorrhage, taste loss, and visual field defect (infrequent).

pegaptanib sodium

(peg-apt'i-nib)

Rx: Macugen

Drug Class: Ophthalmics; Vascular endothelial growth factor antagonist

Pregnancy Category: B

CLINICAL PHARMACOLOGY

Mechanism of Action: A selective vascular endothelial growth factor (VEGF) antagonize that selectively binds and activates receptors located on the surface of vascular endothelial cells. *Therapeutic Effect:* Blocks angiogenesis and vascular permeability and inflammation which contribute to the progression of the neovascular (wet) form of age-related macular degeneration (AMD).

Pharmacokinetics

Human pharmacokinetic data is limited. Based on preclinical data, it is slowly absorbed into systemic circulation from the eye after intravitreous administration. Metabolized by endo- and exonucleases. Excreted in urine. **Half-life:** 10 days (plasma).

AVAILABLE FORMS

- *Syringe for injection:* 0.3 mg (Macugen).

INDICATIONS AND DOSAGES

Neovascular (wet) age-related macular degeneration

Injection, intravitreous

Adults, Elderly. 0.3 mg every 6 weeks.

CONTRAINDICATIONS: Ocular or periocular infections, hypersensitivity to pegaptanib or any component of the formulation

INTERACTIONS

Drug

None known.

Herbal

None known.

Food

None known.

DIAGNOSTIC TEST EFFECTS: *None known.*

SIDE EFFECTS

Occasional

Corneal edema, eye discharge, eye irritation, eye pain, increased intraocular pressure, ocular discomfort, punctate keratitis, reduced visual acuity, reduced visual acuity, visual disturbance, vitreous floater, vitreous opacities

Rare

Dizziness, dull nervousness, eye pain, fainting, tachycardia, bradycardia, itching, redness or other eye irritation, pale skin, pounding in ears, trouble breathing on exertion, weakness

SERIOUS REACTIONS

- Endophthalmitis, retinal detachment, and iatrogenic traumatic cataract have been reported.

Pemirolast Potassium

(pe-meer'oh-last poe-tass'ee-um)

Rx: Alamast

Drug Class: Mast cell stabilizers; Ophthalmics

Pregnancy Category: C

CLINICAL PHARMACOLOGY

Mechanism of Action: An antiallergic agent that prevents activation and release of mediators of inflammation (e.g. mast cells). *Therapeutic Effect:* Reduces symptoms of allergic conjunctivitis.

Pharmacokinetics

Detected in plasma. Excreted in urine. **Half-life:** 4.5 hrs.

AVAILABLE FORMS

• *Ophthalmic Solution:* 0.1% (Alamast).

INDICATIONS AND DOSAGES

Allergic conjunctivitis

Ophthalmic

Adults, Elderly, Children 3 yr and older. 1-2 drops in affected eye(s) 4 times/day.

CONTRAINDICATIONS: Hypersensitivity to pemirolast potassium or any other component of the formulation

INTERACTIONS

Drug

None known.

Herbal

None known.

Food

None known.

DIAGNOSTIC TEST EFFECTS: *None known.*

SIDE EFFECTS

Frequent

Headache, rhinitis, cold and flu symptoms

Occasional

Transient ocular stinging, burning, itching, dry eye, foreign body sensation, tearing

Rare

Sinusitis, sneezing/nasal congestion

SERIOUS REACTIONS

• None reported.

SPECIAL CONSIDERATIONS

PATIENT INFORMATION

• Advise patients not to wear contact lenses if their eyes are red. Pemirolast potassium should not be used to treat contact lens–related irritation. The preservative in Alamast, lauralkonium chloride, may be absorbed by soft contact lenses. Instruct patients who wear soft contact lenses and whose eyes are not red to wait at least 10 minutes after drug instillation before they insert their contact lenses.

PREGNANCY AND LACTATION

• Pregnancy Category C. Increased incidence of fetal anomalies occurred when rats were given oral doses. Fetal harm is not known with topical administration. Pemirolast potassium is excreted in the milk of lactating rats. Excretion into human milk is not known.

penbutolol

(pen-beaut-oh-lol)

Rx: Levatol

Drug Class: Antiadrenergics, beta blocking

Pregnancy Category: C

Do not confuse with pindolol

CLINICAL PHARMACOLOGY

Mechanism of Action: An antihypertensive that possesses nonselective beta-blocking. Has moderate intrinsic sympathomimetic activity. *Therapeutic Effect:* Reduces cardiac output, decreases blood pressure (BP), increases airway resistance, and decreases myocardial ischemia severity.

Pharmacokinetics

Rapidly and extensively absorbed from the gastrointestinal (GI) tract. Protein binding: 80%-90%. Metabolized in liver. Excreted primarily via urine. **Half-life:** 17-26 hrs.

AVAILABLE FORMS

• *Tablets:* 20 mg (Levatol).

INDICATIONS AND DOSAGES

Hypertension

PO

Adults. Initially, 20 mg/day as a single dose. May increase to 40-80 mg/day.

Elderly. Initially, 10 mg/day.

CONTRAINDICATIONS: Bronchial asthma or related bronchospastic conditions, cardiogenic shock, pulmonary edema, second- or third-degree atrioventricular (AV) block, severe bradycardia, overt cardiac failure, hypersensitivity to penbutolol or any component of the formulation

INTERACTIONS

Drug

Calcium blockers: Increase risk of conduction disturbances.
Clonidine: May potentiate blood pressure (BP) effects.
Cimetidine: May increase penbutolol concentrations.
Digoxin: Increases concentrations of this drug.
Diuretics, other hypotensives: May increase hypotensive effect.
Fentanyl: May cause severe hypotension.
Insulin, oral hypoglycemics: May mask symptoms of hypoglycemia and prolong hypoglycemic effect of these drugs.
Lidocaine: May prolong the elimination of lidocaine
NSAIDs: May decrease antihypertensive effect.
Verapamil: May increase risk of hypotension and bradycardia.
Sympathomimetics, xanthines: May mutually inhibit effects.

Herbal

Dong quai: May decrease blood pressure.
St. John's wort, yohimbine: May decrease effectiveness of penbutolol.

Food

None known.

DIAGNOSTIC TEST EFFECTS: May increase ANA titer, SGOT (AST), SGPT (ALT), alkaline phosphatase, LDH, bilirubin, BUN, creatinine, potassium, uric acid, lipoproteins, triglycerides

SIDE EFFECTS

Frequent

Decreased sexual ability, drowsiness, trouble sleeping, unusual tiredness/weakness

Occasional

Diarrhea, bradycardia, depression, cold hands/feet, constipation, anxiety, nasal congestion, nausea, vomiting

Rare

Altered taste, dry eyes, itching, numbness of fingers, toes, scalp

SERIOUS REACTIONS

- Abrupt withdrawal may result in sweating, palpitations, headache, and tremulousness.
- Hypoglycemia may occur in patients with previously controlled diabetes.

SPECIAL CONSIDERATIONS

PRECAUTIONS

- Sympathetic stimulation may be a vital component supporting circulatory function in patients with congestive heart failure, and its inhibition by beta-blockade may precipitate more severe failure. Hypersensitivity to catecholamines has been observed in patients who were withdrawn from therapy with beta-blocking agents Penbutolol sulfate may prevent the appearance of signs and symptoms of acute hypoglycemia, such as tachycardia and blood pressure changes. Penbutolol sulfate may mask certain clinical signs (e.g., tachycardia) of hyperthyroidism. Penbutolol sulfate is contraindicated in bronchial asthma. Patients with bronchospastic diseases should not receive beta-blockers. Patients with a history of severe anaphylactic reactions to a variety of allergens may be more reactive to repeated challenge. Such patients may be unresponsive to the usual doses of epinephrine used to treat allergic reactions.

PATIENT INFORMATION

• Warn patients, especially those with evidence of coronary artery insufficiency, against interruption or discontinuation of penbutolol sulfate without the physician's advice. Although cardiac failure rarely occurs in properly selected patients, advise those being treated with beta-adrenergic receptor antagonists of the symptoms of heart failure and to report such symptoms immediately, should they develop.

PREGNANCY AND LACTATION

• Pregnancy Category C. In a perinatal and postnatal study in rats, the pup body weight and pup survival rate were reduced at the highest dose level. Fetal harm is not known. Whether penbutolol sulfate is excreted in human milk is not known.

penicillin G potassium

(pen-ih-sil'-lin G)

Drug Class: Antibiotics, penicillins

Pregnancy Category: B

Do not confuse penicillin G potassium with penicillin G benzathine or penicillin G procaine.

CLINICAL PHARMACOLOGY

Mechanism of Action: A penicillin that inhibits bacterial cell wall synthesis by binding to one or more of the penicillin-binding proteins of bacteria. *Therapeutic Effect:* Bactericidal.

AVAILABLE FORMS

• *Injection:* 5 million units.

• *Premixed Dextrose Solution:* 1 million units, 2 million units, 3 million units.

INDICATIONS AND DOSAGES

Sepsis, meningitis, pericarditis, endocarditis, pneumonia due to susceptible gram-positive organisms (not* Staphylococcus aureus*) and some gram-negative organisms

IV, IM

Adults, Elderly. 2-24 million units/day in divided doses q4-6h.

Children. 100,000-400,000 units/kg/day in divided doses q4-6h.

Dosage in renal impairment

Dosage interval is modified based on creatinine clearance.

Creatinine Clearance	*Dosage Interval*
10-30 ml/min	Usual dose q8-12h
less than 10 ml/min	Usual dose q12-18h

CONTRAINDICATIONS: Hypersensitivity to any penicillin

INTERACTIONS

Drug

Erythromycin: May antagonize effects of penicillin.

Probenecid: Increases serum concentration of penicillin.

Herbal

None known.

Food

Food, milk: Decrease penicillin absorption.

DIAGNOSTIC TEST EFFECTS: May cause a positive Coombs' test.

IV INCOMPATIBILITIES: Amikacin (Amikin), aminophylline, amphotericin B, dopamine (Intropin)

IV COMPATIBILITIES: Amiodarone (Cordarone), calcium gluconate, diltiazem (Cardizem), diphenhydramine (Benadryl), furosemide (Lasix), heparin, hydromorphone (Dilaudid), lidocaine, magnesium sulfate, methylprednisolone (Solu-Medrol), morphine, potassium chloride

SIDE EFFECTS

Occasional

Lethargy, fever, dizziness, rash, electrolyte imbalance, diarrhea, thrombophlebitis

Rare

Seizures, interstitial nephritis

SERIOUS REACTIONS

- Hypersensitivity reactions ranging from rash, fever, and chills to anaphylaxis occur.

SPECIAL CONSIDERATIONS

PRECAUTIONS

- Use penicillin G potassium with caution in individuals with histories of significant allergies and/or asthma. Do not rely on the oral route of administration in patients with severe illness or with nausea, vomiting gastric dilation, cardiospasm, or intestinal hypermotility. Prolonged use may promote the overgrowth of nonsusceptible organisms, including fungi.

PREGNANCY AND LACTATION

- Pregnancy Category B. Reproduction studies performed in the mouse, rat, and rabbit have revealed no evidence of impaired fertility or harm to the fetus from penicillin G. Penicillins are excreted in human milk.

penicillin V potassium

(pen-ih-sil'-in V)

Drug Class: Antibiotics, penicillins

Pregnancy Category: B

CLINICAL PHARMACOLOGY

Mechanism of Action: A penicillin that inhibits cell wall synthesis by binding to bacterial cell membranes. *Therapeutic Effect:* Bactericidal.

Pharmacokinetics

Moderately absorbed from the GI tract. Protein binding: 80%. Widely distributed. Metabolized in the liver. Primarily excreted in urine. **Half-life:** 1 hr (increased in impaired renal function).

AVAILABLE FORMS

- *Tablets:* 250 mg, 500 mg.
- *Powder for Oral Solution:* 125 mg/5 ml, 250 mg/5 ml.

INDICATIONS AND DOSAGES

Mild to moderate respiratory tract or skin or skin-structure infections, otitis media, necrotizing ulcerative gingivitis

PO

Adults, Elderly, Children 12 yr and older. 125-500 mg q6-8h.

Children younger than 12 yr. 25-50 mg/kg/day in divided doses q6-8h. Maximum: 3 g/day.

Primary prevention of rheumatic fever

PO

Adults, Elderly. 500 mg 2-3 times/day for 10 days.

Children. 250 mg 2-3 times/day for 10 days.

Primary prevention of rheumatic fever

PO

Adults, Elderly, Children. 250 mg twice a day.

CONTRAINDICATIONS: Hypersensitivity to any penicillin

INTERACTIONS

Drug

Probenecid: May increase penicillin blood concentration and risk of toxicity.

Herbal

None known.

Food

None known.

DIAGNOSTIC TEST EFFECTS: May cause positive a Coombs' test.

SIDE EFFECTS

Frequent

Mild hypersensitivity reaction (chills, fever, rash), nausea, vomiting, diarrhea

Rare

Bleeding, allergic reaction

SERIOUS REACTIONS

- Severe hypersensitivity reactions, including anaphylaxis, may occur.
- Nephrotoxicity, antibiotic-associated colitis, and other superinfections may result from high dosages or prolonged therapy.

SPECIAL CONSIDERATIONS

PRECAUTIONS

- Serious and occasionally fatal hypersensitivity (anaphylactic) reactions have been reported in patients receiving penicillin therapy. Pseudomembranous colitis has been reported with nearly all antibacterial agents including penicillins and may range in severity from mild to life threatening. Prolonged use of antibiotics may promote the overgrowth of nonsusceptible organisms, including fungi.

PREGNANCY AND LACTATION

- Pregnancy Category B. Fetal harm is not known. Excretion into human milk is not known.

pentazocine hydrochloride; naloxone hydrochloride

Rx: Talwin NX

Drug Class: Analgesics, narcotic agonist-antagonist

Pregnancy Category: C

DEA Class: Schedule IV

CLINICAL PHARMACOLOGY

Mechanism of Action: Naloxone is a narcotic antagonist that displaces opiates at opiate-occupied receptor sites in the central nervous system (CNS). Pentazocine is both a narcotic agonist and antagonist that induces analgesia by stimulating the kappa and sigma opioid receptors. *Therapeutic Effect:* Naloxone: blocks narcotic effects; reverses opiate-induced sleep or sedation; increases respiratory rate, returns depressed blood pressure (BP) to normal rate. Pentazocine: induces analgesia.

Pharmacokinetics

Well absorbed. Metabolized in liver. Primarily excreted in urine. Minimal excretion in bile and feces. **Half-life:** 2-3 hrs.

AVAILABLE FORMS

- *Tablets:* 50 mg pentazocine hydrochloride/0.5 mg naloxone hydrochloride (Talwin Nx).

INDICATIONS AND DOSAGES

Pain, moderate to severe

PO

Adults, Elderly, Children 12 yr and older. 1 tablet every 3-4 hrs. May be increased to 2 tablets when needed. Maximum: 12 tablets/day.

CONTRAINDICATIONS: Hypersensitivity to pentazocine or naloxone or any component on the formulation

INTERACTIONS

Drug

Alcohol: May increase sedation.
Clonidine: May cause hypertension.
Fluoxetine, sibutramine: May increase risk of serotonin syndrome.
Methohexital, thiopental: May increase the risk of CNS depression.
Opioid analgesics: May cause precipitation of withdrawal symptoms.
Tobacco: May decrease pentazocine concentrations.

Herbal

Yohimbine: May increase adverse effects, such as nervousness, anxiety, palpitations, nausea, and hot and cold flashes.

Food

None known.

DIAGNOSTIC TEST EFFECTS: *None known.*

SIDE EFFECTS

Occasional

Confusion, dizziness, fatigue, lightheadedness, drowsiness, mood changes, headache, GI upset, vomiting, constipation, stomach pain, rash, difficulty urinating

SERIOUS REACTIONS

- Respiratory depression and serious skin reactions, such as Stevens-Johnson syndrome, have been reported but occur rarely.

SPECIAL CONSIDERATIONS

PRECAUTIONS

- Pentazocine can cause a physical and psychological dependence. As in the case of other potent analgesics, the potential of pentazocine for elevating cerebrospinal fluid pressure may be attributed to carbon dioxide retention caused by the respiratory depressant effects of the drug. These effects may be exaggerated greatly in the presence of head injury, other intracranial lesions, or a preexisting increase in intracranial pressure. Because of the potential for increased central nervous system depressant effects, advise cautious use of alcohol in patients who currently are receiving pentazocine. Administer pentazocine with caution to patients with respiratory depression from any cause, severely limited respiratory reserve, severe bronchial asthma, and other obstructive respiratory conditions, or cyanosis. Patients receiving therapeutic doses of pentazocine have experienced hallucinations (usually visual), disorientation, and confusion, effects that have cleared spontaneously within a period of hours. Use caution when administering pentazocine to patients prone to seizures; seizures have occurred in a few such patients in association with the use of pentazocine.
- Decreased metabolism of pentazocine by the liver in extensive liver disease may predispose the patient to accentuation of side effects. Narcotic drug products generally are considered to elevate biliary tract pressure for varying periods. Use pentazocine with caution in patients with myocardial infarction who have nausea or vomiting.

PATIENT INFORMATION

- Because sedation, dizziness, and occasional euphoria have been noted, warn ambulatory patients not to operate machinery, drive cars, or unnecessarily expose themselves to hazards. Pentazocine may cause physical and psychological dependence when taken alone and may have additive central nervous system depressant properties when taken in combination with alcohol or other central nervous system depressants.

PREGNANCY AND LACTATION

- Pregnancy Category C. Fetal harm is not known. Excretion into human milk is not known.

OCULAR CONSIDERATIONS

• Ocular Adverse Reactions: Visual blurring and focusing difficulty; hypotension, tachycardia, and syncope; hallucinations (usually visual), disorientation, and confusion; dizziness, light-headedness, sedation, euphoria, headache, confusion. sweating, nausea, vomiting, constipation, diarrhea, anorexia, and edema of the face; dermatitis, including pruritus; flushed skin, including plethora; and depression of white blood cells

---

perindopril erbumine

(per-in'doh-pril)

Rx: Aceon

Drug Class: Angiotensin converting enzyme inhibitors

Pregnancy Category: C, 1st; D, 2nd / 3rd

CLINICAL PHARMACOLOGY

Mechanism of Action: An ACE inhibitor that suppresses the renin-angiotensin-aldosterone system and prevents conversion of angiotensin I to angiotensin II, a potent vasoconstrictor; may also inhibit angiotensin II at local vascular and renal sites. *Therapeutic Effect:* Reduces peripheral arterial resistance and BP.

AVAILABLE FORMS

• *Tablets:* 2 mg, 4 mg, 8 mg.

INDICATIONS AND DOSAGES

Hypertension

PO

Adults, Elderly. 2-8 mg/day as single dose or in 2 divided doses. Maximum: 16 mg/day.

UNLABELED USES: Management of heart failure

CONTRAINDICATIONS: History of angioedema from previous treatment with ACE inhibitors

INTERACTIONS

Drug

Alcohol, antihypertensives, diuretics: May increase the effects of perindopril.

Lithium: May increase lithium blood concentration and risk of lithium toxicity.

NSAIDs: May decrease the effects of perindopril.

Potassium-sparing diuretics, potassium supplements: May cause hyperkalemia.

Herbal

None known.

Food

None known.

DIAGNOSTIC TEST EFFECTS: May increase BUN, serum alkaline phosphatase, serum bilirubin, serum creatinine, serum potassium, AST (SGOT), and ALT (SGPT) levels. May decrease serum sodium levels. May cause positive antinuclear antibody titer.

SIDE EFFECTS

Occasional (5%-1%)

Cough, back pain, sinusitis, upper extremity pain, dyspepsia, fever, palpitations, hypotension, dizziness, fatigue, syncope

SERIOUS REACTIONS

• Excessive hypotension ("first-dose syncope") may occur in patients with CHF and in those who are severely salt or volume depleted.

• Angioedema (swelling of face and lips) and hyperkalemia occur rarely.

• Agranulocytosis and neutropenia may be noted in those with collagen vascular disease, including scleroderma and systemic lupus erythematosus, and impaired renal function.

• Nephrotic syndrome may be noted in those with history of renal disease.

SPECIAL CONSIDERATIONS

PRECAUTIONS

• Anticipate changes in renal function in susceptible individuals. Hypertensive patients with congestive heart failure may have associated oliguria and/or progressive azotemia and, rarely, acute renal failure and/or death. Elevations of serum potassium have been observed in some patients treated with angiotensin-converting enzyme (ACE) inhibitors. Cough has been reported with all ACE inhibitors. In patients undergoing major surgery or during anesthesia with agents that produce hypotension, enalapril may block angiotensin II formation following compensatory renin release.

PATIENT INFORMATION

• Angioedema: Angioedema, including laryngeal edema, can occur with ACE inhibitor therapy, especially following the first dose. Advise patients to report immediately signs or symptoms suggesting angioedema (swelling of face, extremities, eyes, lips, tongue, and hoarseness or difficulty in swallowing or breathing) and to take no more drug before consulting a physician.

• Symptomatic Hypotension: As with any antihypertensive therapy, caution patients that light-headedness can occur, especially during the first few days of therapy and that it should be reported promptly. Instruct patients that if fainting occurs, they should discontinue perindopril erbumine therapy and consult a physician.

• Caution all patients that inadequate fluid intake or excessive perspiration, diarrhea, or vomiting can lead to an excessive fall in blood pressure in association with ACE inhibitor therapy.

• Hyperkalemia: Advise patients not to use potassium supplements or salt substitutes containing potassium without a physician's advice.

• Neutropenia: Instruct patients to report promptly any indication of infection (e.g., sore throat or fever), which could be a sign of neutropenia.

• Pregnancy: Advise female patients of childbearing age about the consequences of second- and third-trimester exposure to ACE inhibitors, and advise them that these consequences do not appear to have resulted from intrauterine ACE inhibitor exposure that has been limited to the first trimester. Ask these patients to report pregnancies to their physicians as soon as possible.

PREGNANCY AND LACTATION

• Pregnancy Categories C (first trimester) and D (second and third trimesters). The use of ACE inhibitors during the second and third trimesters of pregnancy has been associated with fetal and neonatal injury, including hypotension, neonatal skull hypoplasia, anuria, reversible or irreversible renal failure, and death. Excretion into human milk is not known.

phenobarbital

(fee-noe-bar′bi-tal)

Rx: Luminal

Drug Class: Anticonvulsants; Barbiturates; Preanesthetics; Sedatives/hypnotics

Pregnancy Category: D

DEA Class: Schedule IV

Do not confuse phenobarbital with pentobarbital, or Luminal with Tuinal.

CLINICAL PHARMACOLOGY

Mechanism of Action: A barbiturate that enhances the activity of gamma-aminobutyric acid (GABA) by binding to the GABA receptor complex. *Therapeutic Effect:* Depresses CNS activity.

Pharmacokinetics

Route	Onset	Peak	Duration
PO	20-60 min	N/A	6-10 hr
IV	5 min	30 min	4-10 hr

Well absorbed after PO or parenteral administration. Protein binding: 35%-50%. Rapidly and widely distributed. Metabolized in the liver. Primarily excreted in urine. Removed by hemodialysis. **Half-life:** 53-118 hr.

AVAILABLE FORMS

- *Elixir:* 20 mg/5 ml.
- *Tablets:* 30 mg, 100 mg.
- *Injection:* 60 mg/ml, 130 mg/ml.

INDICATIONS AND DOSAGES

Status epilepticus

IV

Adults, Elderly, Children, Neonates. Loading dose of 15-20 mg/kg as a single dose or in divided doses.

Seizure control

PO, IV

Adults, Elderly, Children older than 12 yr. 1-3 mg/kg/day.

Children 6-12 yr. 4-6 mg/kg/day.

Children 1-5 yr. 6-8 mg/kg/day.

Children younger than 1 yr. 5-6 mg/kg/day.

Neonates. 3-4 mg/kg/day.

Sedation

PO, IM

Adults, Elderly. 30-120 mg/day in 2-3 divided doses.

Children. 2 mg/kg 3 times a day.

Hypnotic

PO, IV, IM, Subcutaneous

Adults, Elderly. 100-320 mg at bedtime.

Children. 3-5 mg/kg at bedtime.

UNLABELED USES: Prevention and treatment of hyperbilirubinemia

CONTRAINDICATIONS: Porphyria, pre-existing CNS depression, severe pain, severe respiratory disease

INTERACTIONS

Drug

Alcohol, other CNS depressants: May increase the effects of phenobarbital.

Carbamazepine: May increase the metabolism of carbamazepine.

Digoxin, glucocorticoids, metronidazole, oral anticoagulants, quinidine, tricyclic antidepressants: May decrease the effects of these drugs.

Valproic acid: Increases the blood concentration and risk of toxicity of phenobarbital.

Herbal

None known.

Food

None known.

DIAGNOSTIC TEST EFFECTS: May decrease serum bilirubin level. Therapeutic serum level is 10-40 mcg/ml; toxic serum level is greater than 40 mcg/ml.

IV INCOMPATIBILITIES: Amphotericin B complex (Abelcet, AmBisome, Amphotec), hydrocortisone (Solu-Cortef), hydromorphone (Dilaudid), insulin

IV COMPATIBILITIES: Calcium gluconate, enalapril (Vasotec), fentanyl (Sublimaze), fosphenytoin (Cerebyx), morphine, propofol (Diprivan)

SIDE EFFECTS

Occasional (3%-1%)

Somnolence

Rare (less than 1%)

Confusion; paradoxical CNS reactions, such as hyperactivity or nervousness in children and excitement or restlessness in the elderly (generally noted during first 2 weeks of therapy, particularly in presence of uncontrolled pain)

SERIOUS REACTIONS

- Abrupt withdrawal after prolonged therapy may produce increased dreaming, nightmares, insomnia, tremor, diaphoresis, and vomiting, hallucinations, delirium, seizures, and status epilepticus.
- Skin eruptions may be a sign of a hypersensitivity reaction.
- Blood dyscrasias, hepatic disease, and hypocalcemia occur rarely.
- Overdose produces cold or clammy skin, hypothermia, severe CNS depression, cyanosis, tachycardia, and Cheyne-Stokes respirations.
- Toxicity may result in severe renal impairment.

SPECIAL CONSIDERATIONS

PRECAUTIONS

- Barbiturates may be habit forming. Tolerance and psychological and physical dependence may occur with continuing use. Administer barbiturates with caution, if at all, to patients who are mentally depressed, have suicidal tendencies, or have a history of drug abuse. Elderly or debilitated patients may react to barbiturates with marked excitement, depression, and confusion. In some persons, barbiturates repeatedly produce excitement rather than depression. In patients with hepatic damage, administer barbiturates with caution and initially in reduced doses. Do not administer barbiturates to patients showing the premonitory signs of hepatic coma. Untoward reactions may occur in the presence of fever, hyperthyroidism, diabetes mellitus, and severe anemia. Intramuscular injection should be confined to a total of 5 ml and made in a large muscle to avoid possible tissue irritation. Parenteral solutions of barbiturates are highly alkaline; therefore, take extreme care to avoid perivascular extravasation or intraarterial injection. Extravascular injection may cause local tissue damage with subsequent necrosis; consequences of intraarterial injection may vary from transient pain to gangrene of the limb. Any complaint of pain in the limb warrants stopping the injection.

PATIENT INFORMATION

- The use of barbiturates carries with it an associated risk of psychological and/or physical dependence. Warn the patient against increasing the dose of the drug without consulting a physician. Barbiturates may impair mental and/or physical abilities required for the performance of potentially hazardous tasks (e.g., driving and operating machinery). Advise the patient not to consume alcohol while taking barbiturates. Concurrent use of the barbiturates with other central nervous system depressants (e.g., alcohol, narcotics, tranquilizers, and antihistamines) may result in additional central nervous system depressant effects.

PREGNANCY AND LACTATION

- Pregnancy Category D. Barbiturates can cause fetal damage when administered to a pregnant woman. Exercise caution when administering a barbiturate to a nursing woman because small amounts of barbiturates are excreted in the milk.

OCULAR CONSIDERATIONS

• Phenobarbital may affect extraocular muscles.

phenylephrine hydrochloride

(fen-ill-eh'-frin)

Rx: AK-Dilate, Despec-SF, Mydfrin, Neofrin, Neo-Synephrine Ophthalmic, Ocu-Phrin, Phenoptic, Rectasol

Drug Class: Adrenergic agonists; Decongestants, ophthalmic; Ophthalmics

Pregnancy Category: C

CLINICAL PHARMACOLOGY

Mechanism of Action: A sympathomimetic, alpha receptor stimulant that acts on the alpha-adrenergic receptors of vascular smooth muscle. Causes vasoconstriction of arterioles of nasal mucosa or conjunctiva, activates dilator muscle of the pupil to cause contraction, produces systemic arterial vasoconstriction. *Therapeutic Effect:* Decreases mucosal blood flow and relieves congestion and increases systolic BP.

Pharmacokinetics

Route	*Onset*	*Peak*	*Duration*
IV	Immediate	N/A	15-20 min
IM	10-15 min	N/A	0.5-2 hr
Subcutaneous	10-15 min	N/A	1 hr

Minimal absorption after intranasal and ophthalmic administration. Metabolized in the liver and GI tract. Primarily excreted in urine. **Half-life:** 2.5 hr.

AVAILABLE FORMS

• *Injection:* 1% (10 mg/ml).
• *Nasal Solution Drops (Neosynephrine):* 0.5%, 1%.
• *Nasal Spray (Neosynephrine):* 0.25%, 0.5%, 1%.
• *Ophthalmic Solution (Ak-Nephrin):* 0.12%.
• *Ophthalmic Solution (AK-Dilate):* 2.5%, 10%.
• *Ophthalmic Solution (Mydfrin, Neosynephrine):* 2.5%.

INDICATIONS AND DOSAGES

Nasal decongestant

Nasal Spray, Nasal Solution

Adults, Elderly, Children 12 yr and older. 2-3 drops or 1-2 sprays of 0.25%-0.5% solution into each nostril.

Children 6-11 yr. 2-3 drops or 1-2 sprays of 0.25% solution into each nostril.

Children younger than 6 yr. 2-3 drops of 0.125% solution (dilute 0.5% solution with 0.9% NaCl to achieve 0.125%) in each nostril. Repeat q4h as needed. Do not use for more than 3 days.

Conjunctival congestion, itching, and minor irritation; whitening of sclera

Ophthalmic

Adults, Elderly, Children 12 yr and older. 1-2 drops of 0.12% solution q3-4h.

Hypotension, shock

IM, Subcutaneous

Adults, Elderly. 2-5 mg/dose q1-2h.

Children. 0.1 mg/kg/dose q1-2h.

IV Bolus

Adults, Elderly. 0.1-0.5 mg/dose q10-15min as needed.

Children. 5-20 mcg/kg/dose q10-15min.

IV Infusion

Adults, Elderly. 100-180 mcg/min.

Children. 0.1-0.5 mcg/kg/min. Titrate to desired effect.

CONTRAINDICATIONS: Acute pancreatitis, heart disease, hepatitis, narrow-angle glaucoma, pheochromocytoma, severe hypertension, thrombosis, ventricular tachycardia

INTERACTIONS

Drug

Beta-blockers: May have mutually inhibitory effects.

Digoxin: May increase risk of arrhythmias.

Ergonovine, oxytocin: May increase vasoconstriction.

MAOIs: May increase vasopressor effects.

Maprotiline, tricyclic antidepressants: May increase cardiovascular effects.

Methyldopa: May decrease effects of methyldopa.

Herbal

None known.

Food

None known.

DIAGNOSTIC TEST EFFECTS: *None known.*

IV INCOMPATIBILITIES: Thiopentothal (Pentothal)

IV COMPATIBILITIES: Amiodarone (Cordarone), dobutamine (Dobutrex), lidocaine, potassium chloride, propofol (Diprivan)

SIDE EFFECTS

Frequent

Nasal: Rebound nasal congestion due to overuse, especially when used longer than 3 days

Occasional

Mild CNS stimulation (restlessness, nervousness, tremors, headache, insomnia, particularly in those hypersensitive to sympathomimetics, such as elderly patients)

Nasal: Stinging, burning, drying of nasal mucosa

Ophthalmic: Transient burning or stinging, brow ache, blurred vision

SERIOUS REACTIONS

- Large doses may produce tachycardia and palpitations (particularly in those with cardiac disease), lightheadedness, nausea, and vomiting.
- Overdose in those older than 60 years may result in hallucinations, CNS depression, and seizures.
- Prolonged nasal use may produce chronic swelling of nasal mucosa and rhinitis.

SPECIAL CONSIDERATIONS

PRECAUTIONS

- 2.5%/10% Solution: Phenylephrine hydrochloride occasionally may raise intraocular pressure. However, when temporary dilation of the pupil may free adhesions, this advantage temporarily may outweigh the danger from coincident dilation of the pupil. Rebound miosis has been reported.
- Older individuals also may develop transient pigment floaters in the aqueous humor 40 to 45 minutes following the administration. The appearance may be similar to anterior uveitis or to a microscopic hyphema. To prevent pain, apply a drop of suitable topical anesthetic before using the drug. Prolonged exposure to air or strong light may cause oxidation and discoloration. Do not use if solution is brown or contains a precipitate.
- Additional Information for the 10% Solution: Significant elevation in blood pressure is rare but has been reported. Exercise caution in administering phenylephrine hydrochloride to children of low body weight, the elderly, and patients with insulin-dependent diabetes, hypertension, hyperthyroidism, generalized arteriosclerosis, or cardiovascular disease. Closely monitor the post-

treatment blood pressure of these patients and any patients who develop symptoms.

• To prevent pain, apply a drop of suitable topical anesthetic before using the 10% eye solution.

• Concomitant use with systemically effective beta-blockers has causes acute hypertension and, in one case, the rupture of a congenital cerebral aneurysm. This drug may potentiate the cardiovascular depressant effects of potent inhalation anesthetic agents.

• Vasopressors, particularly metaraminol, may cause serious cardiac arrhythmias during administration of halothane anesthesia. The pressor effect of sympathomimetic pressor amines is greatly potentiated in patients receiving monoamine oxidase inhibitors and also may be potentiated by tricyclic antidepressants.

PREGNANCY AND LACTATION

• Pregnancy Category C. Fetal harm is not known with topical administration. Excretion into human milk is not known.

phenylephrine hydrochloride; sulfacetamide sodium

(fen-ill-eh'-frin hye-droh-klor'-ide; sul-fa-see'-ta-mide soe'-dee-um)

Drug Class: Anti-infectives, ophthalmic; Decongestants, ophthalmic; Ophthalmics

Pregnancy Category: C

CLINICAL PHARMACOLOGY

Mechanism of Action: Phenylephrine is a sympathomimetic that acts on alpha-adrenergic receptors of vascular smooth muscle. Sulfacetamide is a sulfonamide that interferes with synthesis of folic acid that bacteria require for growth. *Therapeutic Effect:* Increases systolic/diastolic blood pressure (BP), produces constriction of blood vessels, conjunctival arterioles, nasal arterioles. Prevents bacterial growth.

Pharmacokinetics

Minimal absorption following ophthalmic administration.

AVAILABLE FORMS

• *Ophthalmic Solution:* 0.125% phenylephrine hydrochloride and 15% sulfacetamide sodium (Vasosulf).

INDICATIONS AND DOSAGES

Topical application to conjunctiva relieves congestion, itching, minor irritation; whitens sclera of eye

Ophthalmic

Adults, Elderly, Children 12 yr and older. Instill 1-2 drops of q3-4h.

CONTRAINDICATIONS: Angle-closure glaucoma, those with soft contact lenses, hypersensitivity to phenylephrine, sulfacetamide, or any component of the formulation

INTERACTIONS

Drug

None known.

Herbal

None known.

Food

None known.

DIAGNOSTIC TEST EFFECTS: *None known.*

SIDE EFFECTS

Occasional

Transient burning/stinging, brow ache, blurred vision

SERIOUS REACTIONS

• None reported.

SPECIAL CONSIDERATIONS

PRECAUTIONS

• Phenylephrine hydrochloride and sulfacetamide sodium are incompatible with silver preparations. Local anesthetics related to p-aminobenzoic acid may antagonize the action of the sulfonamides. Bacteria initially sensitive to sulfonamides may acquire resistance to the drug. Fungi may proliferate with the use of this preparation. Sulfonamides are inactivated by the p-aminobenzoic acid present in purulent exudates. If signs of hypersensitivity or other untoward reactions occur, discontinue use of the preparation. Keep bottle tightly closed when not in use and protect from light. Do not use if the solution has darkened or contains a precipitate.

PREGNANCY AND LACTATION

• Pregnancy Category C. Fetal harm is not known with topical administration. Excretion into human milk is not known.

phenytoin sodium

(fen'-i-toyn soe'-dee-um)

Drug Class: Anticonvulsants; Hydantoins

Pregnancy Category: D

Do not confuse with Dilaudid or mephenytoin.

CLINICAL PHARMACOLOGY

Mechanism of Action: An anticonvulsant and antiarrhythmic agent that stabilizes neuronal membranes in motor cortex, and decreases abnormal ventricular automaticity. *Therapeutic Effect:* Limits spread of seizure activity. Stabilizes threshold against hyperexcitability. Decreases posttetanic potentiation and repetitive discharge. Shortens refractory period, QT interval, and action potential duration.

Pharmacokinetics

Slowly, variably absorbed after PO administration; slow but completely absorbed after IM administration. Protein binding: 90%-95%. Widely distributed. Metabolized in liver. Primarily excreted in urine. Not removed by hemodialysis. **Half-life:** 22 hrs.

AVAILABLE FORMS

• *Capsules (extended-release): 30 mg (Dilantin), 100 mg (Dilantin), 200 mg (Phenytek), 300 mg (Phenytek).*

• *Capsules (immediate-release): 100 mg.*

• *Injection: 50 mg/ml.*

INDICATIONS AND DOSAGES

Status epilepticus

IV

Adults, Elderly, Children. Loading dose: 15-18 mg/kg. Maintenance dose: 300 mg/day in 2-3 divided doses.

Children 10-16 yr. Loading dose: 15-18 mg/kg. Maintenance dose: 6-7 mg/kg/day.

Children 7-9 yr. Loading dose: 15-18 mg/kg. Maintenance dose 7-8 mg/kg/day.

Children 4-6 yr. Loading dose: 15-18 mg/kg. Maintenance dose: 7.5-9 mg/kg/day

Children 6 mo-3 yr. Loading dose 15-18 mg/kg. Maintenance dose: 8-10 mg/kg/day.

Neonates. Loading dose: 15-20 mg/kg. Maintenance dose: 5-8 mg/kg/day.

Anticonvulsant

PO

Adults, Elderly, Children. Loading dose: 15-20 mg/kg in 3 divided doses 2-4 hrs apart. Maintenance dose: 300 mg/day in 2-3 divided doses.

Arrhythmias

IV

Adults, Elderly, Children. Loading dose: 1.25 mg/kg q5min. May repeat up to total dose of 15 mg/kg.

PO

Adults, Elderly. Maintenance dose: 250 mg 4 times/day for 1 day, then 250 mg 2 times/day for 2 days, then 300-400 mg/day in divided doses 1-4 times/day.

PO/IV

Children. Maintenance dose: 5-10 mg/kg/day in 2-3 divided doses.

UNLABELED USES: Adjunct in treatment of tricyclic antidepressant toxicity, muscle relaxant in treatment of muscle hyperirritability, treatment of digoxin-induced arrhythmias and trigeminal neuralgia.

CONTRAINDICATIONS: Hydantoin hypersensitivity, seizures due to hypoglycemia

IV: Adam-Stokes syndrome, second- and third-degree heart block, sinoatrial block, sinus bradycardia

INTERACTIONS

Drug

Alcohol, central nervous system (CNS) depressants: May increase CNS depression.

Amiodarone, anticoagulants, cimetidine, disulfiram, fluoxetine, isoniazid, sulfonamides: May increase phenytoin blood concentration, effects, and risk of toxicity.

Antacids: May decrease the absorption of phenytoin.

Fluconazole, ketoconazole, miconazole: May increase phenytoin blood concentration.

Glucocorticoids: May decrease the effects of glucocorticoids.

Lidocaine, propranolol: May increase cardiac depressant effects.

Valproic acid: May increase phenytoin blood concentration and decrease the metabolism of phenytoin.

Xanthine: May increase the metabolism of xanthine.

Herbal

None known.

Food

None known.

DIAGNOSTIC TEST EFFECTS: May increase blood glucose levels, serum gamma glutamyl transferase (GGT) levels, and serum alkaline phosphatase levels. Therapeutic serum level is 10-20 mcg/ml; toxic serum level is greater than 20 mcg/ml.

IV INCOMPATIBILITIES: Diltiazem (Cardizem), dobutamine (Dobutrex), enalapril (Vasotec), heparin, hydromorphone (Dilaudid), insulin, lidocaine, morphine, nitroglycerin, norepinephrine (Levophed), potassium chloride, propofol (Diprivan)

SIDE EFFECTS

Frequent

Drowsiness, lethargy, confusion, slurred speech, irritability, gingival hyperplasia, hypersensitivity reaction, including fever, rash, and lymphadenopathy, constipation, dizziness, nausea

Occasional

Headache, hair growth, insomnia, muscle twitching

SERIOUS REACTIONS

- Abrupt withdrawal may precipitate status epilepticus.
- Blood dyscrasias, lymphadenopathy, and osteomalacia, caused by interference of vitamin D metabolism, may occur.
- Toxic phenytoin blood concentration of 25 mcg/ml may produce ataxia, characterized by muscular incoordination, nystagmus or rhythmic oscillation of eyes, and double vision. As level increases, extreme lethargy to comatose states occur.

SPECIAL CONSIDERATIONS

PRECAUTIONS

- Patients with impaired liver function, elderly patients, or those who are gravely ill may show early signs of toxicity. Discontinue phenytoin sodium therapy if a skin rash appears.

• Phenytoin and other hydantoins are contraindicated in patients who have experienced phenytoin hypersensitivity. Hyperglycemia, resulting from the inhibitory effects of the drug on insulin release, has been reported. Osteomalacia has been associated with phenytoin therapy. Phenytoin sodium is not indicated for seizures because of hypoglycemic or other metabolic causes. The drug is not effective for absence (petit mal) seizures.

PATIENT INFORMATION

• Advise patients taking phenytoin of the importance of adhering strictly to the prescribed dosage regimen. Also caution patients on the use of other drugs or alcoholic beverages without first seeking the physician's advice. Instruct patients to call their physician if skin rash develops. Stress the importance of good dental hygiene to minimize the development of gingival hyperplasia and its complications. Instruct the patient not to use capsules that are discolored.

PREGNANCY AND LACTATION

• Pregnancy Category D. A number of reports suggest an association between the use of antiepileptic drugs by women with epilepsy and a higher incidence of birth defects in children born to these women. Infant breast-feeding is not recommended for women taking this drug because phenytoin appears to be secreted in low concentrations in human milk.

OCULAR CONSIDERATIONS

• Phenytoin sodium can affect extraocular muscles.

phytonadione; vitamin K_1

(vight'-ah-myn K)

Rx: Aquamephyton, Mephyton, Vitamin K1

Drug Class: Hemostatics; Vitamins/minerals

Pregnancy Category: C

Do not confuse Mephyton with melphalan or mephenytoin.

CLINICAL PHARMACOLOGY

Mechanism of Action: A fat-soluble vitamin that promotes hepatic formation of coagulation factors II, VII, IX, and X. *Therapeutic Effect:* Essential for normal clotting of blood.

Pharmacokinetics

Readily absorbed from the GI tract (duodenum) after IM or subcutaneous administration. Metabolized in the liver. Excreted in urine; eliminated by biliary system. Onset of action: with PO form, 6-10 hr; with parenteral form, hemorrhage controlled in 3-6 hr and PT returns to normal in 12-14 hr.

AVAILABLE FORMS

• *Tablets (Mephyton):* 5 mg.
• *Injection (AquaMephyton):* 2 mg/ml, 10 mg/ml.

INDICATIONS AND DOSAGES

Oral anticoagulant overdose

PO, IV, Subcutaneous

Adults, Elderly. 2.5-10 mg/dose. May repeat in 12-48 hr if given orally and in 6-8 hr if given by IV or subcutaneous route.

Children. 0.5-5 mg depending on need for further anticoagulation and severity of bleeding.

Vitamin K deficiency

PO

Adults, Elderly. 2.5-25 mg/24 hr.
Children. 2.5-5 mg/24 hr.

IV, IM, Subcutaneous
Adults, Elderly. 10 mg/dose.
Children. 1-2 mg/dose.
Hemorrhagic disease of newborn
IM, Subcutaneous
Neonates. Treatment: 1-2 mg/dose/day. Prophylaxis: 0.5-1 mg within 1 hr of birth; may repeat in 6-8 hr if necessary.

CONTRAINDICATIONS: None known.

INTERACTIONS

Drug

Broad-spectrum antibiotics, high-dose salicylates: May increase vitamin K requirements.

Cholestyramine, colestipol, mineral oil, sucralfate: May decrease the absorption of vitamin K.

Oral anticoagulants: May decrease the effects of these drugs.

Herbal

None known.

Food

None known.

DIAGNOSTIC TEST EFFECTS: *None known.*

IV INCOMPATIBILITIES: No known incompatibilities for Y-site administration.

IV COMPATIBILITIES: Heparin, potassium chloride

SIDE EFFECTS

Occasional

Pain, soreness, and swelling at IM injection site; pruritic erythema (with repeated injections); facial flushing; unusual taste

SERIOUS REACTIONS

- Newborns (especially premature infants) may develop hyperbilirubinemia.
- A severe reaction (cramplike pain, chest pain, dyspnea, facial flushing, dizziness, rapid or weak pulse, rash, diaphoresis, hypotension progressing to shock, cardiac arrest) occurs rarely just after IV administration.

SPECIAL CONSIDERATIONS

PRECAUTIONS

- An immediate coagulant effect should not be expected. Konakion does not directly counteract the effects of oral anticoagulants, but it promotes the synthesis of prothrombin by the liver. Phytonadione will not counteract the anticoagulant action of heparin. Phytonadione is not a clotting agent, but overzealous therapy with vitamin K_1 may restore conditions that originally permitted thromboembolic phenomena.

PREGNANCY AND LACTATION

- Pregnancy Category C. Fetal harm is not known with topical administration. A study has shown that vitamin K is excreted in human milk.

---

pilocarpine hydrochloride

(pye-loe-kar'peen)

Rx: Adsorbocarpine, Akarpine, Isopto Carpine, Ocu-Carpine, Ocusert, Pilagan with C Cap, Pilocar, Pilopine-HS, Piloptic-1, Piloptic-1/2, Piloptic-2, Piloptic-3, Piloptic-4, Piloptic-6, Pilostat, Salagen
Drug Class: Cholinergics; Miotics; Ophthalmics
Pregnancy Category: C

CLINICAL PHARMACOLOGY

Mechanism of Action: A cholinergic that increases exocrine gland secretions by stimulating cholinergic receptors. *Therapeutic Effect:* Improves symptoms of dry mouth in patients with salivary gland hypofunction.

Pharmacokinetics

Route	*Onset*	*Peak*	*Duration*
PO	20 min	1 hr	3-5 hrs

Absorption decreased if taken with a high-fat meal. Inactivation of pilocarpine thought to occur at neuronal synapses and probably in plasma. Excreted in urine. **Half-life:** 4-12 hr.

AVAILABLE FORMS

- *Tablets:* 5 mg.

INDICATIONS AND DOSAGES

Dry mouth associated with radiation treatment for head and neck cancer

PO

Adults, Elderly. 5 mg three times a day. Range: 15-30 mg/day. Maximum: 2 tablets/dose.

Dry mouth associated with Sjögren's syndrome

PO

Adults, Elderly. 5 mg four times a day. Range: 20-40 mg/day.

Dosage in hepatic impairment

Dosage decreased to 5 mg twice a day for adults and elderly with hepatic impairment.

CONTRAINDICATIONS: Conditions in which miosis is undesirable, such as acute iritis and angle-closure glaucoma; uncontrolled asthma

INTERACTIONS

Drug

Anticholinergics: May antagonize the effects of anticholinergics.

Beta-blockers: May produce conduction disturbances.

Herbal

None known.

Food

High-fat meals: May decrease the absorption rate of pilocarpine.

DIAGNOSTIC TEST EFFECTS: *None known.*

SIDE EFFECTS

Frequent (29%)

Diaphoresis

Occasional (11%-05%)

Headache, dizziness, urinary frequency, flushing, dyspepsia, nausea, asthenia, lacrimation, visual disturbances

Rare (less than 4%)

Diarrhea, abdominal pain, peripheral edema, chills

SERIOUS REACTIONS

- Patients with diaphoresis who don't drink enough fluids may develop dehydration.

SPECIAL CONSIDERATIONS

PRECAUTIONS

- Ocular formulations of pilocarpine have been reported to cause visual blurring that may result in decreased visual acuity, especially at night and in patients with central lens changes, and to cause impairment of depth perception. Advise patients to be cautious while driving at night.
- Tablets: Headache, visual disturbance, lacrimation, sweating, respiratory distress, gastrointestinal spasm, nausea, vomiting, diarrhea, atrioventricular block, tachycardia, bradycardia, hypotension, hypertension, shock, mental confusion, cardiac arrhythmia, and tremors may occur.
- Use caution in patients with cholelithiasis or biliary tract disease. Theoretically pilocarpine could precipitate renal colic (or "ureteral reflux"), particularly in patients with nephrolithiasis.
- Cardiovascular Disease: Patients may be unable to compensate for transient changes in hemodynamics or rhythm induced by pilocarpine. Pulmonary edema has been reported as a complication of pilocarpine toxicity from high ocular doses given for acute angle-closure glaucoma.

• Pulmonary Disease: Increased airway resistance, bronchial smooth muscle tone, and bronchial secretions may occur. Administer pilocarpine with caution to patients with controlled asthma, chronic bronchitis, or chronic obstructive pulmonary disease requiring pharmacotherapy.
• Central Nervous System Effects: Use caution in patients with underlying cognitive or psychiatric disturbances.

PATIENT INFORMATION

• Pilocarpine may cause visual disturbances, especially when one is driving at night. If a patient sweats excessively and cannot drink enough liquid, the patient should consult an eye care practitioner. Dehydration may develop.

PREGNANCY AND LACTATION

• Pregnancy Category C. Pilocarpine administration is associated with a reduction in the mean fetal body weight and an increase in the incidence of skeletal variations when given to pregnant rats orally. Excretion into human milk is not known.

pindolol

(pin'doe-loll)
Drug Class: Antiadrenergics, beta blocking
Pregnancy Category: B

CLINICAL PHARMACOLOGY

Mechanism of Action: A nonselective beta-blocker that blocks $beta_1$- and $beta_2$-adrenergic receptors. *Therapeutic Effect:* Slows heart rate, decreases cardiac output, decreases blood pressure (BP), and exhibits antiarrhythmic activity. Decreases myocardial ischemia severity by decreasing oxygen requirements.

Pharmacokinetics

Completely absorbed from GI tract. Metabolized in liver. Primarily excreted in urine. **Half-life:** 3-4 hrs (half-life increased with imparied renal function, elderly).

AVAILABLE FORMS

• *Capsules:* 5 mg, 10 mg (Visken).

INDICATIONS AND DOSAGES

Mild to moderate hypertension

PO

Adults. Initially, 5 mg 2 times/day. Gradually increase dose by 10 mg/day at 2- to 4-week intervals. Maintenance: 10-30 mg/day in 2-3 divided doses. Maximum: 60 mg/day.

Usual elderly dosage:

PO

Initially, 5 mg/day. May increase by 5 mg q3-4 wks.

UNLABELED USES: Treatment of chronic angina pectoris, hypertrophic cardiomyopathy, tremors, and mitral valve prolapse syndrome. Increases antidepressant effect with fluoxetine and other SSRIs.

CONTRAINDICATIONS: Bronchial asthma, COPD, uncontrolled cardiac failure, sinus bradycardia, heart block greater than first degree, cardiogenic shock, CHF (unless secondary to tachyarrhythmias)

INTERACTIONS

Drug

Diuretics, other hypotensives: May increase hypotensive effect of pindolol.

Sympathomimetics, xanthines: May mutually inhibit effects of pindolol.

Insulin and oral hypoglycemics: May mask symptoms of hypoglycemia and/or prolong hypoglycemic effect.

Herbal

None known.

Food

None known.

DIAGNOSTIC TEST EFFECTS: May increase ANA titer, SGOT (AST), SGPT (ALT), alkaline phosphatase, LDH, bilirubin, BUN, creatinine, potassium, uric acid, lipoproteins, and triglycerides.

SIDE EFFECTS

Frequent

Decreased sexual ability, drowsiness, trouble sleeping, unusual tiredness/weakness

Occasional

Bradycardia, depression, cold hands/feet, diarrhea, constipation, anxiety, nasal congestion, nausea, vomiting

Rare

Altered taste, dry eyes, itching, numbness of fingers, toes, and scalp

SERIOUS REACTIONS

- Overdosage may produce profound bradycardia and hypotension.
- Abrupt withdrawal may result in sweating, palpitations, headache, and tremulousness.
- May precipitate congestive heart failure (CHF) or myocardial infarction (MI) in patients with heart disease; thyroid storm in those with thyrotoxicosis; or peripheral ischemia in those with existing peripheral vascular disease.
- Hypoglycemia may occur in previously controlled diabetics.
- Signs of thrombocytopenia, such as unusual bleeding or bruising, occur rarely.

SPECIAL CONSIDERATIONS

PRECAUTIONS

- Sympathetic stimulation may be a vital component supporting circulatory function in patients with congestive heart failure, and its inhibition by beta-blockade may precipitate more severe failure. Hypersensitivity to catecholamines has been observed in patients who were withdrawn from therapy with beta-blocking agents. Pindolol may prevent the appearance of signs and symptoms of acute hypoglycemia, such as tachycardia and blood pressure changes. Pindolol may mask certain clinical signs (e.g., tachycardia) of hyperthyroidism. Pindolol is contraindicated in patients with bronchial asthma. Patients with bronchospastic diseases should not receive beta-blockers. Patients with a history of severe anaphylactic reactions to a variety of allergens may be more reactive to repeated challenge. Such patients may be unresponsive to the usual doses of epinephrine used to treat allergic reactions. Use pindolol with caution in patients with impaired hepatic or renal function.

PATIENT INFORMATION

- Warn patients, especially those with evidence of coronary artery insufficiency, against interruption or discontinuation of pindolol therapy without the physician's advice. Although cardiac failure rarely occurs in properly selected patients, advise patients being treated with beta-adrenergic blocking agents to consult the physician at the first sign or symptom of impending failure.

PREGNANCY AND LACTATION

- Pregnancy Category B. Studies in rats and rabbits exceeding 100 times the maximum recommended human doses revealed no embryotoxicity or teratogenicity. Fetal harm is not known. Because pindolol is secreted in human milk, mothers receiving the drug should not nurse.

pioglitazone

(pye-oh-gli'ta-zone)
Rx: Actos
Drug Class: Antidiabetic agents; Thiazolidinediones
Pregnancy Category: C

CLINICAL PHARMACOLOGY

Mechanism of Action: An antidiabetic that improves target-cell response to insulin without increasing pancreatic insulin secretion. Decreases hepatic glucose output and increases insulin-dependent glucose utilization in skeletal muscle. *Therapeutic Effect:* Lowers blood glucose concentration.

Pharmacokinetics

Rapidly absorbed. Highly protein bound (99%), primarily to albumin. Metabolized in the liver. Excreted in urine. Unknown if removed by hemodialysis. **Half-life:** 16-24 hr.

AVAILABLE FORMS

• *Tablets:* 15 mg, 30 mg, 45 mg.

INDICATIONS AND DOSAGES

Diabetes mellitus, combination therapy

PO

Adult, Elderly. With insulin: Initially, 15-30 mg once a day. Initially continue current insulin dosage; then decrease insulin dosage by 10% to 25% if hypoglycemia occurs or plasma glucose level decreases to less than 100 mg/dl. Maximum: 45 mg/day. With sulfonylureas: Initially, 15-30 mg/day. Decrease sulfonylurea dosage if hypoglycemia occurs. Wtih metformin: Initially, 15-30 mg/day. As monotherapy: Monotherapy is not to be used if patient is well controlled with diet and exercise alone. Initially, 15-30 mg/day. May increase dosage in increments until 45 mg/day is reached.

CONTRAINDICATIONS: Active hepatic disease; diabetic ketoacidosis; increased serum transaminase levels, including ALT (SGPT) greater than 2.5 times normal serum level; type 1 diabetes mellitus

INTERACTIONS

Drug

Gemfibrizol: May increase the effect and toxicity of pioglitazone.
Ketoconazole: May significantly inhibit metabolism of pioglitazone.
Oral contraceptives: May alter the effects of oral contraceptives.

Food

None known.

Herbal

None known.

DIAGNOSTIC TEST EFFECTS: May increase creatine kinase (CK) level. May decrease Hgb levels by 2% to 4% and serum alkaline phosphatase, bilirubin, and ALT (SGOT) levels. Less than 1% of patients experience ALT values 3 times the normal level.

SIDE EFFECTS

Frequent (13%-9%)
Headache, upper respiratory tract infection
Occasional (6%-5%)
Sinusitis, myalgia, pharyngitis, aggravated diabetes mellitus

SERIOUS REACTIONS

• None known.

SPECIAL CONSIDERATIONS

PRECAUTIONS

• Do not use pioglitazone hydrochloride in patients with type 1 diabetes or to treat diabetic ketoacidosis. Patients receiving pioglitazone hydrochloride in combination with insulin or oral hypoglycemic agents may be at risk for hypoglycemia, and a reduction in the dose of the concomitant agent may be necessary. In premenopausal anovulatory patients with insulin resistance, treatment with thiazolidinediones, including pioglitazone hydrochloride, may result in resumption of ovulation. Pioglitazone hydrochloride may cause decreases in hemoglobin and hematocrit. Use the drug with caution in patients with edema. In double blind clinical trials of patients with type 2 diabetes, mild to moderate edema was reported. Pioglitazone hydrochloride can cause plasma volume expansion and preload-induced cardiac hypertrophy. Do not initiate therapy with pioglitazone hydrochloride if the patient exhibits clinical evidence of active liver disease or the alanine transaminase levels exceed 2.5 times the upper limit of normal.

PATIENT INFORMATION

- It is important to instruct patients to adhere to dietary instructions and to have blood glucose and glycosylated hemoglobin tested regularly. During periods of stress such as fever, trauma, infection, or surgery, medication requirements may change, and patients should be reminded to seek medical advice promptly.
- Inform patients that blood tests for liver function will be performed before the start of therapy, every 2 months for the first year, and periodically thereafter. Instruct patients to seek immediate medical advice for unexplained nausea, vomiting, abdominal pain, fatigue, anorexia, or dark urine.
- Instruct patients to take pioglitazone hydrochloride once daily. Pioglitazone hydrochloride can be taken with or without meals. If a dose is missed on one day, the dose should not be doubled the following day.
- When using combination therapy with insulin or oral hypoglycemic agents, explain the risks of hypoglycemia, its symptoms and treatment, and conditions that predispose to its development to patients and their family members.
- In anovulatory, premenopausal women with insulin resistance, therapy with pioglitazone hydrochloride may cause resumption of ovulation, and contraceptive measures may need to be considered.

PREGNANCY AND LACTATION

- Pregnancy Category C. Pioglitazone was not teratogenic in rats at oral doses. Pioglitazone is secreted in the milk of lactating rats. Excretion into human milk is not known.

polymyxin B sulfate; trimethoprim sulfate

(pol-ee-mix'-in bee sul'-fate; trye-meth'-oh-prim sul'-fate)

Rx: Polytrim

Drug Class: Anti-infectives, ophthalmic; Antibiotics, folate antagonists; Antibiotics, polymyxins; Antibiotics, sulfonamides; Ophthalmics

Pregnancy Category: C

CLINICAL PHARMACOLOGY

Mechanism of Action: Polymyxin B damages bacterial cytoplasmic membrane which causes leakage of intracellular components. Trimethoprim is a folate antagonist that blocks bacterial biosynthesis of nucleic acids and proteins by interfering with metabolism of folinic acid *Therapeutic Effect:* Prevents inflammatory process. Interferes with bacterial protein synthesis. Produces antibacterial activity.

Pharmacokinetics

Absorption through intact skin and mucous membranes is insignificant.

AVAILABLE FORMS

• *Solution, ophthalmic:* 1 mg trimethoprim sulfate and 10,000 units polymyxin B sulfate per ml (Polytrim).

INDICATIONS AND DOSAGES

Treatment of surface ocular bacterial conjunctivitis and blepharoconjunctivitis

Ophthalmic

Adults, Elderly, Children. Instill 1-2 drops in eye(s) every 3 hours for 7-10 days. Maximum: 6 doses/day.

CONTRAINDICATIONS: Hypersensitivity to polymyxin B, trimethoprim sulfate, or any component of the formulation

INTERACTIONS

Drug

None known.

Herbal

None known.

Food

None known.

DIAGNOSTIC TEST EFFECTS: *None known.*

SIDE EFFECTS

Occasional

Local irritation, redness, burning, stinging, itching

SERIOUS REACTIONS

• Prolonged use may result in overgrowth of nonsusceptible organisms, including superinfection.

• Hypersensitivity reactions consisting of lid edema, itching, increased redness, tearing, and/or circumocular rash have been reported.

• Photosensitivity has been reported in patients taking oral trimethoprim.

SPECIAL CONSIDERATIONS

PRECAUTIONS

• Fungal infections and superinfections may occur.

PREGNANCY AND LACTATION

• Pregnancy Category C. Fetal harm not known with topical administration. Polymyxin B sulfate and trimethoprim sulfate may interfere with folic acid metabolism. Excretion into human milk is not known.

polyvinyl alcohol

(pol-i-vine'il alk'o-hol)

CLINICAL PHARMACOLOGY

Mechanism of Action: Not reported.

Pharmacokinetics

Not reported.

AVAILABLE FORMS

• *Ophthalmic solution:* 0.5 % (Murine Tears), 1% (Hypotears, Hypotears PF [preservative free]), 1.4% (Akwa Tears, Tears Again).

INDICATIONS AND DOSAGES

Relief of dry eye and eye irritation

Ophthalmic

Adults, Elderly. Instill 1 or 2 drops in affected eye(s) as needed.

CONTRAINDICATIONS: Hypersensitivity to polyvinyl alcohol or any component of the formulation

INTERACTIONS

Drug

None known.

Herbal

None known.

Food

None known.

DIAGNOSTIC TEST EFFECTS: *None known.*

SIDE EFFECTS

Blurred vision for a short time

SERIOUS REACTIONS

• None reported.

SPECIAL CONSIDERATIONS

PATIENT INFORMATION

• Give patients the following instructions:

• To avoid contamination, do not touch the tip of the container to any surface. Replace cap after using. If solution changes color or becomes cloudy, do not use it. If you experience eye pain, changes in vision, or continued redness or irritation of the eye, or if the condition worsens or persists for more than 72 hours, discontinue use and consult an eye care practitioner. Keep this and all drugs out of the reach of children. Keep container tightly closed. Remove contact lenses before using.

potassium chloride

(poe-tass'ee-um klor'ide)

Rx: Cena K, Ed K+10, K+Care, K-10, K-8, Kaochlor, Kaochlor S-F, Kaon-Cl, Kaon-CL 10, Kaon-CL 20%, Kato, Kay Ciel, KCl-20, KCl-40, K-Dur 10, K-Dur 20, K-Lor, Klor-Con, Klor-Con/25, Klor-Con 10, Klor-Con 8, Klor-Con M10, Klor-Con M15, Klor-Con M20, Klotrix, K-Lyte Cl, K-Norm, K-Sol, K-Tab, Micro-K, Micro-K 10, Rum-K

Drug Class: Electrolyte replacements; Vitamins/minerals

Pregnancy Category: C

Do not confuse with Cardura or Slow-FE.

CLINICAL PHARMACOLOGY

Mechanism of Action: An electrolyte that is necessary for multiple cellular metabolic processes. Primary action is intracellular. *Therapeutic Effect:* Necessary for nerve impulse conduction, contraction of cardiac, skeletal, and smooth muscle; maintains normal renal function and acid-base balance.

Pharmacokinetics

Well absorbed from the gastrointestinal (GI) tract. Enters cells via active transport from extracellular fluid. Primarily excreted in urine.

AVAILABLE FORMS

- *Capsules, Extended-Release:* 8 mEq (Micro-K), 10 mEq (K-Norm).
- *Intravenous Solution:* 2 mEq/ml, 30 mEq/100 ml, 40 mEq/100 ml, 10 mEq/100 ml, 20 mEq/100 ml.
- *Liquid:* 20 mEq/15 ml (Cena-K, KCl-20, Kay Ciel, Kaochlor S-F), 30 mEq/ 15 ml (Rum-K), 40 mEq/15 ml (Cena K, Kaon-CL 20%, KCl-40).
- *Powder for Compounding:* 100%.
- *Powder for Reconstitution:* 15 mEq (K+Care), 20 mEq (K+ Care, K-Sol, Kay Ciel, Kato, K-Lor, Klor-Con), 25 mEq (Klor-Con/25).
- *Tablets:* 500 mg, 595 mg.
- *Tablets, Effervescent:* 25 mEq (K-Lyte Cl), 50 mEq (K-Lyte Cl)
- *Tablets, Extended-Release:* 8 mEq (Kaon-Cl, K-8, Klor-Con 8), 10 mEq (Ed K+10, K-10, K-Dur 10, Kaon-CL 10, Klor-Con M10, K-Tab, Klotrix), 15 mEq (Klor-Con M15) 20 mEq (K-Dur 20, Klor-Con M20).

INDICATIONS AND DOSAGES

Prevention of hypokalemia (on diuretic therapy)

PO

Adults, Elderly. 20-40 mEq/day in 1-2 divided doses.

Children. 1-2 mEq/kg in 1-2 divided doses.

Treatment of hypokalemia

IV

Adults, Elderly. 5-10 mEq/hr. Maximum: 400 mEq/day.

Children. 1 mEq/kg over 1-2 hrs.

PO

Adults, Elderly. 40-80 mEq/day further doses based on laboratory values.

Children. 1-2 mEq/day, further doses based on laboratory values.

CONTRAINDICATIONS: Digitalis toxicity, heat cramps, hyperkalemia, patients receiving potassium-sparing diuretics, postoperative oliguria, severe burns, severe renal impairment, shock with dehydration or hemolytic reaction, untreated Addison's disease, hypersensitivity to any component of the formulation.

INTERACTIONS

Drug

Anticholinergics: May increase the risk of gastrointestinal (GI) lesions.

Angiotensin-converting enzyme inhibitors (ACE) inhibitors, beta-adrenergic blockers, heparin, NSAIDs, potassium-containing medications, potassium-sparing diuretics, salt substitutes: May increase potassium blood concentration.

Herbal

None known.

Food

None known.

DIAGNOSTIC TEST EFFECTS: *None known.*

SIDE EFFECTS

Occasional

Nausea, vomiting, diarrhea, flatulence, abdominal discomfort with distention, phlebitis with IV administration (particularly when potassium concentration of greater than 40 mEq/L is infused).

Rare

Rash

SERIOUS REACTIONS

- Hyperkalemia (observed particularly in elderly or in patients with impaired renal function) manifested as paresthesia of extremities, heaviness of legs, cold skin, grayish pallor, hypotension, mental confusion, irritability, flaccid paralysis, and cardiac arrhythmias.

SPECIAL CONSIDERATIONS

PRECAUTIONS

- In patients with impaired mechanisms for excreting potassium, the administration of potassium salts can produce hyperkalemia and cardiac arrest. Do not treat hypokalemia by the concomitant adinistration of potassium salts and a potassium-sparing diuretic. Angiotensin-converting enzyme inhibitors (e.g., captopril and enalapril) will produce some potassium retention by inhibiting aldosterone production. Solid oral dosage forms of potassium chloride can produce ulcerative and/or stenotic lesions of the gastrointestinal tract and death.

PATIENT INFORMATION

Give patients the following instructions:

- Take this medicine following the frequency and amount prescribed by the physician. This is especially important if you also are taking diuretics and/or digitalis preparations. Check with the physician at once if you notice tarry stools or other evidence of gastrointestinal bleeding.
- Extended-Release Capsules and Tablets: Take each dose with meals and with a full glass of water or other liquid. Check with the physician if you have trouble swallowing capsules or if the capsules seem to stick in the throat.
- Extended-Release Formulation for Liquid Suspension: Take each dose with meals mixed in water or other suitable liquid. Inform patients that this product contains as a dispersing agent the stool softener docusate sodium, which may change stool consistency or, rarely, produce diarrhea or cramps.

PREGNANCY AND LACTATION

• Pregnancy Category C. Potassium supplementation that does not lead to hyperkalemia likely would not have an adverse effect on the fetus and would not affect reproductive capacity. The normal potassium ion content of human milk is about 13 mEq/L. Because orally administered potassium becomes part of the (body) potassium pool, so long as body potassium is not excessive, the contribution of potassium chloride supplementation should have little or no effect on the level in human milk.

---

pravastatin

(prav-i-sta'tin)

Rx: Pravachol

Drug Class: Antihyperlipidemics; HMG CoA reductase inhibitors

Pregnancy Category: X

Do not confuse pravastatin with Prevacid, or Pravachol with propranolol.

CLINICAL PHARMACOLOGY

Mechanism of Action: An HMG-CoA reductase inhibitor that interferes with cholesterol biosynthesis by preventing the conversion of HMG-CoA reductase to mevalonate, a precursor to cholesterol. *Therapeutic Effect:* Lowers serum LDL and VLDL cholesterol and plasma triglyceride levels; increases serum HDL concentration.

Pharmacokinetics

Poorly absorbed from the GI tract. Protein binding: 50%. Metabolized in the liver (minimal active metabolites). Primarily excreted in feces via the biliary system. Not removed by hemodialysis. **Half-life:** 2.7 hr.

AVAILABLE FORMS

• *Tablets:* 10 mg, 20 mg, 40 mg, 80 mg.

INDICATIONS AND DOSAGES

Hyperlipidemia, primary and secondary prevention of cardiovascular events in patient with elevated cholesterol levels

PO

Adults, Elderly. Initially, 40 mg/day. Titrate to desired response. Range: 10-80 mg/day.

Children 14-18 yr. 40 mg/day.

Children 8-13 yr. 20 mg/day.

Dosage in hepatic and renal impairment

For adults, give 10 mg/day initially. Titrate to desired response.

CONTRAINDICATIONS: Active hepatic disease or unexplained, persistent elevations of liver function test results

INTERACTIONS

Drug

Cyclosporine, erythromycin, gemfibrozil, immunosuppressants, niacin: Increases the risk of acute renal failure and rhabdomyolysis.

Herbal

None known.

Food

None known.

DIAGNOSTIC TEST EFFECTS: May increase serum CK and transaminase concentrations.

SIDE EFFECTS

Pravastatin is generally well tolerated. Side effects are usually mild and transient.

Occasional (7%-4%)

Nausea, vomiting, diarrhea, constipation, abdominal pain, headache, rhinitis, rash, pruritus

Rare (3%-2%)

Heartburn, myalgia, dizziness, cough, fatigue, flu-like symptoms

SERIOUS REACTIONS

- Malignancy and cataracts may occur.
- Hypersensitivity occurs rarely.

SPECIAL CONSIDERATIONS

PRECAUTIONS

- Pravastatin may elevate creatine phosphokinase and transaminase levels. 3-Hydroxy-3-methylglutaryl–coenzyme A (HMG-CoA) reductase inhibitors interfere with cholesterol synthesis and lower circulating cholesterol levels and, as such, theoretically might blunt adrenal or gonadal steroid hormone production. Central nervous system vascular lesions were seen in dogs treated with pravastatin.

PATIENT INFORMATION

- Advise patients to report promptly unexplained muscle pain, tenderness, or weakness, particularly if accompanied by malaise or fever.

PREGNANCY AND LACTATION

- Pregnancy Category X. Because HMG-CoA reductase inhibitors decrease cholesterol synthesis and possibly the synthesis of other biologically active substances derived from cholesterol, they may cause fetal harm when administered to pregnant women. Therefore, HMG-CoA reductase inhibitors are contraindicated during pregnancy and in nursing mothers. Administer pravastatin to women of childbearing age only when such patients are highly unlikely to conceive and have been informed of the potential hazards. If the patient becomes pregnant while taking this class of drug, discontinue therapy and apprise the patient of the potential hazard to the fetus. A small amount of pravastatin is excreted in human breast milk.

OCULAR CONSIDERATIONS

- A chemically similar drug in this class produced optic nerve degeneration (Wallerian degeneration of retinogeniculate fibers) in clinically normal dogs in a dose-dependent fashion starting at 60 mg/kg per day, a dose that produced mean plasma drug levels about 30 times higher than the mean drug level in human beings taking the highest recommended dose (as measured by total enzyme inhibitory activity). This same drug also produced vestibulocochlear Wallerian-like degeneration and retinal ganglion cell chromatolysis in dogs treated for 14 weeks at 180 mg/kg per day, a dose that resulted in a mean plasma drug level similar to that seen with the 60 mg/kg per day dose.

---

prazosin hydrochloride

(pra'zoe-sin)

Rx: Minipress

Drug Class: Antiadrenergics, alpha blocking; Antiadrenergics, peripheral

Pregnancy Category: C

CLINICAL PHARMACOLOGY

Mechanism of Action: An antidote, antihypertensive, and vasodilator that selectively blocks alpha$_1$-adrenergic receptors, decreasing peripheral vascular resistance. *Therapeutic Effect:* Produces vasodilation of veins and arterioles, decreases total peripheral resistance, and relaxes smooth muscle in bladder neck and prostate.

AVAILABLE FORMS

- *Capsules:* 1 mg, 2 mg, 5 mg.

INDICATIONS AND DOSAGES
Mild to moderate hypertension
PO
Adults, Elderly. Initially, 1 mg 2-3 times a day. Maintenance: 3-15 mg/day in divided doses. Maximum: 20 mg/day.
Children. 5 mcg/kg/dose q6h. Gradually increase up to 25 mcg/kg/dose.
UNLABELED USES: Treatment of benign prostate hyperplasia, CHF, ergot alkaloid toxicity, pheochromocytoma, Raynaud's phenomenon
CONTRAINDICATIONS: None known.
INTERACTIONS
Drug
Estrogen, NSAIDs, other sympathomimetics: May decrease the effects of prazosin.
Hypotension-producing medications, such as antihypertensives and diuretics: May increase the effects of prazosin.
Herbal
Licorice: Causes sodium and water retention and potassium loss.
Food
None known.
DIAGNOSTIC TEST EFFECTS: *None known.*
SIDE EFFECTS
Frequent (10%-7%)
Dizziness, somnolence, headache, asthenia (loss of strength, energy)
Occasional (5%-4%)
Palpitations, nausea, dry mouth, nervousness
Rare (less than 1%)
Angina, urinary urgency
SERIOUS REACTIONS
- First-dose syncope (hypotension with sudden loss of consciousness) may occur 30 to 90 minutes following initial dose of more than 2 mg, a too-rapid increase in dosage, or addition of another antihypertensive agent to therapy. First-dose syncope may be preceded by tachycardia (pulse rate of 120-160 beats/minute).

SPECIAL CONSIDERATIONS

PATIENT INFORMATION
Give patients the following instructions:
- Dizziness or drowsiness may occur after the first dose of this medicine. Avoid driving or performing hazardous tasks for the first 24 hours after taking this medicine or when the dose is increased. Dizziness, light-headedness, or fainting may occur, especially when rising from a lying or sitting position. Getting up slowly may help lessen the problem. These effects also may occur if you drink alcohol, stand for long periods of time, and exercise or if the weather is hot. While taking prazosin hydrochloride, be careful in the amount of alcohol you drink. Also, use extra care during exercise or hot weather or if standing for long periods. Check with your physician if you have any questions.

PREGNANCY AND LACTATION
- Pregnancy Category C. Prazosin hydrochloride has been shown to be associated with decreased litter size in rats. Fetal harm is not known with topical administration. Prazosin hydrochloride has been shown to be excreted in small amounts in human milk.

prednisolone acetate

(pred-niss'-oh-lone as'-i-tate)

Rx: AK-Pred, Econopred Plus, Inflamase Forte, Inflamase Mild, Ocu-Pred, Ocu-Pred-A, Ocu-Pred Forte, Pred Forte, Pred Mild, Prednisol

Drug Class: Corticosteroids; Corticosteroids, ophthalmic; Ophthalmics

Pregnancy Category: C

CLINICAL PHARMACOLOGY

Mechanism of Action: An adrenal corticosteroid that inhibits accumulation of inflammatory cells at inflammation sites, phagocytosis, lysosomal enzyme release and synthesis, and release of mediators of inflammation. *Therapeutic Effect:* Prevents or suppresses cell-mediated immune reactions. Decreases or prevents tissue response to inflammatory process.

Pharmacokinetics

Absorbed into aqueous humor, cornea, iris, choroids, ciliary body, and retina. Systemic absorption may occur, but significant only at high dosages.

AVAILABLE FORMS

- *Ophthalmic solution:* 0.125% (AK-Pred, Inflamase Mild, Ocu-Pred), 1% (AK-Pred, Inflamase Forte, Ocu-Pred Forte, Prednisol).
- *Ophthalmic suspension:* 0.12% (Pred Mild), 0.125%, 1% (Econopred Plus, Ocu-Pred-A, Pred Forte).

INDICATIONS AND DOSAGES

Conjunctivitis

Ophthalmic

Adults, Elderly, Children. 1- 2 drops 2-4 times/day.

CONTRAINDICATIONS: Fungal, mycobacterial, or viral infections of the eye, hypersensitivity to prednisolone acetate or any component of the formulation

INTERACTIONS

Drug

None known.

Herbal

None known.

Food

None known.

DIAGNOSTIC TEST EFFECTS: *None known.*

SIDE EFFECTS

Occasional

Stinging or burning

SERIOUS REACTIONS

- Prolonged use of corticosteroids may result in glaucoma with damage to the optic nerve, defects in visual acuity and fields of vision, posterior subcapsular cataract formation, and delayed wound healing.
- Long-term use may cause corneal and scleral thinning.
- Systemic effects are uncommon, but systemic hypercorticoidism have been reported.
- Acute anterior uveitis and perforation of the globe, keratitis, conjunctivitis, corneal ulcers, mydriasis, conjunctival hyperemia, loss of accommodation and ptosis have occasionally been reported.
- The development of secondary ocular infection has occurred. Fungal and viral infections of the cornea may develop with long-term applications of steroid.

SPECIAL CONSIDERATIONS

PRECAUTIONS

- Fungal infections may occur. Check intraocular pressure frequently.

PREGNANCY AND LACTATION

• Pregnancy Category C. Safety of intensive or protracted use of topical steroids during pregnancy has not been substantiated. Systemically administered corticosteroids appear in human milk. Excretion into human milk is not known.

prednisolone acetate; sulfacetamide sodium

(pred-niss'-oh-lone ass'-eh-tate; sul-fa-see'-ta-mide soe'-dee-um)

Rx: AK-Cide, Blephamide, Blephamide S.O.P., Medasulf, Metimyd, Ocu-Lone C, Vasocidin

Drug Class: Anti-infectives, ophthalmic; Antibiotics, sulfonamides; Corticosteroids, ophthalmic; Ophthalmics

CLINICAL PHARMACOLOGY

Mechanism of Action: Prednisolone is an adrenal corticosteroid that inhibits accumulation of inflammatory cells at inflammation sites, phagocytosis, lysosomal enzyme release and synthesis, and release of mediators of inflammation. Sulfacetamide is a sulfonamide that interferes with synthesis of folic acid that bacteria require for growth. *Therapeutic Effect:* Prevents or suppresses cell-mediated immune reactions. Decreases or prevents tissue response to inflammatory process. Prevents further bacterial growth; bacteriostatic.

Pharmacokinetics

None reported.

AVAILABLE FORMS

• *Ophthalmic ointment:* 0.2% prednisolone acetate and 10% sulfacetamide sodium (Blephamide, Blephamide S.O.P.), 0.5% prednisolone acetate and 10% sulfacetamide sodium (AK-Cide, Ocu-Lone C, Medasulf, Metimyd).

• *Ophthalmic solution:* 0.25% prednisolone acetate and 10% sulfacetamide sodium (Vasocidin).

• *Ophthalmic suspension:* 0.2% prednisolone acetate and 10% sulfacetamide sodium (Blephamide), 0.5% prednisolone acetate and 10% sulfacetamide sodium (AK-Cide, Metimyd, Ocu-Lone C, Vasocidin).

INDICATIONS AND DOSAGES

Steroid-responsive inflammatory ocular conditions for which a corticosteroid is indicated and where superficial bacterial ocular infection or a risk of bacterial ocular infection exists

Ophthalmic ointment

Adults, Elderly, Children. Apply 3 or 4 times/day and once at bedtime.

Ophthalmic suspension

Adults, Elderly, Children. Instill 2-3 drops every 1-2 hours while awake.

CONTRAINDICATIONS: Epithelial herpes simplex keratitis (dendritic keratitis), vaccinia, varicella, and other viral diseases of the cornea or conjunctiva, mycobacterial infection of the eye, and fungal diseases of ocular structure, known or suspected hypersensitivity to other sulfonamides or other corticosteroids or any component of the formulation.

INTERACTIONS

Drug

Silver preparations: This drug is incompatible with silver preparations.

Local anesthetics (related to p-amino benzoic acid): May antagonize the action of sulfonamides.

Herbal

None known.

Food

None known.

DIAGNOSTIC TEST EFFECTS: *None known.*

SIDE EFFECTS

Occasional

Local irritation

Rare

Elevation of intraocular pressure

SERIOUS REACTIONS

- Prolonged use of corticosteroids may result in glaucoma with damage to the optic nerve, defects in visual acuity and fields of vision, posterior subcapsular cataract formation, and delayed wound healing.
- Long-term use may cause corneal and scleral thinning.
- Systemic effects are uncommon, but systemic hypercorticoidism have been reported.
- Acute anterior uveitis and perforation of the globe, keratitis, conjunctivitis, corneal ulcers, mydriasis, conjunctival hyperemia, loss of accommodation, and ptosis have occasionally been reported.
- The development of secondary ocular infection has occurred. Fungal and viral infections of the cornea may develop with long-term applications of steroid.
- Fatalities due to reactions to sulfonamides including Stevens-Johnson syndrome, toxic epidermal necrolysis, fulminant hepatic necrosis, agranulocytosis, aplastic anemia, and other blood dyscrasias have occurred.

SPECIAL CONSIDERATIONS

PRECAUTIONS

- Renew the medication order beyond 20 ml of solution or beyond 8 g of the ointment after slit-lamp examination and fluorescein staining. Consider the possibility of fungal infections of the cornea after prolonged corticosteroid dosing. Cross-sensitivity among different sulfonamides may occur. Cross-allergenicity among corticosteroids has been demonstrated. The p-aminobenzoic acid present in purulent exudates competes with sulfonamides and can reduce their effectiveness.

PATIENT INFORMATION

- If inflammation or pain persists longer than 48 hours or becomes aggravated, advise the patient to discontinue use of the medication and consult an eye care practitioner.
- Protect the drug from light. Sulfonamide solutions darken on prolonged standing and exposure to heat and light. Do not use if solution has darkened. Yellowing does not affect activity. Clumping may occur on long standing at high temperatures. Shake well before using.

PREGNANCY AND LACTATION

- Pregnancy Category C. Prednisolone has been shown to be teratogenic in rabbits, hamsters, and mice. Kernicterus may be precipitated in infants by sulfonamides being given systemically during the third trimester of pregnancy. Whether sulfacetamide sodium can cause fetal harm is not known. Systemically administered corticosteroids appear in human milk. Excretion into human milk is not known.

prednisolone sodium phosphate

(pred-nis'-oh-lone soe'-dee-um foss'-fate)

Drug Class: Corticosteroids; Corticosteroids, ophthalmic; Ophthalmics

Pregnancy Category: C

CLINICAL PHARMACOLOGY

Mechanism of Action: An adrenal corticosteroid that inhibits accumulation of inflammatory cells at inflammation sites, phagocytosis, lysosomal enzyme release and synthesis, and release of mediators of inflammation. *Therapeutic Effect:* Prevents or suppresses cell-mediated immune reactions. Decreases or prevents tissue response to inflammatory process.

Pharmacokinetics

Rapidly and well absorbed from the gastrointestinal (GI tract) following oral administration. Protein binding: 90%-95%. Widely distributed. Metabolized in the liver. Excreted in the urine as sulfate and glucuronide conjugates. **Half-life:** 2-4 hrs.

Absorbed into aqueous humor, cornea, iris, choroid, ciliary body, and retina following ocular administration. Systemic absorption occurs, but may be significant only at higher dosages or in extended pediatric therapy.

AVAILABLE FORMS

- *Ophthalmic solution:* 1% (AK-Pred, Inflamase Forte), 0.125% (Inflamase Mild).
- *Oral solution:* 20 mg/5 ml (Orapred), 6.7 mg/5 ml (Pediapred).

INDICATIONS AND DOSAGES

Asthma

PO

Children. 1-2 mg/kg/day in single or divided doses for 3-10 days.

Endocrine disorders, hematologic and neoplastic disorders, inflammatory conditions

PO

Adults, Elderly. 5-60 mg/day.

Children. 0.14-2 mg/kg/day divided into 3 or 4 doses.

Multiple sclerosis exacerbations

PO

Adults, Elderly. 200 mg/day for 1 week, followed by 80 mg every other day for 1 month.

Nephrotic syndrome

PO

Children. 60 mg/m^2 daily. Maximum: 80 mg/day divided 3 times/day for 4 weeks, then 40 mg/m^2 every other day for 4 weeks.

Ophthalmic disorders

Ophthalmic suspension

Adults, Elderly, Children. Instill 1 or 2 drops up to 6 times/day.

CONTRAINDICATIONS: Systemic fungal infections, live or live attenuated vaccines, hypersensitivity to prednisolone sodium phosphate or any component of the formulation

INTERACTIONS

Drug

Amphotericin: May increase hypokalemia.

Digoxin: May increase the risk of toxicity of this drug caused by hypokalemia.

Diuretics, insulin, oral hypoglycemics, potassium supplements: May decrease the effects of diuretics, insulin, oral hypoglycemics, and potassium supplements.

Liver enzyme inducers: May decrease the effects of prednisolone.

Live-virus vaccines: May decrease the patient's antibody response to vaccine, increase vaccine side effects, and potentiate virus replication.

Herbal

None known.

Food

None known.

DIAGNOSTIC TEST EFFECTS: *None known.*

SIDE EFFECTS

Frequent

Insomnia, heartburn, nervousness, abdominal distention, increased sweating, acne, mood swings, increased appetite, facial flushing, delayed wound healing, increased susceptibility to infection, diarrhea or constipation

Occasional

Headache, edema, change in skin color, frequent urination

Rare

Tachycardia, allergic reaction, such as rash and hives, psychic changes, hallucinations, depression

Ophthalmic: stinging or burning, posterior subcapsular cataracts

SERIOUS REACTIONS

- Prolonged use of corticosteroids may result in glaucoma with damage to the optic nerve, defects in visual acuity and fields of vision, posterior subcapsular cataract formation, and delayed wound healing.
- Long-term use may cause corneal and scleral thinning.
- Systemic effects are uncommon, but systemic hypercorticoidism have been reported.
- Acute anterior uveitis and perforation of the globe, keratitis, conjunctivitis, corneal ulcers, mydriasis, conjunctival hyperemia, loss of accommodation and ptosis have occasionally been reported.
- The development of secondary ocular infection has occurred. Fungal and viral infections of the cornea may develop with long-term applications of steroid.

SPECIAL CONSIDERATIONS

PRECAUTIONS

- Fungal infections of the cornea may occur. Check intraocular pressure frequently.

PATIENT INFORMATION

- Do not touch dropper tip to any surface as this may contaminate the solution.

PREGNANCY AND LACTATION

- Pregnancy Category C. Fetal harm not known with topical administration. Excretion into human milk is not known.

prednisolone sodium phosphate; sulfacetamide sodium

(pred-nis'oh-lone soe'dee-um; sul-fa-see'ta-mide soe'dee-um)

Drug Class: Anti-infectives, ophthalmic; Antibiotics, sulfonamides; Corticosteroids, ophthalmic; Ophthalmics

Pregnancy Category: C

CLINICAL PHARMACOLOGY

Mechanism of Action: Prednisolone is an adrenal corticosteroid that inhibits accumulation of inflammatory cells at inflammation sites, phagocytosis, lysosomal enzyme release and synthesis, and release of mediators of inflammation. Sulfacetamide is a sulfonamide that interferes with synthesis of folic acid that bacteria require for growth. *Therapeutic Effect:* Prevents or suppresses cell-mediated immune reactions. Decreases or prevents tissue response to inflammatory process. Prevents further bacterial growth; bacteriostatic.

Pharmacokinetics

None reported.

AVAILABLE FORMS

- *Ophthalmic suspension:* 0.25% prednisolone sodium phosphate and 10% sulfacetamide sodium.

INDICATIONS AND DOSAGES

Steroid-responsive inflammatory ocular conditions for which a corticosteroid is indicated and where superficial bacterial ocular infection or a risk of bacterial ocular infection exists

Ophthalmic

Adults, Elderly, Children. Instill 1-3 drops every 2-3 hours while awake.

CONTRAINDICATIONS: Viral diseases of the cornea and conjunctiva including epithelial herpes simplex keratitis (dendritic keratitis), vaccinia, and varicella, mycobacterial infection of the eye, fungal diseases of ocular structures, hypersensitivity to prednisolone sodium phosphate, sulfacetamide sodium, or any component of the formulation.

INTERACTIONS

Drug

Silver preparations: This drug is not compatible with silver preparations.

Local anesthetics (related to p-amino benzoic acid): May antagonize the action of sulfonamides.

Herbal

None known.

Food

None known.

DIAGNOSTIC TEST EFFECTS: *None known.*

SIDE EFFECTS

Occasional

Local irritation

Rare

Elevation of intraocular pressure

SERIOUS REACTIONS

• Prolonged use of corticosteroids may result in glaucoma with damage to the optic nerve, defects in visual acuity and fields of vision, posterior subcapsular cataract formation, and delayed wound healing.

• Long-term use may cause corneal and scleral thinning.

• Systemic effects are uncommon, but systemic hypercorticoidism have been reported.

• Acute anterior uveitis and perforation of the globe, keratitis, conjunctivitis, corneal ulcers, mydriasis, conjunctival hyperemia, loss of accommodation and ptosis have occasionally been reported.

• The development of secondary ocular infection has occurred. Fungal and viral infections of the cornea may develop with long-term applications of steroid.

• Fatalities due to reactions to sulfonamides including Stevens-Johnson syndrome, toxic epidermal necrolysis, fulminant hepatic necrosis, agranulocytosis, aplastic anemia, and other blood dyscrasias have occurred.

SPECIAL CONSIDERATIONS

PRECAUTIONS

• Renew the medication order beyond 20 ml only after slit-lamp examination and fluorescein staining. Consider the possibility of fungal infections of the cornea after prolonged corticosteroid dosing. The p-aminobenzoic acid present in purulent exudates competes with sulfonamides and can reduce their effectiveness.

PATIENT INFORMATION

• If inflammation or pain persists longer than 48 hours or becomes aggravated, advise the patient to discontinue use of the medication and consult an eye care practitioner.

• Keep bottle tightly closed when not in use. Protect the drug from light. Sulfonamide solutions darken on prolonged standing and exposure to heat and light. Do not use if solution has darkened. Yellowing does not effect activity. Keep out of reach of children.

PREGNANCY AND LACTATION

• Pregnancy Category C. Prednisolone has been shown to be teratogenic when given in doses 1 to 10 times the human ocular dose. Systemically administered corticosteroid appears in human milk. Excretion into human milk is not known.

prednisone

(pred′ni-sone)

Rx: Deltasone, Liquid Pred, Meticorten, Prednicen-M, Prednicot, Sterapred, Sterapred DS

Drug Class: Corticosteroids

Pregnancy Category: B

Do not confuse prednisone with prednisolone or primidone.

CLINICAL PHARMACOLOGY

Mechanism of Action: An adrenocortical steroid that inhibits accumulation of inflammatory cells at inflammation sites, phagocytosis, lysosomal enzyme release and synthesis, and release of mediators of inflammation. *Therapeutic Effect:* Prevents or suppresses cell-mediated immune reactions. Decreases or prevents tissue response to inflammatory process.

Pharmacokinetics

Well absorbed from the GI tract. Protein binding: 70%-90%. Widely distributed. Metabolized in the liver and converted to prednisolone. Primarily excreted in urine. Not removed by hemodialysis. **Half-life:** 3.4-3.8 hr.

AVAILABLE FORMS

- *Oral Concentrate (Prednisone Intensol):* 5 mg/ml.
- *Oral Solution:* 5 mg/5 ml.
- *Tablets (Deltasone):* 2.5 mg, 5 mg, 10 mg, 20 mg, 50 mg.
- *Tablets (Sterapred):* 5 mg, 10 mg.

INDICATIONS AND DOSAGES

Substitution therapy in deficiency states: acute or chronic adrenal insufficiency, congenital adrenal hyperplasia, and adrenal insufficiency secondary to pituitary insufficiency; nonendocrine disorders: arthritis; rheumatic carditis; allergic, collagen, intestinal tract, liver, ocular, renal, skin diseases; bronchial asthma; cerebral edema; malignancies

PO

Adults, Elderly. 5-60 mg/day in divided doses.

Children. 0.05-2 mg/kg/day in 1-4 divided doses.

CONTRAINDICATIONS: Acute superficial herpes simplex keratitis, systemic fungal infections, varicella

INTERACTIONS

Drug

Amphotericin: May increase hypokalemia.

Digoxin: May increase the risk of digoxin toxicity caused by hypokalemia

Diuretics, insulin, oral hypoglycemics, potassium supplements: May decrease the effects of these drugs.

Hepatic enzyme inducers: May decrease the effects of prednisone.

Live-virus vaccines: May decrease the patient's antibody response to vaccine, increase vaccine side effects, and potentiate virus replication.

Herbal

None known.

Food

None known.

DIAGNOSTIC TEST EFFECTS: May increase blood glucose and serum lipid, amylase, and sodium levels. May decrease serum calcium, potassium, and thyroxine levels.

SIDE EFFECTS

Frequent

Insomnia, heartburn, nervousness, abdominal distention, increased sweating, acne, mood swings, increased appetite, facial flushing, delayed wound healing, increased susceptibility to infection, diarrhea or constipation

Occasional

Headache, edema, change in skin color, frequent urination

Rare

Tachycardia, allergic reaction (including rash and hives), psychological changes, hallucinations, depression

SERIOUS REACTIONS

- Long-term therapy may cause muscle wasting in the arms and legs, osteoporosis, spontaneous fractures, amenorrhea, cataracts, glaucoma, peptic ulcer disease, and CHF.
- Abruptly withdrawing the drug following long-term therapy may cause anorexia, nausea, fever, headache, sudden or severe joint pain, rebound inflammation, fatigue, weakness, lethargy, dizziness, and orthostatic hypotension.
- Suddenly discontinuing prednisone may be fatal.

SPECIAL CONSIDERATIONS

PRECAUTIONS

- Corticosteroids may mask some signs of infection, and new infections may appear during their use. Infections with any pathogen—including viral, bacterial, fungal, protozoan or helminthic infections, in any location of the body—may be associated with the use of corticosteroids alone or in combination with other immunosuppressive agents that affect cellular immunity, humoral immunity, or neutrophil function.
- Average and large doses of hydrocortisone or cortisone can cause elevation of blood pressure, salt and water retention, and increased excretion of potassium. These effects are less likely to occur with the synthetic derivatives except when used in large doses. Dietary salt restriction and potassium supplementation may be necessary. All corticosteroids increase calcium excretion.
- Administration of live or live attenuated vaccines is contraindicated in patients receiving immunosuppressive doses of corticosteroids.
- The use of prednisone tablets in patients with active tuberculosis should be restricted to those cases of fulminating or disseminated tuberculosis in which the corticosteroid is used for the management of the disease along with an appropriate antituberculous regimen.
- If corticosteroids are indicated in patients with latent tuberculosis or tuberculin reactivity, close observation is necessary because reactivation of the disease may occur. During prolonged corticosteroid therapy, these patients should receive chemoprophylaxis. Persons who are taking drugs that suppress the immune system are more susceptible to infections than healthy individuals. Chickenpox and measles, for example, can have a more serious or even fatal course in nonimmune children or adults taking corticosteroids. In such children or adults who have not had these diseases, instruct them to take particular care to avoid exposure.
- Drug-induced secondary adrenocortical insufficiency may be minimized by gradual reduction of dosage.
- An enhanced effect of corticosteroids occurs in patients with hypothyroidism and in those with cirrhosis.
- Psychic derangements may appear when corticosteroids are used, ranging from euphoria, insomnia, mood swings, personality changes, and severe depression to frank psychotic manifestations.

• Use steroids with caution in patients with nonspecific ulcerative colitis, if there is a probability of impending perforation, abscess, or other pyogenic infection; diverticulitis; fresh intestinal anastomoses; active or latent peptic ulcer; renal insufficiency; hypertension; osteoporosis; and myasthenia gravis.

• Carefully observe growth and development of infants and children receiving prolonged corticosteroid therapy.

• Kaposi sarcoma has been reported to occur in patients receiving corticosteroid therapy. Although controlled clinical trials have shown corticosteroids to be effective in speeding the resolution of acute exacerbations of multiple sclerosis, they do not show that corticosteroids affect the ultimate outcome or natural history of the disease.

• Convulsions have been reported with concurrent use of methylprednisolone and cyclosporine.

PATIENT INFORMATION

• Warn persons who are taking immunosuppressant doses of corticosteroids to avoid exposure to chickenpox or measles. Also advise patients that if they are exposed, they should seek medical advice without delay.

PREGNANCY AND LACTATION

• Pregnancy Category B. Because adequate human reproduction studies have not been done with corticosteroids, the use of these drugs in pregnancy, nursing mothers, or women of childbearing potential requires that the possible benefits of the drug be weighed against the potential hazards to the mother and embryo or fetus. Carefully observe infants born of mothers who have received substantial doses of corticosteroids during pregnancy for signs of hypoadrenalism.

OCULAR CONSIDERATIONS

PRECAUTION:

• Prolonged use of corticosteroids may produce posterior subcapsular cataracts and glaucoma with possible damage to the optic nerves and may enhance the establishment of secondary ocular infections caused by fungi or viruses. Use corticosteroids cautiously in patients with ocular herpes simplex because of possible corneal perforation.

• Ocular Adverse Reactions: Posterior subcapsular cataracts, increased intraocular pressure, glaucoma, and exophthalmos may occur.

OCULAR DOSAGE AND ADMINISTRATION

• Optic Neuritis: Vision 20/50 or worse, methylprednisolone 250 mg IV given over 30 minutes q6h for 12 doses, followed by prednisone 1 mg/kg per day PO for 11 days, then 20 mg for one day, and then 15 mg every other day for doses

• Sympathetic Ophthalmia: Prednisone 60 to 80 mg PO daily and an antacid or histamine$_2$ blocker (e.g., rantidine 150 mg PO bid)

• Acute Retinal Necrosis: Some administer methylprednisolone 250 mg IV qid for 3 days followed by prednisone 60 mg PO bid for 1 to 2 weeks. Others wait 1 to 2 weeks until retinitis clears and administer prednisone 60 to 80 mg/day for 1 to 2 weeks followed by taper over 2 to 6 weeks.

• Mooren's ulcer: Prednisone 60 to 100 mg orally once per day and ranitidine 150 mg orally bid

promethazine hydrochloride

(proe-meth'a-zeen)

Rx: Adgan, Anergan 50, Antinaus 50, Pentazine, Phenergan, Phenoject-50, Promacot, Promethegan

Drug Class: Antiemetics/antivertigo; Antihistamines, H1; Phenothiazines

Pregnancy Category: C

DEA Class: Schedule V

Do not confuse promethazine with promazine.

CLINICAL PHARMACOLOGY

Mechanism of Action: A phenothiazine that acts as an antihistamine, antiemetic, and sedative-hypnotic. As an antihistamine, inhibits histamine at histamine receptor sites. As an antiemetic, diminishes vestibular stimulation, depresses labyrinthine function, and act on the chemoreceptor trigger zone. As a sedative-hypnotic, produces CNS depression by decreasing stimulation to the brain stem reticular formation. *Therapeutic Effect:* Prevents allergic responses mediated by histamine, such as rhinitis, urticaria, and pruritus. Prevents and relieves nausea and vomiting.

Pharmacokinetics

Route	*Onset*	*Peak*	*Duration*
PO	20 min	N/A	2-8 hr
IV	3-5 min	N/A	2-8 hr
IM	20 min	N/A	2-8 hr
Rectal	20 min	N/A	2-8 hr

Well absorbed from the GI tract after IM administration. Widely distributed. Metabolized in the liver. Primarily excreted in urine. Not removed by hemodialysis. **Half-life:** 16-19 hr.

AVAILABLE FORMS

- *Syrup (Phenergan):* 6.25 mg/ml.
- *Tablets (Phenergan):* 12.5 mg, 25 mg, 50 mg.
- *Injection (Phenergan):* 25 mg/ml, 50 mg/ml.
- *Suppositories (Phenergan):* 12.5 mg, 25 mg, 50 mg.
- *Suppositories (Phenadoz):* 25 mg.

INDICATIONS AND DOSAGES

Allergic symptoms

PO

Adults, Elderly. 6.25-12.5 mg 3 times a day plus 25 mg at bedtime.

Children. 0.1 mg/kg/dose (maximum: 12.5 mg) 3 times a day plus 0.5 mg/kg/dose (maximum: 25 mg) at bedtime.

IV, IM

Adults, Elderly. 25 mg. May repeat in 2 hr.

Motion sickness

PO

Adults, Elderly. 25 mg 30-60 min before departure; may repeat in 8-12 hr, then every morning on rising and before evening meal.

Children. 0.5 mg/kg 30-60 min before departure; may repeat in 8-12 hr, then every morning on rising and before evening meal.

Prevention of nausea, and vomiting

PO, IV, IM, Rectal

Adults, Elderly. 12.5-25 mg q4-6h as needed.

Children. 0.25-1 mg/kg q4-6h as needed.

Preoperative and postoperative sedation; adjunct to analgesics

IV, IM

Adults, Elderly. 25-50 mg.

Children. 12.5-25 mg.

Sedative

PO, IV, IM, Rectal

Adults, Elderly. 25-50 mg/dose. May repeat q4-6h as needed.

Children. 0.5-1 mg/kg/dose q6h as needed. Maximum: 50 mg/dose.

CONTRAINDICATIONS: Angle-closure glaucoma, GI or GU obstruction, severe CNS depression or coma

INTERACTIONS

Drug

Alcohol, other CNS depressants: May increase CNS depressant effects.

Anticholinergics: May increase anticholinergic effects.

MAOIs: May intensify and prolong the anticholinergic and CNS depressant effects of promethazine.

Herbal

None known.

Food

None known.

DIAGNOSTIC TEST EFFECTS: May suppress wheal and flare reactions to antigen skin testing unless the drug is discontinued 4 days before testing.

IV INCOMPATIBILITIES: Allopurinol (Aloprim), amphotericin B complex (Abelcet, AmBisome, Amphotec), heparin, ketorolac (Toradol), nalbuphine (Nubain), piperacillin and tazobactam (Zosyn)

IV COMPATIBILITIES: Atropine, diphenhydramine (Benadryl), glycopyrrolate (Robinul), hydromorphone (Dilaudid), hydroxyzine (Vistaril), meperidine (Demerol), midazolam (Versed), morphine, prochlorperazine (Compazine)

SIDE EFFECTS

Expected

Somnolence, disorientation; in elderly, hypotension, confusion, syncope

Frequent

Dry mouth, nose, or throat; urine retention; thickening of bronchial secretions

Occasional

Epigastric distress, flushing, visual disturbances, hearing disturbances, wheezing, paraesthesia, diaphoresis, chills

Rare

Dizziness, urticaria, photosensitivity, nightmares

SERIOUS REACTIONS

- Children may experience paradoxical reactions, such as excitation, nervousness, tremor, hyperactive reflexes, and seizures.
- Infants and young children have experienced CNS depression manifested as respiratory depression, sleep apnea, and sudden infant death syndrome.
- Long-term therapy may produce extrapyramidal symptoms, such as dystonia (abnormal movements), pronounced motor restlessness (most frequently in children), and parkinsonian (most frequently in elderly patients).
- Blood dyscrasias, particularly agranulocytosis, occur rarely.

SPECIAL CONSIDERATIONS

PRECAUTIONS

- Use promethazine hydrochloride with caution in patients with asthmatic attack, narrow-angle glaucoma, prostatic hypertrophy, stenosing peptic ulcer, pyloroduodenal obstruction, and bladder-neck obstruction. Use the drug with caution in patients with bone-marrow depression. Leukopenia and agranulocytosis have been reported. Promethazine hydrochloride may cause marked drowsiness. Promethazine hydrochloride may lower seizure threshold. Avoid administering this drug to patients with a history of sleep apnea. Promethazine hydrochloride has been associated with reported cholestatic jaundice. Use the drug cautiously in persons with cardiovascular disease or with impairment of liver function. Antiemetics are not recommended for treatment of uncomplicated vomiting in children.

PATIENT INFORMATION

• Promethazine hydrochloride may cause marked drowsiness or impair the mental and/or physical abilities required for the performance of potentially hazardous tasks, such as driving a vehicle or operating machinery. Advise ambulatory patients to avoid engaging in such activities until they know that they do not become drowsy or dizzy from promethazine hydrochloride therapy. Children require supervision to avoid potential harm in bike riding or in other hazardous activities.

• The concomitant use of alcohol or other central nervous system depressants, including narcotic analgesics, sedatives, hypnotics, and tranquilizers, may have an additive effect and should be avoided or their dosage reduced.

• Advise patients to report any involuntary muscle movements or unusual sensitivity to sunlight.

PREGNANCY AND LACTATION

• Pregnancy Category C. The safe use of promethazine has not been established with respect to the possible adverse effects on fetal development. Therefore weigh the need to use this drug during pregnancy against the possible but unknown hazards to the developing fetus. Promethazine taken within 2 weeks of delivery may inhibit platelet aggregation in the newborn. Excretion into human milk is not known.

proparacaine hydrochloride

(proe-pare'a-kane)

Rx: Alcaine, Ocu-Caine, Ophthetic

Drug Class: Anesthetics, ophthalmic; Ophthalmics

Pregnancy Category: C

CLINICAL PHARMACOLOGY

Mechanism of Action: A local anesthetic that prevents initiation and transmission of impulses at nerve cell membranes by decreasing ion permeability through stabilizing. *Therapeutic Effect:* Local anesthetic effect.

Pharmacokinetics

Onset of action occurs in about 20 seconds. Duration of action is 15-20 minutes.

AVAILABLE FORMS

• *Ophthalmic Solution:* 0.5% (Alcaine, Ocu-Caine, Ophthetic)

INDICATIONS AND DOSAGES

Ophthalmic surgery

Ophthalmic

Adults, Elderly, Children. Instill 1 drop in each eye every 5-10 minutes for 5-7 doses.

Tonometry, gonioscopy, suture removal

Ophthalmic

Adults, Elderly. Instill 1-2 drops in each eye just prior to procedure.

CONTRAINDICATIONS: Hypersensitivity to proparacaine or any component of the formulation

INTERACTIONS

Drug

Phenylephrine, tropicamide (ophthalmics): May increase the effects of these drugs.

Herbal

None known.

Food

None known.

DIAGNOSTIC TEST EFFECTS: *None known.*

SIDE EFFECTS

Occasional

Burning, stinging, redness

Rare

Allergic contact dermatitis, blurred vision

SERIOUS REACTIONS

• Allergic contact dermatitis, conjunctival congestion and hemorrhage, corneal opacification, erosion of the corneal epithelium, iritis, irritation, keratitis, and sensitization have been reported.

SPECIAL CONSIDERATIONS

PRECAUTIONS

• Allergies, cardiac disease, or hyperthyroidism may occur. Proparacaine hydrochloride possibly may delay wound healing. Rare systemic toxicity (manifested by central nervous system stimulation followed by depression) may occur.

PREGNANCY AND LACTATION

• Pregnancy Category C. Fetal harm is not known with topical administration. Excretion into human milk is not known.

propoxyphene hydrochloride/ propoxyphene napsylate

(pro-pox'-ih-feen)

Rx: Darvon, Darvon-N, PP-Cap

Drug Class: Analgesics, narcotic

Pregnancy Category: C

DEA Class: Schedule IV

Do not confuse Darvon with Diovan.

CLINICAL PHARMACOLOGY

Mechanism of Action: An opioid agonist that binds with opioid receptors in the CNS. *Therapeutic Effect:* Alters the perception of and emotional response to pain.

Pharmacokinetics

Route	*Onset*	*Peak*	*Duration*
PO	15-60 min	N/A	4-6 hr

Well absorbed from the GI tract. Protein binding: High. Widely distributed. Metabolized in the liver. Primarily excreted in urine. Not removed by hemodialysis. **Half-life:** 6-12 hr; metabolite: 30-36 hr.

AVAILABLE FORMS

• *Capsules (Hydrochloride):* 65 mg.

• *Tablets (Napsylate):* 100 mg.

INDICATIONS AND DOSAGES

Mild to moderate pain

PO (propoxyphene hydrochloride)

Adults, Elderly. 65 mg q4h as needed. Maximum: 390 mg/day.

PO (propoxyphene napsylate)

Adults, Elderly. 100 mg q4h as needed. Maximum: 600 mg/day.

CONTRAINDICATIONS: None known.

INTERACTIONS

Drug

Alcohol, other CNS depressants: May increase CNS or respiratory depression and risk of hypotension.

Buprenorphine: May decrease the effects of propoxyphene.

Carbamazepine: May increase the blood concentration and risk of toxicity of carbamazepine.

MAOIs: May produce a severe, sometimes fatal reaction; plan to administer 25% of usual propoxyphene dose.

Herbal

None known.

Food

None known.

DIAGNOSTIC TEST EFFECTS: May increase serum alkaline phosphatase, lipase, amylase, bilirubin, LDH, AST (SGOT), and ALT (SGPT) levels. Therapeutic serum drug level is 100-400 ng/ml; toxic serum drug level is greater than 500 ng/ml.

SIDE EFFECTS

Frequent

Dizziness, somnolence, dry mouth, euphoria, hypotension (including orthostatic hypotension), nausea, vomiting, fatigue

Occasional

Allergic reaction (including decreased BP), diaphoresis, flushing, and wheezing), trembling, urine retention, vision changes, constipation, headache

Rare

Confusion, increased BP, depression, abdominal cramps, anorexia

SERIOUS REACTIONS

• Overdose results in respiratory depression, skeletal muscle flaccidity, cold or clammy skin, cyanosis, and extreme somnolence progressing to seizures, stupor, and coma.

• Hepatotoxicity may occur with overdose of the acetaminophen component of fixed-combination products.

• The patient who uses propoxyphene repeatedly may develop a tolerance to the drug's analgesic effect and physical dependence.

propoxyphene napsylate

(proe-pox'-i-feen nap'-seh-late)

Drug Class: Analgesics, narcotic

DEA Class: Schedule IV

CLINICAL PHARMACOLOGY

Mechanism of Action: An opioid agonist that binds with opioid receptors within the central nervous system (CNS). *Therapeutic Effect:* Alters processes affecting pain perception, emotional response to pain.

Pharmacokinetics

Route	*Onset*	*Peak*	*Duration*
PO	15-60 min	N/A	4-6 hrs

Well absorbed from the gastrointestinal (GI) tract. Protein binding: High. Widely distributed. Metabolized in liver. Primarily excreted in urine. Not removed by hemodialysis. **Half-life:** 6-12 hrs.

AVAILABLE FORMS

• *Tablets:* 100 mg (Darvon-N).

INDICATIONS AND DOSAGES

Relief of mild to moderate pain

PO

Adults, Elderly. 100 mg q4h, as needed. Maximum: 600 mg/day.

CONTRAINDICATIONS: Hypersensitivity to propoxyphene napsylate or any component of the formulation

INTERACTIONS

Drug

Alcohol, CNS depressants: May increase CNS or respiratory depression and risk of hypotension.
Buprenorphine: Effects may be decreased with buprenorphine.
Carbamazepine: May increase the blood concentration and risk of toxicity of carbamazepine.
MAOIs: May produce severe, fatal reaction; plan to reduce to one quarter usual dose.

Herbal

None known.

Food

None known.

DIAGNOSTIC TEST EFFECTS: May increase serum alkaline phosphatase, amylase, bilirubin, LDH, lipase, SGOT (AST), and SGPT (ALT) levels. Therapeutic blood serum level is 100-400 ng/ml; toxic blood serum level is greater than 500 ng/ml.

SIDE EFFECTS

Frequent

Dizziness, drowsiness, dry mouth, euphoria, hypotension, nausea, vomiting, unusual tiredness

Occasional

Histamine reaction, including decreased blood pressure (BP), increased sweating, flushing, and wheezing, trembling, decreased urination, altered vision, constipation, headache

Rare

Confusion, increased BP, depression, stomach cramps, anorexia

SERIOUS REACTIONS

- Overdosage results in respiratory depression, skeletal muscle flaccidity, cold or clammy skin, cyanosis, extreme somnolence progressing to convulsions, stupor, and coma.
- Liver toxicity may occur with overdosage of acetaminophen component of fixed-combination.
- Tolerance to propoxyphene's analgesic effect and physical dependence may occur with repeated use.

SPECIAL CONSIDERATIONS

PRECAUTIONS

- Do not prescribe propoxyphene for patients who are suicidal or addiction prone. Prescribe propoxyphene with caution for patients taking tranquilizers or antidepressant drugs and patients who use alcohol in excess. Tell patients not to exceed the recommended dose and to limit their intake of alcohol. Propoxyphene products in excessive doses—alone or in combination with other central nervous system depressants, including alcohol—are a major cause of drug-related deaths. Administer propoxyphene with caution to patients with hepatic or renal impairment because higher serum concentrations or delayed elimination may occur.

PREGNANCY AND LACTATION

- Pregnancy Category C. Safe use in pregnancy has not been established relative to possible adverse effects on fetal development. Low levels of propoxyphene have been detected in human milk.

propranolol hydrochloride

(proe-pran'oh-lole)

Rx: Inderal, Inderal LA, InnoPran XL

Drug Class: Antiadrenergics, beta blocking; Antiarrhythmics, class II

Pregnancy Category: C

Do not confuse Inderal with Adderall or Isordil, or propranolol with Pravachol.

CLINICAL PHARMACOLOGY

Mechanism of Action: An antihypertensive, antianginal, antiarrhythmic, and antimigraine agent that blocks $beta_1$- and $beta_2$-adrenergic receptors. Decreases oxygen requirements. Slows AV conduction and increases refractory period in AV node. Large doses increase airway resistance. *Therapeutic Effect:* Slows sinus heart rate; decreases cardiac output, BP, and myocardial ischemia severity. Exhibits antiarrhythmic activity.

Pharmacokinetics

Route	*Onset*	*Peak*	*Duration*
PO	1-2 hr	N/A	6 hr

Well absorbed from the GI tract. Protein binding: 93%. Widely distributed. Metabolized in the liver. Primarily excreted in urine. Not removed by hemodialysis. **Half-life:** 3-5 hr.

AVAILABLE FORMS

- *Tablets (Inderal):* 10 mg, 20 mg, 40 mg, 60 mg, 80 mg.
- *Capsules (Extended-Release [Inderal LA]):* 60 mg, 80 mg, 120 mg, 160 mg.
- *Capsules (Extended-Release [InnoPran XL]):* 80 mg, 120 mg.
- *Oral Solution (Inderal):* 4 mg/ml.
- *Oral Concentrate (Propranolol Intensol):* 80 mg/ml.
- *Injection (Inderal):* 1 mg/ml.

INDICATIONS AND DOSAGES

Hypertension

PO

Adults, Elderly. Initially, 40 mg twice a day. May increase dose q3-7 days. Range: Up to 320 mg/day in divided doses. Maximum: 640 mg/day.

Children. Initially, 0.5-1 mg/kg/day in divided doses q6-12h. May increase at 3- to 5-day intervals. Usual dose: 1-5 mg/kg/day. Maximum: 16 mg/kg/day.

Angina

PO

Adults, Elderly. 80-320 mg/day in divided doses. (long acting): Initially, 80 mg/day. Maximum: 320 mg/day.

Arrhythmias

IV

Adults, Elderly. 1 mg/dose. May repeat q5min. Maximum: 5 mg total dose.

Children. 0.01-0.1 mg/kg. Maximum: infants, 1 mg; children, 3 mg.

PO

Adults, Elderly. Initially, 10-20 mg q6-8h. May gradually increase dose. Range: 40-320 mg/day.

Children. Initially, 0.5-1 mg/kg/day in divided doses q6-8h. May increase q3-5 days. Usual dosage: 2-4 mg/kg/day. Maximum: 16 mg/kg/day or 60 mg/day.

Life-threatening arrhythmias

IV

Adults, Elderly. 0.5-3 mg. Repeat once in 2 min. Give additional doses at intervals of at least 4 hr.

Children. 0.01-0.1 mg/kg.

Hypertrophic subaortic stenosis

PO

Adults, Elderly. 20-40 mg in 3-4 divided doses. Or 80-160 mg/day as extended-release capsule.

Adjunct to alpha-blocking agents to treat pheochromocytoma
PO
Adults, Elderly. 60 mg/day in divided doses with alpha-blocker for 3 days before surgery. Maintenance (inoperable tumor): 30 mg/day with alpha-blocker.
Migraine headache
PO
Adults, Elderly. 80 mg/day in divided doses. Or 80 mg once daily as extended-release capsule. Increase up to 160-240 mg/day in divided doses.
Children. 0.6-1.5 mg/kg/day in divided doses q8h. Maximum: 4 mg/kg/day.
Reduction of cardiovascular mortality and reinfarction in patients with previous MI
PO
Adults, Elderly. 180-240 mg/day in divided doses.
Essential tremor
PO
Adults, Elderly. Initially, 40 mg twice a day increased up to 120-320 mg/day in 3 divided doses.
UNLABELED USES: Treatment adjunct for anxiety, mitral valve prolapse syndrome, thyrotoxicosis
CONTRAINDICATIONS: Asthma, bradycardia, cardiogenic shock, COPD, heart block, Raynaud's syndrome, uncompensated CHF
INTERACTIONS
Drug
Diuretics, other antihypertensives: May increase hypotensive effect.
Insulin, oral hypoglycemics: May mask symptoms of hypoglycemia and prolong the hypoglycemic effect of insulin and oral hypoglycemics.
IV phenytoin: May increase cardiac depressant effect.
NSAIDs: May decrease antihypertensive effect.
Sympathomimetics, xanthines: May mutually inhibit effects.
Herbal
None known.
Food
None known.
DIAGNOSTIC TEST EFFECTS: May increase serum antinuclear antibody titer and BUN, serum LDH, serum lipoprotein, serum alkaline phosphatase, serum bilirubin, serum creatinine, serum potassium, serum uric acid, AST (SGOT), ALT (SGPT), and serum triglyceride levels.
IV INCOMPATIBILITIES: Amphotericin B complex (Abelcet, AmBisome, Amphotec)
IV COMPATIBILITIES: Alteplase (Activase), heparin, milrinone (Primacor), potassium chloride, propofol (Diprivan)
SIDE EFFECTS
Frequent
Diminished sexual ability, drowsiness, difficulty sleeping, unusual fatigue or weakness
Occasional
Bradycardia, depression, sensation of coldness in extremities, diarrhea, constipation, anxiety, nasal congestion, nausea, vomiting
Rare
Altered taste, dry eyes, pruritus, paraesthesia
SERIOUS REACTIONS
- Overdose may produce profound bradycardia and hypotension.
- Abrupt withdrawal may result in sweating, palpitations, headache, and tremors.
- Propranolol administration may precipitate CHF and MI in patients with cardiac disease; thyroid storm in those with thyrotoxicosis; and peripheral ischemia in those with existing peripheral vascular disease.

• Hypoglycemia may occur in patients with previously controlled diabetes.

SPECIAL CONSIDERATIONS

PRECAUTIONS

• Sympathetic stimulation may be a vital component supporting circulatory function in patients with congestive heart failure, and its inhibition by beta-blockade may precipitate more severe failure. Hypersensitivity to catecholamines has been observed in patients who were withdrawn from therapy with beta-blocking agents. Propranolol hydrochloride may prevent the appearance of signs and symptoms of acute hypoglycemia, such as tachycardia and blood pressure changes. Propranolol hydrochloride may mask certain clinical signs (e.g., tachycardia) of hyperthyroidism. Propranolol hydrochloride is contraindicated in bronchial asthma. Patients with bronchospastic diseases should not receive beta-blockers. Patients with a history of severe anaphylactic reactions to a variety of allergens may be more reactive to repeated challenge. Such patients may be unresponsive to the usual doses of epinephrine used to treat allergic reactions. Use propranolol hydrochloride with caution in patients with impaired hepatic or renal function. Use this drug with caution in patients with impaired hepatic or renal function. Propranolol hydrochloride is not indicated for the treatment of hypertensive emergencies.

PREGNANCY AND LACTATION

• Pregnancy Category C. Fetal harm is not known. Propranolol is excreted in human milk. Exercise caution when administering propranolol to a nursing woman.

OCULAR CONSIDERATIONS

• Beta-adrenoreceptor blockade can cause reduction of intraocular pressure. Inform patients that propranolol may interfere with the glaucoma screening test. Withdrawal may lead to a return of increased intraocular pressure.

propylene glycol

(pro'pil-een gli'kol)

CLINICAL PHARMACOLOGY

Mechanism of Action: A lubricating eye drop that contains a polymer system formulated to adjust to the tear film pH. *Therapeutic Effect:* Lubricates and creates an ocular shield allowing epithelial repair.

Pharmacokinetics

Not reported.

AVAILABLE FORMS

• *Ophthalmic solution:* 0.3% (Systane), 1% (Moisture Eyes).

INDICATIONS AND DOSAGES

Relief of dry eye and eye irritation

Ophthalmic

Adults, Elderly. Instill 1 or 2 drops in affected eye(s) as needed.

CONTRAINDICATIONS: Hypersensitivity to propylene glycol or any component of the formulation

INTERACTIONS

Drug

None known.

Herbal

None known.

Food

None known.

DIAGNOSTIC TEST EFFECTS: *None known.*

SIDE EFFECTS

Blurred vision for a short time

SERIOUS REACTIONS

• None reported.

SPECIAL CONSIDERATIONS

PATIENT INFORMATION

Give patients the following instructions:

- To avoid contamination, do not touch the tip of the container to any surface. Replace cap after using. If solution changes color or becomes cloudy, do not use it. If you experience eye pain, changes in vision, or continued redness or irritation of the eye, or if the condition worsens or persists for more than 72 hours, discontinue use and consult an eye care practitioner. Keep this and all drugs out of the reach of children. Keep container tightly closed. Remove contact lenses before using.

---

pyridoxine hydrochloride (vitamin B_6)

(peer-i-dox'een)

Rx: Vitamin B6

Drug Class: Vitamins/minerals

Pregnancy Category: A

Do not confuse pyridoxine with paroxetine, pralidoxime, or Pyridium.

CLINICAL PHARMACOLOGY

Mechanism of Action: Acts as a coenzyme for various metabolic functions, including metabolism of proteins, carbohydrates, and fats. Aids in the breakdown of glycogen and in the synthesis of gamma-aminobutyric acid in the CNS. *Therapeutic Effect:* Prevents pyridoxine deficiency. Increases the excretion of certain drugs, such as isoniazid, that are pyridoxine antagonists.

Pharmacokinetics

Readily absorbed primarily in jejunum. Stored in the liver, muscle, and brain. Metabolized in the liver. Primarily excreted in urine. Removed by hemodialysis. **Half-life:** 15-20 days.

AVAILABLE FORMS

- *Capsules:* 250 mg.
- *Tablets:* 20 mg, 25 mg, 50 mg, 100 mg, 250 mg, 500 mg.
- *Injection:* 100 mg/ml.

INDICATIONS AND DOSAGES

Pyridoxine deficiency

PO

Adults, Elderly. Initially, 2.5-10 mg/day; then 2.5 mg/day when clinical signs are corrected.

Children. Initially, 5-25 mg/day for 3 wk, then 1.5-2.5 mg/day.

Pyridoxine dependent seizures

PO, IV, IM

Infants. Initially, 10-100 mg/day. Maintenance: PO: 50-100 mg/day.

Drug-induced neuritis

PO (treatment)

Adults, Elderly. 100-300 mg/day in divided doses

Children. 10-50 mg/day.

PO (prophylaxis)

Adults, Elderly. 25-100 mg/day.

Children. 1-2 mg/kg/day.

CONTRAINDICATIONS: None known.

INTERACTIONS

Drug

Immunosuppressants, isoniazid, penicillamine: May antagonize pyridoxine, causing anemia or peripheral neuritis.

Levodopa: Reverses the effects of levodopa.

Herbal

None known.

Food

None known.

DIAGNOSTIC TEST EFFECTS: *None known.*

IV INCOMPATIBILITIES: Don't mix pyridoxine with any other medications.

SIDE EFFECTS

Occasional

Stinging at IM injection site

Rare

Headache, nausea, somnolence; sensory neuropathy (paraesthesia, unstable gait, clumsiness of hands) with high doses

SERIOUS REACTIONS

- Long-term megadoses (2-6 g over more than 2 mo) may produce sensory neuropathy (reduced deep tendon reflexes, profound impairment of sense of position in distal limbs, gradual sensory ataxia). Toxic symptoms subside when drug is discontinued.
- Seizures have occurred after IV megadoses.

SPECIAL CONSIDERATIONS

PRECAUTIONS

- Single deficiency, as of pyridoxine alone, is rare. Multiple vitamin deficiency is to be expected in any inadequate diet. Patients treated with levodopa should avoid supplemental vitamins that contain more than 5 mg pyridoxine in the daily dose. Women taking oral contraceptives may exhibit increased pyridoxine requirements.

PREGNANCY AND LACTATION

- Pregnancy Category A. The requirement for pyridoxine appears to be increased during pregnancy. Pyridoxine is sometimes of value in the treatment of nausea and vomiting of pregnancy. The need for pyridoxine is increased during lactation. Excretion into human milk is not known.

pyrimethamine

(pye-ri-meth'-a-meen)

Rx: Daraprim

Drug Class: Antiprotozoals

Pregnancy Category: C

Do not confuse with Dantrium, Daranide.

CLINICAL PHARMACOLOGY

Mechanism of Action: An antiprotozoal with blood and some tissue schizonticidal activity against malaria parasites of humans. Highly selective activity against plasmodia and *Toxoplasma gondii. Therapeutic Effect:* Inhibition of tetrahydrofolic acid synthesis.

Pharmacokinetics

Well absorbed, peak levels occurring between 2-6 hours following administration. Protein binding: 87%. Eliminated slowly. **Half-life:** approximately 96 hours.

AVAILABLE FORMS

- *Tablets:* 25 mg (Daraprim)

INDICATIONS AND DOSAGES

Toxoplasmosis

PO

Adults. Initially, 50-75 mg daily, with 1-4 g daily of a sulfonamide of the sulfapyrimidine type (e.g., sulfadoxine). Continue for 1-3 weeks, depending on response of patient and tolerance to therapy then reduce dose to half that previously given for each drug and continue for additional 4-5 weeks.

Children. 1 mg/kg/day divided into 2 equal daily doses; after 2-4 days reduce to one-half and continue for approximately 1 month. The usual pediatric sulfonamide dosage is used in conjunction with pyrimethamine.

Acute malaria

PO

Adults (in combination with sulfonamide). 25 mg daily for 2 days with a sulfonamide

Adults (without concomitant sulfonamide). 50 mg for 2 days

Children 4-10 yr. 25 mg daily for 2 days.

Chemoprophylaxis of malaria

PO

Adults and pediatric patients over 10 yr. 25 mg once weekly.

Children 4-10 yr. 12.5 mg once weekly.

Infants and children under 4 yr. 6.25 mg once weekly.

UNLABELED USES: Prophylaxis for first episode and recurrence of *Pneumocystis carinii* pneumonia and *Toxoplasma gondii* in HIV-infected patients.

CONTRAINDICATIONS: Hypersensitivity to pyrimethamine, megaloblastic anemia due to folate deficiency, monotherapy for treatment of acute malaria.

INTERACTIONS

Drug

Antifolic drugs: Pyrimethamine may be used with sulfonamides, quinine, and other antimalarials, and with other antibiotics. However, the concomitant use of other antifolic drugs, such as sulfonamides or trimethoprim-sulfamethoxazole combinations, while the patient is receiving pyrimethamine, may increase the risk of bone marrow suppression. If signs of folate deficiency develop, pyrimethamine should be discontinued. Folinic acid (leucovorin) should be administered until normal hematopoiesis is restored.

Benzodiazepines: Mild hepatotoxicity has been reported in some patients when lorazepam and pyrimethamine were administered concomitantly.

Herbal

None known.

Food

None known.

DIAGNOSTIC TEST EFFECTS: *None known.*

SIDE EFFECTS

Frequent

Anorexia, vomiting

Occasional

Hypersensitivity reactions, Stevens-Johnson syndrome, toxic epidermal necrolysis, erythema multiforme, anaphylaxis, hyperphenylalaninemia, megaloblastic anemia, leukopenia, thrombocytopenia, pancytopenia, atrophic glossitis, hematuria, and disorders of cardiac rhythm

Rare

Pulmonary eosinophilia

SERIOUS REACTIONS

- None known.

SPECIAL CONSIDERATIONS

PRECAUTIONS

- Do not exceed the recommended dosage for chemoprophylaxis of malaria. A small starting dose for toxoplasmosis is recommended in patients with convulsive disorders to avoid the potential nervous system toxicity of pyrimethamine. Use pyrimethamine with caution in patients with impaired renal or hepatic function or in patients with possible folate deficiency, such as individuals with malabsorption syndrome, alcoholism, or pregnancy and those receiving therapy, such as phenytoin, that affects folate levels.

PATIENT INFORMATION

- Warn patients that at the first appearance of a skin rash, they should stop use of pyrimethamine and seek medical attention immediately. Also warn patients that the appearance of sore throat, pallor, purpura, or glossitis may be an early indication of a serious disorder that requires prophylactic treatment to be stopped and to seek medical treatment. Warn patients to keep pyrimethamine out of the reach of children. Warn patients that if anorexia and vomiting occur, to take the drug with meals to minimize these effects.

PREGNANCY AND LACTATION

- Pregnancy Category C. Pyrimethamine has been shown to be teratogenic in rats, hamsters, and Goettingen miniature pigs. Pyrimethamine is excreted in human milk.

OCULAR CONSIDERATIONS

- The action of pyrimethamine against *Toxoplasma gondii* is enhanced greatly when used along with sulfonamides. This was demonstrated in the treatment of experimental toxoplasmosis in the mouse. The combination of the two drugs effectively prevented the development of severe uveitis in most rabbits following the inoculation of the anterior chamber of the eye with *Toxoplasma*.

quinacrine hydrochloride

(kwin′ah-kreen hye-droh-klor′ide)

Drug Class: Antihelmintics; Antiprotozoals

Pregnancy Category: C

Do not confuse with quinine or quinidine.

CLINICAL PHARMACOLOGY

Mechanism of Action: An acridine derivative that inhibits the synthesis of parasite nucleic acid. *Therapeutic Effect:* Interferes with parasite metabolism.

Pharmacokinetics

Well absorbed from the gastrointestinal (GI) tract. Protein binding: highly bound. Widely distributed. Excreted unchanged in the urine. Small amounts are excreted in sweat, saliva, breath, bile and feces. **Half-life:** 5 days.

AVAILABLE FORMS

- *Tablets:* 100 mg (Atabrine).

INDICATIONS AND DOSAGES

Giardiasis

PO

Adults, Elderly. 100 mg 3 times/day for 5-7 days.

Children. 7 mg/kg/day in 3 divided doses for 5 days. Maximum: 300 mg/day.

Malaria, treatment

PO

Adults, Elderly, Children 8 yr and older. 200 mg with 1 gram sodium bicarbonate q6h for 5 doses, followed by 100 mg 3 times/day for 6 days. Maximum total dose: 2.8 g in 7 days.

Children 4-8 yr. 200 mg 3 times the first day, then 100 mg 2 times/day for 6 days.

Children 1-4 yr. 100 mg 3 times the first day, then 100 mg once daily for 6 days.

Malaria, suppression

PO

Adults, Elderly. 100 mg once daily.

Children. 50 mg. Maintenance: Maintain for 1 to 3 months.

Tapeworm (beef, pork, fish)

PO

Adults, Elderly. 4 doses of 200 mg 10 min apart for a total of 800 mg. Sodium bicarbonate 600 mg with each dose to reduce the nausea and vomiting.

Children 11-14 yr. 3 or 4 divided doses administered 10 min apart for a total of 600 mg. Sodium bicarbonate 300 mg with each dose. Saline purge 1-2 hrs later.

Children 5-10 yr. Total dose of 400 mg.

Tapeworm (dwarf)

PO

Adults. One first day, 900 mg of antimalarial compound, in 3 portions 20 min apart, with sodium sulfate purge 1 and 1½ hrs later. On the following 3 days, 100 mg 3 times/day.

Children 11-14 yr. Initially, 400 mg, followed by 100 mg 3 times/day for 3 days.

Children 8-10 yr. Initially, 300 mg, followed by 100 mg twice/day for 3 days.

Children 4-8 yr. Initially, 200 mg, followed by 100 mg after breakfast for 3 days.

UNLABELED USES: Pleural effusions, pneumothorax, non-surgical female sterilization, systemic lupus erythematosus

CONTRAINDICATIONS: Porphyria, psoriasis, concomitant use of primaquine, hypersensitivity to quinacrine or any component of the formulation

INTERACTIONS

Drug

Alcohol: May cause drug-induced disulfiram-like reactions.

Aurothioglucose: May increase the risk of blood dyscrasias.

Primaquine: May increase the toxicity of primaquine.

Herbal

None known.

Food

None known.

DIAGNOSTIC TEST EFFECTS: *None known.*

SIDE EFFECTS

Frequent

Yellowish discoloration of skin, headache, dizziness, nausea, diarrhea, abdominal cramps, anorexia, vomiting

Occasional

Nightmares, irritability, nervousness, blurred vision, visual halos

Rare

Convulsions, reversible corneal edema and deposits

SERIOUS REACTIONS

• Toxic psychosis, aplastic anemia, and hepatitis have been reported.

SPECIAL CONSIDERATIONS

PRECAUTIONS

• Because quinacrine hydrochloride is known to concentrate in the liver, use it with caution in patients with hepatic disease or alcoholism or along with known hepatotoxic drugs. Periodically obtain complete blood cell counts if patients are given prolonged therapy. If any severe blood disorder appears that is not attributable to the disease under treatment, consider discontinuance of the drug. Administer the drug with caution to patients having glucose-6-phosphate dehydrogenase deficiency. Instruct patients receiving prolonged quinacrine therapy to report promptly any visual disturbances and to receive periodic complete eye examinations.

PREGNANCY AND LACTATION

- Pregnancy Category C. Avoid use of this drug in the suppression or treatment of malaria during pregnancy except when in the judgment of the physician the benefit outweighs the possible hazard.

OCULAR CONSIDERATIONS

- Cases of reversible corneal edema or deposits, manifested by visual halos, focusing difficulty and blurred vision, have been reported in patients taking quinacrine as long-term suppressive therapy for malaria.
- Retinopathy has been reported rarely in patients who received relatively high doses of quinacrine hydrochloride for prolonged periods in the treatment of certain chronic diseases. Retinopathy has not been reported as a result of quinacrine hydrochloride use in malaria suppression or in the short-term treatment of parasitic diseases.

quinapril

(kwin'na-pril)

Rx: Accupril

Drug Class: Angiotensin converting enzyme inhibitors

Pregnancy Category: D

Do not confuse Accupril with Accolate or Accutane.

CLINICAL PHARMACOLOGY

Mechanism of Action: An ACE inhibitor that suppresses the renin-angiotensin-aldosterone system and prevents the conversion of angiotensin I to angiotensin II, a potent vasoconstrictor; may also inhibit angiotensin II at local vascular and renal sites. *Therapeutic Effect:* Reduces peripheral arterial resistance, BP, and pulmonary capillary wedge pressure; improves cardiac output.

Pharmacokinetics

Route	Onset	Peak	Duration
PO	1 hr	N/A	24 hr

Readily absorbed from the GI tract. Protein binding: 97%. Metabolized in the liver, GI tract, and extravascular tissue to active metabolite. Primarily excreted in urine. Minimal removal by hemodialysis. **Half-life:** 1-2 hr; metabolite, 3 hr (increased in those with impaired renal function).

AVAILABLE FORMS

- *Tablets:* 5 mg, 10 mg, 20 mg, 40 mg.

INDICATIONS AND DOSAGES

Hypertension (monotherapy)

PO

Adults. Initially, 10-20 mg/day. May adjust dosage at intervals of at least 2 wk or longer. Maintenance: 20-80 mg/day as single dose or 2 divided doses. Maximum: 80 mg/day.

Elderly. Initially, 2.5-5 mg/day. May increase by 2.5-5 mg q1-2wk.

Hypertension (combination therapy)

PO

Adults. Initially, 5 mg/day titrated to patient's needs.

Elderly. Initially, 2.5-5 mg/day. May increase by 2.5-5 mg q1-2wk.

Adjunct to manage heart failure

PO

Adults, Elderly. Initially, 5 mg twice a day. Range: 20-40 mg/day.

Dosage in renal impairment

Dosage is titrated to the patient's needs after the following initial doses:

Creatinine Clearance	*Initial Dose*
more than 60 ml/min	10 mg
30-60 ml/min	5 mg
10-29 ml/min	2.5 mg

UNLABELED USES: Treatment of hypertension and renal crisis in scleroderma

CONTRAINDICATIONS: Bilateral renal artery stenosis

INTERACTIONS

Drug

Alcohol, antihypertensives, diuretics: May increase the effects of quinapril.

Lithium: May increase lithium blood concentration and risk of lithium toxicity.

NSAIDs: May decrease the effects of quinapril.

Potassium-sparing diuretics, potassium supplements: May cause hyperkalemia.

Herbal

Garlic: May increase antihypertensive effect.

Ginseng, yohimbe: May worsen hypertension.

Food

None known.

DIAGNOSTIC TEST EFFECTS: May increase BUN, serum alkaline phosphatase, serum bilirubin, serum creatinine, serum potassium, AST (SGOT), and ALT (SGPT) levels. May decrease serum sodium levels. May cause positive antinuclear antibody titer.

SIDE EFFECTS

Frequent (7%-5%)

Headache, dizziness

Occasional (4%-2%)

Fatigue, vomiting, nausea, hypotension, chest pain, cough, syncope

Rare (less than 2%)

Diarrhea, cough, dyspnea, rash, palpitations, impotence, insomnia, drowsiness, malaise

SERIOUS REACTIONS

- Excessive hypotension ("first-dose syncope") may occur in patients with CHF and in those who are severely salt or volume depleted.
- Angioedema and hyperkalemia occur rarely.
- Agranulocytosis and neutropenia may be noted in those with collagen vascular disease, including scleroderma and systemic lupus erythematosus, and impaired renal function.
- Nephrotic syndrome may be noted in those with history of renal disease.

SPECIAL CONSIDERATIONS

PRECAUTIONS

- Anticipate changes in renal function in susceptible individuals. In hypertensive patients with unilateral or bilateral renal artery stenosis, increases in blood urea nitrogen and serum creatinine have been observed in some patients following angiotensin-converting enzyme (ACE) inhibitor therapy. Hyperkalemia occurred in patients receiving quinapril hydrochloride. Cough has been reported with all ACE inhibitors. In patients undergoing major surgery or during anesthesia with agents that produce hypotension, enalapril may block angiotensin II formation following compensatory renin release.

PATIENT INFORMATION

- Pregnancy: Inform female patients of childbearing age about the consequences of second- and third-trimester exposure to ACE inhibitors, and advise them that these consequences do not appear to have resulted from intrauterine ACE-inhibitor exposure that has been limited to the first trimester. Ask these patients to report pregnancies to their physicians as soon as possible.

• Angioedema: Angioedema, including laryngeal edema can occur with treatment with ACE inhibitors, especially following the first dose.

• Advise patients to report immediately any signs or symptoms suggesting angioedema (swelling of face, extremities, eyes, lips, and tongue or difficulty in swallowing or breathing) and to stop taking the drug until they have consulted with their physician.

• Symptomatic Hypotension: Caution patients that light-headedness can occur, especially during the first few days of quinapril hydrochloride therapy and to report it to a physician. If actual syncope occurs, instruct patients not to take the drug until they have consulted with their physician.

• Caution all patients that inadequate fluid intake or excessive perspiration, diarrhea, or vomiting can lead to an excessive fall in blood pressure because of reduction in fluid volume, with the same consequences of light-headedness and possible syncope.

• Instruct patients planning to undergo any surgery and/or anesthesia to inform their physician that they are taking an ACE inhibitor.

• Hyperkalemia: Advise patients not to use potassium supplements or salt substitutes containing potassium without consulting their physician.

• Neutropenia: Instruct patients to report promptly any indication of infection (e.g., sore throat or fever), which could be a sign of neutropenia.

• NOTE: As with many other drugs, certain advice to patients being treated with quinapril hydrochloride is warranted. This information is intended to aid in the safe and effective use of this medication. Such advice is not a disclosure of all possible adverse or intended effects.

PREGNANCY AND LACTATION

• Pregnancy Categories C (first trimester) and D (second and third trimesters). The use of ACE inhibitors during the second and third trimesters of pregnancy has been associated with fetal and neonatal injury, including hypotension, neonatal skull hypoplasia, anuria, reversible or irreversible renal failure, and death. Because quinapril hydrochloride is secreted in human milk, exercise caution when administering this drug to a nursing woman.

quinine

(kwye'-nine)

Rx: QM-260

Drug Class: Antiprotozoals

Pregnancy Category: X

Do not confuse with quinidine.

CLINICAL PHARMACOLOGY

Mechanism of Action: A cinchone alkaloid that relaxes skeletal muscle by increasing the refractory period, decreasing excitability of motor end plates (curarelike), and affecting distribution of calcium with muscle fiber. Antimalaria: Depresses oxygen uptake, carbohydrate metabolism, elevates pH in intracellular organelles of parasites. *Therapeutic Effect:* Relaxes skeletal muscle; produces parasite death.

Pharmacokinetics

Rapidly absorbed mainly from upper small intestine. Protein binding: 70%-95%. Metabolized in liver. Excreted in feces, saliva, and urine. **Half-life:** 8-14 hrs (adults), 6-12 hrs (children).

AVAILABLE FORMS

- *Capsules:* 200 mg, 325 mg (Quinine).
- *Tablets:* 260 mg (Quinine).

INDICATIONS AND DOSAGES

Nocturnal leg cramps

PO

Adults, Elderly. 260-300 mg at bedtime as needed.

Treatment of malaria

PO

Adults, Elderly. 260-650 mg 3 times a day for 6-12 days.

Children. 10 mg/kg q8h for 5-7 days.

Dosage in renal impairment

Creatinine Clearance	Dosage Interval
10-50 ml/min	75% of normal dose or q12h
Less than 10 ml/min	30%-50% of normal dose or q24h

CONTRAINDICATIONS: Hypersensitivity to quinine (possible cross-sensitivity to quinidine), G-6-PD deficiency, tinnitus, optic neuritis, history of thrombocytopenia during previous quinine therapy, blackwater fever

INTERACTIONS

Drug

Amiodarone, alkalinizing agents, cimetidine, verapamil: May increase quinine serum concentrations.

Beta-blockers: May increase bradycardia.

Digoxin: May increase blood concentration of digoxin.

Mefloquine: May increase risk of seizures and EKG abnormalities.

Phenobarbital, phenytoin, rifampin: May decrease quinine serum concentrations.

Warfarin: May increase anticoagulant effect.

Herbal

St. John's wort: May decrease quinine levels.

Food

None known.

DIAGNOSTIC TEST EFFECTS: May interfere with 17-OH steroid determinations. May result in positive Coombs' test.

SIDE EFFECTS

Frequent

Nausea, headache, tinnitus, slight visual disturbances (mild cinchonism)

Occasional

Extreme flushing of skin with intense generalized pruritus is most typical hypersensitivity reaction; also rash, wheezing, dyspnea, angioedema.

Prolonged therapy: cardiac conduction disturbances, decreased hearing

SERIOUS REACTIONS

- Overdosage (severe cinchonism) may result in cardiovascular effects, severe headache, intestinal cramps with vomiting and diarrhea, apprehension, confusion, seizures, blindness, and respiratory depression.
- Hypoprothrombinemia, thrombocytopenic purpura, hemoglobinuria, asthma, agranulocytosis, hypoglycemia, deafness, and optic atrophy occur rarely.

SPECIAL CONSIDERATIONS

PRECAUTIONS

- Discontinue quinine sulfate if there is any evidence of hypersensitivity. Cutaneous flushing, pruritus, skin rashes, fever, gastric distress, dyspnea, ringing in the ears, and visual impairment are the usual expressions of hypersensitivity. Hemoglobinuria and asthma from quinine sulfate are rare types of idiosyncrasy. In patients with atrial fibrillation the administration of quinine sulfate requires the same precautions as those for quinidine.

PREGNANCY AND LACTATION

• Pregnancy Category X. Quinine sulfate may cause fetal harm when administered to a pregnant woman. Congenital malformations in the human being have been reported. Exercise caution when giving quinine sulfate to nursing women because quinine sulfate is excreted in breast milk (in small amounts).

OCULAR CONSIDERATIONS

• Adverse reactions include visual disturbances, blurred vision with scotomata, photophobia, diplopia, diminished visual fields, and disturbed color vision.

raloxifene

(ra-lox'-i-feen)

Rx: Evista

Drug Class: Estrogen receptor modulators, selective; Hormones/hormone modifiers

Pregnancy Category: X

Do not confuse raloxifene with propoxyphene.

CLINICAL PHARMACOLOGY

Mechanism of Action: A selective estrogen receptor modulator that affects some receptors like estrogen. *Therapeutic Effect:* Like estrogen, prevents bone loss and improves lipid profiles.

Pharmacokinetics

Rapidly absorbed after PO administration. Highly bound to plasma proteins (greater than 95%) and albumin. Undergoes extensive first-pass metabolism in liver. Excreted mainly in feces and, to a lesser extent, in urine. Unknown if removed by hemodialysis. **Half-life:** 27.7 hr.

AVAILABLE FORMS

• *Tablets:* 60 mg.

INDICATIONS AND DOSAGES

Prevention or treatment of osteoporosis

PO

Adults, Elderly. 60 mg a day.

UNLABELED USES: Treatment of breast cancer in postmenopausal women, prevention of fractures

CONTRAINDICATIONS: Active or history of venous thromboembolic events, such as deep vein thrombosis, pulmonary embolism, and retinal vein thrombosis; women who are or may become pregnant

INTERACTIONS

Drug

Ampicillin, cholestyramine: Reduce raloxifene absorption.

Hormone replacement therapy, systemic estrogen: Don't use raloxifene concurrently with these drugs.

Warfarin: May decrease PT and the effects of warfarin.

Herbal

None known.

Food

None known.

DIAGNOSTIC TEST EFFECTS: Lowers serum total cholesterol and LDL levels, but does not affect HDL or triglyceride levels. Slightly decreases platelet count and serum inorganic phosphate, albumin, calcium, and protein levels.

SIDE EFFECTS

Frequent (25%-10%)

Hot flashes, flu-like symptoms, arthralgia, sinusitis

Occasional (9%-5%)

Weight gain, nausea, myalgia, pharyngitis, cough, dyspepsia, leg cramps, rash, depression

Rare (4%-3%)

Vaginitis, UTI, peripheral edema, flatulence, vomiting, fever, migraine, diaphoresis

SERIOUS REACTIONS

- Pneumonia, gastroenteritis, chest pain, vaginal bleeding, and breast pain occur rarely.

SPECIAL CONSIDERATIONS

PRECAUTIONS

- Women treated with raloxifene hydrochloride had an increased risk of venous thromboembolism (deep vein thrombosis and pulmonary embolism). Raloxifene hydrochloride lowers serum total and low-density lipoprotein cholesterol.

PATIENT INFORMATION

For safe and effective use of raloxifene hydrochloride, the physician should inform patients about the following:

- Patient Immobilization: Patients should discontinue raloxifene hydrochloride at least 72 hours before and during prolonged immobilization (e.g., postsurgical recovery and prolonged bed rest), and patients should avoid prolonged restrictions of movement during travel because of the increased risk of venous thromboembolic events.
- Hot Flashes or Flushes: Raloxifene hydrochloride may increase the incidence of hot flashes and is not effective in reducing hot flashes or flushes associated with estrogen deficiency. In some asymptomatic patients, hot flashes may occur on beginning raloxifene hydrochloride therapy.
- Other Osteoporosis Treatment and Prevention Measures: Instruct patients to take supplemental calcium and/or vitamin D if daily dietary intake is inadequate.
- Consider weight-bearing exercise along with the modification of certain behavioral factors, such as cigarette smoking and/or alcohol consumption, if these factors exist.

PREGNANCY AND LACTATION

- Pregnancy Category X. Do not use raloxifene hydrochloride in women who are or may become pregnant. Raloxifene hydrochloride may cause fetal harm. Raloxifene hydrochloride should not be used by lactating women. Whether raloxifene is excreted in human milk is not known.

---

ramipril

(ram'i-pril)

Rx: Altace

Drug Class: Angiotensin converting enzyme inhibitors

Pregnancy Category: D

Do not confuse Altace with Alteplase or Artane.

CLINICAL PHARMACOLOGY

Mechanism of Action: An ACE inhibitor that suppresses the renin-angiotensin-aldosterone system. Decreases plasma angiotensin II, increases plasma renin activity, and decreases aldosterone secretion. *Therapeutic Effect:* Reduces peripheral arterial resistance and BP.

Pharmacokinetics

Route	*Onset*	*Peak*	*Duration*
PO	1-2 hr	3-6 hr	24 hr

Well absorbed from the GI tract. Protein binding: 73%. Metabolized in the liver to active metabolite. Primarily excreted in urine. Not removed by hemodialysis. **Half-life:** 5.1 hr.

AVAILABLE FORMS

- *Capsules:* 1.25 mg, 2.5 mg, 5 mg, 10 mg.

INDICATIONS AND DOSAGES

Hypertension (monotherapy)

PO

Adults, Elderly. Initially, 2.5 mg/day. Maintenance: 2.5-20 mg/day as single dose or in 2 divided doses.

Hypertension (in combination with other antihypertensives)

PO

Adults, Elderly. Initially, 1.25 mg/day titrated to patient's needs.

CHF

PO

Adults, Elderly. Initially, 1.25-2.5 mg twice a day. Maximum: 5 mg twice a day.

Risk reduction for myocardial infarction stroke

PO

Adults, Elderly. Initially, 2.5 mg/day for 7 days, then 5 mg/day for 21 days, then 10 mg/day as a single dose or in divided doses.

Dosage in renal impairment

Creatinine clearance equal to or less than 40 ml/min. 25% of normal dose.

Hypertension. Initially, 1.25 mg/day titrated upward.

CHF. Initially, 1.25 mg/day, titrated up to 2.5 mg twice a day.

UNLABELED USES: Treatment of hypertension and renal crisis in scleroderma

CONTRAINDICATIONS: Bilateral renal artery stenosis

INTERACTIONS

Drug

Alcohol, antihypertensives, diuretics: May increase the effects of ramipril.

Lithium: May increase lithium blood concentration and risk of lithium toxicity.

NSAIDs: May decrease the effects of ramipril.

Potassium-sparing diuretics, potassium supplements: May cause hyperkalemia.

Herbal

Garlic: May increase antihypertensive effect.

Ginseng, yohimbe: May worsen hypertension.

Food

None known.

DIAGNOSTIC TEST EFFECTS: May increase BUN, serum alkaline phosphatase, serum bilirubin, serum creatinine, serum potassium, AST (SGOT), and ALT (SGPT) levels. May decrease serum sodium levels. May cause positive antinuclear antibody titer.

SIDE EFFECTS

Frequent (12%-5%)

Cough, headache

Occasional (4%-2%)

Dizziness, fatigue, nausea, asthenia (loss of strength)

Rare (less than 2%)

Palpitations, insomnia, nervousness, malaise, abdominal pain, myalgia

SERIOUS REACTIONS

- Excessive hypotension ("first-dose syncope") may occur in patients with CHF and and in those who are severely salt or volume depleted.
- Angioedema and hyperkalemia occur rarely.
- Agranulocytosis and neutropenia may be noted in those with collagen vascular disease, including scleroderma and systemic lupus erythematosus, and impaired renal function.
- Nephrotic syndrome may be noted in those with history of renal disease.

SPECIAL CONSIDERATIONS

PRECAUTIONS

- Anticipate changes in renal function in susceptible individuals. In hypertensive patients with unilateral or bilateral renal artery stenosis, increases in blood urea nitrogen and serum creatinine have been observed in some patients following angiotensin-converting enzyme (ACE) inhibitor therapy. Hyperkalemia occurred in hypertensive patients receiving ramipril. Cough has been reported with all ACE inhibitors. Patients with impaired liver function could develop greatly elevated plasma levels of ramipril. In patients undergoing major surgery or during anesthesia with agents that produce hypotension, enalapril may block angiotensin II formation following compensatory renin release.

PATIENT INFORMATION

• Pregnancy: Advise female patients of childbearing age about the consequences of second- and third-trimester exposure to ACE inhibitors, and inform them that these consequences do not appear to have resulted from intrauterine ACE-inhibitor exposure that has been limited to the first trimester. Ask these patients to report pregnancies to their physicians as soon as possible.

• Angioedema: Angioedema, including laryngeal edema, can occur with treatment with ACE inhibitors, especially following the first dose. Advise patients to report immediately any signs or symptoms suggesting angioedema (swelling of face, eyes, lips, or tongue or difficulty in breathing) and to take no more drug until they have consulted with the prescribing physician.

• Symptomatic Hypotension: Caution patients that light-headedness can occur, especially during the first days of therapy and to report it. Instruct patients that if syncope occurs, to discontinue ramipril until they have consulted their physician. Caution all patients that inadequate fluid intake or excessive perspiration, diarrhea, or vomiting can lead to an excessive fall in blood pressure, with the same consequences of light-headedness and possible syncope.

• Hyperkalemia: Advise patients not to use salt substitutes containing potassium without consulting their physician.

• Neutropenia: Instruct patients promptly to report any indication of infection (e.g., sore throat or fever), which could be a sign of neutropenia.

PREGNANCY AND LACTATION

• Pregnancy Categories C (first trimester) and D (second and third trimesters). The use of ACE inhibitors during the second and third trimesters of pregnancy has been associated with fetal and neonatal injury, including hypotension, neonatal skull hypoplasia, anuria, reversible or irreversible renal failure, and death. Ingestion of single 10-mg oral dose of ramipril resulted in undetectable amounts of ramipril and its metabolites in breast milk. However, because multiple doses may produce low milk concentrations that are not predictable from single doses, women receiving ramipril should not breast-feed.

ranitidine hydrochloride/ ranitidine bismuth citrate

(ra-ni'ti-deen)

Rx: Zantac, Zantac 150, Zantac 300, Zantac EFFERdose

Drug Class: Antihistamines, H2; Gastrointestinals

Pregnancy Category: B

Do not confuse Zantac with Xanax, Ziac, or Zyrtec.

CLINICAL PHARMACOLOGY

Mechanism of Action: An antiulcer agent that inhibits histamine action at histamine 2 receptors of gastric parietal cells. *Therapeutic Effect:* Inhibits gastric acid secretion when fasting, at night, or when stimulated by food, caffeine, or insulin. Reduces volume and hydrogen ion concentration of gastric juice.

Pharmacokinetics

Rapidly absorbed from the GI tract. Protein binding: 15%. Widely distributed. Metabolized in the liver. Primarily excreted in urine. Not removed by hemodialysis. **Half-life:** PO, 2.5 hr; IV, 2-2.5 hr (increased with impaired renal function).

AVAILABLE FORMS

- *Tablets (Effervescent [Zantac EFFERdose]):* 25 mg, 150 mg.
- *Capsules:* 150 mg, 300 mg.
- *Granules (Zantac EFFERdose):* 150 mg.
- *Syrup (Zantac):* 15 mg/ml.
- *Tablets (Zantac 75):* 75 mg.
- *Tablets (Zantac):* 150 mg, 300 mg.
- *Injection (Zantac):* 25 mg/ml.

INDICATIONS AND DOSAGES

Duodenal ulcers, gastric ulcers, gastroesophageal reflux disease

PO

Adults, Elderly. 150 mg twice a day or 300 mg at bedtime. Maintenance: 150 mg at bedtime.

Children. 2-4 mg/kg/day in divided doses twice a day. Maximum: 300 mg/day.

Erosive esophagitis

PO

Adults, Elderly. 150 mg 4 times a day. Maintenance: 150 mg 2 times/day or 300 mg at bedtime.

Children. 4-10 mg/kg/day in 2 divided doses. Maximum: 600 mg/day.

Hypersecretory conditions

PO

Adults, Elderly. 150 mg twice a day. May increase up to 6 g/day.

Usual parenteral dosage

IV, IM

Adults, Elderly. 50 mg/dose q6-8h. Maximum: 400 mg/day.

Children. 2-4 mg/kg/day in divided doses q6-8h. Maximum: 200 mg/day.

Usual neonatal dosage

PO

Neonates. 2 mg/kg/day in divided doses q12h.

IV

Neonates. Initially, 1.5 mg/kg/dose; then 1.5-2 mg/kg/day in divided doses q12h.

Dosage in renal impairment

For patients with creatinine clearance less than 50 ml/min, give 150 mg PO q24h or 50 mg IV or IM q18-24h.

UNLABELED USES: Prevention of aspiration pneumonia

CONTRAINDICATIONS: History of acute porphyria

INTERACTIONS

Drug

Antacids: May decrease the absorption of ranitidine.

Ketoconazole: May decrease the absorption of ketoconazole.

Herbal

None known.

Food

None known.

DIAGNOSTIC TEST EFFECTS: Interferes with skin tests using allergen extracts. May increase hepatic function enzyme, gamma-glutamyl transpeptidase, and serum creatinine levels.

IV INCOMPATIBILITIES: Amphotericin B complex (Abelcet, AmBisome, Amphotec)

IV COMPATIBILITIES: Diltiazem (Cardizem), dobutamine (Dobutrex), dopamine (Intropin), heparin, hydromorphone (Dilaudid), insulin, lidocaine, lorazepam (Ativan), morphine, norepinephrine (Levophed), potassium chloride, propofol (Diprivan)

SIDE EFFECTS

Occasional (2%)

Diarrhea

Rare (1%)

Constipation, headache (may be severe)

SERIOUS REACTIONS

- Reversible hepatitis and blood dyscrasias occur rarely.

SPECIAL CONSIDERATIONS

PRECAUTIONS

- Adjust dosage in patients with impaired renal function. Use caution in patients with hepatic dysfunction because ranitidine hydrochloride is metabolized in the liver. Avoid use of ranitidine hydrochloride in patients with a history of acute porphyria.

PREGNANCY AND LACTATION

- Pregnancy Category B. Reproduction studies revealed no evidence of impaired fertility or harm to the fetus from ranitidine hydrochloride. Fetal harm is not known. Ranitidine hydrochloride is secreted in human milk.

OCULAR CONSIDERATIONS

- For intraocular foreign body and traumatic optic neuropathy in the presence of sinus wall fracture or penetrating orbital injury, consider methylprednisolone 250 mg IV q6h for 12 doses plus ranitidine 150 mg orally bid (treatment is controversial).

---

repaglinide

(re-pag′lih-nide)

Rx: Prandin

Drug Class: Antidiabetic agents; Meglitinides

Pregnancy Category: C

CLINICAL PHARMACOLOGY

Mechanism of Action: An antihyperglycemic that stimulates release of insulin from beta cells of the pancreas by depolarizing beta cells, leading to an opening of calcium channels. Resulting calcium influx induces insulin secretion. *Therapeutic Effect:* Lowers blood glucose concentration.

Pharmacokinetics

Rapidly, completely absorbed from the GI tract. Protein binding: 98%. Metabolized in the liver to inactive metabolites. Excreted primarily in feces with a lesser amount in urine. Unknown if removed by hemodialysis. **Half-life:** 1 hr.

AVAILABLE FORMS

- *Tablets:* 0.5 mg, 1 mg, 2 mg.

INDICATIONS AND DOSAGES

Diabetes mellitus

PO

Adults, Elderly. 0.5-4 mg 2-4 times a day. Maximum: 16 mg/day.

CONTRAINDICATIONS: Diabetic ketoacidosis, type 1 diabetes mellitus

INTERACTIONS

Drug

Beta-blockers, chloramphenicol, gemfibrozil, MAOIs, NSAIDs, probenecid, salicylates, sulfonamides, warfarin: May increase the effects of repaglinide.

Herbal

None known.

Food

Food: Decreases repaglinide plasma concentration.

DIAGNOSTIC TEST EFFECTS: *None known.*

SIDE EFFECTS

Frequent (10%-6%)

Upper respiratory tract infection, headache, rhinitis, bronchitis, back pain

Occasional (5%-3%)

Diarrhea, dyspepsia, sinusitis, nausea, arthralgia, urinary tract infection

Rare (2%)

Constipation, vomiting, paresthesia, allergy

SERIOUS REACTIONS

- Hypoglycemia occurs in 16% of patients.
- Chest pain occurs rarely.

SPECIAL CONSIDERATIONS

PRECAUTIONS

- Repaglinide administration is associated with increased cardiovascular mortality compared with treatment with diet alone or diet plus insulin. Hepatic insufficiency may cause elevated repaglinide blood levels and may diminish gluconeogenic capacity. Elderly or debilitated patients or patients with pituitary or hepatic insufficiency are particularly susceptible to the hypoglycemic action of glucose-lowering drugs. Hypoglycemia may be difficult to recognize in the elderly and in persons taking beta-adrenergic blocking drugs. When a patient stabilized on any diabetic regimen is exposed to stress such as fever, trauma, infection, or surgery, a loss of glycemic control may occur.

PATIENT INFORMATION

- Inform patients of the potential risks and advantages of repaglinide and of alternative modes of therapy. Also inform patients about the importance of adherence to dietary instructions, of a regular exercise program, and of regular testing of blood glucose and hemoglobin A1c. Explain the risks of hypoglycemia, its symptoms and treatment, and conditions that predispose to its development and concomitant administration of other glucose-lowering drugs to patients and responsible family members. Also explain primary and secondary failure.
- Instruct patients to take repaglinide before meals (2, 3, or 4 times a day preprandially). Doses are usually taken within 15 minutes of the meal, but time may vary from immediately preceding the meal to as long as 30 minutes before the meal.
- Instruct patients who skip a meal (or add an extra meal) to skip (or add) a dose for that meal.

PREGNANCY AND LACTATION

- Pregnancy Category C. Offspring of rat dams exposed to repaglinide at 15 times clinical exposure developed nonteratogenic skeletal deformities consisting of shortening, thickening, and bending of the humerus during the postnatal period. Fetal harm is not known. Measurable levels of repaglinide were detected in the breast milk of the dams, and lowered blood glucose levels were observed in the rats. Excretion into human milk is not known.

reserpine

(reh-zer′-peen)

Drug Class: Antiadrenergics, peripheral

Pregnancy Category: C

Do not confuse with Risperdal, risperidone

CLINICAL PHARMACOLOGY

Mechanism of Action: An antihypertensive that depletes stores of catecholamines and 5-hydroxytryptamine in many organs, including the brain and adrenal medulla. Depression of sympathetic nerve function results in a decreased heart rate and a lowering of arterial blood pressure. Depletion of catecholamines and 5-hydroxytryptamine from the brain is thought to be the mechanism of the sedative and tranquilizing properties. *Therapeutic Effects:* Decrease blood pressure and heart rate; sedation.

Pharmacokinetics

Characterized by slow onset of action and sustained effects. Both cardiovascular and central nervous system effects may persist for a period of time following withdrawal of the drug. Mean maximum plasma levels were attained after a median of 3.5 hours. Bioavailability was approximately 50% of that of a corresponding intravenous dose. Protein binding: 96%. **Half life:** 33 hours.

AVAILABLE FORMS

- *Tablets:* 0.25 mg, 0.1 mg (reserpine)

INDICATIONS AND DOSAGES

Hypertension

PO

Adults: Usual initial dosage 0.5 mg daily for 1 or 2 weeks. For maintenance, reduce to 0.1 to 0.25 mg daily.

Children: Reserpine is not recommended for use in children. If it is to be used in treating a child, the usual recommended starting dose is 20 mcg/kg daily. The maximum recommended dose is 0.25 mg (total) daily.

Psychiatric Disorders

PO

Adults: Initial dosage 0.5 mg daily, may range from 0.1-1.0 mg. Adjust dosage upward or downward according to response.

UNLABELED USES: Cerebral vasospasm, migraines, Raynaud's syndrome, reflex sympathetic dystrophy, refractory depression, tardive dyskinesia, thyrotoxic crisis.

CONTRAINDICATIONS: Hypersensitivity, mental depression or history of mental depression (especially with suicidal tendencies), active peptic ulcer, ulcerative colitis, patients receiving electroconvulsive therapy.

INTERACTIONS

Drug

MAO inhibitors: May cause hypertensive reactions.

Beta-blockers: Resrpine may increase effect.

CNS depressants/ethanol: Reserpine may increase effects.

Levodopa, quinidine, procainamide, digitalis glycosides: Reserpine may increase effects/toxicity.

Tricyclic antidepressants: May increase antihypertensive effects.

Herbal

Dong quai: Has estrogenic activity

Ephedra/yohimbe: May worsen hypertension

Valerian, St John's wort, kava kava, gotu kola: May increase CNS depression

Garlic: May have increased antihypertensive effects

Food

Ethanol: May increase CNS depression.

DIAGNOSTIC TEST EFFECTS: *None known.*

SIDE EFFECTS

Occasional

Burning in the stomach, nausea, vomiting, diarrhea, dry mouth, nosebleed, stuffy nose, dizziness, headache, nervousness, nightmares, drowsiness, muscle aches, weight gain, redness of the eyes

Rare

Irregular heartbeat, difficulty breathing, heart problems, feeling faint, swelling, gynecomastia, decreased libido

SERIOUS REACTIONS

• None known.

SPECIAL CONSIDERATIONS

PRECAUTIONS

• Reserpine may cause mental depression. Use reserpine cautiously in patients with a history of peptic ulcer, ulcerative colitis, or gallstones. Exercise caution when treating hypertensive patients with renal insufficiency. Hypotension has occurred in patients receiving rauwolfia preparations.

PATIENT INFORMATION

• Inform patients of possible side effects and advise them to take the mediation regularly and continuously as directed.

PREGNANCY AND LACTATION

• Pregnancy Category C. Reserpine crosses the placental barrier, and increased respiratory tract secretions, nasal congestion, cyanosis, and anorexia may occur in neonates of mothers treated with reserpine. Fetal harm is not known. Reserpine is excreted in maternal breast milk, and increased respiratory tract secretions, nasal congestion, cyanosis, and anorexia may occur in breastfed infants.

rimexolone

(rye-mex'o-lone)

Rx: Vexol

Drug Class: Corticosteroids, ophthalmic; Ophthalmics

Pregnancy Category: C

Do not confuse with riluzole.

CLINICAL PHARMACOLOGY

Mechanism of Action: An ophthalmic agent that suppresses migration of polymorphoneclear leukocytes and reverses increased capillary permeability. *Therapeutic Effect:* Decreases inflammation.

Pharmacokinetics

Absorbed through aqueous humor. Metabolized in liver. Excreted in urine and feces.

AVAILABLE FORMS

• *Ophthalmic Suspension:* 1% (Vexol).

INDICATIONS AND DOSAGES

Inflammation after ocular surgery, treatment of anterior uveitis

Ophthalmic

Adults, Elderly. Instill 1 drop 2-4 times/day up to q4h. May use q1-2h during the first 1-2 days.

CONTRAINDICATIONS: Fungal, viral, or untreated pus-forming bacterial ocular infections, hypersensitivity to rimexolone or any component of the formulation

INTERACTIONS

Drug

None known.

Herbal

None known.

Food
None known.
DIAGNOSTIC TEST EFFECTS: *None known.*
SIDE EFFECTS
Occasional
Temporary mild blurred vision
Rare
Burning/stinging eyes
SERIOUS REACTIONS
• Prolonged has been associated with the development of corneal or scleral perforation and posterior subcapsular cataracts.
• Cataracts, corneal thinning, glaucoma, increased intraocular pressure, optic nerve damage, secondary ocular infection, and visual acuity defects occur rarely.

SPECIAL CONSIDERATIONS
PRECAUTIONS
• Fungal infections of the cornea may occur.
PREGNANCY AND LACTATION
• Pregnancy Category C. Teratogenic and embryotoxic in rabbits occurred following subcutaneous administration at the lowest dose tested. Excretion into human milk is not known.

risedronate sodium
(rye-se-droe'nate)
Rx: Actonel
Drug Class: Bisphosphonates
Pregnancy Category: C

CLINICAL PHARMACOLOGY
Mechanism of Action: A bisphosphonate that binds to bone hydroxyapatite and inhibits osteoclasts. *Therapeutic Effect:* Reduces bone turnover (the number of sites at which bone is remodeled) and bone resorption.
AVAILABLE FORMS
• *Tablets:* 5 mg, 30 mg, 35 mg.
INDICATIONS AND DOSAGES
Paget's disease
PO
Adults, Elderly. 30 mg/day for 2 mo. Retreatment may occur after 2-mo post-treatment observation period.
Prevention and treatment of postmenopausal osteoporosis
PO
Adults, Elderly. 5 mg/day or 35 mg once weekly.
Glucocorticoid-induced osteoporosis
PO
Adults, Elderly. 5 mg/day.
CONTRAINDICATIONS: Hypersensitivity to other bisphosphonates, including etidronate, tiludronate, risedronate, and alendronate; hypocalcemia; inability to stand or sit upright for at least 20 minutes; renal impairment when serum creatinine clearance is greater than 5 mg/dl
INTERACTIONS
Drug
Antacids containing aluminum, calcium, magnesium; vitamin D: May decrease the absorption of risedronate.
Herbal
None known.
Food
None known.
DIAGNOSTIC TEST EFFECTS: *None known.*
SIDE EFFECTS
Frequent (30%)
Arthralgia
Occasional (12%-8%)
Rash, flu-like symptoms, peripheral edema
Rare (5%-3%)
Bone pain, sinusitis, asthenia, dry eye, tinnitus
SERIOUS REACTIONS
• Overdose causes hypocalcemia, hypophosphatemia, and significant GI disturbances.

SPECIAL CONSIDERATIONS

PRECAUTIONS

- Adverse reactions reported are cataract (5.9%), conjunctivitis (3.1%), amblyopia (3.3%), and dry eye (3.3%).
- Cataract was reported to be higher in daily dosing (5 mg; 2.9%) than weekly dosing (35 mg; 1.9%).

---

risperidone

(ris-per'i-done)

Rx: Risperdal, Risperdal Consta, Risperdal M-Tab

Drug Class: Antipsychotics

Pregnancy Category: C

Do not confuse risperidone with reserpine.

CLINICAL PHARMACOLOGY

Mechanism of Action: A benzisoxazole derivative that may antagonize dopamine and serotonin receptors. *Therapeutic Effect:* Suppresses psychotic behavior.

Pharmacokinetics

Well absorbed from the GI tract; unaffected by food. Protein binding: 90%. Extensively metabolized in the liver to active metabolite. Primarily excreted in urine. **Half-life:** 3-20 hr; metabolite: 21-30 hr (increased in elderly).

AVAILABLE FORMS

- *Oral Solution (Risperdal):* 1 mg/ml.
- *Tablets (Risperdal):* 0.25 mg, 0.5 mg, 1 mg, 2 mg, 3 mg, 4 mg.
- *Tablets (Orally-Disintegrating [Risperdal M-Tabs]):* 0.5 mg, 1 mg, 2 mg.
- *Injection (Risperdal Consta):* 25 mg, 37.5 mg, 50 mg.

INDICATIONS AND DOSAGES

Psychotic disorder

PO

Adults. 0.5-1 mg twice a day. May increase dosage slowly. Range: 2-6 mg/day.

Elderly. Initially, 0.25-2 mg/day in 2 divided doses. May increase dosage slowly. Range: 2-6 mg/day.

IM

Adults, Elderly. 25 mg q2wk. Maximum: 50 mg q2wk.

Mania

PO

*Adults, Elderly.*Initially, 2-3 mg as a single daily dose. May increase at 24-hour intervals of 1 mg/day. Range: 2-6 mg/day.

Dosage in renal impairment

Initial dosage for adults and elderly patients is 0.25-0.5 mg twice a day. Dosage is titrated slowly to desired effect.

UNLABELED USES: Autism in children, behavioral symptoms associated with dementia, Tourette's disorder

CONTRAINDICATIONS: None known.

INTERACTIONS

Drug

Alcohol, other CNS depressants: May increase CNS depression.

Carbamazepine: May decrease the risperidone blood concentration.

Clozapine: May increase the risperidone blood concentration.

Dopamine agonists, levodopa: May decrease the effects of these drugs.

Paroxetine: May increase the risperidone blood concentration and the risk of extrapyramidal symptoms.

Herbal

None known.

Food

None known.

DIAGNOSTIC TEST EFFECTS: May increase serum prolactin, creatinine, alkaline phosphatase, uric acid, AST (SGOT), ALT (SGPT), and triglyceride levels. May decrease blood glucose and serum potassium, protein, and sodium levels. May cause EKG changes.

SIDE EFFECTS

Frequent (26%-13%)

Agitation, anxiety, insomnia, headache, constipation

Occasional (10%-4%)

Dyspepsia, rhinitis, somnolence, dizziness, nausea, vomiting, rash, abdominal pain, dry skin, tachycardia

Rare (3%-2%)

Visual disturbances, fever, back pain, pharyngitis, cough, arthralgia, angina, aggressive behavior, orthostatic hypotension, breast swelling

SERIOUS REACTIONS

• Rare reactions include tardive dyskinesia (characterized by tongue protrusion, puffing of the cheeks, and chewing or puckering of the mouth) and neuroleptic malignant syndrome (marked by hyperpyrexia, muscle rigidity, change in mental status, irregular pulse or BP, tachycardia, diaphoresis, cardiac arrhythmias, rhabdomyolysis, and acute renal failure).

SPECIAL CONSIDERATIONS

PRECAUTIONS

• A potentially fatal symptom complex sometimes referred to as neuroleptic malignant syndrome has been reported in association with antipsychotic drugs. Tardive dyskinesia may develop in patients treated with antipsychotic drugs. A potential exists for proarrhythmic effects. Risperidone may induce orthostatic hypotension associated with dizziness and tachycardia. Use risperidone cautiously in patients with a history of seizures. Esophageal dysmotility and aspiration have been associated with antipsychotic drug use. Risperidone elevates prolactin levels, and the elevation persists during chronic administration. Somnolence was a commonly reported adverse event associated with risperidone treatment. Rare cases of priapism have been reported. Risperidone has an antiemetic effect in animals; this effect also may occur in human beings. The possibility of a suicide attempt is inherent in schizophrenia, and close supervision of high-risk patients should accompany drug therapy.

PATIENT INFORMATION

• Physicians are advised to discuss the following issues with patients for whom they prescribe risperidone.

• Orthostatic Hypotension: Advise patients of the risk of orthostatic hypotension, especially during the period of initial dose titration.

• Interference with Cognitive and Motor Performance: Because risperidone has the potential to impair judgment, thinking, or motor skills, caution patients about operating hazardous machinery, including automobiles, until they are reasonably certain that risperidone therapy does not affect them adversely.

• Pregnancy: Advise patients to notify their physician if they become pregnant or intend to become pregnant during therapy.

• Nursing: Advise patients not to breast-feed an infant if they are taking risperidone.

• Concomitant Medication: Advise patients to inform their physicians if they are taking, or plan to take, any prescription or over-the-counter drugs, because a potential exists for interactions.

• Alcohol: Advise patients to avoid alcohol while taking risperidone.

PREGNANCY AND LACTATION

• Pregnancy Category C. Placental transfer of risperidone occurs in rat pups. Fetal harm is not known. Whether risperidone is excreted in human milk is not known. In animal studies, risperidone was excreted in breast milk. Therefore women receiving risperidone should not breast-feed.

OCULAR CONSIDERATIONS

• Vision Disorders: abnormal accommodation and xerophthalmia (infrequent); diplopia, eye pain, blepharitis, photopsia, photophobia, and abnormal lacrimation (rare)

rofecoxib

(ro-fe-coks′ib)

Rx: Vioxx

Drug Class: Analgesics, nonnarcotic; COX-2 inhibitors; Nonsteroidal antiinflammatory drugs

Pregnancy Category: C

Alert

Rofecoxib has been withdrawn from the market. Do not confuse with Zyvox.

CLINICAL PHARMACOLOGY

Mechanism of Action: A nonsteroidal antiinflammatory that produces analgesic and antiinflammatory effect by inhibiting prostaglandin synthesis. *Therapeutic Effect:* Reduces inflammatory response and intensity of pain stimulus reaching sensory nerve endings.

Pharmacokinetics

Rapid, complete absorption from the gastrointestinal (GI) tract. Protein binding: 87%. Primarily metabolized in liver. Primarily eliminated in urine with a lesser amount excreted in feces. Not removed by hemodialysis. **Half-life:** 17 hr.

AVAILABLE FORMS

• *Tablets:* 12.5 mg, 25 mg, 50 mg.
• *Suspension*: 12.5 mg/5 ml, 25 mg/5 ml.

INDICATIONS AND DOSAGES

Osteoarthritis

PO

Adults. Initially, 12.5 mg/day. May increase dosage to 25 mg/day. Maximum is 25 mg/day.

Rheumatoid arthritis

PO

Adults, Elderly. 25 mg/day.

Acute pain, dysmenorrhea

PO

Adults. Initially, 50 mg/day.

CONTRAINDICATIONS: Hypersensitivity to aspirin and NSAIDs

INTERACTIONS

Drug

Anticoagulants: May increase the effects of anticoagulants.

Aspirin: May increase the risk of GI bleeding and side effects.

Herbal

Feverfew: May decrease the effects of this herb.

Ginkgo biloba: May increase the risk of bleeding.

Food

None known.

DIAGNOSTIC TEST EFFECTS: May prolong bleeding time. May increase LDH, liver function tests, and serum alkaline phosphatase. May decrease blood Hgb, Hct, and serum sodium levels.

SIDE EFFECTS

Frequent (6%-5%)

Nausea (with or without vomiting), diarrhea, abdominal distress

Occasional (3%)

Dyspepsia, including heartburn, indigestion, epigastric pain

Rare (less than 2%)
Constipation, flatulence

SERIOUS REACTIONS

• None known.

SPECIAL CONSIDERATIONS

PRECAUTIONS

• Rofecoxib poses the risk of gastrointestinal ulceration, bleeding, and perforation and of anaphylactoid reactions. Treatment is not recommended in patients with advanced kidney disease. Rofecoxib cannot be expected to substitute for corticosteroids or to treat corticosteroid insufficiency.

• Borderline elevations of one or more liver tests may occur in up to 15% of patients taking nonsteroidal antiinflammatory drugs. Use of rofecoxib is not recommended in patients with moderate or severe hepatic insufficiency. Long-term administration of nonsteroidal antiinflammatory drugs has resulted in renal papillary necrosis and other renal injury. Use caution when initiating treatment with rofecoxib in patients with considerable dehydration. Anemia sometimes occurs in patients receiving rofecoxib. Fluid retention and edema have been observed in some patients taking rofecoxib. Patients with asthma may have aspirin-sensitive asthma. The use of aspirin in patients with aspirin-sensitive asthma has been associated with severe bronchospasm, which can be fatal.

PATIENT INFORMATION

• Rofecoxib can cause discomfort and, rarely, more serious side effects, such as gastrointestinal bleeding, which may result in hospitalization and even fatal outcomes. Although serious gastrointestinal tract ulcerations and bleeding can occur without warning symptoms, patients should be alert for the signs and symptoms of ulcerations and bleeding and should ask for medical advice when observing any indicative signs or symptoms. Apprise patients of the importance of this follow-up.

• Patients should report promptly signs or symptoms of gastrointestinal ulceration or bleeding, skin rash, unexplained weight gain, or edema to their physicians.

• Inform patients of the warning signs and symptoms of hepatotoxicity (e.g., nausea, fatigue, lethargy, pruritus, jaundice, right upper quadrant tenderness, and flu-like symptoms). If these occur, instruct patients to stop therapy and seek immediate medical therapy.

• Also instruct patients to seek immediate emergency help in the case of an anaphylactoid reaction.

• In late pregnancy, avoid administration of rofecoxib because it may cause premature closure of the ductus arteriosus.

PREGNANCY AND LACTATION

• Pregnancy Category C. Rofecoxib produced periimplantation and postimplantation losses and reduced embryo/fetal survival in rats and rabbits. In late pregnancy, avoid administration of rofecoxib because it may cause premature closure of the ductus arteriosus. Fetal harm is not known. Rofecoxib is excreted in the milk of lactating rats at concentrations similar to those in plasma. Excretion into human milk is not known.

OCULAR CONSIDERATIONS

• Adverse reactions include allergic rhinitis, blurred vision, conjunctivitis, dry throat, and ocular injection.

rosiglitazone maleate

(roz-ih-gli'ta-zone)

Rx: Avandia

Drug Class: Antidiabetic agents; Thiazolidinediones

Pregnancy Category: C

Do not confuse Avandia with Avalide, Avinza, or Prandin.

CLINICAL PHARMACOLOGY

Mechanism of Action: An antidiabetic that improves target-cell response to insulin without increasing pancreatic insulin secretion. Decreases hepatic glucose output and increases insulin-dependent glucose utilization in skeletal muscle. *Therapeutic Effect:* Lowers blood glucose concentration.

Pharmacokinetics

Rapidly absorbed. Protein binding: 99%. Metabolized in the liver. Excreted primarily in urine, with a lesser amount in feces. Not removed by hemodialysis. **Half-life:** 3-4 hr.

AVAILABLE FORMS

- *Tablets:* 2 mg, 4 mg, 8 mg.

INDICATIONS AND DOSAGES

Diabetes mellitus, combination therapy

PO

Adults, Elderly. Initially, 4 mg as a single daily dose or in divided doses twice a day. May increase to 8 mg/day after 12 wk of therapy if fasting glucose level is not adequately controlled.

Diabetes mellitus, monotherapy

Adults, Elderly. Initially, 4 mg as single daily dose or in divided doses twice a day. May increase to 8 mg/day after 12 wk of therapy.

CONTRAINDICATIONS: Active hepatic disease, diabetic ketoacidosis, increased serum transaminase levels, including ALT (SGPT) greater than 2.5 times the normal serum level, type 1 diabetes mellitus

INTERACTIONS

Drug

None known.

Herbal

None known.

Food

None known.

DIAGNOSTIC TEST EFFECTS: May decrease Hct and Hgb and serum alkaline phosphatase, bilirubin, and AST (SGOT) levels. Less than 1% of patients experience ALT values that are 3 times the normal level.

SIDE EFFECTS

Frequent (9%)

Upper respiratory tract infection

Occasional (4%-2%)

Headache, edema, back pain, fatigue, sinusitis, diarrhea

SERIOUS REACTIONS

- None known.

SPECIAL CONSIDERATIONS

PRECAUTIONS

- Rosiglitazone maleate can cause fluid retention that may exacerbate or lead to heart failure. Because of its mechanism of action, rosiglitazone maleate is active only in the presence of endogenous insulin. Therefore, do not use rosiglitazone maleate in patients with type 1 diabetes or to treat diabetic ketoacidosis. Risk for hypoglycemia exists when rosiglitazone maleate is used in combination with other hypoglycemic agents. Exercise caution in patients with edema. Dose-related weight gain was seen with rosiglitazone maleate alone and in combination with other hypoglycemic agents. Rosiglitazone maleate administration may result in ovulation in some premenopausal anovulatory women.

PATIENT INFORMATION

• Management of type 2 diabetes should include diet control. Caloric restriction, weight loss, and exercise are essential for the proper treatment of the diabetic patient because they help improve insulin sensitivity. This is important not only in the primary treatment of type 2 diabetes but also in maintaining the efficacy of drug therapy. Adherence to dietary instructions and regular blood glucose and glycosylated hemoglobin testing are important. Advise patients that it can take 2 weeks to see a reduction in blood glucose and 2 to 3 months to see full effect. Inform patients that blood will be drawn to check their liver function before the start of therapy and every 2 months for the first 12 months and periodically thereafter. Patients with unexplained symptoms of nausea, vomiting, abdominal pain, fatigue, anorexia, or dark urine immediately should report these symptoms to their physician. Patients who experience an unusually rapid increase in weight or edema or who develop shortness of breath or other symptoms of heart failure while taking rosiglitazone maleate immediately should report these symptoms to their physician. Rosiglitazone maleate can be taken with or without meals. When administering rosiglitazone maleate in combination with other hypoglycemic agents, explain the risk of hypoglycemia, its symptoms and treatment, and conditions that predispose to its development to patients and their family members. Therapy with rosiglitazone maleate, like other thiazolidinediones, may result in ovulation in some premenopausal anovulatory women. As a result, these patients may be at an increased risk for pregnancy while taking rosiglitazone maleate. Thus, recommend adequate contraception in premenopausal women. This possible effect has not been investigated specifically in clinical studies, so the frequency of this occurrence is not known.

PREGNANCY AND LACTATION

• Pregnancy Category C. No effect on implantation or the embryo was found with rosiglitazone treatment during early pregnancy in rats, but treatment during mid to late gestation was associated with fetal death and growth retardation in rats and rabbits. Drug-related material was detected in milk from lactating rats. Excretion into human milk is not known.

salmeterol

(sal-me'te-rol)

Rx: Serevent, Serevent Diskus

Drug Class: Adrenergic agonists; Bronchodilators

Pregnancy Category: C

Do not confuse Serevent with Serentil.

CLINICAL PHARMACOLOGY

Mechanism of Action: An adrenergic agonist that stimulates beta$_2$-adrenergic receptors in the lungs, resulting in relaxation of bronchial smooth muscle. *Therapeutic Effect:* Relieves bronchospasm and reduces airway resistance.

Pharmacokinetics

Route	Onset	Peak	Duration
Inhalation	10-20 min	3 hr	12 hr

Low systemic absorption; acts primarily in the lungs. Protein binding: 95%. Metabolized by hydroxylation. Primarily eliminated in feces. **Half-life:** 3-4 hr.

AVAILABLE FORMS

- *Powder for Oral Inhalation (Serevent Diskus):* 50 mcg.

INDICATIONS AND DOSAGES

Prevention and maintenance treatment of asthma

Inhalation (Diskus)

Adults, Elderly, Children 4 yr and older. 1 inhalation (50 mcg) q12h.

Prevention of exercise-induced bronchospasm

Inhalation

Adults, Elderly, Children 4 yr and older. 1 inhalation at least 30 min before exercise.

COPD

Inhalation

Adults, Elderly. 1 inhalation q12h.

CONTRAINDICATIONS: History of hypersensitivity to sympathomimetics

INTERACTIONS

Drug

Beta-blockers: May decrease the effects of beta-blockers.

Herbal

None known.

Food

None known.

DIAGNOSTIC TEST EFFECTS: May decrease serum potassium level.

SIDE EFFECTS

Frequent (28%)

Headache

Occasional (7%-3%)

Cough, tremor, dizziness, vertigo, throat dryness or irritation, pharyngitis

Rare (3%)

Palpitations, tachycardia, nausea, heartburn, GI distress, diarrhea

SERIOUS REACTIONS

- Salmeterol may prolong the QT interval, which may precipitate ventricular arrhythmias.
- Hypokalemia and hyperglycemia may occur.

SPECIAL CONSIDERATIONS

PRECAUTIONS

- Use salmeterol xinafoate with caution in patients with cardiovascular disorders, especially coronary insufficiency, cardiac arrhythmias, and hypertension; in patients with convulsive disorders or thyrotoxicosis; and in patients who are unusually responsive to sympathomimetic amines. No effects on glucose have been seen with salmeterol xinafoate at recommended doses.

PATIENT INFORMATION

Give patients the following information:

- Instruct patients to shake the container well before using.
- The action of salmeterol xinafoate inhalation aerosol may last up to 12 hours or longer. Instruct patients not to exceed the recommended dosage (two inhalations twice daily, morning and evening).
- Salmeterol xinafoate inhalation aerosol is not meant to relieve acute asthma or chronic obstructive pulmonary disease symptoms; instruct patients not to use extra doses for that purpose. Acute symptoms should be treated with an inhaled, short-acting beta$_2$-agonist such as albuterol (the physician should provide the patient with such medication and instruct the patient in how it should be used).
- Instruct patients not to stop salmeterol xinafoate inhalation aerosol therapy for chronic obstructive pulmonary disease without physician/provider guidance because symptoms may recur after discontinuation.
- Instruct patients to notify their physician immediately if any of the following situations occur, which may be a sign of seriously worsening asthma: decreasing effective-

ness of inhaled, short-acting beta$_2$-agonists; the need for more inhalations than usual of inhaled, short-acting beta$_2$-agonists; use of four or more inhalations per day of a short-acting beta$_2$-agonist for 2 days or more consecutively; use of more than one 200-inhalation canister of an inhaled, short-acting beta$_2$-agonist (e.g., albuterol) in an 8-week period.

• Instruct patients not to use salmeterol xinafoate inhalation aerosol as a substitute for oral or inhaled corticosteroids. Instruct patients not to change the dosage of these medications and not to stop taking the medication without consulting their physician, even if they feel better after initiating treatment with salmeterol xinafoate inhalation aerosol.

• Caution patients regarding common adverse cardiovascular effects, such as palpitations, chest pain, rapid heart rate, tremor, or nervousness.

• In patients receiving salmeterol xinafoate inhalation aerosol, advise them to use other inhaled medications only as directed by their physician.

• When using salmeterol xinafoate inhalation aerosol to prevent exercise-induced bronchospasm, patients should take the dose at least 30 to 60 minutes before exercise.

• Advise pregnant or nursing women to contact their physician about use of salmeterol xinafoate inhalation aerosol.

• Effective and safe use of salmeterol xinafoate inhalation aerosol includes an understanding of the way that it should be administered.

PREGNANCY AND LACTATION

• Pregnancy Category C. Fetal harm is not known. Plasma levels of salmeterol after inhaled therapeutic doses are very low. In rats, salmeterol xinafoate is excreted in the milk. However, because there no experience with the use of salmeterol xinafoate by nursing mothers, decide whether to discontinue nursing or to discontinue the drug, taking into account the importance of the drug to the mother.

---

scopolamine

(skoe-pol'a-meen)

Rx: Isopto Hyoscine, Scopace, Transderm-Scop

Drug Class: Anticholinergics; Antiemetics/antivertigo; Cycloplegics; Gastrointestinals; Mydriatics; Ophthalmics; Preanesthetics; Sedatives/hypnotics

Pregnancy Category: C

CLINICAL PHARMACOLOGY

Mechanism of Action: An anticholinergic that reduces excitability of labyrinthine receptors, depressing conduction in the vestibular cerebellar pathway. *Therapeutic Effect:* Prevents motion-induced nausea and vomiting.

AVAILABLE FORMS

• *Transdermal System:* 1.5 mg.

INDICATIONS AND DOSAGES

Prevention of motion sickness

Transdermal

Adults. 1 system q72h.

Postoperative nausea or vomiting

Transdermal

Adults, Elderly. 1 system no sooner than 1 hr. before surgery and removed 24 hr. after surgery.

CONTRAINDICATIONS: Angle-closure glaucoma, GI or GU obstruction, myasthenia gravis, paralytic ileus, tachycardia, thyrotoxicosis

INTERACTIONS

Drug

Antihistamines, tricyclic antidepressants: May increase the anticholinergic effects of scopolamine.

CNS depressants: May increase CNS depression.

Herbal

None known.

Food

None known.

DIAGNOSTIC TEST EFFECTS: May interfere with gastric secretion test.

SIDE EFFECTS

Frequent (greater than 15%)

Dry mouth, somnolence, blurred vision

Rare (5%-1%)

Dizziness, restlessness, hallucinations, confusion, difficulty urinating, rash

SERIOUS REACTIONS

• None known.

SPECIAL CONSIDERATIONS

PRECAUTIONS

• Avoid inducing angle-closure glaucoma with gonioscopy.

PATIENT INFORMATION

• Advise patients not to drive or engage in other hazardous activities when drowsy or while pupils are dilated. Patient may experience sensitivity to light and should protect eyes in bright illumination during dilation. Warn parents not to get this preparation in their child's mouth and to wash their own hands and the child's hands following administration.

OCULAR CONSIDERATIONS

• Ocular Adverse Reactions: Irritation, follicular conjunctivitis, photophobia, vascular congestion, edema, exudate, and an eczematoid dermatitis may occur. Somnolence, dryness of the mouth, or visual hallucinations may occur.

OCULAR DOSAGE AND ADMINISTRATION

• Cycloplegic Refraction: 1 or 2 drops 1 hour before refracting

• Uveitis: 1 or 2 drops up to 4 times daily

sertraline

(sir'trall-een)

Rx: Zoloft

Drug Class: Antidepressants, serotonin specific reuptake inhibitors

Pregnancy Category: C

Do not confuse sertraline with Serentil.

CLINICAL PHARMACOLOGY

Mechanism of Action: An antidepressant, anxiolytic, and obsessive-compulsive disorder adjunct that blocks the reuptake of the neurotransmitter serotonin at CNS neuronal presynaptic membranes, increasing its availability at postsynaptic receptor sites. *Therapeutic Effect:* Relieves depression, reduces obsessive-compulsive behavior, decreases anxiety.

Pharmacokinetics

Incompletely and slowly absorbed from the GI tract; food increases absorption. Protein binding: 98%. Widely distributed. Undergoes extensive first-pass metabolism in the liver to active compound. Excreted in urine and feces. Not removed by hemodialysis. **Half-life:** 26 hr.

AVAILABLE FORMS

• *Oral Concentrate:* 20 mg/ml.

• *Tablets:* 25 mg, 50 mg, 100 mg.

INDICATIONS AND DOSAGES

Depression, obsessive-compulsive disorder

PO

Adults, Children 13-17 yr. Initially, 50 mg/day with morning or evening meal. May increase by 50 mg/day at 7-day intervals.

Elderly, Children 6-12 yr. Initially, 25 mg/day. May increase by 25-50 mg/day at 7-day intervals. Maximum: 200 mg/day.

Panic disorder, posttraumatic stress disorder, social anxiety disorder

PO

Adults, Elderly. Initially, 25 mg/day. May increase by 50 mg/day at 7-day intervals. Range: 50-200 mg/day. Maximum: 200 mg/day.

Premenstrual dysphoric disorder

PO

Adults. Initially, 50 mg/day. May increase up to 150 mg/day in 50-mg increments.

CONTRAINDICATIONS: Use within 14 days of MAOIs

INTERACTIONS

Drug

Highly protein-bound medications (such as, digoxin and warfarin): May increase the blood concentration and risk of toxicity of these drugs.

MAOIs: May cause neuroleptic malignant syndrome, hypertensive crisis, hyperpyrexia, seizures, and serotonin syndrome (marked by diaphoresis, diarrhea, fever, mental changes, restlessness, and shivering).

Herbal

St. John's wort: May increase the risk of adverse effects.

Food

None known.

DIAGNOSTIC TEST EFFECTS: May increase serum total cholesterol, triglyceride, AST (SGOT), and ALT (SGPT) levels. May decrease serum uric acid level.

SIDE EFFECTS

Frequent (26%-12%)

Headache, nausea, diarrhea, insomnia, somnolence, dizziness, fatigue, rash, dry mouth

Occasional (6%-4%)

Anxiety, nervousness, agitation, tremor, dyspepsia, diaphoresis, vomiting, constipation, abnormal ejaculation, visual disturbances, altered taste

Rare (less than 3%)

Flatulence, urinary frequency, paraesthesia, hot flashes, chills

SERIOUS REACTIONS

- None known.

SPECIAL CONSIDERATIONS

PRECAUTIONS

- Hypomania or mania occurred in approximately 0.4% of Zoloft-treated patients. Significant weight loss may be an undesirable result of treatment with sertraline for some patients. Zoloft has not been evaluated in patients with a seizure disorder. The possibility of a suicide attempt is inherent in depression and may persist until significant remission occurs. Zoloft is associated with a mean decrease in serum uric acid. Caution is advisable in using Zoloft in patients with diseases or conditions that could affect metabolism or hemodynamic responses. If administering sertraline to patients with liver impairment, use a lower or less frequent dose. In controlled studies, Zoloft did not cause sedation and did not interfere with psychomotor performance. Several cases of hyponatremia have been reported and appeared to be reversible when Zoloft was discontinued.

PATIENT INFORMATION

- Physicians are advised to discuss the following issues with patients for whom they prescribe Zoloft: Inform patients that although Zoloft has not been shown to impair the ability of normal subjects to perform tasks requiring complex motor and mental skills in laboratory experiments, drugs that act on the central nervous system may affect some individuals adversely. Therefore, advise patients that until they learn how they respond to Zoloft, they should be careful doing activities when they need to be alert, such as driving a car or operating machinery. Inform patients that although Zoloft has not been shown in experiments with normal subjects to increase the mental and motor skill impairments caused by alcohol, the concomitant use of Zoloft and alcohol is not advised. Inform patients that although no adverse interaction of Zoloft with over-the-counter drug products is known to occur, the potential for interaction exists. Thus, advise patients against the use of any over-the-counter product. Advise patients to notify their physician if they become pregnant or intend to become pregnant during therapy. Advise patients to notify their physician if they are breastfeeding an infant. Zoloft oral concentrate is contraindicated with disulfiram (Antabuse) because of the alcohol content of the concentrate. Zoloft oral concentrate contains 20 mg/ml of sertraline (as the hydrochloride) as the active ingredient and 12% alcohol. Zoloft oral concentrate must be diluted before use. Instruct patients as follows: Just before taking Zoloft, use the dropper provided to remove the required amount of Zoloft oral concentrate and mix it with 4 oz (½ cup) of water, ginger ale, lemon/lime soda, or lemonade or orange juice only. Do not mix Zoloft oral concentrate with anything other than the liquids listed. Take the dose immediately after mixing. Do not mix in advance. At times, a slight haze may appear after mixing; this is normal. Note that patients with latex sensitivity should exercise caution because the dropper dispenser contains dry natural rubber.

PREGNANCY AND LACTATION

- Pregnancy Category C. When pregnant rats and rabbits were given sertraline during the period of organogenesis, delayed ossification was observed in fetuses. Fetal harm is not known. Excretion into human milk is not known.

OCULAR CONSIDERATIONS

- Adverse Reactions: conjunctivitis, eye pain, and abnormal accommodation (infrequent); xerophthalmia, photophobia, diplopia, abnormal lacrimation, scotoma, and visual field defect (rare)

sildenafil citrate

(sill-den'-a-fill)

Rx: Viagra

Drug Class: Impotence agents; Phosphodiesterase inhibitors

Pregnancy Category: B

Do not confuse Viagra with Vaniqa.

CLINICAL PHARMACOLOGY

Mechanism of Action: An erectile dysfunction agent that inhibits phosphodiesterase type 5, the enzyme responsible for degrading cyclic guanosine monophosphate in the corpus cavernosum of the penis, resulting in smooth muscle relaxation and increased blood flow. *Therapeutic Effect:* Facilitates an erection.

AVAILABLE FORMS

- *Tablets:* 25 mg, 50 mg, 100 mg.

INDICATIONS AND DOSAGES

Erectile dysfunction

PO

Adults. 50 mg (30 min-4 hr before sexual activity). Range: 25-100 mg. Maximum dosing frequency is once daily.

Elderly older than 65 yr. Consider starting dose of 25 mg.

UNLABELED USES: Treatment of diabetic gastroparesis, sexual dysfunction associated with the use of selective serotonin reuptake inhibitors

CONTRAINDICATIONS: Concurrent use of sodium nitroprusside or nitrates in any form

INTERACTIONS

Drug

Cimetidine, erythromycin, itraconazole, ketoconazole: May increase sildenafil plasma concentration.

Nitrates: Potentiates the hypotensive effects of nitrates.

Herbal

None known.

Food

High-fat meals: Delay drug's maximum effectiveness by 1 hour.

DIAGNOSTIC TEST EFFECTS: *None known.*

SIDE EFFECTS

Frequent

Headache (16%), flushing (10%)

Occasional (7%-3%)

Dyspepsia, nasal congestion, UTI, abnormal vision, diarrhea

Rare (2%)

Dizziness, rash

SERIOUS REACTIONS

• Prolonged erections (lasting over 4 hours) and priapism (painful erections lasting over 6 hours) occur rarely.

SPECIAL CONSIDERATIONS

PRECAUTIONS

• The safety of sildenafil citrate is unknown in patients with bleeding disorders and patients with active peptic ulceration. Use sildenafil citrate with caution in patients with anatomic deformation of the penis (such as angulation, cavernosal fibrosis, or Peyronie's disease) or in patients who have conditions that may predispose them to priapism (such as sickle cell anemia, multiple myeloma, or leukemia). The safety and efficacy of combinations of sildenafil citrate with other treatments for erectile dysfunction have not been studied. Therefore the use of such combinations is not recommended. Sildenafil potentiates the antiaggregatory effect of sodium nitroprusside (a nitric oxide donor). The combination of heparin and sildenafil citrate had an additive effect on bleeding time in the anesthetized rabbit, but this interaction has not been studied in human beings.

PATIENT INFORMATION

• Physicians should discuss with patients the contraindication of sildenafil citrate with regular and/or intermittent use of organic nitrates. Physicians also should discuss with patients the potential cardiac risk of sexual activity in patients with preexisting cardiovascular risk factors. Advise patients who experience symptoms (e.g., angina pectoris, dizziness, or nausea) upon initiation of sexual activity to refrain from further activity and to discuss the episode with their physician.

• Physicians should warn patients that prolonged erections greater than 4 hours and priapism (painful erections greater than 6 hours in duration) have been reported infrequently since market approval of sildenafil citrate. In the event of an erection that persists longer than 4 hours, the patient should seek immediate medical assistance. If priapism is not treated immediately, penile tissue damage and permanent loss of potency may result.

- The use of sildenafil citrate offers no protection against sexually transmitted diseases. Consider counseling of patients about the protective measures necessary to guard against sexually transmitted diseases, including the human immunodeficiency virus.

PREGNANCY AND LACTATION

- Pregnancy Category B. Sildenafil citrate is not indicated for use in newborns, children, or women. No evidence of teratogenicity, embryotoxicity, or fetotoxicity was observed in rats and rabbits.

OCULAR CONSIDERATIONS

- Ocular Adverse Effects: Diplopia, temporary vision loss/decreased vision, ocular redness or bloodshot appearance, ocular burning, ocular swelling/pressure, increased intraocular pressure, retinal vascular disease or bleeding, vitreous detachment/traction, and paramacular edema may occur.
- Abnormal vision has been reported (11%): mild and transient, predominantly color tinge to vision, but also increased sensitivity to light or blurred vision. Abnormal vision was more common at 100-mg dose than at lower doses.

silver nitrate

Drug Class: Anti-infectives, ophthalmic; Ophthalmics

CLINICAL PHARMACOLOGY

Mechanism of Action: Free silver ions precipitate bacterial proteins by combining with chloride in tissue forming silver chloride; coagulates cellular protein to form an eschar or scab. The germicidal action is credited to precipitation of bacterial proteins by free silver ions. *Therapeutic Effect:* Inhibits growth of both gram-positive and gram-negative bacteria.

Pharmacokinetics

Minimal gastrointestinal (GI) tract and cutaneous absorption. Minimal excretion in urine.

AVAILABLE FORMS

- *Applicator sticks:* 75% silver nitrate and 25% potassium nitrate.
- *Ophthalmic solution:* 1%.
- *Topical solution:* 10%, 25%, 50%.

INDICATIONS AND DOSAGES

Exuberant granulations

Applicator sticks

Adults, Elderly, Children. Apply to mucous membranes and other moist skin surfaces only on area to be treated 2-3 times/wk for 2-3 wks.

Topical, solution

Adults, Elderly, Children. Apply a cotton applicator dipped in solution on the affected area 2-3 times/wk for 2-3 wks.

Gonococcal ophthalmia neonatorum

Ophthalmic

Children. Instill 2 drops in each eye immediately after delivery.

UNLABELED USES: *Children.* Instill 2 drops in each eye immediately after delivery.

CONTRAINDICATIONS: Broken skin, cuts, or wounds, hypersensitivity to silver nitrate or any of its components

INTERACTIONS

Drug

None known.

Herbal

None known.

Food

None known.

DIAGNOSTIC TEST EFFECTS: *None known.*

SIDE EFFECTS

Occasional

Ophthalmic: Chemical conjunctivitis

Topical: Burning, irritation, staining of the skin

Rare

Hyponatremia, methemoglobinemia

SERIOUS REACTIONS

- Symptoms of overdose include blackening of skin and mucous membranes, pain and burning of the mouth, salivation, vomiting, diarrhea, shock, convulsions, coma, and death.
- Methemoglobinemia is cause by absorbed silver nitrate but occurs rarely.
- Cauterization of the cornea and blindness occur rarely.

SPECIAL CONSIDERATIONS

PRECAUTIONS

- Handle silver nitrate carefully; it can stain skin and utensils. Stains may be removed by applications of iodine tincture followed by sodium thiosulfate solution.

simvastatin

(sim′va-sta-tin)

Rx: Zocor

Drug Class: Antihyperlipidemics; HMG CoA reductase inhibitors

Pregnancy Category: X

Do not confuse Zocor with Cozaar.

CLINICAL PHARMACOLOGY

Mechanism of Action: A HMG-CoA reductase inhibitor that interferes with cholesterol biosynthesis by inhibiting the conversion of the enzyme HMG-CoA to mevalonate. *Therapeutic Effect:* Decreases serum LDL, cholesterol, VLDL, and plasma triglyceride levels; slightly increases serum HDL concentration.

Pharmacokinetics

Route	Onset	Peak	Duration
PO to reduce cholesterol	3 days	14 days	N/A

Well absorbed from the GI tract. Protein binding: 95%. Undergoes extensive first-pass metabolism. Hydrolyzed to active metabolite. Primarily eliminated in feces. Unknown if removed by hemodialysis.

AVAILABLE FORMS

- *Tablets:* 5 mg, 10 mg, 20 mg, 40 mg, 80 mg.

INDICATIONS AND DOSAGES

To decrease elevated total and LDL cholesterol in hypercholesterolemia (types IIa and IIb), lower triglyceride levels, and increase HDL levels; to reduce risk of death and prevent MI in patients with heart disease and elevated cholesterol level; to reduce risk of revascularization procedures; to decrease risk

of stroke or transient ischemic attack; to prevent cardiovascular events.

PO

Adults. Initially, 10-40 mg/day in evening. Dosage adjusted at 4-wk intervals.

Elderly. Initially, 10 mg/day. May increase by 5-10 mg/day q4wk. Range: 5-80 mg/day. Maximum: 80 mg/day.

CONTRAINDICATIONS: Active hepatic disease or unexplained, persistent elevations of liver function test results, age younger than 18 years, pregnancy

INTERACTIONS

Drug

Cyclosporine, erythromycin, gemfibrozil, immunosuppressants, niacin: Increases the risk of acute renal failure and rhabdomyolysis.

Erythromycin, itraconazole, ketoconazole: May increase simvastatin blood concentration and cause muscle inflammation, myalgia, or weakness.

Herbal

None known.

Food

None known.

DIAGNOSTIC TEST EFFECTS: May increase serum CK and serum transaminase concentrations.

SIDE EFFECTS

Simvastatin is generally well tolerated. Side effects are usually mild and transient.

Occasional (3%-2%)

Headache, abdominal pain or cramps, constipation, upper respiratory tract infection

Rare (less than 2%)

Diarrhea, flatulence, asthenia (loss of strength and energy), nausea or vomiting

SERIOUS REACTIONS

• Lens opacities may occur.

• Hypersensitivity reaction and hepatitis occur rarely.

SPECIAL CONSIDEATIONS

PRECAUTIONS

• Simvastatin may cause elevation of creatine kinase and transaminase levels. Simvastatin may cause myopathy. Concomitant administration with verapamil, gemfibrozil, and other fibrates also can cause myopathy.

PATIENT INFORMATION

• Advise patients to report promptly unexplained muscle pain, tenderness, or weakness.

PREGNANCY AND LACTATION

• Pregnancy Category X. Administer simvastatin to women of childbearing age only when such patients are highly unlikely to conceive. Simvastatin is contraindicated during pregnancy and in nursing mothers. Excretion into human milk is not known.

OCULAR CONSIDERATIONS

• Optic nerve degeneration was seen in clinically normal dogs treated with simvastatin for 14 weeks at 180 mg/kg per day, a dose that produced mean plasma drug levels about 12 times higher than the mean plasma drug level in human beings taking 80 mg/day.

• A chemically similar drug in this class also produced optic nerve degeneration (Wallerian degeneration of retinogeniculate fibers) in clinically normal dogs in a dose-dependent fashion starting at 60 mg/kg per day, a dose that produced mean plasma drug levels about 30 times higher than the mean plasma drug level in human beings taking the highest recommended dose (as measured by total enzyme inhibitory activity). This same drug also produced vestibulocochlear Wallerian-like degeneration and retinal ganglion cell chromatolysis in dogs treated for 14 weeks at 180 mg/kg per day, a dose that resulted in a mean plasma drug level similar to that seen with the 60 mg/kg per day dose.

• Central nervous system vascular lesions, characterized by perivascular hemorrhage and edema, mononuclear cell infiltration of perivascular spaces, perivascular fibrin deposits, and necrosis of small vessels were seen in dogs treated with simvastatin at a dose of 360 mg/kg per day, a dose that produced mean plasma drug levels that were about 14 times higher than the mean plasma drug levels in human beings taking 80 mg/day. Similar central nervous system vascular lesions have been observed with several other drugs of this class.

• Female rats developed cataracts after 2 years of treatment with 50 and 100 mg/kg per day (22 and 25 times the human AUC at 80 mg/day, respectively) and in dogs after 3 months at 90 mg/kg per day (19 times) and at 2 years at 50 mg/kg per day (5 times).

---

sodium chloride

(sew'-dee-um klor'-eyed)

Drug Class: Electrolyte replacements; Vitamins/minerals

Pregnancy Category: C

CLINICAL PHARMACOLOGY

Mechanism of Action: Sodium is a major cation of extracellular fluid that controls water distribution, fluid and electrolyte balance, and osmotic pressure of body fluids; it also maintains acid-base balance.

Pharmacokinetics

Well absorbed from the GI tract. Widely distributed. Primarily excreted in urine.

AVAILABLE FORMS

- *Tablets:* 1 g
- *Injection (Concentrate):* 23.4% (4 mEq/ml).
- *Injection:* 0.45%, 0.9%, 3%.
- *Irrigation:* 0.45%, 0.9%.
- *Nasal Gel (Nasal Moist):* 0.65%.
- *Nasal Solution (OTC [SalineX]):* 0.4%.
- *Nasal Solution (OTC [Nasal Moist, SeaMist]):* 0.65%.
- *Ophthalmic Solution (OTC [Muro 128]):* 5%.
- *Ophthalmic Ointment (OTC [Muro 128]):* 5%.

INDICATIONS AND DOSAGES

Prevention and treatment of sodium and chloride deficiencies; source of hydration

IV

Adults, Elderly. 1-2 L/day 0.9% or 0.45% or 100 ml 3% or 5% over 1 hr; assess serum electrolyte levels before giving additional fluid.

Prevention of heat prostration and muscle cramps from excessive perspiration

PO

Adults, Elderly. 1-2 g 3 times a day.

Relief of dry and inflamed nasal membranes

Intranasal

Adults, Elderly. Use as needed.

Diagnostic aid in ophthalmoscopic exam, treatment of corneal edema

Ophthalmic solution

Adults, Elderly. Apply 1-2 drops q3-4h.

Ophthalmic ointment

Adults, Elderly. Apply once a day or as directed.

CONTRAINDICATIONS: Fluid retention, hypernatremia

INTERACTIONS

Drug

Hypertonic saline solution, oxytocics: May cause uterine hypertonus, ruptures, or lacerations.

Herbal

None known.

Food

None known.

DIAGNOSTIC TEST EFFECTS: *None known.*

SIDE EFFECTS

Frequent

Facial flushing

Occasional

Fever; irritation, phlebitis, or extravasation at injection site

Ophthalmic: Temporary burning or irritation

SERIOUS REACTIONS

• Too-rapid administration may produce peripheral edema, CHF, and pulmonary edema.

• Excessive dosage may cause hypokalemia, hypervolemia, and hypernatremia.

SPECIAL CONSIDERATIONS

PATIENT INFORMATION

Give patients the following instructions:

• Sodium chloride is for external use only. To avoid contamination, do not touch the tip of the container to any surface. Replace cap after using. Do not use if the solution changes color and becomes cloudy. Stop use and ask an eye care practitioner if you experience eye pain, changes in vision, or continued redness or irritation of the eye or if the condition worsens or persists for more than 72 hours. Keep out of reach of children.

OCULAR CONSIDERATIONS

• Ocular Indications and Usage: Temporary relief of corneal edema, Fuch's endothelial dystrophy, and bullous keratopathy

• Ocular Adverse Reactions: Burning and stinging

OCULAR DOSAGE AND ADMINISTRATION

• Solution: Instill 1 or 2 drops in the affected eye(s) every 3 to 4 hours.

• Ointment: Pull down lower lid and apply ¼ inch of ointment to the inside of the eyelid every 3 to 4 hours.

---

sodium hyaluronate

(soe'-dee-um hye-a-loo-roe'-nate)

Rx: Amvisc, Amvisc Plus, AQuify Long-Lasting Comfort Drops (OTC), Biolon, blink Contacts Lubricant Eye Drops, Duovisc, Healon, Healon5, Hyalgan, Provisc, Viscoat, Vitrax

Drug Class: Hyaluronic acid derivatives; Ophthalmics

CLINICAL PHARMACOLOGY

Mechanism of Action: A polysaccharide that maintains viscosity of synovial fluid and supports lubricating/shock-absorbing properties of auricular cartilage when used intra-articularly. As an aid in ophthalmic surgery, sodium hyaluronate protects corneal endothelial tissues, decreases the chances for formation of adhesions and synechiae, replaces aqueous humor, maintains a deep anterior chamber during the operative procedure, and helps push back the iris and vitreous. *Therapeutic Effect:* Intra-articular: Decreases pain intensity, joint pain, and morning stiffness. Ophthalmic: Maintains deep anterior chamber during surgical procedures; lessens corneal endothelial damage.

Pharmacokinetics

Intra-articular: Onset of action occurs in 1 to 2 weeks. The peak response occurs in 5 to 9 weeks and may persist for a few months.

Ophthalmic: Excreted via canal of schlemm after intraocular administration.

AVAILABLE FORMS

- *Contact Lens Rewetter:* 0.1%, 0.15%
- *Intra-articular Solution:* 10 mg/ml (Hyalgan, Supartz).
- *Intraocular Kit:* (Duovisc).
- *Intraocular Liquid:* 10 mg/ml (Biolon, Healon, Provisc), 12 mg/ml (Amvisc), 14 mg/ml (Healon), 14 mg (Healon), 16 mg/ml (Amvisc Plus), 23 mg/ml (Healon5), 30 mg/ml (Vitrax).
- *Ophthalmic Solution:* 40 mg-30 mg/ml (Viscoat).

INDICATIONS AND DOSAGES

Contact lens rewetter

1 or 2 drops to each eye as needed. Blink several times.

Treatment of pain in osteoarthritis in knee

Intra-articular

Adults, Elderly. 5 injections/treatment cycle (1 week apart).

Surgical aid, ophthalmic procedures

Intraocular

Adults, Elderly. Depends on procedure.

UNLABELED USES: Rheumatoid arthritis of the knee, painful shoulder, degenerative temporomandibular joint disorders, hip osteoarthritis, wound healing, and in combination with corticosteroids for osteoarthritis of the knee.

CONTRAINDICATIONS: Hypersensitivity to sodium hyaluronate or any component of the formulation, active knee joint infection, skin infection at injection site.

INTERACTIONS

Drug

None known.

Herbal

None known.

Food

None known.

DIAGNOSTIC TEST EFFECTS: *None known.*

SIDE EFFECTS

Occasional

Injection-site pain, skin reaction (ecchymosis, rash), pruritus, headache, gastrointestinal discomfort

Rare

Ophthalmic: Increase in intraocular pressure.

SERIOUS REACTIONS

- Postoperative elevated intraocular pressure may occur.
- Postoperative inflammatory reactions, such as iritis, hypopyon, endophthalmitis, occurs rarely.
- Pseudogout and septic arthritis occur rarely.

SPECIAL CONSIDERATIONS

PRECAUTIONS

- Use caution when injecting sodium hyaluronate into patients who are allergic to avian proteins, feathers, and egg products.

PREGNANCY AND LACTATION

- Pregnancy Category not listed. Reproductive toxicity studies in rats and rabbits have revealed no evidence of impaired fertility or harm to the experimental animal fetus from intraarticular injections of sodium hyaluronate. Excretion into human milk is not known.

OCULAR CONSIDERATIONS

- Ocular Indications and Usage: Surgical adjunct for cataract extraction, intraocular lens implantation (IOL), corneal transplant, glaucoma filtration, retinal attachment surgery, posterior segment surgery, and contact lens rewetter
- Ocular Adverse Reactions: For intraocular use, transient rise in intraocular pressure has been reported. Iritis, hypopyon, corneal

edema, and corneal decompensation may occur.

Contact lens rewetter: Eyes stinging, burning, or itching; excessive watering; unusual eye secretions; redness; reduced sharpness or blurred vision; photophobia; foreign body sensation; rainbows or halos around objects; dry eyes.

OCULAR DOSAGE AND ADMINISTRATION

• Cataract and IOL Surgery: Inject sodium hyaluronate slowly before delivery of IOL to protect corneal endothelium from damage. Sodium hyaluronate may be used to coat the IOL and surgical instruments before insertion. Additional amounts can be injected during surgery for replacement.

• Trabeculectomy: Inject sodium hyaluronate slowly through the corneal paracentesis to reconstitute the anterior chamber. Additional amounts can be allowed to extrude into the subconjunctival filtration site through and around the sutured outer scleral flap.

• Penetrating Keratoplasty: Sodium hyaluronate can be injected into the anterior chamber of the donor eye before transplantation to protect the corneal endothelium from damage. After the corneal button is removed, the anterior chamber of the host eye can be filled. The donor cornea is sutured into place. Additional amounts can be injected during surgery for replacement.

• Retinal Surgery: Inject sodium hyaluronate slowly into the vitreous cavity. Sodium hyaluronate can separate membranes from the retina for safe excision and release of traction, can be used to maneuver tissues into proper position, and can hold the retina against the sclera for reattachment.

• Dry Eyes: Off-label uses include the lubrication and protection of the ocular surface. A 0.1% topical solution in saline up to 4 times a day has been used to reduce symptoms.

sulfacetamide

(sul-fa-see'ta-mide)

Rx: AK-Sulf, Bleph-10, Isopto Cetamide, Klaron, Ocu-Sul 10, Ocu-Sul 15, Ocu-Sul 30, Ocusulf-10, Ovace, S.O.S.S., Sebizon, Sodium Sulamyd, Sulf-10, Sulfac 10%, Sulfacet Sodium

Drug Class: Anti-infectives, ophthalmic; Antibiotics, sulfonamides; Ophthalmics

Pregnancy Category: C

CLINICAL PHARMACOLOGY

Mechanism of Action: Interferes with synthesis of folic acid that bacteria require for growth. *Therapeutic Effect:* Prevents further bacterial growth. Bacteriostatic.

Pharmacokinetics

Small amounts may be absorbed into the cornea. Excreted rapidly in urine. **Half-life:** 7-13 hrs.

AVAILABLE FORMS

• *Lotion:* 10% (Carmol, Klaron, Ovace).

• *Ophthalmic Ointment:* 10% (AK-Sulf).

• *Ophthalmic Solution:* 10% (Bleph-10, Ocusulf, Sulf-10).

INDICATIONS AND DOSAGES

Treatment of corneal ulcers, conjunctivitis and other superficial infections of the eye, prophylaxis after injuries to the eye/removal of foreign bodies, adjunctive therapy for trachoma and inclusion conjunctivitis

Ophthalmic

Adults, Elderly. Ointment: Apply small amount in lower conjunctival sac 1-4 times/day and at bedtime. Solution: 1-3 drops to lower conjunctival sac q2-3h. Seborrheic dermatitis, seborrheic sicca (dandruff), secondary bacterial skin infections

Topical

Adults, Elderly. Apply 1-4 times/day.

UNLABELED USES: Treatment of bacterial blepharitis, blepharoconjunctivitis, bacterial keratitis, keratoconjunctivitis

CONTRAINDICATIONS: Hypersensitivity to sulfonamides or any component of preparation (some products contain sulfite), use in combination with silver-containing products

INTERACTIONS

Drug

Silver-containing preparations: These products are incompatible together.

Herbal

None known.

Food

None known.

DIAGNOSTIC TEST EFFECTS: *None known.*

SIDE EFFECTS

Frequent

Transient ophthalmic burning, stinging

Occasional

Headache

Rare

Hypersensitivity (erythema, rash, itching, swelling, photosensitivity)

SERIOUS REACTIONS

• Superinfection, drug-induced lupus erythematosus, Stevens-Johnson syndrome occur rarely; nephrotoxicity with high dermatologic concentrations.

SPECIAL CONSIDERATIONS

PRECAUTIONS

• Fungal infection may occur. Bacterial resistance to sulfonamides also may develop. Effectiveness may be reduced by the p-aminobenzoic acid present in purulent exudates. Cross-sensitivity between different sulfonamides may occur. Discontinue use at the first sign of hypersensitivity, increase in purulent discharge, or aggravation of inflammation or pain.

PATIENT INFORMATION

Give patients the following instructions:

• Keep bottle tightly closed. Store medication at controlled room temperature: 15° to 30° C (59° to 86° F). Sulfonamide solutions darken on prolonged standing and exposure to heat and light. Do not use if solution has darkened. Yellowishness does not affect activity.

PREGNANCY AND LACTATION

• Pregnancy Category C. Kernicterus may occur in the newborn with orally administered sulfonamides. Fetal harm is not known with topical administration. Systemically administered sulfonamides are capable of producing kernicterus in infants of lactating women.

sulfadiazine

(sul-fa-dye'-a-zeen)

Rx: Sulfadiazine Sodium

Drug Class: Antibiotics, sulfonamides

Pregnancy Category: C

Do not confuse with azathioprine, sulfasalazine, or sulfisoxazole.

CLINICAL PHARMACOLOGY

Mechanism of Action: A sulfonamide derivative that interferes with bacterial growth by inhibiting bacterial folic acid synthesis through competitive antagonism of PABA. *Therapeutic Effect:* Inhibits bacterial growth.

Pharmacokinetics

Well absorbed. Widely distributed throughout body tissues and fluids including pleural, peritoneal, synovial, and ocular fluids and readily diffused into CSF. Metabolized in liver. Excreted in urine. **Half-life:** 10 hrs.

AVAILABLE FORMS

- *Tablets:* 500 mg (Sulfadiazine Sodium).

INDICATIONS AND DOSAGES

Asymptomatic meningococcal carriers

PO

Adults, Elderly. 1 g twice daily for 2 days.

Children 1-12 yr. 500 mg twice daily for 2 days.

Infants 1-12 months. 500 mg once daily for 2 days.

Congenital toxoplasmosis

PO

Children 2 months and older. 25-50 mg/kg/dose 4 times/day.

Children younger than 2 months, Newborns. 100 mg/kg/day divided q6h in conjunction with pyrimethamine 1 mg/kg/day once daily and supplemental folinic ancid 5 mg every 3 days for 6 months.

Nocardiosis

PO

Adults, Elderly. 4-8 g/day for a minimum of 6 weeks.

Rheumatic fever prophylaxis

PO

Adults, Elderly, Children more than 30 kg. 1 g/day.

Children less than 30 kg. 0.5 g/day.

Toxoplasmosis

PO

Adults, Elderly. 2-6 g/day in divided doses q6h in conjunction with pyrimethamine 50-75 mg/day and with supplemental folinic acid.

Children 2 months and older. Loading dose: 75 mg/kg. Maintenance: 120-150 mg/kg/day. Maximum: 6 g/day divided q4-6h in conjunction with pyrimethamine 2 mg/kg/day divided q12h for 3 days followed by 1 mg/kg/day once daily with supplemental folinic acid.

CONTRAINDICATIONS: Porphyria, children less than 2 months of age unless indicated for the treatment of congenital toxoplasmosis, sunscreens containing PABA, pregnancy (at term), hypersensitivity to any sulfa drug or any component of the formulation.

INTERACTIONS

Drug

Oral anticoagulants, oral hypoglycemics: May increase the effects of these drugs.

PABA, PABA metabolites (e.g., procaine, proparacaine, tetracaine, sunblock): May decrease the effect of these drugs.

Herbal

Dong quai, St. John's wort: May cause photosensitization.

Food

Vitamin C, acidifying agents (e.g. cranberry juice): May cause crystalluria.

DIAGNOSTIC TEST EFFECTS: *None known.*

SIDE EFFECTS

Occasional

Fever, dizziness, headache, anorexia, nausea, vomiting, diarrhea, rash, itching, photosensitivity

SERIOUS REACTIONS

- Stevens-Johnson syndrome, hematologic toxicity (leukopenia, agranulocytosis), liver toxicity, and thyroid function disturbance occur rarely.
- Overdosage symptoms include drowsiness, dizziness, anorexia, abdominal pain, nausea, vomiting, he-

molytic anemia, acidosis, jaundice, fever, and agranulocytosis.

SPECIAL CONSIDERATIONS

PRECAUTIONS

• General: Give sulfonamides with caution to patients with impaired renal of hepatic function and to those with severe allergy or bronchial asthma.

• Hemolysis may occur in individuals deficient in glucose-6-phosphate dehydrogenase. This reaction is dose related.

• Advise patient to maintain adequate fluid intake to prevent crystalluria and stone formation.

• Information for the Patient: Instruct patients to drink an 8-oz glass of water with each dose of medication and at frequent intervals throughout the day. Caution patients to report promptly the onset of sore throat, fever, pallor, purpura, or jaundice when taking this drug, because these may be early indications of serious blood disorders.

• Carcinogenesis, Mutagenesis, and Impairment of Fertility: The sulfonamides bear certain chemical similarities to some goitrogens. Rats appear to be especially susceptible to the goitrogenic effects of sulfonamides, and long-term administration has produced thyroid malignancies in rats.

PREGNANCY AND LACTATION

• Pregnancy Category C. The teratogenic potential of most sulfonamides has not been thoroughly investigated in animals or human beings. However, a significant increase in the incidence of cleft palate and other bony abnormalities in offspring has been observed when certain sulfonamides of the short-, intermediate-, and long-acting types were given to pregnant rats and mice in high oral doses. Sulfadiazine is contraindicated for use in nursing mothers because the sulfonamides cross the placenta, are excreted in breast milk, and may cause kernicterus.

sulfamethoxazole; trimethoprim

(koe-trye-mox'a-zole)

Rx: Bactrim, Bactrim DS, Bactrim Pediatric, Bethaprim, Bethaprim Pediatric, Septra, Septra DS, Septra I.V., Septra Infusion, SMX-TMP Plain, Sulfatrim, Sulfatrim Pediatric, Sulfatrim Suspension, Uroplus, Uroplus DS

Drug Class: Antibiotics, folate antagonists; Antibiotics, sulfonamides

Pregnancy Category: C

Do not confuse Bactrim with bacitracin, co-trimoxazole with clotrimazole, or Septra with Sectral or Septa.

CLINICAL PHARMACOLOGY

Mechanism of Action: A sulfonamide and folate antagonist that blocks bacterial synthesis of essential nucleic acids. *Therapeutic Effect:* Bactericidal in susceptible microorganisms.

Pharmacokinetics

Rapidly and well absorbed from the GI tract. Protein binding: 45%-60%. Widely distributed. Metabolized in the liver. Excreted in urine. Minimally removed by hemodialysis. **Half-life:** sulfamethoxazole 6-12 hr, trimethoprim 8-10 hr (increased in impaired renal function).

AVAILABLE FORMS

• **Alert:** All dosage forms have same 5:1 ratio of sulfamethoxazole (SMX) to trimethoprim (TMP).

• *Oral Suspension (Septra, Sulfatrim Pediatric):* SMX 200 mg and TMP 40 mg per 5 ml.

• *Tablets (Bactrim, Septra):* SMX 400 mg and TMP 80 mg.
• *Tablets (Double Strength [Bactrim DS, Septra DS]):* SMX 800 mg and TMP 160 mg.
• *Injection (Septra):* SMX 80 mg and TMP 16 mg per ml.

INDICATIONS AND DOSAGES

Mild to moderate infections

PO, IV

Adults, Elderly, Children older than 2 mo. 6-12 mg/kg/day in divided doses q12h.

Serious infections,* Pneumocystis carinii *pneumonia (PCP)

PO, IV

Adults, Elderly, Children older than 2 mo. 15-20 mg/kg/day in divided doses q6-8 h.

Prevention of PCP

PO

Adults. One double-strength tablet each day.

Children. 150 mg/m^2/day on 3 consecutive days/wk.

Traveler's diarrhea

PO

Adults, Elderly. One double-strength tablet q12h for 5 days.

Acute exacerbation of chronic bronchitis

PO

Adults, Elderly. One double-strength tablet q12h for 14 days.

Prevention of UTIs

PO

Adults, Elderly, children older than 2 mo. 2 mg/kg/dose once a day.

Dosage in renal impairment

Dosage and frequency are modified based on creatinine clearance, the severity of the infection and the serum concentration of the drug. For those with creatinine clearance of 15-30 ml/min, a 50% dosage reduction is recommended.

UNLABELED USES: Treatment of bacterial endocarditis; gonorrhea; meningitis; septicemia; sinusitis; and biliary tract, bone, joint, chancroid, chlamydial, intra-abdominal, skin and soft-tissue infections

CONTRAINDICATIONS: Hypersensitivity to trimethoprim or any sulfonamides, infants younger than 2 months old, megaloblastic anemia due to folate deficiency.

INTERACTIONS

Drug

Hemolytics: May increase the risk of toxicity.

Hepatotoxic medications: May increase the risk of hepatotoxicity.

Hydantoin anticonvulsants, oral antidiabetics, warfarin: May increase or prolong the effects of these drugs and increase their risk of toxicity.

Methenamine: May form a precipitate.

Methotrexate: May increase the effects of methotrexate.

Herbal

None known.

Food

None known.

DIAGNOSTIC TEST EFFECTS: May increase BUN and serum alkaline phosphatase, creatinine, potassium, AST (SGOT), and ALT (SGPT) levels.

IV INCOMPATIBILITIES: Fluconazole (Diflucan), foscarnet (Foscavir), midazolam (Versed), vinorelbine (Navelbine)

IV COMPATIBILITIES: Diltiazem (Cardizem), heparin, hydromorphone (Dilaudid), lorazepam (Ativan), magnesium sulfate, morphine

SIDE EFFECTS

Frequent

Anorexia, nausea, vomiting, rash (generally 7-14 days after therapy begins), urticaria

Occasional

Diarrhea, abdominal pain, pain or irritation at the IV infusion site

Rare
Headache, vertigo, insomnia, seizures, hallucinations, depression

SERIOUS REACTIONS

- Rash, fever, sore throat, pallor, purpura, cough, and shortness of breath may be early signs of serious adverse reactions.
- Fatalities have occasionally occurred after Stevens-Johnson syndrome, toxic epidermal necrolysis, fulminant hepatic necrosis, agranulocytosis, aplastic anemia, and other blood dyscrasias in patients taking sulfonamides.
- Myelosuppression, decreased platelet count and severe dermatologic reactions may occur, especially in the elderly.

SPECIAL CONSIDERATIONS

PRECAUTIONS

- Rare fatalities have been associated with the administration of sulfonamides that caused severe reactions including Stevens-Johnson syndrome, toxic epidermal necrolysis, fulminant hepatic necrosis, agranulocytosis, aplastic anemia, and other blood dyscrasias. Discontinue use at the first appearance of skin rash or any sign of adverse reaction. Clinical signs such as rash, sore throat, fever, arthralgia, pallor, purpura, or jaundice may be early indications of serious reactions. Cough, shortness of breath, and pulmonary infiltrates are hypersensitivity reactions of the respiratory tract in association with sulfonamide treatment. Pseudomembranous colitis has been reported and may range in severity from mild to life threatening. Give sulfamethoxazole with caution to patients with impaired renal or hepatic function, to those with possible folate deficiency, and to those with severe allergies or bronchial asthma. In individuals deficient in glucose-6-phosphate dehydrogenase, hemolysis may occur. Trimethoprim has been noted to impair phenylalanine metabolism. Caution is advisable in patients with porphyria or thyroid dysfunction.

PREGNANCY AND LACTATION

- Pregnancy Category C. Sulfamethoxazole and trimethoprim are contraindicated in pregnant patients and nursing mothers, because sulfonamides pass the placenta and are excreted in the milk and may cause kernicterus.

OCULAR CONSIDERATIONS

Ocular Indications and Usage

- Preseptal cellulitis; urinary tract infections, acute otitis media, chronic bronchitis, shigellosis, *Pneumocystis carinii* pneumonia, and traveler's diarrhea

OCULAR DOSAGE AND ADMINISTRATION

- In preseptal cellulitis, for patients allergic to penicillin (mild): Adults, 800 mg sulfamethoxazole and 160 mg trimethoprim orally; children over 5 years, 40 mg/kg per day sulfamethoxazole and 8 mg/kg per day trimethoprim orally in two divided doses
- This drug combination is not recommended for use in pediatric patients less than 2 months of age. The usual adult dosage in the treatment of urinary tract infections is 1 sulfamethoxazole/trimethoprim DS (double-strength) tablet, 2 sulfamethoxazole/trimethoprim tablets, or 4 teaspoonfuls (20 ml) of sulfamethoxazole/trimethoprim pediatric suspension every 12 hours for 10 to 14 days.
- The usual adult dosage in the treatment of acute exacerbations of chronic bronchitis is 1 sulfamethoxazole/trimethoprim DS tablet, 2 sulfamethoxazole/trimethoprim tablets, or 4 teaspoonfuls (20 ml) of

sulfamethoxazole/trimethoprim pediatric suspension every 12 hours for 14 days.

• The recommended dosage for treatment of patients with documented *Pneumocystis carinii* pneumonia is 15 to 20 mg/kg trimethoprim and 75 to 100 mg/kg sulfamethoxazole per 24 hours given in equally divided doses every 6 hours for 14 to 21 days.

• For the treatment of traveler's diarrhea, the usual adult dosage is 1 sulfamethoxazole/trimethoprim DS tablet, 2 sulfamethoxazole/trimethoprim tablets, or 4 teaspoonfuls (20 ml) of pediatric suspension every 12 hours for 5 days.

---

suprofen

(soo-proe'-fen)

Drug Class: Nonsteroidal antiinflammatory drugs; Ophthalmics

Pregnancy Category: C

CLINICAL PHARMACOLOGY

Mechanism of Action: A nonsteroidal antiinflammatory that inhibits prostaglandin synthesis and the intensity of pain stimulus reaching sensory nerve endings. Constricts iris sphincter. *Therapeutic Effect:* Produces analgesic and antiinflammatory effect. Prevents miosis during cataract surgery.

Pharmacokinetics

No data available on systemic absorption.

AVAILABLE FORMS

• *Ophthalmic Solution:* 1% (Profenal).

INDICATIONS AND DOSAGES

Miosis inhibitor in ophthalmic surgery

OphthalmicAdults, Elderly. Apply 2 drops 3, 2, and 1 hour prior to surgery. If desired, 2 drops may be applied q4h while the patient is awake on the day prior to surgery.

CONTRAINDICATIONS: Rhinitis, urticaria, asthma, allergic reactions to aspirin or other antiinflammatory agents, epithelial herpes keratitis, hypersensitivity to suprofen or any component of the formulation.

INTERACTIONS

Drug

None known.

Herbal

None known.

Food

None known.

DIAGNOSTIC TEST EFFECTS: *None known.*

SIDE EFFECTS

Frequent

Burning, stinging on instillation, ocular discomfort

Occasional

Itching, tearing

Rare

Headache, trouble sleeping, weakness

SERIOUS REACTIONS

• Nausea or vomiting, pain, sensitivity to light, trouble breathing, and shortness of breath occur rarely.

SPECIAL CONSIDERATIONS

PRECAUTIONS

• Suprofen is contraindicated in patients with active herpes simplex keratitis. Consider the possibility of increased ocular bleeding during surgery associated with use of nonsteroidal antiinflammatory drugs.

PREGNANCY AND LACTATION

• Pregnancy Category C. Oral doses in rats and rabbits resulted in stillbirths and a decrease in postnatal survival. Fetal harm is not known with topical administration. Suprofen is excreted in human milk after a single oral dose.

OCULAR CONSIDERATIONS

• Off-label uses include treatment of giant papillary conjunctivitis. Suprofen provides reduction of papillae and mucous strands.

tacrolimus

(tak-roe-leem′us)

Rx: Prograf, Protopic

Drug Class: Dermatologics; Immunosuppressives

Pregnancy Category: C

Do not confuse Protopic with Protonix, Protopam, Protopin.

CLINICAL PHARMACOLOGY

Mechanism of Action: An immunologic agent that inhibits T-lymphocyte activation by binding to intracellular proteins, forming a complex, and inhibiting phosphatase activity. *Therapeutic Effect:* Suppresses the immunologically mediated inflammatory response; prevents organ transplant rejection.

Pharmacokinetics

Variably absorbed after PO administration (food reduces absorption). Protein binding: 75%-97%. Extensively metabolized in the liver. Excreted in urine. Not removed by hemodialysis. **Half-life:** 11.7 hr.

AVAILABLE FORMS

• *Capsules (Prograf):* 0.5 mg, 1 mg, 5 mg.

• *Injection (Prograf):* 5 mg/ml.

• *Ointment (Protopic):* 0.03%, 0.1%.

INDICATIONS AND DOSAGES

Prevention of liver transplant rejection

PO

Adults, Elderly. 0.1-0.15 mg/kg/day in 2 divided doses 12 hr apart.

Children. 0.15-0.2 mg/kg/day in 2 divided doses 12 hr apart.

IV

Adults, Elderly, Children. 0.03-0.15 mg/kg/day as a continuous infusion.

Prevention of kidney transplant rejection

PO

Adults, Elderly. 0.2 mg/kg/day in 2 divided doses 12 hr apart

IV

Adults, Elderly. 0.03-0.15 mg/kg/day as continuous infusion.

Atopic dermatitis

Topical

Adults, Elderly, Children 2 yr and older. Apply 0.03% ointment to affected area twice a day. 0.1% ointment may be used in adults and the elderly. Continue until 1 wk after symptoms have cleared.

UNLABELED USES: Prevention of organ rejection in patients receiving allogeneic bone marrow, heart, pancreas, pancreatic island cell, or small-bowel transplant, treatment of autoimmune disease, severe recalcitrant psoriasis

CONTRAINDICATIONS: Concurrent use with cyclosporine (increases the risk of nephrotoxicity), hypersensitivity to HCO-60 polyoxyl 60 hydrogenated castor oil (used in solution for injection), hypersensitivity to tacrolimus

INTERACTIONS

Drug

Aminoglycosides, amphotericin B, cisplatin: Increase the risk of renal dysfunction.

Antacids: Decrease the absorption of tacrolimus.

Antifungals, bromocriptine, calcium channel blockers, cimetidine, clarithromycin, cyclosporine, danazol, diltiazem, erythromycin, methylprednisolone, metoclopramide: Increase tacrolimus blood concentration.

Carbamazepine, phenobarbital, phenytoin, rifamycin: Decrease tacrolimus blood concentration.
Cyclosporine: Increases the risk of nephrotoxicity.
Live-virus vaccines: May potentiate virus replication, increase vaccine side effects, and decrease the patient's antibody response to the vaccine.
Other immunosuppressants: May increase the risk of infection or lymphomas.

Herbal

Echinacea: May decrease the effects of tacrolimus.

Food

Grapefruit, grapefruit juice: May alter the effects of the drug.

DIAGNOSTIC TEST EFFECTS: May increase blood glucose, BUN, and serum creatinine levels, as well as WBC count. May decrease serum magnesium level and RBC and thrombocyte counts. May alter serum potassium level.

IV INCOMPATIBILITIES: No known drug incompatibilities. Do not mix tacrolimus with other medications if possible.

IV COMPATIBILITIES: Calcium gluconate, dexamethasone (Decadron), diphenhydramine (Benadryl), dobutamine (Dobutrex), dopamine (Intropin), furosemide (Lasix), heparin, hydromorphone (Dilaudid), insulin, leucovorin, lorazepam (Ativan), morphine, nitroglycerin, potassium chloride

SIDE EFFECTS

Frequent (greater than 30%)

Headache, tremor, insomnia, paresthesia, diarrhea, nausea, constipation, vomiting, abdominal pain, hypertension

Occasional (29%-10%)

Rash, pruritus, anorexia, asthenia, peripheral edema, photosensitivity

SERIOUS REACTIONS

- Nephrotoxicity (characterized by increased serum creatinine level and decreased urine output), neurotoxicity (including tremor, headache, and mental status changes), and pleural effusion are common adverse reactions.
- Thrombocytopenia, leukocytosis, anemia, atelectasis, sepsis, and infection occur occasionally.

SPECIAL CONSIDERATIONS

OCULAR CONSIDERATIONS

- Tacrolimus (Prograf) is being evaluated for the treatment of dry eye and seasonal allergic conjunctivitis. (Bonner H: Ocular drug preview: spotlight on emerging pharmaceuticals, *Rev Optometry* vol 141, issue 12, 2004. http://www.revoptom.com/index.asp?page=2_1309.htm.)

---

tamoxifen citrate

(ta-mox'i-fen)

Rx: Nolvadex

Drug Class: Antineoplastics, antiestrogens; Estrogen receptor modulators, selective; Hormones/hormone modifiers

Pregnancy Category: D

CLINICAL PHARMACOLOGY

Mechanism of Action: A nonsteroidal antiestrogen that competes with estradiol for estrogen-receptor binding sites in the breasts, uterus, and vagina. *Therapeutic Effect:* Inhibits DNA synthesis and estrogen response.

Pharmacokinetics

Well absorbed from the GI tract. Metabolized in the liver. Primarily eliminated in feces by biliary system. **Half-life:** 7 days.

AVAILABLE FORMS

- *Tablets:* 10 mg, 20 mg.

INDICATIONS AND DOSAGES

Adjunctive treatment of breast cancer

PO

Adults, Elderly. 20-40 mg/day. Give doses greater than 20 mg/day in divided doses.

Prevention of breast cancer in high-risk women

PO

Adults, Elderly. 20 mg/day.

UNLABELED USES: Induction of ovulation

CONTRAINDICATIONS: None known.

INTERACTIONS

Drug

Estrogens: May decrease the effects of tamoxifen.

Herbal

None known.

Food

None known.

DIAGNOSTIC TEST EFFECTS: May increase serum cholesterol, calcium, and triglyceride levels.

SIDE EFFECTS

Frequent

Women (greater than 10%): Hot flashes, nausea, vomiting

Occasional

Women (9%-1%): Changes in menstruation, genital itching, vaginal discharge, endometrial hyperplasia or polyps

Men: Impotence, decreased libido

Men and women: Headache, nausea, vomiting, rash, bone pain, confusion, weakness, somnolence

SERIOUS REACTIONS

• Retinopathy, corneal opacity, and decreased visual acuity have been noted in patients receiving extremely high dosages (240-320 mg/day) for longer than 17 months.

SPECIAL CONSIDERATIONS

PRECAUTIONS

• In patients with significant thrombocytopenia, rare hemorrhagic episodes have occurred, but it is uncertain if these episodes are due to tamoxifen citrate therapy. Leukopenia has been observed, sometimes in association with anemia and/or thrombocytopenia.

• Reports of neutropenia and pancytopenia in patients receiving tamoxifen citrate have been rare; this condition sometimes can be severe.

PATIENT INFORMATION

• Reduction in Invasive Breast Cancer and Ductal Carcinoma in Situ in Women: Women with ductal carcinoma in situ treated with lumpectomy and radiation therapy who are considering tamoxifen citrate to reduce the incidence of a second breast cancer event should assess the risks and benefits of therapy, because treatment with tamoxifen citrate decreased the incidence of invasive breast cancer but has not been shown to affect survival.

• Reduction in Breast Cancer Incidence in High-Risk Women: Women should understand that tamoxifen citrate reduces the incidence of breast cancer but may not eliminate risk. Tamoxifen citrate decreased the incidence of small estrogen receptor positive tumors but did not alter the incidence of estrogen receptor negative tumors or larger tumors. Advise women with breast cancer who are at high risk of developing a second breast cancer that treatment with about 5 years of tamoxifen citrate reduced the annual incidence rate of a second breast cancer by approximately 50%.

• Women who are pregnant or who plan to become pregnant should not take tamoxifen citrate to reduce their risk of breast cancer.

• Monitoring during Tamoxifen Citrate Therapy: Instruct women taking or having previously taken tamoxifen citrate to seek prompt medical attention for new breast lumps, vaginal bleeding, gynecologic symptoms (menstrual irregularities, changes in vaginal discharge, or pelvic pain or pressure), symptoms of leg swelling or tenderness, unexplained shortness of breath, or changes in vision. Women should inform all health care providers, regardless of the reason for evaluation, that they take tamoxifen citrate.

• Women taking tamoxifen citrate to reduce the incidence of breast cancer should have a breast examination, a mammogram, and a gynecologic examination before the initiation of therapy. These studies should be repeated at regular intervals while the women are receiving therapy, in keeping with good medical practice. Women taking tamoxifen citrate as adjuvant breast cancer therapy should follow the same monitoring procedures as for women taking tamoxifen citrate for the reduction in the incidence of breast cancer. Women taking tamoxifen citrate as treatment for metastatic breast cancer should review this monitoring plan with their health care provider and select the appropriate modalities and schedule of evaluation.

PREGNANCY AND LACTATION

• Pregnancy Category D. Tamoxifen citrate may cause fetal harm when administered to a pregnant woman. Advise women not to become pregnant while taking tamoxifen citrate and to use barrier or nonhormonal contraceptive measures if they are sexually active. Excretion into human milk is not known.

OCULAR CONSIDERATIONS

• Ocular disturbances, including corneal changes, cataracts, decrement in color vision perception, retinal vein thrombosis, and retinopathy have been reported in patients receiving tamoxifen citrate. An increased incidence of cataracts and the need for cataract surgery have been reported in patients receiving tamoxifen citrate.

• In the NSABP P-1 trial, an increased risk of borderline significance of developing cataracts among those women without cataracts at baseline (540, tamoxifen citrate; 483, placebo; RR = 1.13, 95% CI: 1.00 to 1.28) was observed. Among these same women, tamoxifen citrate was associated with an increased risk of having cataract surgery. Among all women on the trial (with or without cataracts at baseline), tamoxifen citrate was associated with an increased risk of having cataract surgery (210, tamoxifen citrate; 129, placebo; RR = 1.51, 95% CI: 1.21 to 1.89). Eye examinations were not required during the study. No other conclusions regarding noncataract ocular events can be made.

tamsulosin hydrochloride

(tam-sool'o-sin)
Rx: Flomax
Drug Class: Antiadrenergics, alpha blocking
Pregnancy Category: B
Do not confuse Flomax with Fosamax or Volmax.

CLINICAL PHARMACOLOGY
Mechanism of Action: An $alpha_1$ antagonist that targets receptors around bladder neck and prostate capsule. *Therapeutic Effect:* Relaxes smooth muscle and improves urinary flow and symptoms of prostatic hyperplasia.
Pharmacokinetics
Well absorbed and widely distributed. Protein binding: 94%-99%. Metabolized in the liver. Primarily excreted in urine. Unknown if removed by hemodialysis. **Half-life:** 9-13 hr.
AVAILABLE FORMS
• *Capsules:* 0.4 mg.
INDICATIONS AND DOSAGES
Benign prostatic hyperplasia
PO
Adults. 0.4 mg once a day, approximately 30 min after same meal each day. May increase dosage to 0.8 mg if inadequate response in 2-4 wk.
CONTRAINDICATIONS: History of sensitivity to tamsulosin
INTERACTIONS
Drug
Other alpha-adrenergic blocking agents (such as cimetidine, doxazosin, prazosin, terazosin): May increase the alpha-blockade effects of both drugs.
Warfarin: May alter the effects of warfarin.
Herbal
None known.
Food
None known.
DIAGNOSTIC TEST EFFECTS: *None known.*
SIDE EFFECTS
Frequent (9%-7%)
Dizziness, somnolence
Occasional (5%-3%)
Headache, anxiety, insomnia, orthostatic hypotension
Rare (less than 2%)
Nasal congestion, pharyngitis, rhinitis, nausea, vertigo, impotence
SERIOUS REACTIONS
• First-dose syncope (hypotension with sudden loss of consciousness) may occur within 30 to 90 minutes after administration of initial dose and may be preceded by tachycardia (pulse rate of 120-160 beats/minute).

SPECIAL CONSIDERATIONS

PRECAUTIONS
• Amblyopia was reported in one patient with 0.4-mg dosing (0.2%) and in 10 patients (2.0%) with the 0.8-mg dosing.

telmisartan

(tel-meh-sar'-tan)
Rx: Micardis
Drug Class: Angiotensin II receptor antagonists
Pregnancy Category: C, 1st; D, 2nd / 3rd

CLINICAL PHARMACOLOGY
Mechanism of Action: An angiotensin II receptor, type AT_1, antagonist that blocks vasoconstrictor and aldosterone-secreting effects of angiotensin II, inhibiting the binding of angiotensin II to the AT_1 receptors. *Therapeutic Effect:* Causes vasodilation, decreases peripheral resistance, and decreases BP.

Pharmacokinetics

Rapidly and completely absorbed after PO administration. Protein binding: greater than 99%. Undergoes metabolism in the liver to inactive metabolite. Excreted in feces. Unknown if removed by hemodialysis. **Half-life:** 24 hr.

AVAILABLE FORMS

- *Tablets:* 20 mg, 40 mg, 80 mg.

INDICATIONS AND DOSAGES

Hypertension

PO

Adults, Elderly. 40 mg once a day. Range: 20-80 mg/day.

UNLABELED USES: Treatment of CHF

CONTRAINDICATIONS: None known.

INTERACTIONS

Drug

Digoxin: Increases digoxin plasma concentration.

Warfarin: Slightly decreases warfarin plasma concentration.

Herbal

None known.

Food

None known.

DIAGNOSTIC TEST EFFECTS: May increase serum creatinine level. May decrease blood Hgb and Hct levels.

SIDE EFFECTS

Occasional (7%-3%)

Upper respiratory tract infection, sinusitis, back or leg pain, diarrhea

Rare (1%)

Dizziness, headache, fatigue, nausea, heartburn, myalgia, cough, peripheral edema

SERIOUS REACTIONS

- Overdosage may manifest as hypotension and tachycardia. Bradycardia occurs less often.

SPECIAL CONSIDERATIONS

PRECAUTIONS

- Patients with biliary obstructive disorders or hepatic insufficiency can be expected to have reduced clearance. Changes in renal function have been reported in susceptible individuals. In patients with unilateral or bilateral renal artery stenosis, increases in serum creatinine or blood urea nitrogen have been reported.

PATIENT INFORMATION

- Pregnancy: Inform female patients of childbearing age about the consequences of second- and third-trimester exposure to drugs that act on the renin-angiotensin system, and inform them that these consequences do not appear to have resulted from intrauterine drug exposure that has been limited to the first trimester. Ask these patients to report pregnancies to their physicians as soon as possible.

PREGNANCY AND LACTATION

- Pregnancy Categories C (first trimester) and D (second and third trimesters). The use of drugs that act directly on the renin-angiotensin system during the second and third trimesters of pregnancy has been associated with fetal and neonatal injury, including hypotension, neonatal skull hypoplasia, anuria, reversible or irreversible renal failure, and death. Whether telmisartan is excreted in human milk is not known, but telmisartan was shown to be present in the milk of lactating rats.

terazosin hydrochloride

(ter-a'zoe-sin)

Rx: Hytrin

Drug Class: Antiadrenergics, alpha blocking; Antiadrenergics, peripheral

Pregnancy Category: C

CLINICAL PHARMACOLOGY

Mechanism of Action: An antihypertensive and benign prostatic hyperplasia agent that blocks alpha-adrenergic receptors. Produces vasodilation, decreases peripheral resistance, and targets receptors around bladder neck and prostate. *Therapeutic Effect:* In hypertension, decreases BP. In benign prostatic hyperplasia, relaxes smooth muscle and improves urine flow.

Pharmacokinetics

Route	Onset	Peak	Duration
PO	15 min	1-2 hr	12-24 hr

Rapidly, completely absorbed from the GI tract. Protein binding: 90%-94%. Metabolized in the liver to active metabolite. Primarily eliminated in feces via biliary system; excreted in urine. Not removed by hemodialysis. **Half-life:** 12 hr.

AVAILABLE FORMS

- *Capsules:* 1 mg, 2 mg, 5 mg, 10 mg.
- *Tablets:* 1 mg, 2 mg, 5 mg, 10 mg.

INDICATIONS AND DOSAGES

Mild to moderate hypertension

PO

Adults, Elderly. Initially, 1 mg at bedtime. Slowly increase dosage to desired levels. Range: 1-5 mg/day as single or 2 divided doses. Maximum: 20 mg.

Benign prostatic hyperplasia

PO

Adults, Elderly. Initially, 1 mg at bedtime. May increase up to 10 mg/day. Maximum: 20 mg/day.

CONTRAINDICATIONS: None known.

INTERACTIONS

Drug

Estrogen, NSAIDs, other sympathomimetics: May decrease the effects of terazosin.

Hypotension-producing medications, such as antihypertensives and diuretics: May increase the effects of terazosin.

Herbal

Dong quai, ginseng, garlic, yohimbe: May decrease the effects of terazosin.

Food

None known.

DIAGNOSTIC TEST EFFECTS: May decrease blood Hgb and Hct levels, serum albumin level, total serum protein level, and WBC count.

SIDE EFFECTS

Frequent (9%-5%)

Dizziness, headache, unusual tiredness

Rare (less than 2%)

Peripheral edema, orthostatic hypotension, myalgia, arthralgia, blurred vision, nausea, vomiting, nasal congestion, somnolence

SERIOUS REACTIONS

- First-dose syncope (hypotension with sudden loss of consciousness) may occur 30 to 90 minutes after initial dose of 2 mg or more, a too rapid increase in dosage, or addition of another antihypertensive agent to therapy. First-dose syncope may be preceded by tachycardia (pulse rate of 120-160 beats/minute).

SPECIAL CONSIDERATIONS

PRECAUTIONS

• Carcinoma of the prostate and benign prostatic hypertrophy cause many of the same symptoms. These two diseases frequently coexist. Although syncope is the most severe orthostatic effect of terazosin, other symptoms of lowered blood pressure such as dizziness, light-headedness, and palpitations are more common.

PATIENT INFORMATION

• (See the prescribing information received with the prescription for further information.) Make patients aware of the possibility of syncopal and orthostatic symptoms, especially at the initiation of therapy, and advise them to avoid driving or hazardous tasks for 12 hours after the first dose, after a dosage increase, and after interruption of therapy when treatment is resumed. Caution patients to avoid situations where injury could result should syncope occur during initiation of terazosin therapy. Also advise patients of the need to sit or lie down when symptoms of lowered blood pressure occur, although these symptoms are not always orthostatic, and to be careful when rising from a sitting or lying position. If dizziness, lightheadedness, or palpitations are bothersome, patients should report these to the physician so that dose adjustment can be considered. Inform patients that drowsiness or somnolence can occur with terazosin, requiring caution in persons who must drive or operate heavy machinery.

• Advise patients about the possibility of priapism as a result of treatment with terazosin and other similar medications. Patients should know that this reaction to terazosin is rare, but that if it is not brought to immediate medical attention, it can lead to permanent erectile dysfunction (impotence).

PREGNANCY AND LACTATION

• Pregnancy Category C. Terazosin was not teratogenic in rats or rabbits that were administered oral doses. Fetal harm is not known with topical administration. Excretion into human milk is not known.

---

tetracaine

(tet'ra-cane)

Rx: AK-T-Caine, Dextrose-Pontocaine HCl, Pontocaine, Pontocaine HCl, Pontocaine Ophthalmic

Drug Class: Anesthetics, local; Anesthetics, spinal

Pregnancy Category: C

Do not confuse with procaine, lidocaine.

CLINICAL PHARMACOLOGY

Mechanism of Action: Tetracaine causes a reversible blockade of nerve conduction by decreasing nerve membrance permeability to sodium. *Therapeutic effect:* Local anesthetic.

Pharmacokinetics

Systemic absorption of tetracaine is variable. Metabolized by plasma pseudocholinesterasis. Excreted in the urine.

AVAILABLE FORMS

• *Solution for injection:* 0.2%, 0.3%, 1%, 2% (Pontocaine)
• *Cream:* 1%
• *Ointment:* 0.5%

INDICATIONS AND DOSAGES

Anesthetize lower abdomen

Spinal

Adults. 3-4 ml (9-12 mg) of a 0.3% solution

T

Anesthetize perineum
Spinal
Adults. 1-2 ml (3-6 mg) of a 0.3% solution
Anesthetize upper abdomen
Spinal
Adults. 5 ml (15 mg) of a 0.3% solution
Obstetric anesthesia, low spinal (saddle block) anesthesia
Spinal
Adults. 1-2 ml (2-14 mg) of a 0.2% solution
Anesthesia of the perineum
Intrathecal
Adults. 0.5 ml (5 mg) as a 1% solution, diluted with equal amount of CSF or 10% dextrose injection.
Anesthesia of the perineum and lower extremeties
Intrathecal
Adults. 1 ml (10 mg) as a 1% solution, diluted with equal amount of CSF or 10% dextrose injection.
Anesthesia up to the costal margin
Intrathecal
Adults. 1.5-2 ml (15-20 mg) as a 1% solution, diluted with equal amount of CSF.
Topical anesthesia
Topical
Adults. Apply to the affected areas as needed. Maximum dosage is 28 g per 24 hours.
Children. Apply to the affected areas as needed. Maximum dosage is 7 g in a 24-hour period.
Topical anesthesia of nose and throat, abolish laryngeal and esophageal reflexes prior to diagnostic procedure
Topical
Adults. Direct application of a 0.25% or 0.5% topical solution or by oral inhalation of a nebulized 0.5% solution. Total dose should not exceed 20 mg.
Mild pain, burning and/or pruritus associated with herpes labialis (cold sores or fever blisters)
Topical
Adults and children 2 years and older. Apply to the affected area no more than 3-4 times a day.
Ophthalmic anesthesia
Topical
Adults. 1-2 drops of a 0.5% solution.

CONTRAINDICATIONS: Hypersensitivity, to esther local anesthetics, sulfites, PABA, infection or inflammation at the injection site, bactermia, platelet abnormalities, thrombocytopenia, increased bleeding time, uncontrolled coagulopathy, or anticoagulant therapy, sulfonamide therapy.

INTERACTIONS

Drug

Local anesthetics: The toxic effects are additive.

Cholinesterase inhibitors: Local anesthetics can antagonize the effects of these medications.

Neuromuscular blockers: Local anesthetics prolong and enhance the effects of these medications.

Anihypertensives, nitrates, vasodilators: Additive hypotensive effects.

Opiate agonists: lay lead to increased depression of the CNS

Class IA and III antiarrhythmics, macrolide and ketolide antibiotics, quinolone antibiotics, alfuzosin, arsenic trioxide, astemizole, beta agonists, amoxapine, bepridil, cisapride, chloroquine, clozapine, cyclobenzaprine, dolasetron, droperidol, flecainide, halofantrine, haloperidol, halogenated anesthetics, levomethadyl, maprotiline, methadone, octreotide, palonosetron, pentamidine, chlorpromazine, fluphenazine, mesoridazine, pimozide, probucol, propafenone, risperidone, sertindole, tacrolimus, ter-

fenadine, vardenafil, ziprasidone: May increase the risk of cardiotoxicity, including QT prolongation.

MAOIs: Increased risk of hypotension.

Herbal

None known.

Food

None known.

DIAGNOSTIC TEST EFFECTS: *None known.*

IV COMPATIBILITIES: Water, physiologic saline solution, dextrose solution, CSF

SIDE EFFECTS

Frequent

Burning stinging, or tenderness, skin rash, itching, redness, or inflammation, numbness or tingling of the face or mouth, pain at the injection site, sensitivity to light, swelling of the eye or eyelid, watering or the eyes, acute ocular pain and ocular irritation (burning, stinging, or redness)

Occasional

Paresthesias, weakness and paralysis of lower extremity, hypotension, high or total spinal block, urinary retention or incontinence, fecal incontinence, headache, back pain, septic meningitis, meningismus, arachnoiditis, shivering cranial nerve palsies due to traction on nerves from loss of CSF, and loss of perineal sensation and sexual function

Rare

Anxiety, restlessness, difficulty breathing shortness of breath, dizziness, drowsiness, lightheadedness, nausea, vomiting, seizures (convulsions), slow, irregular heartbeat (palpitations), swelling of the face or mouth, skin rash, itching (hives), tremors, visual impairment.

SERIOUS REACTIONS

• Tetracaine induced CNS toxicity usually presents with symptoms of a CNS stimulation such as anxiety, apprehension, restlessness, nervousness, disorientation, confusion, dizziness, tinnitus, blurred vision, tremor, and/or seizures. Subsequently, depressive symptoms may occur including drowsiness, respiratory arrest, or coma.

• Depression or cardiac excitability and contractility may cause AV block, ventricular arrhythmias, or cardiac arrest. Symptoms of local anesthetic CNS toxicity, such as dizziness, tongue numbness, visual impairment or disturbances, and muscular twitching appear to occur before cardiotoxic effects. Cardiotoxic effects include angina, QT prolongation, PR prolongation, atrial fibrillation, sinus bradycardia, hypotension, palpitations, and cardiovascular collapse. Maternal seizures and cardiovascular collapse may occur following paracervical block in early pregnancy due to rapid systemic absorption.

Alert

• Tetracaine is more likely than any other topical anesthetic to cause contact reactions including, skin rash (unspecified), mucous membrane irritation, erythema, pruritis, urticaria, burning, stinging, edema, or tenderness.

Alert

• During labor and obstetric delivery, local anesthetics can cause varying degrees of maternal, fetal, and neonatal toxicities. Fetal heart rate should be monitored continuously because fetal bradycardia may occur in patients receiving tetracaine anesthesia and may be associated with fetal acidosis. Maternal hypotension can result from regional anesthesia; patient position can alleviate this problem. Spinal tetracaine may cause decreased uterine contractility or maternal expulsion efforts and alter the forces of parturition.

SPECIAL CONSIDERATIONS

PRECAUTIONS

• Resuscitative equipment and drugs should be immediately available whenever any local anesthetic drug is used. Do not use tetracaine hydrochloride in patients with heart block. Tetracaine hydrochloride contains acetone sodium bisulfite, a sulfite that may cause allergic-type reactions including anaphylactic symptoms and life-threatening or less severe asthmatic episodes in certain susceptible persons. The overall prevalence of sulfite sensitivity in the general population is unknown and probably low. Sulfite sensitivity is seen more frequently in asthmatic than in nonasthmatic persons.

PREGNANCY AND LACTATION

• Pregnancy Category C. Animal reproduction studies have not been conducted with tetracaine hydrochloride. Whether tetracaine hydrochloride can cause fetal harm is not known. Excretion into human milk is not known.

OCULAR CONSIDERATIONS

• Ocular Indications and Usage: Tetracaine hydrochloride is indicated for ocular procedures such as tonometry. Eye ointment is used for electroretinography. Tetracaine hydrochloride is indicated for the production of spinal anesthesia for procedures requiring 2 to 3 hours.

tetracycline hydrochloride

(tet-ra-sye'kleen)

Rx: Ala-Tet, Brodspec, Panmycin, Sumycin, Tetracon

Drug Class: Anti-infectives, ophthalmic; Anti-infectives, topical; Antibiotics, tetracyclines; Dermatologics; Ophthalmics

Pregnancy Category: D

CLINICAL PHARMACOLOGY

Mechanism of Action: A tetracycline antibiotic that inhibits bacterial protein synthesis by binding to ribosomes. *Therapeutic Effect:* Bacteriostatic.

Pharmacokinetics

Readily absorbed from the GI tract. Protein binding: 30%-60%. Widely distributed. Excreted in urine; eliminated in feces through biliary system. Not removed by hemodialysis. **Half-life:** 6-11 hr (increased in impaired renal function).

AVAILABLE FORMS

- *Capsules:* 250 mg, 500 mg.
- *Oral Suspension:* 125 mg/5 ml.
- *Tablets:* 250 mg, 500 mg.
- *Topical Solution.* 2.2 mg/ml.
- *Topical Ointment:* 3%.

INDICATIONS AND DOSAGES

Inflammatory acne vulgaris, Lyme disease, mycoplasmal disease,* Legionella *infections, Rocky Mountain spotted fever, chlamydial infections in patients with gonorrhea

PO

Adults, Elderly. 250-500 mg q6-12h.

Children 8 yr and older. 25-50 mg/kg/day in 4 divided doses. Maximum: 3 g/day.

Helicobacter pylori ***infections***
PO
Adults, Elderly. 500 mg 2-4 times a day (in combination).
Topical
Adults, Elderly. Apply twice a day (once in the morning, once in the evening).
Dosage in renal impairment
Dosage interval is modified based on creatinine clearance.

Creatinine Clearance	*Dosage Interval*
50-80 ml/min	Usual dose q8-12h
10-50 ml/min	Usual dose q12-24h
less than 10 ml/min	Usual dose q24h

CONTRAINDICATIONS: Children 8 years and younger, hypersensitivity to tetracyclines or sulfites
INTERACTIONS
Drug
Carbamazepine, phenytoin: May decrease tetracycline blood concentration.
Cholestyramine, colestipol: May decrease tetracycline absorption.
Oral contraceptives: May decrease the effects of oral contraceptives.
Herbal
St. John's wort: May increase the risk of photosensitivity.
Food
Dairy products: Inhibit tetracycline absorption.
DIAGNOSTIC TEST EFFECTS: May increase BUN and serum alkaline phosphatase, amylase, bilirubin, AST (SGOT), and ALT (SGPT) levels.
SIDE EFFECTS
Frequent
Dizziness, light-headedness, diarrhea, nausea, vomiting, abdominal cramps, possibly severe photosensitivity
Topical: Dry, scaly skin; stinging or burning sensation
Occasional
Pigmentation of skin or mucous membranes, rectal or genital pruritus, stomatitis
Topical: Pain, redness, swelling, or other skin irritation.
SERIOUS REACTIONS
- Superinfection (especially fungal), anaphylaxis, and benign intracranial hypertension may occur.
- Bulging fontanelles occur rarely in infants.

SPECIAL CONSIDERATIONS

PATIENT INFORMATION
- Store drug at controlled room temperature between 15° and 30° C (59° and 86° F).

PRECAUTIONS
- Capsules: Fungal infections may occur. Superinfection of the bowel by staphylococci may be life-threatening. Anticoagulant therapy may require downward adjustment of the dosage. Perform renal and hepatic studies. Treat infections from group A beta-hemolytic streptococci for at least 10 days. Avoid giving tetracycline along with penicillin. Sensitivity reactions are more likely in patients with a history of allergy.
- Ocular Suspension: Superinfection may occur.

PREGNANCY AND LACTATION
- Pregnancy Category C. Fetal harm is not known. Excretion into human milk is not known.

OCULAR CONSIDERATIONS
OCULAR DOSAGE AND ADMINISTRATION
- Ocular Rosacea: 250 mg orally qid for 3 to 6 weeks; taper dose slowly. Some patients are on maintenance dose (250 mg/day) indefinitely if active disease recurs when patient is not taking medication.
- Staphylococcal Hypersensitivity, Corneal: Moderate to severe recurrent episodes not prevented by lid

hygiene alone, 250 mg orally qid for 1 month, then bid for 1 month, then once per day.

- Trachoma: 2 drops 4 times daily. Continued for 1 to 3 months. Concomitant oral tetracycline is helpful.
- Adult Inclusion (chalmydial) Conjunctivitis: 500 mg orally 3 times daily. Treat for 3 weeks or more.

tetrahydrozoline hydrochloride

(tet-ra-hi-droz'o-leen)

Rx: Tyzine Nasal

Drug Class: Decongestants, nasal; Decongestants, ophthalmic; Ophthalmics

Pregnancy Category: C

CLINICAL PHARMACOLOGY

Mechanism of Action: A vasoconstrictor that stimulates alpha-adrenergic receptors in sympathetic nervous system. Constricts arterioles. *Therapeutic Effect:* Reduces redness, irritation, and congestion.

Pharmacokinetics

May be systemically absorbed. Metabolic, elimination rates unknown.

AVAILABLE FORMS

- *Nasal solution:* 0.05%, 0.1% (Tyzine).
- *Ophthalmic solution:* 0.05% (Visine).

INDICATIONS AND DOSAGES

Relief of itching, minor irritation and to control hyperemia with superficial corneal vascularity

Ophthalmic

Adults, Elderly, Children. 1-2 drops 2-4 times/day.

Relief of nasal congestion of rhinitis, the common cold, sinusitis, hay fever, or other allergies; reduces swelling and improves visualization for surgery or diagnostic procedures; opens obstructed eustachian ostia with ear inflammation

Intranasal

Adults, Elderly, Children older than 6 yr. 2-4 drops (0.1% solution) to each nostril q4-6h (no sooner than q3h).

Children 2-6 yr. 2-3 drops (0.05% solution) to each nostril q4-6h (no sooner than q3h).

CONTRAINDICATIONS: Children less than 2 years of age, the 0.1% nasal solution is contraindicated in children less than 6 years of age, angle-closure glaucoma or other serious eye diseases, hypersensitivity to tetrahydrozyline or any component of the formulation

INTERACTIONS

Drug

Maprotiline, tricyclic antidepressants: May increase pressor effects.

MAOIs: May cause severe hypertensive reaction.

Herbal

Ma huang: May increase CNS stimulation.

Food

None known.

DIAGNOSTIC TEST EFFECTS: *None known.*

SIDE EFFECTS

Occasional

Intranasal: Transient burning, stinging, sneezing, dryness of mucosa

Ophthalmic: Irritation, blurred vision, mydriasis

Systemic sympathomimetic effects may occur with either route: headache, hypertension, weakness, sweating, palpitations, tremors. Prolonged use may result in rebound congestion.

SERIOUS REACTIONS

• Overdosage may result in CNS depression with drowsiness, decreased body temperature, bradycardia, hypotension, coma, and apnea.

SPECIAL CONSIDERATIONS

PRECAUTIONS

• Remove contact lenses before using.

thiamine hydrochloride (vitamin B_1)

(thy'a-min)

Rx: Vitamin B_1

Drug Class: Vitamins/minerals

Pregnancy Category: A

CLINICAL PHARMACOLOGY

Mechanism of Action: A water-soluble vitamin that combines with adenosine triphosphate in the liver, kidneys, and leukocytes to form thiamine diphosphate, a coenzyme that is necessary for carbohydrate metabolism. *Therapeutic Effect:* Prevents and reverses thiamine deficiency.

Pharmacokinetics

Readily absorbed from the GI tract, primarily in duodenum, after IM administration. Widely distributed. Metabolized in the liver. Primarily excreted in urine.

AVAILABLE FORMS

• *Tablets:* 50 mg, 100 mg, 250 mg, 500 mg.

• *Injection:* 100 mg/ml.

INDICATIONS AND DOSAGES

Dietary supplement

PO

Adults, Elderly. 1-2 mg/day.

Children. 0.5-1 mg/day.

Infants. 0.3-0.5 mg/day.

Thiamine deficiency

PO

Adults, Elderly. 5-30 mg/day, as a single dose or in 3 divided doses, for 1 mo.

Children. 10-50 mg/day in 3 divided doses.

Thiamine deficiency in patients who are critically ill or have malabsorption syndrome

IV, IM

Adults, Elderly. 5-100 mg, 3 times a day.

Children. 10-25 mg/day.

Metabolic disorders

PO

Adults, Elderly, Children. 10-20 mg/day; increased up to 4 g/day in divided doses.

CONTRAINDICATIONS: None known.

INTERACTIONS

Drug

None known.

Herbal

None known.

Food

None known.

DIAGNOSTIC TEST EFFECTS: *None known.*

IV INCOMPATIBILITIES: Sodium bicarbonate

IV COMPATIBILITIES: Famotidine (Pepcid), multivitamins

SIDE EFFECTS

Frequent

Pain, induration, and tenderness at IM injection site

SERIOUS REACTIONS

• IV administration may result in a rare, severe hypersensitivity reaction marked by a feeling of warmth, pruritus, urticaria, weakness, diaphoresis, nausea, restlessness, tightness in throat, angioedema, cyanosis, pulmonary edema, GI tract bleeding, and cardiovascular collapse.

SPECIAL CONSIDERATIONS

PRECAUTIONS

• Simple vitamin B_1 deficiency is rare. Suspect multiple vitamin deficiencies in any case of dietary inadequacy.

PATIENT INFORMATION

• Advise the patient as to proper dietary habits during treatment so that relapses will be less likely to occur with reduction in dosage or cessation of injection therapy.

PREGNANCY AND LACTATION

• Pregnancy Category A. Studies in pregnant women have not shown that thiamine hydrochloride increases the risk of fetal abnormalities if administered during pregnancy. Excretion into human milk is not known.

---

thioridazine

(thye-or-rid'a-zeen)

Rx: Mellaril

Drug Class: Antipsychotics; Phenothiazines

Pregnancy Category: C

Do not confuse thioridazine with thiothixene or Thorazine, or Mellaril with Mebaral.

CLINICAL PHARMACOLOGY

Mechanism of Action: A phenothiazine that blocks dopamine at postsynaptic receptor sites. Possesses strong anticholinergic and sedative effects. *Therapeutic Effect:* Suppresses behavioral response in psychosis; reduces locomotor activity and aggressiveness.

AVAILABLE FORMS

• *Oral Solution (Concentrate [Thioridazine Intensol]):* 30 mg/ml.

• *Tablets (Melleril):* 10 mg, 15 mg, 25 mg, 50 mg, 100 mg, 150 mg, 200 mg.

INDICATIONS AND DOSAGES

Psychosis

PO

Adults, Elderly, Children 12 yr and older. Initially, 25-100 mg 3 times a day; dosage increased gradually. Maximum: 800 mg/day.

Children 2-11 yr. Initially, 0.5 mg/kg/day in 2-3 divided doses. Maximum: 3 mg/kg/day.

UNLABELED USES: Treatment of behavioral problems in children, dementia, depressive neurosis

CONTRAINDICATIONS: Angle-closure glaucoma, blood dyscrasias, cardiac arrhythmias, cardiac or hepatic impairment, concurrent use of drugs that prolong QT interval, severe CNS depression

INTERACTIONS

Drug

Alcohol, other CNS depressants: May increase respiratory depression and the hypotensive effects of thioridazine.

Antithyroid agents: May increase the risk of agranulocytosis.

Extrapyramidal symptom–producing medications: May increase the risk of extrapyramidal symptoms.

Hypotension-producing agents: May increase hypotension.

Levodopa: May decrease the effects of levodopa.

Lithium: May decrease the absorption of thioridazine and produce adverse neurologic effects.

MAOIs, tricyclic antidepressants: May increase the anticholinergic and sedative effects of thioridazine.

Herbal

None known.

Food

None known.

DIAGNOSTIC TEST EFFECTS: May cause EKG changes. Therapeutic serum level is 0.2-2.6 mcg/ml; toxic serum level is not established.

SIDE EFFECTS

Occasional

Drowsiness during early therapy, dry mouth, blurred vision, lethargy, constipation or diarrhea, nasal congestion, peripheral edema, urine retention

Rare

Ocular changes, altered skin pigmentation (in those taking high doses for prolonged periods), photosensitivity, darkening of urine

SERIOUS REACTIONS

• Prolonged QT interval may produce torsades de pointes, a form of ventricular tachycardia, and sudden death.

SPECIAL CONSIDERATIONS

PRECAUTIONS

• Leukopenia and/or agranulocytosis and convulsive seizures have been reported but are infrequent. In schizophrenic patients with epilepsy, maintain anticonvulsant medication during treatment with thioridazine hydrochloride.

• Where patients are participating in activities requiring complete mental alertness (e.g., driving), it is advisable to administer the phenothiazines cautiously and to increase the dosage gradually. Female patients appear to have a greater tendency to orthostatic hypotension than male patients. Avoid the administration of epinephrine to treat drug-induced hypotension in view of the fact that phenothiazines may induce a reversed epinephrine effect on occasion. If a vasoconstrictor is required, the most suitable are levarterenol and phenylephrine.

• Antipsychotic drugs elevate prolactin levels; the elevation persists during chronic administration.

PATIENT INFORMATION

• Inform patients that thioridazine hydrochloride has been associated with potentially fatal heart rhythm disturbances. The risk of such events may be increased when certain drugs are given together with thioridazine hydrochloride. Therefore, advise patients to inform the prescriber that they are receiving thioridazine hydrochloride treatment before taking any new medication.

• Given the likelihood that some patients exposed chronically to antipsychotics will develop tardive dyskinesia, give all patients in whom chronic use is contemplated full information about this risk, if possible. The decision to inform patients and/or their guardians obviously must take into account the clinical circumstances and the competency of the patient to understand the information provided.

PREGNANCY AND LACTATION

• Pregnancy Category C

OCULAR CONSIDERATIONS

• Pigmentary retinopathy, which has been observed primarily in patients taking larger than recommended doses, is characterized by diminution of visual acuity, brownish coloring of vision, and impairment of night vision; examination of the fundus discloses deposits of pigment. The possibility of this complication may be reduced by remaining within the recommended limits of dosage.

timolol maleate

(tim'oh-lole)

Rx: Betimol, Blocadren, Timolol, Ophthalmic, Timoptic Ocudose, Timoptic Ocumeter, Timoptic Ocumeter Plus, Timoptic-XE

Drug Class: Antiadrenergics, beta blocking; Ophthalmics

Pregnancy Category: C

Do not confuse timolol with atenolol, or Timoptic with Viroptic.

CLINICAL PHARMACOLOGY

Mechanism of Action: An antihypertensive, antimigraine, and antiglaucoma agent that blocks $beta_1$- and $beta_2$-adrenergic receptors. *Therapeutic Effect:* Reduces intraocular pressure (IOP) by reducing aqueous humor production, lowers BP, slows the heart rate, and decreases myocardial contractility.

Pharmacokinetics

Route	Onset	Peak	Duration
PO	15-45 min	0.5-2.5 hr	4 hr
Ophthalmic	30 min	1-2 hr	12-24 hr

Well absorbed from the GI tract. Protein binding: 60%. Minimal absorption after ophthalmic administration. Metabolized in the liver. Primarily excreted in urine. Not removed by hemodialysis. **Half-life:** 4 hr. Systemic absorption may occur with ophthalmic administration.

AVAILABLE FORMS

- *Tablets (Blocadren):* 5 mg, 10 mg, 20 mg.
- *Ophthalmic Gel (Timoptic-XE):* 0.25%, 0.5%.
- *Ophthalmic Solution (Betimol, Timoptic, Timoptic OccuDose):* 0.25%, 0.5%.

INDICATIONS AND DOSAGES

Mild to moderate hypertension

PO

Adults, Elderly. Initially, 10 mg twice a day, alone or in combination with other therapy. Gradually increase at intervals of not less than 1 wk. Maintenance: 20-60 mg/day in 2 divided doses.

Reduction of cardiovascular mortality in definite or suspected acute MI

PO

Adults, Elderly. 10 mg twice a day, beginning 1-4 wk after infarction.

Migraine prevention

PO

Adults, Elderly. Initially, 10 mg twice a day. Range: 10-30 mg/day.

Reduction of IOP in open-angle glaucoma, aphakic glaucoma, ocular hypertension, and secondary glaucoma

Ophthalmic

Adults, Elderly, Children. 1 drop of 0.25% solution in affected eye(s) twice a day. May be increased to 1 drop of 0.5% solution in affected eye(s) twice a day. When IOP is controlled, dosage may be reduced to 1 drop once a day. If patient is switched to timolol from another antiglaucoma agent, administer concurrently for 1 day. Discontinue other agent on following day.

Ophthalmic (Timoptic-XE)

Adults, Elderly. 1 drop/day

Ophthalmic (Istalol)

Adults, Elderly. Apply once daily.

UNLABELED USES: Systemic: Treatment of anxiety, cardiac arrhythmias, chronic angina pectoris, hypertrophic cardiomyopathy, migraine, pheochromocytoma, thyrotoxicosis, tremors

Ophthalmic: To decrease IOP in acute or chronic angle-closure glaucoma, treatment of angle-closure glaucoma during and after iridectomy, malignant glaucoma, secondary glaucoma

CONTRAINDICATIONS: Bronchial asthma, cardiogenic shock, CHF unless secondary to tachyarrhythmias, COPD, patients receiving MAOI therapy, second- or third-degree heart block, sinus bradycardia, uncontrolled cardiac failure

INTERACTIONS

Drug

Diuretics, other antihypertensives: May increase hypotensive effect.

Insulin, oral hypoglycemics: May mask symptoms of hypoglycemia and prolong hypoglycemic effects of these drugs.

NSAIDs: May decrease antihypertensive effect.

Sympathomimetics, xanthines: May mutually inhibit effects.

Herbal

None known.

Food

None known.

DIAGNOSTIC TEST EFFECTS: May increase antinuclear antibody titer and BUN, serum LDH, serum lipoprotein, serum alkaline phosphatase, serum bilirubin, serum creatinine, serum potassium, serum uric acid, AST (SGOT), ALT (SGPT), and serum triglyceride levels.

SIDE EFFECTS

Frequent

Diminished sexual function, drowsiness, difficulty sleeping, unusual tiredness or weakness

Ophthalmic: Eye irritation, visual disturbances

Occasional

Depression, cold hands or feet, diarrhea, constipation, anxiety, nasal congestion, nausea, vomiting

Rare

Altered taste, dry eyes, itching, numbness of fingers, toes, or scalp

SERIOUS REACTIONS

- Overdose may produce profound bradycardia, hypotension, and bronchospasm.
- Abrupt withdrawal may result in diaphoresis, palpitations, headache, and tremors.
- Timolol administration may precipitate CHF and MI in patients with cardiac disease; thyroid storm in those with thyrotoxicosis; and peripheral ischemia in those with existing peripheral vascular disease.
- Hypoglycemia may occur in patients with previously controlled diabetes.
- Ophthalmic overdose may produce bradycardia, hypotension, bronchospasm, and acute cardiac failure.

SPECIAL CONSIDERATIONS

PRECAUTIONS

- Use caution in patients with cerebrovascular insufficiency. After filtration procedures, a risk of choroidal detachment exists.
- Angle-Closure Glaucoma: Do not use timolol alone to treat angle-closure glaucoma.
- Anaphylaxis: A history of atopy or a history of severe anaphylactic reactions may make a patient unresponsive to the usual doses of epinephrine used to treat anaphylactic reactions.
- Muscle Weakness: Timolol potentiates muscle weakness (e.g., diplopia, ptosis, and generalized weakness) in myasthenia gravis.

PATIENT INFORMATION

- Timoptic Ophthalmic Solution and Timoptic Preservative-Free Ophthalmic Solution: Advise patients with bronchial asthma, a history of bronchial asthma, severe chronic obstructive pulmonary disease, sinus bradycardia, second- or third-degree atrioventricular block, or cardiac failure not to take this product. Timoptic ophthalmic solution contains benzalkonium chloride, which may be absorbed by soft contact lenses. Lenses may be reinserted 15 minutes following timolol administration.

• Timoptic-XE Sterile Ophthalmic Gel-Forming Solution: Instruct patients to invert the closed container and shake once before each use. Shaking the container more than once is unnecessary. Instruct patients requiring concomitant topical medications to administer these at least 10 minutes before instilling Timoptic-XE. Advise patients with bronchial asthma, a history of bronchial asthma, severe chronic obstructive pulmonary disease, sinus bradycardia, second- or third-degree atrioventricular block, or cardiac failure not to take this product.

• Transient blurred vision can last from 30 seconds to 5 minutes. Potential visual disturbances may impair the ability to perform hazardous tasks such as operating machinery or driving a motor vehicle.

PREGNANCY AND LACTATION

• Pregnancy Category C. Increased fetal resorptions were seen in rats and rabbits with oral doses. Fetal harm is not known with topical administration. Excretion into human milk has been detected.

tobramycin

(toe-bra-mye'sin)

Rx: AK-Tob, Tobrasol, Tobrex

Drug Class: Anti-infectives, ophthalmic; Antibiotics, aminoglycosides; Ophthalmics

Pregnancy Category: B

CLINICAL PHARMACOLOGY

Mechanism of Action: An aminoglycoside antibiotic that irreversibly binds to protein on bacterial ribosomes. *Therapeutic Effect:* Interferes in protein synthesis of susceptible microorganisms.

Pharmacokinetics

Rapid, complete absorption after IM administration. Protein binding: less than 30%. Widely distributed but does not cross the blood-brain barrier and is in low concentrations in cerebrospinal fluid (CSF). Excreted unchanged in urine. Removed by hemodialysis. **Half-life:** 2 hrs. Half-life is increased with impaired renal function and in neonates. Half-life is decreased in cystic fibrosis, febrile, or burn patients.

AVAILABLE FORMS

• *Inhalation solution:* 60 mg/ml (Tobi).

• *Injection:* 10 mg/ml, 40 mg/ml (Nebcin).

• *Powder for Injection:* 1.2 g (Nebcin).

INDICATIONS AND DOSAGES

Skin/skin structure, bone, joint, respiratory tract infections, postoperative, burn, intraabdominal infections, complicated urinary tract infections, septicemia, meningitis

IM/IV

Adults, Elderly. 3mg/kg/day in 3 divided doses. May use up to 5 mg/kgday in 3 to 4 equal doses.

Cystic fibrosis

Inhalation

Adult, Elderly, Children 6 yr and older. 1 ampule (300mg) via nebulizer twice daily (28 days on, 28 days off). Consider starting elderly patients at 3 mg/kg IV q8h.

Dosage in Renal Impairment

Dosage and frequency are modified based on degree of renal impairment and the serum concentration of the drug. After a loading dose of 1-2 mg/kg, the maintenance dose and frequency are based on serum creatinine levels and creatinine clearance. Dosage should be reduced to 3 mg/kg/day as soon as clinically indicated. Dosage should not exceed 5 mg/kg/day.

CONTRAINDICATIONS: Hypersensitivity to aminoglycosides (cross-sensitivity)

INTERACTIONS

Drug

Other aminoglycosides, nephrotoxic and ototoxic-producing medications: May increase the risk of tobramycin toxicity.

Neuromuscular blocking agents: May increase the effects of neuromuscular blocking agents.

Herbal

None known.

Food

None known.

DIAGNOSTIC TEST EFFECTS: May increase serum bilirubin, BUN, serum creatinine, serum LDH concentrations, SGOT (AST), and SGPT (ALT) levels. May decrease serum calcium, magnesium, potassium, and sodium concentrations. Therapeutic blood level: Peak is 5-20 mcg/ml; trough is 0.5-2 mcg/ml. Toxic blood level: Peak is greater than 20 mcg/ml; trough is greater than 2 mcg/ml.

IV INCOMPATIBILITIES: Amphotericin B complex (Abelcet, AmBisome, Amphotec), heparin, hetastarch (Hespan), indomethacin (Indocin), propofol (Diprivan), sargramostim (Leukine, Prokine)

IV COMPATIBILITIES: Amiodarone (Cordarone), calcium gluconate, diltiazem (Cardizem), furosemide (Lasix), hydromorphone (Dilaudid), insulin, magnesium sulfate, midazolam (Versed), morphine, theophylline

SIDE EFFECTS

Occasional

IM: Pain, induration at IM injection site

IV: Phlebitis, thrombophlebitis

Rare

Hypotension, nausea, vomiting

SERIOUS REACTIONS

- Nephrotoxicity, as evidenced by increased BUN and serum creatinine and decreased creatinine clearance, may be reversible if the drug is stopped at the first sign of nephrotoxic symptoms.
- Irreversible ototoxicity, manifested as tinnitus, dizziness, ringing or roaring in ears, impaired hearing and neurotoxicity, as evidenced by headache, dizziness, lethargy, tremors, and visual disturbances, occur occasionally. The risk of irreversible neurotoxicity and ototoxicity is greater with higher dosages, prolonged therapy, or if the solution is applied directly to the mucosa.
- Superinfections, particularly with fungi, may result from bacterial imbalance with any route of administration.
- Anaphylaxis may occur.

SPECIAL CONSIDERATIONS

PRECAUTIONS

• Fungal infections may occur. Eye ointments may retard corneal wound healing. Cross-sensitivity to other aminoglycoside antibiotics may occur.

PREGNANCY AND LACTATION

• Pregnancy Category B. No evidence exists of impaired fertility or harm to the fetus in animal studies with oral doses. Fetal harm is not known with topical administration. Excretion into human milk is not known.

tolazamide

(tole-az′-a-mide)

Rx: Tolinase

Drug Class: Antidiabetic agents; Sulfonylureas, first generation

Pregnancy Category: C

Do not confuse with tolubutamide, tocainide, or tolazine.

CLINICAL PHARMACOLOGY

Mechanism of Action: A first-generation sulfonylurea that promotes release of insulin from beta cells of pancreas. *Therapeutic Effect:* Lowers blood glucose concentration.

Pharmacokinetics

Well absorbed from the gastrointestinal (GI) tract. Extensively metabolized in liver to five metabolites, three which are active. Primarily excreted in urine. Unknown if removed by hemodialysis. **Half-life:** 7 hrs.

AVAILABLE FORMS

• *Tablets:* 100 mg, 250 mg, 500 mg; 100 mg, 250 mg (Tolinase).

INDICATIONS AND DOSAGES

Diabetes mellitus

PO

Adults, Elderly. Initially, 100-250 mg once a day, with breakfast or first main meal. Maintenance: 100-1000 mg once a day. May increase by increments of 100-250 mg at weekly, based on blood glucose response. May increase by 100-250 mg/day at weekly intervals. Maximum: 1000 mg/day. Doses more than 500 mg/day should be given in 2 divided doses with meals.

UNLABELED USES: *None known.*

CONTRAINDICATIONS: Diabetic complications, such as ketosis, acidosis, and diabetic coma, sole therapy for type 1 diabetes mellitus, hypersensitivity to tolazamide or its components

INTERACTIONS

Drug

Beta-blockers: May increase hypoglycemic effect and mask signs of hypoglycemia.

Cimetidine, fluoroquinolones, fluconazole, MAOIs, quinidine, ranitidine, large doses of salicylates: May increase effects of tolazamide.

Corticosteroids, lithium, thiazide diuretics: May decrease effects of tolazamide.

Oral anticoagulants: May increase effects of oral anticoagulants.

Herbal

Bitter melon, fenugreek, ginseng, glucomannan, glucosamine, gymnema extracts, licorice, psyllium, St. John's wort: May increase risk of hypoglycemia.

Food

None known.

DIAGNOSTIC TEST EFFECTS: May increase BUN, LDH concentrations, serum alkaline phosphatase, creatinine, and SGOT (AST) levels.

IV INCOMPATIBILITIES: *None known.*

IV COMPATIBILITIES: *None known.*

SIDE EFFECTS

Frequent

Altered taste sensation, dizziness, drowsiness, weight gain, constipation, diarrhea, heartburn, nausea, vomiting, stomach fullness, headache

Occasional

Increased sensitivity of skin to sunlight, peeling of skin, itching, rash

SERIOUS REACTIONS

• Severe hypoglycemia may occur due to overdosage and insufficient food intake, especially with increased glucose demands.

• GI hemorrhage, cholestatic hepatic jaundice, leukopenia, thrombocytopenia, pancytopenia, agranulocytosis and aplastic or hemolytic anemia occurs rarely.

SPECIAL CONSIDERATIONS

PRECAUTIONS

• Tolazamide administration is associated with increased cardiovascular mortality compared with treatment with diet alone or diet plus insulin. All sulfonylurea drugs are capable of producing severe hypoglycemia. Renal or hepatic insufficiency may cause elevated blood levels of tolazamide, and the latter also may diminish gluconeogenic capacity, both of which increase the risk of serious hypoglycemic reactions. Elderly, debilitated, or malnourished patients and those with adrenal or pituitary insufficiency are particularly susceptible to the hypoglycemic action of glucose-lowering drugs. Hypoglycemia may be difficult to recognize in the elderly and in persons who are taking beta-adrenergic blocking drugs. When a patient stabilized on any diabetic regimen is exposed to stress such as fever, trauma, infection, or surgery, loss of control of blood glucose may occur.

PATIENT INFORMATION

• Inform patients of the potential risks and advantages of tolazamide and of alternative modes of therapy. Also inform them about the importance of adherence to dietary instructions, of a regular exercise program, and of regular testing of urine and/or blood glucose. Explain the risks of hypoglycemia, its symptoms and treatment, and conditions that predispose to its development to patients and responsible family members. Also explain primary and secondary failure.

PREGNANCY AND LACTATION

• Pregnancy Category C. Because recent information suggests that abnormal blood glucose levels during pregnancy are associated with a higher incidence of congenital abnormalities, many experts recommend that insulin be used during pregnancy to maintain blood glucose levels as close to normal as possible. Although whether tolazamide is excreted in human milk is not known, some sulfonylurea drugs are known to be excreted in human milk.

tolbutamide

(tole-byoo′ta-mide)

Rx: Tol-Tab

Drug Class: Antidiabetic agents; Sulfonylureas, first generation

Pregnancy Category: C

Do not confuse with tolazamide, tocainide, or tolazine.

CLINICAL PHARMACOLOGY

Mechanism of Action: A first-generation sulfonylurea that promotes the release of insulin from beta cells of pancreas. *Therapeutic Effect:* Lowers blood glucose concentration.

Pharmacokinetics

Route	*Onset*	*Peak*	*Duration*
PO	1 hr	5-8 hrs	12-24 hrs
IV	N/A	30-45 min	90-181 min

Well absorbed from the gastrointestinal (GI) tract. Protein binding: 80%-99%. Extensively metabolized in liver to 2 inactive metabolites, primarily via oxidation. Excreted in urine. Removed by hemodialysis. **Half-life:** 4.5-6.5 hrs.

AVAILABLE FORMS

• *Tablets:* 500 mg (Orinase, Tol-Tab).

• *Injection, Powder for Reconstitution:* 1 g (Orinase Diagnostic).

INDICATIONS AND DOSAGES

Diabetes mellitus

PO

Adults. Initially, 1 g daily, with breakfast or first main meal, or in divided doses. Maintenance: 0.25-3 g once a day. After dose of 2 g is reached, dosage should be increased in increments of up to 2 mg q1-2wks, based on blood glucose response. Maximum: 3 g/day.

Endocrine tumor diagnosis

IV

Adults. 1 g infused over 2-3 minutes.

CONTRAINDICATIONS: Diabetic ketoacidosis with or without coma, sole therapy for type 1 diabetes mellitus, use in children, hypersensitivity to tolbutamide or any component of its formulation

INTERACTIONS

Drug

Beta-blockers: May increase the hypoglycemic effect and mask signs of hypoglycemia.

Cimetidine, fluoroquinolones, fluconazole, MAOIs, quinidine, ranitidine, large doses of salicylates: May increase the effects of tolbutamide.

Corticosteroids, lithium, thiazide diuretics: May decrease the effects of tolbutamide.

Oral anticoagulants: May increase the effects of oral anticoagulants.

Fosphenytoin, phenytoin: May increase the risk of phenytoin toxicity.

Rifampin: May decrease effectiveness of tolbutamide.

Sertraline: May decrease the clearance of tolbutamide.

Herbal

Bitter melon, fenugreek, ginseng, glucomannan, glucosamine, gymnema extracts, licorice, psyllium, St. John's wort: May increase the risk of hypoglycemia.

Food

None known.

DIAGNOSTIC TEST EFFECTS: May increase BUN, LDH concentrations, serum alkaline phosphatase, creatinine, and SGOT (AST) levels.

SIDE EFFECTS

Frequent

Increased sensitivity of skin to sunlight, peeling of skin, itching, rash, dizziness, drowsiness, weight gain, constipation, diarrhea, heartburn, nausea, headache, pain at injection site

Occasional

Altered taste sensation, constipation, vomiting, stomach fullness

SERIOUS REACTIONS

• Severe hypoglycemia may occur because of overdosage or insufficient food intake, especially with increased glucose demands.

• Cardiovascular mortality has been reported higher in patients treated with tolbutamide.

• GI hemorrhage, cholestatic hepatic jaundice, leukopenia, thrombocytopenia, pancytopenia, agranulocytosis and aplastic or hemolytic anemia occurs rarely.

SPECIAL CONSIDERATIONS

PRECAUTIONS

• Tolbutamide administration is associated with increased cardiovascular mortality compared with treatment with diet alone or diet plus insulin. All sulfonylurea drugs are capable of producing severe hypoglycemia. Renal or hepatic insufficiency may cause elevated blood levels of tolbutamide, and the latter also may diminish gluconeogenic capacity, both of which increase the risk of serious hypoglycemic reactions. Elderly, debilitated, or malnourished patients and those with adrenal or pituitary insufficiency are particularly susceptible to the hypoglycemic action of glucose-lowering drugs. Hypoglycemia may be difficult to recognize in the elderly and persons who are taking beta-adrenergic blocking drugs. When a patient stabilized on any diabetic regimen is exposed to stress such as fever, trauma, infection, or surgery, loss of blood glucose control may occur. The effectiveness of any hypoglycemic drug, including tolbutamide, in lowering blood glucose to a desired level decreases in patients over a period of time, which may be due to progression of the severity of the diabetes or to diminished responsiveness to the drug. This phenomenon is known as secondary drug failure to distinguish it from primary failure in which the drug is ineffective in an individual patient when first given.

PATIENT INFORMATION

• Inform patients of the potential risks and advantages of tolbutamide and of alternative modes of therapy. Also inform patients about the importance of adherence to dietary instructions, of a regular exercise program, and of regular testing of urine and blood glucose. Explain the risks of hypoglycemia, its symptoms and treatment, and conditions that predispose to its development to patients and responsible family members. Also explain primary and secondary failure.

PREGNANCY AND LACTATION

• Pregnancy Category C. Tolbutamide has been shown to be teratogenic in rats given doses 25 to 100 times the human dose. Tolbutamide is not recommended for the treatment of pregnant diabetic patients. Because recent information suggests that abnormal blood glucose levels during pregnancy are associated with a higher incidence of congenital abnormalities, many experts recommend that insulin be used during pregnancy to maintain blood glucose levels as close to normal as possible. Excretion into human milk is not known.

topiramate

(toe-peer'a-mate)

Rx: Topamax, Topamax Sprinkle

Drug Class: Anticonvulsants

Pregnancy Category: C

Do not confuse topiramate or Topamax with Toprol XL.

CLINICAL PHARMACOLOGY

Mechanism of Action: An anticonvulsant that blocks repetitive, sustained firing of neurons by enhancing the ability of gamma-aminobutyric acid to induce an influx of chloride ions into the neurons; may also block sodium channels. *Therapeutic Effect:* Decreases seizure activity.

Pharmacokinetics

Rapidly absorbed after PO administration. Protein binding: 13%-17%. Not extensively metabolized. Primarily excreted unchanged in urine. Removed by hemodialysis. **Half-life:** 21 hr.

AVAILABLE FORMS

- *Capsules (Sprinkle):* 15 mg, 25 mg.
- *Tablets:* 25 mg, 50 mg, 100 mg, 200 mg.

INDICATIONS AND DOSAGES

Adjunctive treatment of partial seizures, Lennox-Gastant syndrome

PO

Adults, Elderly, Children older than 17 yr. Initially, 25-50 mg for 1 wk. May increase by 25-50 mg/day at weekly intervals. Maximum: 1,600 mg/day.

Children 2-16 yr. Initially, 1-3 mg/kg/day to maximum of 25 mg.. May increase by 1-3 mg/kg/day at weekly intervals. Maintenance: 5-9 mg/kg/day in 2 divided doses.

Tonic-clonic seizures

PO

Adults, Elderly, Children. Dosage is individualized and titrated.

Migraine prevention

PO

Adults, Elderly. 100 mg/day in 2 divided doses.

Dosage in renal impairment

Expect to reduce drug dosage by 50% in patients with tonic-clonic seizures who have a creatinine clearance of less than 70 ml/min.

UNLABELED USES: Prevention of migraine headaches, treatment of alcohol dependence

CONTRAINDICATIONS: None known.

INTERACTIONS

Drug

Alcohol, other CNS depressants: May increase CNS depression.

Carbamazepine, phenytoin, valproic acid: May decrease topiramate blood concentration.

Carbonic anhydrase inhibitors: May increase the risk of renal calculi.

Oral contraceptives: May decrease the effectiveness of oral contraceptives.

Herbal

None known.

Food

None known.

DIAGNOSTIC TEST EFFECTS: *None known.*

SIDE EFFECTS

Frequent (30%-10%)

Somnolence, dizziness, ataxia, nervousness, nystagmus, diplopia, paresthesia, nausea, tremor

Occasional (9%-3%)

Confusion, breast pain, dysmenorrhea, dyspepsia, depression, asthenia, pharyngitis, weight loss, anorexia, rash, musculoskeletal pain, abdominal pain, difficulty with coordination, sinusitis, agitation, flu-like symptoms

Rare (3%-2%)

Mood disturbances, such as irritability and depression; dry mouth; aggressive behavior

SERIOUS REACTIONS

- Psychomotor slowing, impaired concentration, language problems (such as word-finding difficulties), and memory disturbances occur occasionally. These reactions are generally mild to moderate but may be severe enough to require discontinuation of drug therapy.

SPECIAL CONSIDERATIONS

PRECAUTIONS

- A syndrome consisting of acute myopia associated with secondary angle-closure glaucoma has been reported in patients receiving topiramate. Symptoms include acute onset of decreased visual acuity and/or ocular pain. Ocular findings can include myopia, anterior chamber shallowing, ocular hyperemia (redness), and increased intraocular pressure. Mydriasis may or may not be present. This syndrome may be associated with supraciliary effusion resulting in anterior displacement of the lens and iris, with secondary angle-closure glaucoma. Symptoms typically occur within 1 month of initiating topiramate therapy. In contrast to primary narrow-angle glaucoma, which is rare in persons under 40 years of age, secondary angle-closure glaucoma associated with topiramate has been reported in pediatric patients and in adults. The primary treatment to reverse symptoms is discontinuation of topiramate as rapidly as possible, according to the judgment of the treating eye care practitioner. Other measures, along with discontinuation of topiramate, may be helpful.
- Elevated intraocular pressure of any cause, if left untreated, can lead to serious sequelae, including permanent vision loss.
- Concomitant use of topiramate, a weak carbonic anhydrase inhibitor, with other carbonic anhydrase inhibitors such acetazolamide or dichlorphenamide may create a physiologic environment that increases the risk of renal stone formation and therefore should be avoided.
- Adverse reactions reported are conjunctivitis (frequent); abnormal accommodation, photophobia, strabismus, and mydriasis (infrequent); and iritis (rare).

tramadol hydrochloride

(tray'-mah-doal)

Rx: Ultram

Drug Class: Analgesics, narcotic-like

Pregnancy Category: C

Do not confuse tramadol with Toradol, or Ultram with Ultane.

CLINICAL PHARMACOLOGY

Mechanism of Action: An analgesic that binds to mu-opioid receptors and inhibits reuptake of norepinephrine and serotonin. Reduces the intensity of pain stimuli reaching sensory nerve endings. *Therapeutic Effect:* Alters the perception of and emotional response to pain.

Pharmacokinetics

Route	*Onset*	*Peak*	*Duration*
PO	less than 1 hr	2-3 hr	4-6 hr

Rapidly and almost completely absorbed after PO administration. Protein binding: 20%. Extensively metabolized in the liver to active metabolite (reduced in patients with advanced cirrhosis). Primarily excreted in urine. Minimally removed by hemodialysis. **Half-life:** 6-7 hr.

AVAILABLE FORMS

- *Tablets:* 50 mg.

INDICATIONS AND DOSAGES

Moderate to moderately severe pain

PO

Adults, Elderly. 50-100 mg q4-6h. Maximum: 400 mg/day for patients 75 yr and younger; 300 mg/day for patients older than 75 yr.

Dosage in renal impairment

For patients with creatinine clearance of less than 30 ml/min, increase dosing interval to q12h. Maximum: 200 mg/day.

Dosage in hepatic impairment

Dosage is decreased to 50 mg q12h.

CONTRAINDICATIONS: Acute alcohol intoxication; concurrent use of centrally acting analgesics, hypnotics, opioids, or psychotropic drugs

INTERACTIONS

Drug

Alcohol, other CNS depressants: May increase CNS or respiratory depression and hypotension.

Carbamazepine: Decreases tramadol blood concentration.

MAOIs: Increase tramadol blood concentration.

Herbal

None known.

Food

None known.

DIAGNOSTIC TEST EFFECTS: May increase serum creatinine, AST (SGOT), and ALT (SGPT) hepatic levels. May decrease blood Hgb level. May cause proteinuria.

SIDE EFFECTS

Frequent (25%-15%)

Dizziness or vertigo, nausea, constipation, headache, somnolence

Occasional (10%-5%)

Vomiting, pruritus, CNS stimulation (such as nervousness, anxiety, agitation, tremor, euphoria, mood swings, and hallucinations), asthenia, diaphoresis, dyspepsia, dry mouth, diarrhea

Rare (less than 5%)

Malaise, vasodilation, anorexia, flatulence, rash, blurred vision, urine retention or urinary frequency, menopausal symptoms

SERIOUS REACTIONS

- Overdose results in respiratory depression and seizures.
- Tramadol may have a prolonged duration of action and cumulative effect in patients with hepatic or renal impairment.

SPECIAL CONSIDERATIONS

PRECAUTIONS

- Respiratory Depression: Administer tramadol hydrochloride cautiously in patients at risk for respiratory depression.
- Increased Intracranial Pressure or Head Trauma: Use tramadol with caution in patients with increased intracranial pressure or head injury. Pupillary changes (miosis) from tramadol may obscure the existence, extent, or course of intracranial pathologic conditions.
- Clinicians also should maintain a high index of suspicion for adverse drug reaction when evaluating altered mental status in these patients if they are receiving tramadol.
- Acute Abdominal Conditions: The administration of tramadol may complicate the clinical assessment of patients with acute abdominal conditions.

• Withdrawal: Withdrawal symptoms may occur if tramadol hydrochloride is discontinued abruptly. These symptoms may include anxiety, sweating, insomnia, rigors, pain, nausea, tremors, diarrhoea, upper respiratory symptoms, piloerection, and rarely hallucinations.
• Patients Physically Dependent on Opioids: Tramadol is not recommended for patients who are dependent on opioids.
• Use in Renal and Hepatic Disease: Impaired renal function results in a decreased rate and extent of excretion of tramadol and its active metabolite, M1. Metabolism of tramadol and M1 is reduced in patients with advanced cirrhosis of the liver. In cirrhotic patients, dosing reduction is recommended.
• Seizure Risk: Seizures have been reported in patients receiving tramadol hydrochloride within the recommended dosage range.
• Anaphylactoid Reactions: Serious and rarely fatal anaphylactoid reactions have been reported in patients receiving therapy with tramadol hydrochloride.
• Use in Opioid-Dependent Patients: Do not use tramadol hydrochloride in opioid-dependent patients.
• Use with Central Nervous System Depressants: Use tramadol with caution and in reduced dosages when administered to patients receiving central nervous system depressants such as alcohol, opioids, anesthetic agents, phenothiazines, tranquilizers, or sedative hypnotics.
• Use with Monoamine Oxidase Inhibitors: Use tramadol with great caution in patients taking monoamine oxidase inhibitors because animal studies have shown increased deaths with combined administration.

PATIENT INFORMATION

• Tramadol hydrochloride may impair mental or physical abilities required for the performance of potentially hazardous tasks such as driving a car or operating machinery. Tramadol hydrochloride should not be taken with alcohol-containing beverages. Use tramadol hydrochloride with caution in patients taking medications such as tranquilizers, hypnotics, or other opiate-containing analgesics. Instruct patients to inform the physician if they are pregnant, think they might become pregnant, or are trying to become pregnant. The patient should understand the single-dose and 24-hour dose limit and the time interval between doses because exceeding these recommendations can result in respiratory depression and seizures.

PREGNANCY AND LACTATION

• Pregnancy Category C. Tramadol has been shown to be embryotoxic and fetotoxic in mice, rats, and rabbits at maternally toxic doses. Tramadol is not recommended for obstetric preoperative medication or for postdelivery analgesia in nursing mothers because its safety in infants and newborns has not been studied. Tramadol hydrochloride is not excreted into human milk.

trandolapril

(tran-doe'la-pril)

Rx: Mavik

Drug Class: Angiotensin converting enzyme inhibitors

Pregnancy Category: C, 1st; D, 2nd / 3rd

Do not confuse trandolapril with tramadol.

CLINICAL PHARMACOLOGY

Mechanism of Action: An ACE inhibitor that suppresses the renin-angiotensin-aldosterone system and prevents the conversion of angiotensin I to angiotensin II, a potent vasoconstrictor; may also inhibit angiotensin II at local vascular and renal sites. Decreases plasma angiotensin II, increases plasma renin activity, and decreases aldosterone secretion. *Therapeutic Effect:* Reduces peripheral arterial resistance and pulmonary capillary wedge pressure; improves cardiac output and exercise tolerance.

Pharmacokinetics

Slowly absorbed from the GI tract. Protein binding: 80%. Metabolized in the liver and GI mucosa to active metabolite. Primarily excreted in urine. Removed by hemodialysis. **Half-life:** 24 hr.

AVAILABLE FORMS

- *Tablets:* 1 mg, 2 mg, 4 mg.

INDICATIONS AND DOSAGES

Hypertension (without diuretic)

PO

Adults, Elderly. Initially, 1 mg once a day in nonblack patients, 2 mg once a day in black patients. Adjust dosage at least at 7-day intervals. Maintenance: 2-4 mg/day. Maximum: 8 mg/day.

CHF

PO

Adults, Elderly. Initially, 0.5-1 mg, titrated to target dose of 4 mg/day.

CONTRAINDICATIONS: History of angioedema from previous treatment with ACE inhibitors

INTERACTIONS

Drug

Alcohol, antihypertensives, diuretics: May increase the effects of trandolapril.

Lithium: May increase lithium blood concentration and risk of lithium toxicity.

NSAIDs: May decrease the effects of trandolapril.

Potassium-sparing diuretics, potassium supplements: May cause hyperkalemia.

Herbal

None known.

Food

None known.

DIAGNOSTIC TEST EFFECTS: May increase BUN, serum alkaline phosphatase, serum bilirubin, serum creatinine, serum potassium, AST (SGOT), and ALT (SGPT) levels. May decrease serum sodium levels. May cause positive antinuclear antibody titer.

SIDE EFFECTS

Frequent (35%-23%)

Dizziness, cough

Occasional (11%-3%)

Hypotension, dyspepsia (heartburn, epigastric pain, indigestion), syncope, asthenia (loss of strength), tinnitus

Rare (less than 1%)

Palpitations, insomnia, drowsiness, nausea, vomiting, constipation, flushed skin

SERIOUS REACTIONS

- Excessive hypotension ("first-dose syncope") may occur in patients with CHF and in those who are severely salt or volume depleted.

• Angioedema and hyperkalemia occur rarely.
• Agranulocytosis and neutropenia may be noted in those with collagen vascular disease, including scleroderma and systemic lupus erythematosus, and impaired renal function.
• Nephrotic syndrome may be noted in those with history of renal disease.

SPECIAL CONSIDERATIONS

PRECAUTIONS

• Anticipate changes in renal function in susceptible individuals. In hypertensive patients with unilateral or bilateral renal artery stenosis, increases in blood urea nitrogen and serum creatinine have been observed in some patients following angiotensin-converting enzyme (ACE) inhibitor therapy. Hyperkalemia occurred in hypertensive patients receiving trandolapril. Cough has been reported with all ACE inhibitors. In patients undergoing major surgery or during anesthesia with agents that produce hypotension, trandolapril may block angiotensin II formation following compensatory renin release.

PATIENT INFORMATION

• Angioedema: Angioedema, including laryngeal edema, may occur at any time during treatment with ACE inhibitors, including trandolapril. Advise patients to report immediately any signs or symptoms suggesting angioedema (swelling of face, extremities, eyes, lips, or tongue or difficulty in swallowing or breathing) and to stop taking the drug until they have consulted with their physician.
• Symptomatic Hypotension: Caution patients that light-headedness can occur, especially during the first days of trandolapril therapy, and to report this to a physician. If actual syncope occurs, instruct patients to stop taking the drug until they have consulted with their physician.
• Caution all patients that inadequate fluid intake, excessive perspiration, diarrhea, or vomiting resulting in reduced fluid volume may precipitate an excessive fall in blood pressure with the same consequences of light-headedness and possible syncope.
• Instruct patients planning to undergo any surgery and/or anesthesia to inform their physician that they are taking an ACE inhibitor that has a long duration of action.
• Hyperkalemia: Advise patients not to use potassium supplements or salt substitutes containing potassium without consulting their physician.
• Neutropenia: Instruct patients to report promptly any indication of infection (e.g., sore throat or fever), which could be a sign of neutropenia.
• Pregnancy: Inform female patients of childbearing age about the consequences of second- and third-trimester exposure to ACE inhibitors, and inform them that these consequences do not appear to have resulted from intrauterine ACE-inhibitor exposure that has been limited to the first trimester. Ask these patients to report pregnancies to their physicians as soon as possible.
• NOTE: As with many other drugs, certain advice to patients being treated with trandolapril is warranted. This information is intended to aid in the safe and effective use of this medication. Such advice is not a disclosure of all possible adverse or intended effects.

PREGNANCY AND LACTATION

• Pregnancy Categories C (first trimester) and D (second and third trimesters). The use of ACE inhibitors during the second and third trimesters of pregnancy has been associated with fetal and neonatal injury, including hypotension, neonatal skull hypoplasia, anuria, reversible or irreversible renal failure, and death. Radiolabeled trandolapril or its metabolites are secreted in rat milk. Do not administer trandolapril to nursing mothers.

---

travoprost

(tra'-voe-prost)

Rx: Travatan

Drug Class: Ophthalmics; Prostaglandins

Pregnancy Category: C

CLINICAL PHARMACOLOGY

Mechanism of Action: An ophthalmic agent that is a prostanoid selective FP receptor agonist. *Therapeutic Effect:* Reduces intraocular pressure (IOP) by reducing aqueous humor production.

Pharmacokinetics

Absorbed through the cornea and hydrolyzed to the active free acid form. Metabolized in cornea and liver. Metabolites are inactive. Excreted in urine. **Half-life:** 17-86 min.

AVAILABLE FORMS

• *Ophthalmic Solution:* 0.004% (Travatan).

INDICATIONS AND DOSAGES

Open-angle glaucoma, ocular hypertension

Ophthalmic

Adults, Elderly. 1 drop in affected eye(s) once daily, in the evening.

CONTRAINDICATIONS: Hypersensitivity to travoprost or benzalkonium chloride, or any other component of the formulation

INTERACTIONS

Drug

None known.

Herbal

None known.

Food

None known.

DIAGNOSTIC TEST EFFECTS: *None known.*

SIDE EFFECTS

Frequent

Ocular hyperemia

Occasional

Ocular pain, pruritus, eye discomfort, decreased visual acuity, foreign body sensation

Rare

Abnormal vision, cataract, conjunctivitis, dry eye, eye disorder, flare, iris discoloration, keratitis, lid margin crusting, photophobia, subconjunctival hemorrhage, and tearing

SERIOUS REACTIONS

• Ocular adverse events (including accidental injury), angina pectoris, anxiety, arthritis, back pain, bradycardia, bronchitis, chest pain, cold syndrome, depression, dyspepsia, gastrointestinal disorder, headache, hypercholesterolemia, hypertension, hypotension, infection, pain, prostate disorder, sinusitis, urinary incontinence, and urinary tract infection, occur rarely.

SPECIAL CONSIDERATIONS

PRECAUTIONS

• Patients may slowly develop increased brown pigmentation of the iris. This change may not be noticeable for months to years. Iris pigmentation changes may be more noticeable in patients with mixed colored irides (blue-brown, grey-brown, yellow-brown, and green-brown); however, color change also has been observed in patients with brown eyes. The color change is believed to be due to increased melanin content in the stromal melanocytes of the iris. Typically the brown pigmentation around the pupil spreads concentrically toward the periphery in affected eyes, but the entire iris or parts of it may become more brownish. Use travoprost with caution in patients with iritis/uveitis. Cystoid macular edema has been reported in aphakic patients and pseudophakic patients with a torn posterior lens capsule. Travoprost has not been evaluated for the treatment of angle-closure, inflammatory, or neovascular glaucoma. Use travoprost with caution in patients with renal or hepatic impairment. Instruct patients to remove contact lenses and reinsert them 15 minutes following administration of travoprost.

PATIENT INFORMATION

- If more than one topical ocular drug is being used, administer the drugs at least 5 minutes apart.

PREGNANCY AND LACTATION

- Pregnancy Category C. Travoprost may interfere with the maintenance of pregnancy and should not be used by women during pregnancy or by women attempting to become pregnant. Animal studies demonstrated excretion into milk. Excretion into human milk is not known.

trifluridine

(trye-flure'i-deen)

Rx: Viroptic

Drug Class: Antivirals; Ophthalmics

Pregnancy Category: C

Do not confuse with Zostrix.

CLINICAL PHARMACOLOGY

Mechanism of Action: An antiviral agent that incorporates into DNS causing increased rate of mutation and errors in protein formation. *Therapeutic Effect:* Prevents viral replication.

Pharmacokinetics

Intraocular solution is undetectable in serum. **Half-life:** 12 min.

AVAILABLE FORMS

- *Ophthalmic solution:* 1% (Viroptic).

INDICATIONS AND DOSAGES

Herpes simplex virus ocular infections

Ophthalmic

Adults, Elderly, Children older than 6 yr. 1 drop onto cornea q2h while awake. Maximum: 9 drops/day. Continue until corneal ulcer has completely reepithelialized; then, 1 drop q4h while awake (minimum: 5 drops/day) for an additional 7 days.

CONTRAINDICATIONS: Hypersensitivity to trifluridine or any component of the formulation

INTERACTIONS

Drug

None known.

Herbal

None known.

Food

None known.

DIAGNOSTIC TEST EFFECTS: *None known.*

SIDE EFFECTS

Frequent

Transient stinging or burning with instillation

Occasional

Edema of eyelid

Rare

Hypersensitivity reaction

SERIOUS REACTIONS

• Ocular toxicity may occur if used longer than 21 days.

SPECIAL CONSIDERATIONS

PRECAUTIONS

• Trifluridine may cause mild irritation of the conjunctiva and cornea when instilled.

PREGNANCY AND LACTATION

• Pregnancy Category C. Fetal toxicity occurred in rabbits with oral doses. No teratogenic or fetotoxic effects were found after topical application of trifluridine eye solution 1% to the eyes of rabbits on the sixth to eighteenth days of pregnancy. Excretion of trifluridine in human milk is unlikely after ocular instillation of trifluridine because of the relatively small dosage, its dilution in body fluids, and its extremely short half-life. Excretion into human milk is not known.

tripelennamine hydrochloride

(tri-pel-enn'a-meen hye-droh-klor'-ide)

Drug Class: Antihistamines, H1

Pregnancy Category: B

CLINICAL PHARMACOLOGY

Mechanism of Action: An ethylenediamine antihistamine that exhibits selective peripheral histamine H_1 receptor blocking action. Competes with histamine at receptor site. *Therapeutic Effect:* Relieves allergic conditions, including urticaria and pruritus.

Pharmacokinetics

None reported.

AVAILABLE FORMS

• *Tablets:* 50 mg (PBZ).

• *Tablets (sustained-release):* 100 mg (PBZ-SR).

INDICATIONS AND DOSAGES

Perennial and seasonal allergic rhinitis, dermatographism

PO

Adults, Elderly. 25-50 mg q4-6h. Sustained-release tablets: 100 mg in morning and evening, up to 100 mg q8h.

Children, Infants. 5 mg/kg/day in 4-6 divided doses. Maximum: 300 mg/day.

CONTRAINDICATIONS: Narrow-angle glaucoma, stenosing peptic ulcer, symptomatic prostatic hypertrophy, bladder neck obstruction, pyloroduodenal obstruction, lower respiratory tract symptoms (including asthma), premature infants, neonates and nursing mothers, concomitant therapy with MAOIs, hypersensitivity tripelennamine or related components or any component of the formulation.

INTERACTIONS

Drug

Procarbazine: May increase risk of CNS depression.

Herbal

None known.

Food

None known.

DIAGNOSTIC TEST EFFECTS: *None known.*

SIDE EFFECTS

Frequent

Dizziness, sleepiness, fatigue, headache, dry mouth, difficulty urinating

Rare
Sore throat, unusual bleeding or bruising, unusual tiredness or weakness

SERIOUS REACTIONS

• Hypotension and tachycardia may occur with high doses.

• Leukopenia, hemolytic anemia, and thrombocytopenia may occur.

SPECIAL CONSIDERATIONS

PRECAUTIONS

• Antihistamines often produce drowsiness and may reduce mental alertness in children and adults. Antihistamines may produce excitation, particularly in children. PBZ, like other antihistamines, has atropine-like, anticholinergic activity and should be used with caution in patients with increased intraocular pressure, hyperthyroidism, cardiovascular disease, hypertension, or history of bronchial asthma.

PATIENT INFORMATION

• Warn patients about engaging in activities requiring mental alertness (e.g., driving a car or operating machinery or hazardous appliances). In elderly patients, approximately 60 years or older, antihistamines are more likely to cause dizziness, sedation, and hypotension.

• Warn patients that the central nervous system effects of PBZ may be additive with those of alcohol and other central nervous system depressants (e.g., hypnotics, sedatives, tranquilizers, and antianxiety agents).

PREGNANCY AND LACTATION

• Pregnancy Category C. Although no tripelennamine-related teratogenic potential or other adverse effects on the fetus have been observed in limited animal reproduction studies, the safe use of this drug in pregnancy or during lactation has not been established. Therefore, the drug should not be used during pregnancy or lactation unless, in the judgment of the physician, the expected benefits outweigh the potential hazards.

---

tropicamide

(troe-pik′-a-mide)

Rx: Mydriacyl, Ocu-Tropic, Opticyl, Tropicacyl

Drug Class: Anticholinergics; Cycloplegics; Mydriatics; Ophthalmics

CLINICAL PHARMACOLOGY

Mechanism of Action: An antimuscarininc agent that produces competitive antagonism of the actions of acetylcholine. *Therapeutic Effect:* Produces dilation of pupil (mydriasis); produces paralysis of accommodation (cycloplegia).

Pharmacokinetics

Onset of action occurs within 20 to 40 minutes. The duration is about 6 hours.

AVAILABLE FORMS

• *Ophthalmic Solution:* 0.5% (Mydriacyl, Opticyl, Tropicacyl), 1% (Mydriacyl).

INDICATIONS AND DOSAGES

Ocular diagnostic procedure, examination of fundus

Ophthalmic

Adults, Elderly, Children. 1-2 drops in the eye(s) 15-20 min prior to exam

Ocular diagnostic procedure, refractive procedures

Ophthalmic

Adults, Elderly, Children. 1-2 drops in the eye(s). May be repeated in 5 min.

CONTRAINDICATIONS: Primary glaucoma or tendency toward glaucoma, hypersensitivity to tropicamide or any component of the formulation

INTERACTIONS

Drug

Cisapride: May decrease the efficacy of cisapride.

Herbal

None known.

Food

None known.

DIAGNOSTIC TEST EFFECTS: *None known.*

SIDE EFFECTS

Occasional

Blurred vision, ocular irritation, headache

Rare

Photophobia, increased intraocular pressure

SERIOUS REACTIONS

- Cardiorespiratory collapse has been reported.
- Systemic absorption, including behavioral disturbances, confusion, dry mouth, fast heartbeat, and psychotic reactions, occurs rarely.

SPECIAL CONSIDERATIONS

PRECAUTIONS

- Estimate the depth of the angle of the anterior chamber before use.

PATIENT INFORMATION

- Advise patients not to drive or engage in other hazardous activities while pupils are dilated. Patients may experience sensitivity to light and should protect eyes in bright illumination during dilation. Warn parents not to get this preparation in their child's mouth and to wash their own hands and the child's hands following administration.

Unoprostone Isopropyl

(yoo-noh-prost'ohn eye-se-pro'pel)

Rx: Rescula

Drug Class: Ophthalmics; Prostaglandins

Pregnancy Category: C

CLINICAL PHARMACOLOGY

Mechanism of Action: An ophthalmic agent that increases the outflow of aqueous humor. *Therapeutic Effect:* Decreases intraocular pressure.

Pharmacokinetics

Peak response occurs in 4 to 8 weeks. The duration of a single dose is about 10 hours. Hydrolyzed to unoprostone free acid form in the cornea. Rapidly eliminated from plasma. Excreted as metabolites in urine. **Half-life:** 14 min.

AVAILABLE FORMS

- *Ophthalmic Solution:* 0.15% (Rescula).

INDICATIONS AND DOSAGES

Glaucoma, ocular hypertension

Ophthalmic

Adults, Elderly. Instill 1 drop in affected eye(s) 2 times/day.

CONTRAINDICATIONS: Hypersensitivity to unoprostone isopropyl, benzalkonium chloride or any other component of the formulation

INTERACTIONS

Drug

None known.

Herbal

None known.

Food

None known.

DIAGNOSTIC TEST EFFECTS: *None known.*

SIDE EFFECTS

Frequent (25%-10%)

Burning, stinging, dry eyes, itching, increased eyelash length and redness.

Occasional (less than 10%)

Abnormal vision, eyelid disorder, foreign body sensation.

SERIOUS REACTIONS

• Elevated intraocular pressure occurs rarely.

SPECIAL CONSIDERATIONS

PRECAUTIONS

• Use unoprostone isopropyl with caution in patients with active intraocular inflammation (e.g., uveitis).

• Unoprostone isopropyl has not been evaluated for the treatment of angle-closure, inflammatory, or neovascular glaucoma. Use unoprostone isopropyl with caution in patients with renal or hepatic impairment. Unoprostone isopropyl contains benzalkonium chloride. Soft contact lenses may be reinserted 15 minutes following administration.

PATIENT INFORMATION

• Advise patients that if they develop any ocular reactions, particularly conjunctivitis and eyelid reactions, they immediately should seek their eye care practitioner's advice.

• If the patient is using more than one topical ocular drug, instruct the patient to administer the drugs at least 5 minutes apart.

PREGNANCY AND LACTATION

• Pregnancy Category C. Rats and rabbits studies showed no fetal harm with oral doses but did show fetal harm with subcutaneous doses. Fetal harm is not known with topical administration. Intravenous administration in rats was followed by excretion into milk. Excretion into human milk with topical administration is not known.

urokinase

(you-oh-kine-ace)

Rx: Abbokinase, Abbokinase Open-Cath

Drug Class: Thrombolytics

Pregnancy Category: B

CLINICAL PHARMACOLOGY

Mechanism of Action: A thrombolytic agent that activates fibrinolytic system by converting plasminogen to plasmin (enzyme that degrades fibrin clots). Acts indirectly by forming complex with plasminogen, which converts plasminogen to plasmin. Action occurs within thrombus, on its surface, and in circulating blood. *Therapeutic Effect:* Destroys thrombi.

Pharmacokinetics

Rapidly cleared from circulation by liver. Small amounts eliminated in urine and via bile. **Half-life:** 20 min.

AVAILABLE FORMS

• *Powder for Injection:* 250,000 IU/vial, 5000 IU/ml (Abbokinase).

INDICATIONS AND DOSAGES

Pulmonary embolism

IV

Adults, Elderly. Initially, 4400 IU/kg at rate of 90 ml/hr over 10 min; then, 4400 IU/kg at rate of 15 ml/hr for 12 hrs. Flush tubing. Follow with anticoagulant therapy.

Coronary artery thrombi

Intracoronary

Adults, Elderly. 6000 IU/min for up to 2 hrs.

Occluded IV catheter

Adults, Elderly. Disconnect IV tubing from catheter; attach a 1-ml TB syringe with 5000 U urokinase to catheter; inject urokinase slowly (equal to volume of catheter). Connect empty 5-ml syringe; aspirate residual clot. When patency is restored, irrigate with 0.9% NaCl; reconnect IV tubing to catheter.

CONTRAINDICATIONS: Active internal bleeding, atrioventricular (AV) malformation or aneurysm, bleeding diathesis, intracranial neoplasm, intracranial or intraspinal surgery or trauma, recent (within the past 2 mos) cerebrovascular accident

INTERACTIONS

Drug

Anticoagulants, including cefotetan, heparin, plicamycin, valproic acid: May increase risk of hemorrhage.

Antifibrinolytics, including aminocaproic acid: May antagonize effects.

Platelet aggregation inhibitors, including aspirin, NSAIDs, ticlopidine: May increase risk of bleeding.

Herbal

Ginkgo biloba: May increase risk of bleeding.

Food

None known.

DIAGNOSTIC TEST EFFECTS: Decreases plasminogen and fibrinogen levels during infusion, which decreases clotting time (confirms the presence of lysis). Increases aPTT, PT, TT.

IV INCOMPATIBILITIES: Do not add or mix any other medication with urokinase.

SIDE EFFECTS

Frequent

Superficial or surface bleeding at puncture sites (venous cutdowns, arterial punctures, surgical sites, IM sites, retroperitoneal/intracerebral sites); internal bleeding (GI/GU tract, vaginal).

Rare

Mild allergic reaction such as rash or wheezing

SERIOUS REACTIONS

• Severe internal hemorrhage may occur. Lysis of coronary thrombi may produce atrial/ventricular arrhythmias

SPECIAL CONSIDERATIONS

OCULAR CONSIDERATIONS

• Urokinase has been used to prevent haze after photorefractive keratectomy in rabbits. Urokinase may stimulate migration, facilitate reepithelialization, ensure corneal epithelial cell adhesion, and promote successful wound healing. (Csutak A et al: Urokinase-type plasminogen activator to prevent haze after photorefractive keratectomy, and pregnancy as a risk factor for haze in rabbits, *Invest Ophthalmol Vis Sci* 45[5]:1329-1333, 2004. Wang Z, Sosne G, Kurpakus-Wheater M: Plasminogen activator inhibitor-1 [PAI-1] stimulates human corneal epithelial cell adhesion and migration in vitro, *Exp Eye Res* 80[1]:1-8, 2005.)

valacyclovir

(val-a-sye'kloe-ver)

Rx: Valtrex

Drug Class: Antivirals

Pregnancy Category: B

CLINICAL PHARMACOLOGY

Mechanism of Action: A virustatic antiviral that is converted to acyclovir triphosphate, becoming part of the viral DNA chain. *Therapeutic Effect:* Interferes with DNA synthesis and replication of herpes simplex virus and varicella-zoster virus.

Pharmacokinetics

Rapidly absorbed after PO administration. Protein binding: 13%-18%. Rapidly converted by hydrolysis to the active compound acyclovir. Widely distributed to tissues and body fluids (including CSF). Primarily eliminated in urine. Removed by hemodialysis. **Half-life:** 2.5-3.3 hr (increased in impaired renal function).

AVAILABLE FORMS

• *Caplets:* 500 mg, 1000 mg.

INDICATIONS AND DOSAGES

Herpes zoster (shingles)

PO

Adults, Elderly. 1 g 3 times a day for 7 days.

Herpes simplex (cold sores)

PO

Adults, Elderly. 2 g twice a day for 1 day.

Initial episode of genital herpes

PO

Adults, Elderly. 1 g twice a day for 10 days.

Recurrent episodes of genital herpes

PO

Adults, Elderly. 500 mg twice a day for 3 days.

Prevention of genital herpes

PO

Adults, Elderly. 500-1000 mg/day.

Dosage in renal impairment

Dosage and frequency are modified based on creatinine clearance.

Creatinine Clearance	*Herpes Zoster*	*Genital Herpes*
50 ml/min or higher	1 g q8h	500 mg q12h
30-49 ml/min	1 g q12h	500 mg q12h
10-29 ml/min	1 g q24h	500 mg q24h
less than 10 ml/min	500 mg q24h	500 mg q24h

UNLABELED USES: To reduce the risk of heterosexual transmission of genital herpes

CONTRAINDICATIONS: Hypersensitivity to or intolerance of acyclovir, valacyclovir, or their components

INTERACTIONS

Drug

Cimetidine, probenecid: May increase acyclovir blood concentration.

Herbal

None known.

Food

None known.

DIAGNOSTIC TEST EFFECTS: *None known.*

SIDE EFFECTS

Frequent

Herpes zoster (17%-10%): Nausea, headache

Genital herpes (17%): Headache

Occasional

Herpes zoster (7%-3%): Vomiting, diarrhea, constipation (50 yr or older), asthenia, dizziness (50 yr and older)

Genital herpes (8%-3%): Nausea, diarrhea, dizziness

Rare

Herpes zoster (3%-1%): Abdominal pain, anorexia

Genital herpes (3%-1%): Asthenia, abdominal pain

SERIOUS REACTIONS

• None known.

SPECIAL CONSIDERATIONS

PRECAUTIONS

• Dosage reduction is recommended when administering valacyclovir hydrochloride to patients with renal impairment.

PATIENT INFORMATION

• Herpes Zoster: No data exist on treatment initiated more than 72 hours after onset of the zoster rash. Advise patients to initiate treatment as soon as possible after a diagnosis of herpes zoster.

• Genital Herpes: Inform patients that valacyclovir hydrochloride is not a cure for genital herpes. No data exist that evaluate whether valacyclovir hydrochloride will prevent transmission of infection to others. Because genital herpes is a sexually transmitted disease, patients should avoid contact with lesions or intercourse when lesions and/or symptoms are present to avoid infecting partners. Genital herpes also can be transmitted in the absence of symptoms through asymptomatic viral shedding. If medical management of a genital herpes recurrence is indicated, advise patients to initiate therapy at the first sign or symptom of an episode. No data exist on the effectiveness of treatment initiated more than 72 hours after the onset of signs and symptoms of a first episode of genital herpes or more than 24 hours of the onset of signs and symptoms of a recurrent episode. No data exist on the safety or effectiveness of chronic suppressive therapy of more than 1 year's duration.

PREGNANCY AND LACTATION

• Pregnancy Category B. Valacyclovir was not teratogenic in rats or rabbits. Excretion into human milk is not known.

valsartan

(val-sar'tan)

Rx: Diovan

Drug Class: Angiotensin II receptor antagonists

Pregnancy Category: C, 1st; D, 2nd / 3rd

Do not confuse valsartan with Valstan.

CLINICAL PHARMACOLOGY

Mechanism of Action: An angiotensin II receptor, type AT_1, antagonist that blocks vasoconstrictor and aldosterone-secreting effects of angiotensin II, inhibiting the binding of angiotensin II to the AT_1 receptors. *Therapeutic Effect:* Causes vasodilation, decreases peripheral resistance, and decreases BP.

Pharmacokinetics

Poorly absorbed after PO administration. Food decreases peak plasma concentration. Protein binding: 95%. Metabolized in the liver. Recovered primarily in feces and, to a lesser extent, in urine. Unknown if removed by hemodialysis. **Half-life:** 6 hr.

AVAILABLE FORMS

• *Tablets:* 40 mg, 80 mg, 160 mg, 320 mg.

INDICATIONS AND DOSAGES

Hypertension

PO

Adults, Elderly. Initially, 80-160 mg/day in patients who are not volume depleted. May increase up to a maximum: 320 mg/day.

CHF

PO

Adults, Elderly. Initially, 40 mg twice a day. May increase up to 160 mg twice a day. Maximum: 320 mg/day.

CONTRAINDICATIONS: Bilateral renal artery stenosis, biliary cirrhosis or obstruction, hypoaldosteronism, severe hepatic impairment

INTERACTIONS

Drug

Diuretics: Produces additive hypotensive effects.

Herbal

None known.

Food

All foods: Decreases peak plasma concentration of valsartan.

DIAGNOSTIC TEST EFFECTS: May increase AST (SGOT), ALT (SGPT), and serum bilirubin, creatinine, and potassium levels. May decrease blood Hgb and Hct levels.

SIDE EFFECTS

Rare (2%-1%)

Insomnia, fatigue, heartburn, abdominal pain, dizziness, headache, diarrhea, nausea, vomiting, arthralgia, edema

SERIOUS REACTIONS

- Overdosage may manifest as hypotension and tachycardia. Bradycardia occurs less often.
- Viral infection and upper respiratory tract infection (cough, pharyngitis, sinusitis, rhinitis) occur rarely.

SPECIAL CONSIDERATIONS

PRECAUTIONS

- Patients with biliary obstructive disorders or hepatic insufficiency can be expected to have reduced clearance. Changes in renal function have been reported in susceptible individuals. In patients with unilateral or bilateral renal artery stenosis, increases in serum creatinine or blood urea nitrogen have been reported.

PATIENT INFORMATION

- Pregnancy: Inform female patients of childbearing age about the consequences of second- and third-trimester exposure to drugs that act on the renin-angiotensin system, and inform them that these consequences do not appear to have resulted from intrauterine drug exposure that has been limited to the first trimester. Ask these patients to report pregnancies to their physicians as soon as possible.

PREGNANCY AND LACTATION

- Pregnancy Categories C (first trimester) and D (second and third trimesters). The use of drugs that act directly on the renin-angiotensin system during the second and third trimesters of pregnancy has been associated with fetal and neonatal injury, including hypotension, neonatal skull hypoplasia, anuria, reversible or irreversible renal failure, and death. Whether valsartan is excreted in human milk is not known, but valsartan is excreted in the milk of lactating rats.

---

venlafaxine

(ven-la-fax'een)

Rx: Effexor, Effexor XR

Drug Class: Antidepressants, miscellaneous

Pregnancy Category: C

CLINICAL PHARMACOLOGY

Mechanism of Action: A phenethylamine derivative that potentiates CNS neurotransmitter activity by inhibiting the reuptake of serotonin, norepinephrine and, to a lesser degree, dopamine. *Therapeutic Effect:* Relieves depression.

Pharmacokinetics

Well absorbed from the GI tract. Protein binding: 25%-30%. Metabolized in the liver to active metabolite. Primarily excreted in urine. Not removed by hemodialysis. **Half-life:** 3-7 hr; metabolite, 9-13 hr (increased in hepatic or renal impairment.

AVAILABLE FORMS

- *Capsules (Extended-Release [Effexor XL]):* 37.5 mg, 75 mg, 150 mg.
- *Tablets (Effexor):* 25 mg, 37.5 mg, 50 mg, 75 mg, 100 mg.

INDICATIONS AND DOSAGES

Depression

PO

Adults, Elderly. Initially, 75 mg/day in 2-3 divided doses with food. May increase by 75 mg/day at intervals of 4 days or longer. Maximum: 375 mg/day in 3 divided doses.

PO (Extended-Release)

Adults, Elderly. 75 mg/day as a single dose with food. May increase by 75 mg/day at intervals of 4 days or longer. Maximum: 225 mg/day.

Anxiety disorder

PO (Extended-Release)

Adults. 37.5-225 mg/day.

Dosage in renal and hepatic impairment

Expect to decrease venlafaxine dosage by 50% in patients with moderate hepatic impairment, 25% in patients with mild to moderate renal impairment, and 50% in patients on dialysis (withhold dose until completion of dialysis).

UNLABELED USES: Prevention of relapses of depression; treatment of attention-deficit hyperactivity disorder, autism, chronic fatigue syndrome, obsessive-compulsive disorder

CONTRAINDICATIONS: Use within 14 days of MAOIs

INTERACTIONS

Drug

MAOIs: May cause neuroleptic malignant syndrome, autonomic instability (including rapid fluctuations of vital signs), extreme agitation, hyperthermia, mental status changes, myoclonus, rigidity, and coma.

Herbal

St. John's wort: May increase the sedative-hypnotic effect of venlafaxine.

Food

None known.

DIAGNOSTIC TEST EFFECTS: May increase BUN level and serum alkaline phosphatase, bilirubin, cholesterol, uric acid, AST (SGOT), and ALT (SGPT) levels. May decrease serum phosphate and sodium levels. May alter blood glucose and serum potassium levels.

SIDE EFFECTS

Frequent (greater than 20%)

Nausea, somnolence, headache, dry mouth

Occasional (20%-10%)

Dizziness, insomnia, constipation, diaphoresis, nervousness, asthenia, ejaculatory disturbance, anorexia

Rare (less than 10%)

Anxiety, blurred vision, diarrhea, vomiting, tremor, abnormal dreams, impotence

SERIOUS REACTIONS

• A sustained increase in diastolic BP of 10-15 mm Hg occurs occasionally.

SPECIAL CONSIDERATIONS

PRECAUTIONS

• Tremor, myoclonus, diaphoresis, nausea, vomiting, flushing, dizziness, hyperthermia with features resembling neuroleptic malignant syndrome, seizures, and death have been reported in patients who recently had discontinued monoamine oxidase inhibitor therapy and had started taking venlafaxine. Reports also indicate serious, sometimes fatal, reactions in patients receiving antidepressants with pharmacologic properties similar to venlafaxine in combination with a monoamine oxidase inhibitor. Venlafaxine is associated with sustained increases in blood pressure in some patients. Treatment-emergent insomnia and nervousness and treatment-emergent anorexia were reported. The risk of skin and mucous membrane bleeding may be increased in patients taking venlafaxine.

• The possibility of a suicide attempt is inherent in depression and may persist until significant remission occurs. In patients with renal impairment or cirrhosis of the liver, the clearances of venlafaxine and its active metabolites were decreased.

PATIENT INFORMATION

• Interference with Cognitive and Motor Performance: Clinical studies were performed to examine the effects of venlafaxine on behavioral performance of healthy individuals. The results revealed no clinically significant impairment of psychomotor, cognitive, or complex behavior performance. However, because any psychoactive drug may impair judgment, thinking, or motor skills, caution patients about operating hazardous machinery, including automobiles, until they are reasonably certain that venlafaxine therapy does not adversely affect their ability to engage in such activities.

• Concomitant Modification: Advise patients to inform their physicians if they are taking, or plan to take, any prescription or over-the-counter drugs because of the potential for interactions.

• Alcohol: Although venlafaxine has not been shown to increase the impairment of mental and motor skills caused by alcohol, advise patients to avoid alcohol while taking venlafaxine.

• Allergic Reactions: Advise patients to notify their physician if they develop a rash, hives, or a related allergic phenomenon.

• Pregnancy: Advise patients to notify their physician if they become pregnant or intend to become pregnant during therapy.

• Nursing: Advise patients to notify their physician if they are breast-feeding an infant.

PREGNANCY AND LACTATION

• Pregnancy Category C. Venlafaxine did not cause malformations in offspring of rats or rabbits. However, in rats there was a decrease in pup weight, an increase in stillborn pups, and an increase in pup deaths during the first 5 days of lactation. Fetal harm is not known. Venlafaxine and ODV have been reported to be excreted in human milk.

OCULAR CONSIDERATIONS

• Mydriasis has been reported in association with venlafaxine; therefore, monitor patients with raised intraocular pressure or those at risk of acute narrow-angle glaucoma.

• Adverse reactions include abnormality of accommodation and mydriasis (frequent); cataract, conjunctivitis, corneal lesion, diplopia, dry eyes, exophthalmos, eye pain, photophobia, and visual field defect (infrequent); and blepharitis, chromatopsia, conjunctival edema, glaucoma, retinal hemorrhage, subconjunctival hemorrhage, keratitis, miosis, papilledema, decreased papillary reflex, scleritis, and uveitis (rare).

verapamil hydrochloride

(ver-ap'a-mill)

Rx: Calan, Calan SR, Covera-HS, Isoptin, Isoptin I.V., Isoptin SR, Verelan, Verelan PM

Drug Class: Antiarrhythmics, class IV; Calcium channel blockers

Pregnancy Category: C

Do not confuse Isoptin with Intropin, or Verelan with Virilon, Vivarin, or Voltaren.

CLINICAL PHARMACOLOGY

Mechanism of Action: A calcium channel blocker and antianginal, antiarrhythmic, and antihypertensive agent that inhibits calcium ion entry across cardiac and vascular smooth-muscle cell membranes. This action causes the dilation of coronary arteries, peripheral arteries, and arterioles. *Therapeutic Effect:* Decreases heart rate and myocardial contractility and slows SA and AV conduction. Decreases total peripheral vascular resistance by vasodilation.

Pharmacokinetics

Route	*Onset*	*Peak*	*Duration*
PO	30 min	1-2 hr	6-8 hr
PO (Extended-release)	30 min	N/A	N/A
IV	1-2 min	3-5 min	10-60 min

Well absorbed from the GI tract. Protein binding: 90% (60% in neonates). Undergoes first-pass metabolism in the liver to active metabolite. Primarily excreted in urine. Not removed by hemodialysis. **Half-life:** 2-8 hr.

AVAILABLE FORMS

- *Caplet (Calan SR):* 120 mg, 180 mg, 240 mg.
- *Capsules (Extended-Release [Verelan PM]):* 100 mg, 200 mg, 300 mg.
- *Capsules (Sustained-Release [Verelan]):* 120 mg, 180 mg, 240 mg, 360 mg.
- *Tablets (Calan):* 40 mg, 80 mg, 120 mg.
- *Tablets (Extended-Release [Covera HS]).* 180 mg, 240 mg.
- *Tablets (Sustained-Release [Isoptin SR}):* 120 mg, 180 mg, 240 mg.
- *Injection:* 2.5 mg/ml.

INDICATIONS AND DOSAGES

Supraventricular tachyarrhythmias, temporary control of rapid ventricular rate with atrial fibrillation or flutter

IV

Adults, Elderly. Initially, 5-10 mg; repeat in 30 min with 10-mg dose.

Children 1 to 15 yr. 0.1 mg/kg. May repeat in 30 min up to a maximum second dose of 10 mg. Not recommended in children younger than 1 yr.

Arrhythmias, including prevention of recurrent paroxysmal supraventricular tachycardia and control of ventricular resting rate in chronic atrial fibrillation or flutter (with digoxin)

PO

Adults, Elderly. 240-480 mg/day in 3-4 divided doses.

Vasospastic angina (Prinzmetal's variant), unstable (crescendo or preinfarction) angina, chronic stable (effort-associated) angina

PO

Adults. Initially, 80-120 mg 3 times a day. For elderly patients and those with hepatic dysfunction, 40 mg 3 times a day. Titrate to optimal dose. Maintenance: 240-480 mg/day in 3-4 divided doses.

PO (Covera-HS)

Adults, Elderly. 180-480 mg/day at bedtime.

Hypertension

PO

Adults, Elderly. Initially, 40-80 mg 3 times a day. Maintenance: 480 mg or less a day.

PO (Covera-HS)

Adults, Elderly. 180-480 mg/day at bedtime.

PO (Extended-Release)

Adults, Elderly. 120-240 mg/day. May give 480 mg or less a day in 2 divided doses.

PO (Verelan PM)

Adults, Elderly. 100-300 mg/day.

UNLABELED USES: Treatment of hypertrophic cardiomyopathy, vascular headaches

CONTRAINDICATIONS: Atrial fibrillation or flutter and an accessory bypass tract, cardiogenic shock, heart block, sinus bradycardia, ventricular tachycardia

INTERACTIONS

Drug

Beta-blockers: May have additive effect.

Carbamazepine, quinidine, theophylline: May increase verapamil blood concentration and risk of toxicity.
Digoxin: May increase digoxin blood concentration.
Disopyramide: May increase negative inotropic effect.
Procainamide, quinidine: May increase risk of QT-interval prolongation.

Herbal

None known.

Food

Grapefruit, grapefruit juice: May increase verapamil blood concentration.

DIAGNOSTIC TEST EFFECTS: EKG waveform may show increased PR interval. Therapeutic serum level is 0.08-0.3 mcg/ml.

IV INCOMPATIBILITIES: Amphotericin B complex (Abelcet, AmBisome, Amphotec), nafcillin (Nafcil), propofol (Diprivan), sodium bicarbonate

IV COMPATIBILITIES: Amiodarone (Cordarone), calcium chloride, calcium gluconate, dexamethasone (Decadron), digoxin (Lanoxin), dobutamine (Dobutrex), dopamine (Intropin), furosemide (Lasix), heparin, hydromorphone (Dilaudid), lidocaine, magnesium sulfate, metoclopramide (Reglan), milrinone (Primacor), morphine, multivitamins, nitroglycerin, norepinephrine (Levophed), potassium chloride, potassium phosphate, procainamide (Pronestyl), propranolol (Inderal)

SIDE EFFECTS

Frequent (7%)

Constipation

Occasional (4%-2%)

Dizziness, light-headedness, headache, asthenia (loss of strength, energy), nausea, peripheral edema, hypotension

Rare (less than 1%)

Bradycardia, dermatitis or rash

SERIOUS REACTIONS

- Rapid ventricular rate in atrial flutter or fibrillation, marked hypotension, extreme bradycardia, CHF, asystole, and second- and third-degree AV block occur rarely.

SPECIAL CONSIDERATIONS

PRECAUTIONS

- The contents of the verapamil hydrochloride, extended-release, controlled-onset capsule should not be crushed or chewed. Administer verapamil hydrochloride cautiously to patients with impaired hepatic function. It may be necessary to decrease the dosage of verapamil when it is administered to patients with attenuated neuromuscular transmission. Administer verapamil hydrochloride cautiously to patients with impaired renal function.

PREGNANCY AND LACTATION

- Pregnancy Category C. Oral doses given to rats were embryocidal and retarded fetal growth and development. Fetal harm is not known. Verapamil is excreted in human milk.

OCULAR CONSIDERATIONS

- In chronic animal toxicology studies, verapamil caused lenticular and/or suture line changes at 30 mg/kg per day or greater, and frank cataracts at 62.5 mg/kg per day or greater in the beagle dog, but not in the rat. Development of cataracts from use of verapamil has not been reported in human beings.
- Asymptomatic bradycardia (36 beats/min) with a wandering atrial pacemaker has been observed in a patient receiving concomitant administration of timolol (a beta-adrenergic blocker) eye drops and oral verapamil. Verapamil may increase serum levels of cyclosporin.

• Some patients currently are being put on verapamil (Calan) for vasospasm. Vasospasm may contribute to ocular ischemia and subsequent visual loss in patients with normal-tension glaucoma. Calcium channel blockers reduce vasospasm through the inhibition of calcium influx. The drug relaxes the vascular smooth muscle and reduces vascular tone. The calcium channel blockers have been found to increase blood flow and volume to the optic nerve and to increase trabecular meshwork outflow. (Bonner H: Ocular drug preview: spotlight on emerging pharmaceuticals, *Rev Optometry* vol 141, issue 12, 2004. http://www.revoptom.com/index.asp?page=2_1309.htm.)

Verteporfin

(ver-te-por'fin)
Drug Class: Ophthalmics
Pregnancy Category: C

CLINICAL PHARMACOLOGY

Mechanism of Action: A benzoporphyrin derivative that requires administration of both verteporfin for injection and nonthermal red light. Verteporfin is transported in the plasma by lipoproteins. In the presence of oxygen, photoactivation of verteporfin results in the production of highly reactive, short-lived singlet oxygen and reactive oxygen radicals. The production of these radicals leads to local damage to neovascular endothelium. *Therapeutic Effect:* Results in occlusion of abnormal (leaking) vessels.

Pharmacokinetics

Metabolized in liver to diacid metabolite. Minimal excretion in urine. The extent of excretion is unknown in bile and feces. **Half-life:** 5-6 hrs.

AVAILABLE FORMS

• *Powder for Injection:* 15 mg.

INDICATIONS AND DOSAGES

Age-related macular degeneration

IV

Adults, Elderly. 6 mg/m^2 followed by light therapy 15 min after start of 10 min verteporfin infusion. Light dose in 50 J/cm^2 of neovascular lesion at intensity of 600 mW/cm^2 over 83 sec.

CONTRAINDICATIONS: Porphyria, patients treated with other photosensitizing agents (current of previous in 3 months) hypersensitivity to verteporfin or other porphyrin derivatives (e.g., porfimer)

INTERACTIONS

Drug

None known.

Herbal

None known.

Food

None known.

DIAGNOSTIC TEST EFFECTS: *None known.*

SIDE EFFECTS

Occasional

Headache, injection site reactions, temporary photosensitivity, visual disturbances

Rare

Dizziness, dull nervousness, eye pain, fainting, tachycardia, bradycardia, itching, redness or other eye irritation, pale skin, pounding in ears, trouble breathing on exertion, weakness

SERIOUS REACTIONS

• Anemia, atrial fibrillation, hypertension, peripheral vascular disorder, cataracts, eye hemorrhage, severe vision decrease, elevated liver function tests, and gastrointestinal (GI) cancers occur rarely.

• Overdosage may produce nonperfusion of normal retinal vessels with the possibility of severe decrease in vision that could be permanent, prolongation of the period during which the patient remains photosensitive to bright light. If overdose occurs, it is recommended to extend the photosensitivity precautions for a time proportional to the overdose.

SPECIAL CONSIDERATIONS

PRECAUTIONS

• Take standard precautions during infusion of verteporfin to avoid extravasation. Use verteporfin with caution in patients with moderate to severe hepatic impairment.

PATIENT INFORMATION

• Patients become temporarily photosensitive after the infusion. Patients should wear a wrist band to remind them to avoid direct sunlight for 5 days. During that period, patients should avoid exposure of unprotected skin, eyes, or other body organs to direct sunlight or bright indoor light. Sources of bright light include tanning salons, bright halogen lighting, and high-power lighting used in surgical operating rooms or dental offices. If treated patients must go outdoors in daylight during the first 5 days after treatment, they should protect all parts of their skin and their eyes by wearing protective clothing and dark sunglasses. Ultraviolet sunscreens are not effective in protecting against photosensitivity reactions because photoactivation of the residual drug in the skin can be caused by visible light. Patients should not stay in the dark and should be encouraged to expose their skin to ambient indoor light because it will help inactivate the drug in the skin through a process called photobleaching.

PREGNANCY AND LACTATION

• Pregnancy Category C. Studies in rats and rabbits showed fetal harm with intravenous injection. Excretion into human milk is not known.

vidarabine

(vye-dare'-a-been)

Drug Class: Anti-infectives, ophthalmic; Antivirals; Ophthalmics

Pregnancy Category: C

Do not confuse with Zostrix.

CLINICAL PHARMACOLOGY

Mechanism of Action: An antiviral agent that appears to interfere with viral DNS synthesis. *Therapeutic Effect:* Regenerates corneal epithelium.

Pharmacokinetics

None reported.

AVAILABLE FORMS

• *Ophthalmic ointment:* 3% (Vira-A).

INDICATIONS AND DOSAGES

Treatment of keratitis, keratoconjunctivitis caused by herpes simplex virus, types 1 and 2

Ophthalmic

Adults, Elderly. Apply 0.5 inch into lower conjunctival sac 5 times/day at 3 hr intervals. After re-epithelialization, treat for additional 7 days at dosage of 2 times/day.

CONTRAINDICATIONS: Hypersensitivity to vidarabine or any component of the formulation

INTERACTIONS

Drug

None known.

Herbal

None known.

Food

None known.

DIAGNOSTIC TEST EFFECTS: *None known.*

SIDE EFFECTS

Frequent

Burning, itching, irritation

Occasional
Foreign body sensation, tearing, sensitivity to light, pain, photophobia

SERIOUS REACTIONS
• None significant.

SPECIAL CONSIDERATIONS

PRECAUTIONS
• Vidarabine may produce a temporary visual haze because of the ointment.

PREGNANCY AND LACTATION
• Pregnancy Category C. The possibility of embryonic or fetal damage in pregnant women receiving vidarabine is remote. Breast milk excretion is unlikely because vidarabine is deaminated rapidly in the gastrointestinal tract.

vitamin A

(vight'-ah-myn A)

Rx: Aquasol A
Drug Class: Vitamins/minerals
Pregnancy Category: X
Do not confuse Aquasol A with Anusol.

CLINICAL PHARMACOLOGY

Mechanism of Action: A fat-soluble vitamin that may act as a cofactor in biochemical reactions. *Therapeutic Effect:* Is essential for normal function of retina, visual adaptation to darkness, bone growth, testicular and ovarian function, and embryonic development; preserves integrity of epithelial cells.

Pharmacokinetics

Rapidly absorbed from the GI tract if bile salts, pancreatic lipase, protein, and dietary fat are present. Transported in blood to the liver, where it's metabolized; stored in parenchymal hepatic cells, then transported in plasma as retinol, as needed. Excreted primarily in bile and, to a lesser extent, in urine.

AVAILABLE FORMS
• *Capsules:* 10,000 units, 25,000 units.
• *Injection (Aquasol A):* 50,000 units/ml.
• *Tablets (Palmitate A):* 5000 units, 15,000 units.

INDICATIONS AND DOSAGES

Severe vitamin A deficiency

PO

Adults, Elderly, Children 8 yr and older. 500,000 units/day for 3 days; then 50,000 units/day for 14 days, then 10,000-20,000 units/day for 2 mo.

Children 1-7 yr. 5000 units/kg/day for 5 days, then 5000-10,000 units/day for 2 mo.

Children younger than 1 yr. 5000-10,000 units/day for 2 mo.

IM

Adults, Elderly, Children 8 yr and older. 100,000 units/day for 3 days; then 50,000 units/day for 14 days.

Children 1-7 yr. 17,500-35,000 units/day for 10 days.

Children younger than 1 yr. 7500-15,000 units/day.

Malabsorption syndrome

PO

Adults, Elderly, Children 8 yr and older. 10,000-50,000 units/day.

Dietary supplement

PO

Adults, Elderly. 4000-5000 units/day.

Children 7-10 yr. 3300-3500 units/day.

Children 4-6 yr. 2500 units/day.

Children 6 mo-3 yr. 1500-2000 units/day.

Neonates younger than 5 mo. 1500 units/day.

CONTRAINDICATIONS: Hypervitaminosis A

INTERACTIONS

Drug

Cholestyramine, colestipol, mineral oil: May decrease the absorption of vitamin A.

Isotretinoin: May increase the risk of toxicity.

Herbal

None known.

Food

None known.

DIAGNOSTIC TEST EFFECTS: May increase BUN and serum cholesterol, calcium, and triglyceride levels. May decrease blood erythrocyte and leukocyte counts.

SIDE EFFECTS

None known.

SERIOUS REACTIONS

• Chronic overdose produces malaise, nausea, vomiting, drying or cracking of skin or lips, inflammation of tongue or gums, irritability, alopecia, and night sweats.

• Bulging fontanelles have occurred in infants.

SPECIAL CONSIDERATIONS

PRECAUTIONS

• Prolonged daily dose administration of more than 25,000 units vitamin A should be done under close supervision.

PREGNANCY AND LACTATION

• Pregnancy Category X. Use of vitamin A in excess of the recommended dietary allowance may cause fetal harm when administered to a pregnant woman. The U.S. Recommended Daily Allowance of vitamin A (5000 units) is recommended for nursing mothers.

OCULAR CONSIDERATIONS

• Alternative forms of vitamin A (retinol) such as tretinoin, isotretinoin, etretinate, and acitretin have been shown to cause intracranial hypertension. (Fraunfelder FW: Ocular side effects from herbal medicines and nutritional supplements, *Am J Ophthalmol* 138[4]:639-647, 2004.)

vitamin B complex; vitamin C

(vye'-ta-min bee-kom'-pleks; vye'-ta-min see)

Rx: Cefol, Cerefolin, Cernevit, Cernevit-12, Dialyvite Rx, Foltx, Formula B, Icar C, Infuvite, Infuvite Pediatric, Key-Plex, Lipotriad, M.V.I.-12, M.V.I. Pediatric, Nephplex Rx, Nephrocaps, Nephrolan RX, Nephro-Vite Rx, Renal Caps, Renaphro, Rena-Vite Rx, StressTabs, Therobec, Vitamin B-Plex, Vitaplex

Drug Class: Vitamins/minerals

CLINICAL PHARMACOLOGY

Mechanism of Action: Vitamin B_1 is a water-soluble vitamin that combines with adenosine triphosphate (ATP) in liver, kidney, and leukocytes to form thiamine diphosphate. *Therapeutic Effect:* Is necessary for carbohydrate metabolism.

Vitamin B_6 is a coenzyme for various metabolic functions that maintains metabolism of proteins, carbohydrates, and fats. Aids in release of liver and muscle glycogen and in the synthesis of gamma-aminobutyric acid (GABA) in the central nervous system (CNS).

Vitamin B_{12} is a coenzyme for metabolic functions, including fat and carbohydrate metabolism and protein synthesis. *Therapeutic Effect:* Necessary for growth, cell replication, hematopoiesis, and myelin synthesis.

Vitamin C assists in collagen formation and tissue repair and is involved in oxidation reduction reactions and other metabolic reactions. *Therapeutic Effect:* Involved in carbohydrate utilization, metabolism, and synthesis of carnitine, lipids, and proteins. Preserves blood vessel integrity.

Pharmacokinetics

Vitamin B_1 is readily absorbed from the gastrointestinal (GI) tract. Widely distributed. Metabolized in liver. Primarily excreted in urine.

Vitamin B_6 is readily absorbed primarily in jejunum. Stored in liver, muscle, brain. Metabolized in liver. Primarily excreted in urine. Removed by hemodialysis.

Vitamin B_{12} is absorbed in lower half of ileum in presence of calcium. Initially, bound to intrinsic factor; this complex passes down intestine, binding to receptor sites on ileal mucosa. In presence of calcium, absorbed systemically. Protein binding: High. Metabolized in liver. Primarily eliminated in urine unchanged.

Vitamin C is readily absorbed from the gastrointestinal (GI) tract. Metabolized in liver. Excreted in urine. Removed by hemodialysis.

AVAILABLE FORMS

- *Capsules (vitamin B complex with C and folic acid):* (Nephrocaps, Renal Caps, Renaphro).
- *Powder for injection (pediatric multiple vitamins):* (M.V.I. Pediatric).
- *Intravenous solution (multiple vitamins):* Cernevit, Cernevit, Key-Plex, Infuvite, Infuvite Pediatric, M.V.I.-12).
- *Tablets (vitamin B complex with C and folic acid):* Cefol, Dialyvite Rx, Formula B, Icar C, Nephplex Rx, Nephrolan RX, Nephro-Vite, Rena-Vite Rx, StressTabs, Therobec, Vitamin B-Plex, Vitaplex).
- *Tablets (vitamin B complex with folic acid):* Cerefolin.
- *Tablets (vitamin B complex):* Foltx.
- *Tablets (lipotropic with multivitamins):* Lipotriad.

INDICATIONS AND DOSAGES

Dietary supplement

PO

Adults, Elderly. 1 daily.

CONTRAINDICATIONS: Folate deficient anemia, hereditary optic nerve atrophy, history of allergy to cobalamin, or hypersensitivity to any other component of the formulation.

INTERACTIONS

Drug

Alcohol, colchicines: May decrease the absorption of cyanocobalamin.

Ascorbic acid: May destroy vitamin B_{12}.

Deferoxamine: May increase iron toxicity.

Folic acid (large doses): May decrease vitamin B_{12} blood concentration.

Immunosuppressants, isoniazid, penicillamine: May antagonize vitamin B_6 (may cause anemia or peripheral neuritis).

Levodopa: Vitamin B_6 may reverse the effects of levodopa.

Herbal

None known.

Food

None known.

DIAGNOSTIC TEST EFFECTS: Vitamin C may decrease serum bilirubin and urinary pH. May increase uric acid and urine oxalate.

SIDE EFFECTS

Occasional

Diarrhea, itching

Rare

Abdominal cramps, nausea, vomiting, increased urination with doses of vitamin C exceeding 1 g, headache, somnolence, high dosages of vitamin B_6 cause sensory neuropathy (paresthesia, unstable gait, clumsiness of hands)

SERIOUS REACTIONS

- Long-term megadoses of vitamin B_6 (2 to 6 g over longer than 2 mos) may produce sensory neuropathy (reduced deep tendon reflex, profound impairment of sense of position in distal limbs, gradual sensory ataxia). Toxic symptoms reverse with drug discontinuance.
- Vitamin B_{12} may cause a rare allergic reaction generally due to impurities in preparation.
- Vitamin B_{12} may produce peripheral vascular thrombosis, pulmonary edema, hypokalemia, and congestive heart failure (CHF).
- Vitamin C may produce urine acidification, leading to crystalluria.
- Prolonged use of large doses of vitamin C may result in scurvy when dosage is reduced to normal.

SPECIAL CONSIDERATIONS

PRECAUTIONS

- Patient may require additional nutritional supplementation with fat-soluble vitamins and minerals.

PATIENT INFORMATION

- Because toxic reactions have been reported with injudicious use of certain vitamins, urge patients to follow specific instructions from the physician regarding dosage regimen. As with any medication, advise patients to keep Larobec out of reach of children.

warfarin sodium

(war'far-in)

Rx: Coumadin, Jantoven

Drug Class: Anticoagulants

Pregnancy Category: X

Do not confuse Coumadin with Kemadrin.

CLINICAL PHARMACOLOGY

Mechanism of Action: A coumarin derivative that interferes with hepatic synthesis of vitamin K–dependent clotting factors, resulting in depletion of coagulation factors II, VII, IX, and X. *Therapeutic Effect:* Prevents further extension of formed existing clot; prevents new clot formation or secondary thromboembolic complications.

Pharmacokinetics

Route	Onset	Peak	Duration
PO	1.5-3 days	5-7 days	N/A

Well absorbed from the GI tract. Metabolized in the liver. Primarily excreted in urine. Not removed by hemodialysis. **Half-life:** 1.5-2.5 days.

AVAILABLE FORMS

- *Tablets (Coumadin, Jantoven):* 1 mg, 2 mg, 2.5 mg, 3 mg, 4 mg, 5 mg, 6 mg, 7.5 mg, 10 mg.

INDICATIONS AND DOSAGES

Anticoagulant

PO

Adults, Elderly. Initially, 5-15 mg/day for 2-5 days; then adjust based on International Normalized Ratio (INR). Maintenance: 2-10 mg/day.

Children. Initially, 0.1-0.2 mg/kg (maximum 10 mg). Maintenance: 0.05-0.34 mg/kg/day.

Usual elderly dosage (maintenance)

PO, IV

• *Elderly.* 2-5 mg/day.

UNLABELED USES: Prevention of recurrent cerebral embolism, myocardial reinfarction; treatment adjunct in transient ischemic attacks

CONTRAINDICATIONS: Neurosurgical procedures, open wounds, pregnancy, severe hypertension, severe hepatic or renal damage, uncontrolled bleeding, ulcers

INTERACTIONS

Drug

Acetaminophen, allopurinol, amiodarone, anabolic steroids, androgens, aspirin, cefamandole, cefoperazone, chloral hydrate, chloramphenicol, cimetidine, clofibrate, danazol, dextrothyroxine, diflunisal, disulfiram, erythromycin, fenoprofen, gemfibrozil, indomethacin, methimazole, metronidazole, oral hypoglycemics, phenytoin, plicamycin, propylthiouracil, quinidine, salicylates, sulfinpyrazone, sulfonamides, sulindac: Warfarin increases the effects of these drugs.

Alcohol: May enhance warfarin's anticoagulant effect.

Barbiturates, carbamazepine, cholestyramine, colestipol, estramustine, estrogens, griseofulvin, primidone, rifampin, vitamin K: Warfarin decreases the effects of these drugs.

Herbal

American ginseng, St. John's wort: May decrease the effectiveness of warfarin.

Feverfew, garlic, ginkgo biloba, ginseng, glucosamine-chondroitin: May increase the risk of bleeding.

Food

None known.

DIAGNOSTIC TEST EFFECTS: *None known.*

SIDE EFFECTS

Occasional

GI distress, such as nausea, anorexia, abdominal cramps, diarrhea

Rare

Hypersensitivity reaction, including dermatitis and urticaria, especially in those sensitive to aspirin

SERIOUS REACTIONS

• Bleeding complications ranging from local ecchymoses to major hemorrhage may occur. Drug should be discontinued immediately and vitamin K or phytonadione administered. Mild hemorrhage: 2.5-10 mg PO, IM, or IV. Severe hemorrhage: 10-15 mg IV and repeated q4h, as necessary.

• Hepatotoxicity, blood dyscrasias, necrosis, vasculitis, and local thrombosis occur rarely.

SPECIAL CONSIDERATIONS

PRECAUTIONS

• Observe caution when administering warfarin sodium in any situation or in the presence of any predisposing condition in which added risk of hemorrhage, necrosis, and/or gangrene is present. Use warfarin sodium with caution in patients with heparin-induced thrombocytopenia and deep venous thrombosis. Minor and severe allergic/hypersensitivity reactions and anaphylactic reactions have been reported.

PATIENT INFORMATION

• The objective of anticoagulant therapy is to decrease the clotting ability of the blood to prevent thrombosis while avoiding spontaneous bleeding. Effective therapeutic levels with minimal complications depend in part on cooperative and well-instructed patients who communicate effectively with their physician.

Give patients the following instructions:

• Strict adherence to prescribed dosage schedule is necessary. Do not take or discontinue any other medication, including salicylates (e.g., aspirin and topical analgesics) and other over-the-counter medications except on advice of physician. Avoid alcohol consumption. Do not take warfarin sodium during pregnancy, and do not become pregnant while taking it. Avoid any activity or sport that may result in traumatic injury. Prothrombin time tests and regular visits to the physician or clinic are needed to monitor therapy. Carry identification stating that you are taking warfarin sodium. If you forget to take the prescribed dose of warfarin sodium, notify the physician immediately. Take the dose as soon as possible on the same day but do not take a double dose of warfarin sodium the next day to make up for the missed doses. The amount of vitamin K in food may affect therapy with warfarin sodium. Eat a normal, balanced diet maintaining a consistent amount of vitamin K. Avoid drastic changes in dietary habits, such as eating large amounts of green leafy vegetables. Contact your physician to report any illness, such as diarrhea, infection, or fever. Notify your physician immediately if any unusual bleeding or symptoms occur. Signs and symptoms of bleeding include pain, swelling or discomfort, prolonged bleeding from cuts, increased menstrual flow or vaginal bleeding, nosebleeds or bleeding of gums from brushing, unusual bleeding or bruising, red or dark brown urine, red or tar black stools, headache, dizziness, or weakness.

• If therapy with warfarin sodium is discontinued, caution patients that the anticoagulant effects of warfarin sodium may persist for about 2 to 5 days. Inform patients that all warfarin sodium products represent the same medication and should not be taken concomitantly because overdosage may result.

PREGNANCY AND LACTATION

• Pregnancy Category X. Warfarin sodium is contraindicated in women who are or may become pregnant because the drug passes through the placental barrier and may cause fatal hemorrhage to the fetus in utero. Furthermore, there have been reports of birth malformations in children born to mothers who have been treated with warfarin sodium during pregnancy. Warfarin sodium appears in the milk of nursing mothers in an inactive form. Infants nursed by mothers treated with warfarin sodium had no change in prothrombin times.

white petrolatum; mineral oil

(wite pe-tru-la'tum; min'er oyel)

CLINICAL PHARMACOLOGY

Mechanism of Action: An ocular lubricant that forms an occlusive film on the surface of the eye. *Therapeutic Effect:* Lubricates and protects the eye from drying.

Pharmacokinetics

Not reported.

AVAILABLE FORMS

• *Ophthalmic ointment:* 3.5g (Hypotears, Lacri-Lube, Moisture-Eyes PM, Naurale PM, Puralube, Refresh PM, Tears Naturale, Tears Renewed,), 7 g (Lacri-Lube).

INDICATIONS AND DOSAGES

Dry eye

Ophthalmic

Adults, Elderly, Children. Apply 1/4 inch of ointment to the inside of the lower lid as needed.

CONTRAINDICATIONS: Hypersensitivity to white petrolatum, mineral oil, or any component of the formulation

INTERACTIONS

Drug

None known.

Herbal

None known.

Food

None known.

DIAGNOSTIC TEST EFFECTS: *None known.*

SIDE EFFECTS

Blurred vision for a short time, irritation

SERIOUS REACTIONS

- None reported.

SPECIAL CONSIDERATIONS

PRECAUTIONS

- White petrolatum and mineral oil temporarily can blur vision. This combination is not for use with contact lenses.

PATIENT INFORMATION

Give patients the following instructions:

- This drug combination is for external use only. To avoid contamination, do not touch the tip of the container to any surface. Replace cap after using. Do not use if the solution changes color and becomes cloudy. Stop use and consult an eye care practitioner if you experience eye pain, changes in vision, or continued redness or irritation of the eye or if the condition worsens or persists for more than 72 hours. Keep out of reach of children.

OCULAR CONSIDERATIONS

- Ocular Indications and Usage: This drug combination gives temporary relief of burning, irritation, and discomfort from dryness of the eye or exposure to wind or sun. This drug combination may be used as a protectant against further irritation.

OCULAR DOSAGE AND ADMINISTRATION

- Pull down lower lid of eye and apply small amount (1/4 inch) of ointment to inside of the eyelid. This drug combination is convenient for use at bedtime. Replace cap after using.

Appendix A

Food and Drug Administration Pregnancy Categories

PREGNANCY CATEGORY DEFINITION

A Controlled studies in pregnant women fail to demonstrate a risk to the fetus in the first trimester with no evidence of risk in later trimesters. The possibility of fetal harm appears remote.

B Either animal reproduction studies have not demonstrated a fetal risk but there are no controlled studies in pregnant women, or animal reproduction studies have shown an adverse effect (other than a decrease in fertility) that was not confirmed in controlled studies in women in the first trimester, and there is no evidence of a risk in later trimesters.

C Either studies in animals have revealed adverse effects on the fetus (teratogenic or embryocidal effects or other) and there are no controlled studies in women, or studies in women and animals are not available. Drugs should be given only if the potential benefits justify the potential risk to the fetus.

D There is positive evidence of human fetal risk, but the benefits to treat serious disease in pregnant women may be acceptable despite the risk (e.g., if the drug is needed in a life-threatening situation or for a serious disease for which safer drugs cannot be used or are ineffective.)

X Studies in animals or human beings have demonstrated fetal abnormalities or there is evidence of fetal risk based on human experience, or both, and the risk of the use of the drug in pregnant women clearly outweighs any possible benefit. The drug is contraindictated in women who are or may become pregnant.

Regardless of the designated Pregnancy Category or presumed safety, no drug should be administered during pregnancy unless it is clearly needed and potential benefits outweigh potential risks.

Appendix B

Drug Enforcement Administration Schedules of Controlled Substances

The controlled substances that come under jurisdiction of the Controlled Substances Act are divided into five schedules. Examples of controlled substances and their schedules are as follows:

SCHEDULE I SUBSTANCES

The controlled substances in this schedule are those that have no accepted medical use in the United States and have a high abuse potential. Some examples are heroin, marijuana, LSD (lysergic acid diethylamide), peyote, mescaline, psilocybin, THC (tetrahydrocannabinol), MDA (methylenedioxyamphetamine), ketobemidone, acetylmethadol, fenethylline, tilidine, methaqualone, dihydromorphine, and others.

SCHEDULE II SUBSTANCES

The controlled substances in this schedule have a high abuse potential with severe psychic or physical dependence liability. Schedule II controlled substances consist of certain narcotic, stimulant, and depressant drugs. A written prescription signed by the physician is required for Schedule II drugs. In an emergency situation, oral prescriptions for limited quantities of Schedule II substances may be filled; however, the physician must provide a signed prescription within 72 hours. Schedule II prescriptions cannot be refilled. Some examples of Schedule II controlled narcotic substances are opium, morphine, codeine, hydromorphone, methadone, meperidine, cocaine, oxycodone, fentanyl, etorphine hydrochloride, anileridine, and oxymorphone. Also in Schedule II are amphetamine and methamphetamine, phenmetrazine, methylphenidate, glutethimide, amobarbital, pentobarbital, secobarbital, and phencyclidine.

SCHEDULE III SUBSTANCES

The controlled substances in this schedule have an abuse potential less than those in Schedules I and II and include compounds containing limited quantities of certain narcotic drugs and nonnarcotic drugs such as derivatives of barbituric acid except those that are listed in another schedule, methyprylon, nalorphine, benzphetamine, chlorphentermine, clortermine, phendimetrazine, anabolic steroids, and paregoric. Any suppository dosage form containing amobarbital, secobarbital, or pentobarbital is in this schedule.

SCHEDULE IV SUBSTANCES

The controlled substances in this schedule have an abuse potential less than those listed in Schedule III and include drugs such as barbital, phenobarbital, mephobarbital, chloral hydrate, ethchlorvynol, ethinamate, meprobamate, paraldehyde, methohexital, fenfluramine, diethylpropion, phentermine, chlordiazepoxide, diazepam, oxazepam, clorazepate, flurazepam, clonazepam, prazepam, lorazepam, alprazolam, halazepam, triazolam, mebutamate, dextropropoxyphene, and pentazocine.

SCHEDULE V SUBSTANCES

The controlled substances in this schedule have an abuse potential less than those listed in Schedule IV and consist of preparations containing limited quantities of certain narcotic drugs generally for antitussive and antidiarrheal purposes.

Appendix C

Techniques of Medication Administration

Eye Drops

1. Wash hands.
2. Instruct patient to lie down or tilt head backward and look up.
3. Gently pull lower eyelid down until a pocket (pouch) is formed between eye and lower lid (conjunctival sac).
4. Hold dropper above pocket. Without touching tip of eye dropper to eyelid or conjunctival sac, place prescribed number of drops into the center pocket (placing drops directly onto eye may cause a sudden squeezing of eyelid, with subsequent loss of solution). Continue to hold the eyelid for a moment after the drops are applied (allows medication to distribute along entire conjunctival sac).
5. Instruct patient to close eyes gently so that medication will not be squeezed out of sac. Just closing the eyelids alone will enhance absorption.
6. Apply gentle finger pressure to the lacrimal sac at the inner canthus (bridge of the nose, inside corner of the eye) for 1 to 2 minutes (promotes absorption, minimizes drainage into nose and throat, lessens risk of systemic absorption). This is referred to as *punctal occlusion.*
7. Remove excess solution around eye with a tissue.
8. Wash hands immediately to remove medication on hands. Never rinse eye dropper.

Eye Ointment

1. Wash hands.
2. Instruct patient to lie down or tilt head backward and look up.
3. Gently pull lower eyelid down until a pocket (pouch) is formed between eye and lower lid (conjunctival sac).
4. Hold applicator tube above pocket. Without touching the applicator tip to eyelid or conjunctival sac, place prescribed amount of ointment ($^1/_4$ to $^1/_2$ inch) into the center pocket (placing ointment directly onto eye may cause discomfort).
5. Instruct patient to close eye for 1 to 2 minutes, rolling eyeball in all directions (increases contact area of drug to eye).
6. Inform patient of temporary blurring of vision. If possible, apply ointment just before bedtime.
7. Wash hands immediately to remove medication on hands. Never rinse tube applicator.

Appendix D

Eye and Topical Agents

ANTIGLAUCOMA AGENTS

Uses	*Action*
Antiglaucoma agents are used to reduce elevated intraocular pressure (IOP) in patients with open-angle glaucoma and ocular hypertension.	Some antiglaucoma agents decrease IOP by increasing the outflow of aqueous humor: *Miotics (direct acting)* are cholinergic agents or miotics. They stimulate ciliary muscles, leading to increased contraction of the iris sphincter muscle. *Miotics (indirect acting)* primarily inhibit cholinesterase, allowing acetylcholine to accumulate, which prolongs parasympathetic activity. *Sympathomimetics* increase the rate of fluid flow out of the eyes and decrease the rate of aqueous humor production. Other antiglaucoma agents decrease IOP by decreasing aqueous humor production: *Alpha$_2$-agonists* activate receptors in the ciliary body, inhibiting aqueous secretion and increasing uveoscleral aqueous outflow. *Beta-blockers* reduce the production of aqueous humor. *Carbonic anhydrase inhibitors* reduce fluid flow into the eyes by inhibiting the enzyme carbonic anhydrase. *Prostaglandins* increase the outflow of aqueous fluid by the uveoscleral route.

Type	*Name*	*Availability*	*Dosage Range*	*Side Effects*
Miotics	Carbachol (Isopto Carbachol)	**S:** 0.75%, 1.5%, 2.25%, 3%	1 drop 2 times/day	Ciliary or accommodative spasm, blurred vision, reduced night vision, sweating, increased salivation, urinary frequency, nausea, diarrhea
	Echothiophate (Phospholine Iodide)	**S:** 0.03%, 0.06%, 0.125%, 0.25%	1 drop 2 times/day	Headaches, accommodative spasm, sweating, vomiting, nausea, diarrhea, tachycardia
	Pilocarpine (Isopto-Carpine)	**S:** 0.25%, 0.5%, 1%, 2%, 3%, 4%, 5%, 6%, 8%, 10%	1-2 drops 3-4 times/day	Same as carbachol
	Physostigmine (eserine)	**O:** 0.25%	Apply up to 3 times/day	Blurred vision, eye pain
Sympathomimetics	Dipivefrin (Propine)	**S:** 0.1%	1 drop q12h	Ocular congestion, burning, stinging
	Epinephrine (Epifrin, Epinal)	**S:** 0.5%, 1%, 2%	1 drop 1-2 times/day	Mydriasis, blurred vision, tachycardia, hypertension, tremors, headaches, anxiety
Alpha-agonists	Apraclonidine (Iopidine)	**S:** 0.5%	1-2 drops 3 times/day	Ocular allergic-like reactions, hypersensitivity reaction, change in visual activity, lethargy
	Brimonidine (Alphagan)	**S:** 0.2%	1-2 drops 2-3 times/day	Ocular allergy, headaches, drowsiness, fatigue
Prostaglandins	Bimatoprost (Lumigan)	**S:** 0.03%	1 drop daily in evening	Ocular hyperemia, eyelash growth, pruritus
	Latanoprost (Xalatan)	**S:** 0.005%	1 drop daily in evening	Burning, stinging, iris pigmentation
	Travoprost (Travatan)	**S:** 0.004	1 drop daily in evening	Ocular hyperemia, eye discomfort, foreign body sensation, pain, pruritus

	Unoprostone (Rescula)	**S:** 0.15%	1 drop 2 times/day	Iris pigmentation
Beta-blockers	Betaxolol (Betoptic)	**Suspension:** 0.25% **S:** 0.5%	1-2 drops 1-2 times/day	Transient irritation, burning, tearing, blurred vision
	Carteolol (Ocupress)	**S:** 1%	1 drop 2 times/day	Mild, transient ocular stinging, burning, discomfort
	Levobetaxolol (Betaxon)	**S:** 0.5%	1 drop 2 times/day	Transient irritation, burning, tearing, blurred vision
	Levobunolol (Betagan)	**S:** 0.25%, 0.5%	1 drop 1-2 times/day	Local discomfort, conjunctivitis, brow ache, tearing, blurred vision, headache, anxiety
	Metipranolol (Optipranolol)	**S:** 0.3%	1 drop 2 times/day	Transient irritation, burning, stinging, blurred vision
	Timolol (Timoptic)	**S:** 0.25%, 0.5% **G:** 0.25%, 0.5%	**S:** 1 drop 2 times/day **G:** 1 drop daily	Same as betaxolol
Carbonic anhydrase inhibitors	Acetazolamide (Diamox)	**T:** 125 mg, 250 mg **C:** 500 mg	0.25-1 g/day	Diarrhea, loss of appetite, metallic taste, nausea, tingling in hands and fingers
	Brinzolamide (Azopt)	**Suspension:** 1%	1 drop 3 times/day	Blurred vision, bitter taste
	Dorzolamide (Trusopt)	**S:** 2%	1 drop 2-3 times/day	Burning, stinging, blurred vision, bitter taste

C, Capsules; *G*, gel; *O*, ointment; *S*, solution; *T*, tablets.

MISCELLANEOUS OCULAR AGENTS

Uses	*Action*
Miscellaneous ocular agents are used to prevent and treat mild ocular disorders, such as allergic conjunctivitis, keratitis, and dry eyes.	Miscellaneous ocular agents act in various ways. For example, *hydroxypropyl methylcellulose* stabilizes and thickens precorneal tear film, protecting and lubricating the eyes. *Azelastine, emedastine,* and *levocabastine* antagonize histamine$_1$-receptors, thus inhibiting histamine-stimulated responses in the conjunctiva, such as redness and itching. By stabilizing mast cells, *lodoxamide* prevents antigen-stimulated release of histamine, which inhibits type 1 hypersensitivity reactions. A broad-spectrum antiinfective, *sulfacetamide,* interferes with the synthesis of folic acid that bacteria require for growth. *Vidarabine* blocks DNA polymerase, blocking viral DNA synthesis.

Name	*Indications*	*Dosages*	*Side Effects*
Azelastine (Optivar)	Relief of itching eyes caused by allergic conjunctivitis	1 drop 2 times/day	Transient eye burning or stinging, headache, bitter taste, eye pain, fatigue, flulike symptoms, pharyngitis, rhinitis, blurred vision
Carboxy-methylcellulose (Refresh Plus, Refresh Tears, Refresh Liquigel)	Temporary relief of burning, irritation, and discomfort due to dryness of the eye or exposure to wind and sun	1-2 drops in the affected eye(s) as needed	Transient blurred vision, eyelash stickiness
Emedastine (Emadine)	Treatment of signs and symptoms of allergic conjunctivitis	1-2 drops 2 times/day	Headache, bad taste, blurred vision, eye burning or stinging, dry eyes, tearing

Epinastine (Elestat)	Treatment of allergic conjunctivitis	1 drop 4 times/day	Headache, taste disturbance, drowsiness, blurred vision, eye burning or stinging, dry eyes, foreign body sensation, rhinitis
HP-Guar (Systane)	Temporary relief of burning and irritation caused by dryness of the eye	1-2 drops, as needed	Eye pain, changes in vision, redness, irritation
Hydroxypropyl methylcellulose (Artificial Tears, Isopto Tears, Tears Naturale)	Relief of eye dryness and irritation caused by insufficient tear production	1-2 drops 3-4 times/day	Eye irritation, blurred vision, eyelash stickiness
Ketotifen (Zaditor)	Temporary relief of itching eyes caused by allergic conjunctivitis	1 drop every 8-12 hours	Conjunctival infection, headache, rhinitis, eye burning or stinging, ocular discharge, eye pain
Levocabastine (Livostin)	Treatment of signs and symptoms of seasonal allergic conjunctivitis	1 drop 4 times/day	Transient eye stinging, burning, or discomfort; headache; dry eyes; eyelid edema
Lodoxamide (Alomide)	Treatment of vernal keratoconjunctivitis and keratitis	1 drop 4 times/day	Transient eye stinging or burning, instillation discomfort, itching eyes, blurred vision, dry eyes, tearing, headache
Olopatadine (Patanol)	Treatment of signs and symptoms of allergic conjunctivitis	1-2 drops 2 times/day	Headache, drowsiness, eye burning or stinging, foreign body sensation, pharyngitis, rhinitis, pruritus

Name	*Indications*	*Dosages*	*Side Effects*
Pemirolast (Alamast)	Prevention of itching eyes caused by allergic conjunctivitis	1-2 drops 3-4 times/day	Transient eye stinging or burning, instillation discomfort, itching eyes, blurred vision, tearing, headache
Propylene glycol (Moisture Eyes)	Temporary relief of burning and irritation caused by dryness of the eye; prevents further irritation	1-2 drops in affected eye	Eye pain, changes in vision, redness, irritation
Sodium hyaluronate (AQuify, blink Contacts)	Contact lens rewetter	1-2 drops, as needed. Blink several times	Eye stinging, burning, itching, excessive watering, unusual eye secretions, redness, blurred vision, photophobia, dry eyes.
Sulfacetamide (Sulf-10)	Treatment of corneal ulcers, bacterial conjunctivitis, other superficial eye infections; prevention of infection after eye injury	1-3 drops every 2-3 hours; or 1.25- to 2.5-cm strip of ointment 4 times/day and at bedtime	Transient eye burning or stinging, headache, rash, itching eyes, eye swelling, photosensitivity
Vidarabine (Vira-A)	Treatment of keratitis or keratoconjunctivitis caused by herpes simplex virus, type 1 or 2	$^{1}/_{2}$-inch strip of ointment 5 times/day at 3-hour intervals; after reepithelialization, $^{1}/_{2}$-inch strip of ointment 2 times/day for 7 days	Eye burning or irritation, itching eyes, tearing, eye pain, photophobia

TOPICAL ANTIINFLAMMATORY AGENTS

Uses	*Action*
Topical antiinflammatory agents relieve inflammation and pruritus caused by corticosteroid-responsive disorders such as contact dermatitis, eczema, insect bite reactions, first- and second-degree localized burns, and sunburn.	Topical antiinflammatory agents diffuse across cell membranes and form complexes with cytoplasm. These complexes stimulate the synthesis of inhibitory enzymes that are responsible for the antiinflammatory effects of the agent, which include inhibition of edema, erythema, pruritus, capillary dilation, and phagocyte activity. Topical corticosteroids can be classified based on potency: *Low-potency agents* provide modest antiinflammatory effects. They are safest for long-term application, facial and intertriginous application, use with occlusive dressings, and for infants and young children. *Medium-potency agents* are active against moderate inflammatory conditions, such as chronic eczematous dermatoses. They may be used for facial and intertriginous application for a limited time only. *High-potency agents* are effective in more severe inflammatory conditions, such as lichen simplex chronicus and psoriasis. They may be used for facial and intertriginous application for a short time only and can be used on skin thickened by chronic conditions. *Very-high-potency agents* offer an alternative to systemic therapy for local effects, such as with chronic lesions caused by psoriasis. Because they pose an increased risk of skin atrophy, they should be used only for short periods on small areas without occlusive dressings.

TOPICAL CORTICOSTEROIDS

Name	*Availability*	*Potency*	*Side Effects*
Alclometasone (Aclovate)	**C, O:** 0.05%	Low	Burning, stinging, irritation, itching, rash
Amcinonide (Cyclocort)	**C, O, L:** 0.1%	High	Same as above
Betamethasone dipropionate (Diprosone)	**C, O, G, L:** 0.05%	High	Same as above
Betamethasone valerate (Valisone)	**C:** 0.01%, 0.05%, 0.1% **O:** 0.1% **L:** 0.1%	High	Same as above
Clobetasol (Temovate)	**C, O:** 0.05%	High	Same as above
Desonide (Tridesilon)	**C, O, L:** 0.05%	Low	Same as above
Desoximetasone (Topicort)	**C:** 0.25%, 0.5% **O:** 0.25% **G:** 0.05%	High	Same as above
Dexamethasone (Decadron)	**C:** 0.1%	Medium	Same as above
Fluocinolone (Synalar)	**C:** 0.01%, 0.025%, 0.2% **O:** 0.025%	High	Same as above
Fluocinonide (Lidex)	**C, O, G:** 0.05%	High	Same as above
Fluticasone (Cutivate)	**C:** 0.05% **O:** 0.005%	Medium	Same as above
Halobetasol (Ultravate)	**C, O:** 0.05%	High	Same as above
Hydrocortisone (Cort-Dome, Hytone)	**C, O:** 0.5%, 1%, 2.5%	Medium	Same as above
Mometasone (Elocon)	**C, O, L:** 0.1%	Medium	Same as above
Prednicarbate (Dermatop)	**C:** 0.1%	—	Same as above
Triamcinolone (Aristocort, Kenalog)	**C, O, L:** 0.025%, 0.1%, 0.5%	Medium	Same as above

C, Cream; *G,* gel; *L,* lotion; *O,* ointment.

MISCELLANEOUS TOPICAL AGENTS

Uses	*Action*
Miscellaneous topical agents are used to treat dermatologic disorders, such as acne, dermatitis, and infections. Some also are used to prevent certain dermatologic disorders and to relieve localized pain.	Miscellaneous topical agents act in various ways. Some *antiinfectives,* such as *docosanol, mupirocin,* and *penciclovir,* prevent viral or bacterial replication; *silver sulfadiazine* acts on bacterial cell walls, producing bactericidal effects. *Becaplermin* is a platelet-derived growth factor that stimulates new tissue growth to heal open wounds. *Capsaicin* depletes and prevents the accumulation of substance P (a mediator of pain impulses) from peripheral sensory neurons to the central nervous system, relieving pain. *Pimecrolimus* is an antiinflammatory agent that inhibits the release of cytokine, an enzyme that produces inflammatory reactions. *Tretinoin* decreases the cohesiveness of follicular epithelial cells and increases their turnover.

Name	*Indications*	*Dosages*	*Side Effects*
Azelaic acid (Azelex)	Treatment of mild to moderate acne vulgaris	Apply to affected area 2 times/day.	Pruritus, stinging, burning, tingling
Becaplermin (Regranex)	Treatment of lower leg diabetic neuropathic ulcers extending into subcutaneous tissue or beyond	Apply once daily. After 12 hours, rinse ulcer and re-cover with saline gauze.	Local rash near ulcer
Capsaicin (Zostrix)	Treatment of neuralgia, osteoarthritis, and rheumatoid arthritis	Apply directly to affected area 3-4 times/day.	Burning, stinging, erythema at application site

Name	*Indications*	*Dosages*	*Side Effects*
Collagenase (Santyl)	Débridement of necrotic tissue in chronic dermal ulcers and severe burns	Apply once daily, or more frequently if dressing becomes soiled.	Transient erythema
Docosanol (Abreva)	Treatment of cold sores or fever blisters caused by herpes simplex virus, type 1 or 2	Apply to lesions 5 times/day at onset of symptoms and until lesions are healed, up to a maximum of 10 days.	Headache, skin irritation
Eflornithine (Vaniqa)	Reduction of unwanted facial and chin hair	Apply to affected area 2 times/day at least 8 hours apart.	Anemia, leukopenia, thrombocytopenia, dizziness, alopecia, vomiting, diarrhea, hearing impairment
Imiquimod (Aldara)	Treatment of external genital and perianal warts (condylomata acuminata)	Apply 3 times/week before normal sleeping hours. Leave on skin for 6-10 hours and then remove. Continue for a maximum of 16 weeks.	Local skin reactions, erythema, itching, burning, excoriation, flaking, fungal infection
Mupirocin (Bactroban)	*Topical:* Treatment of impetigo and infected traumatic skin lesions *Nasal:* Reduction of spread of methicillin-resistant *Staphylococcus aureus*	*Topical:* Apply 3 times/day. *Nasal:* Apply 2 times/day for 5 days.	*Topical:* Pain, burning, stinging, itching *Nasal:* Headache, rhinitis, upper respiratory congestion, pharyngitis, altered taste
Penciclovir (Denavir)	Treatment of recurrent herpes labialis (cold sores)	Apply every 2 hours while awake for 4 days.	Headache, mild erythema, altered taste, rash

Pimecrolimus (Elidel)	Treatment of mild to moderate atopic dermatitis (eczema)	Apply 2 times/day.	Upper respiratory tract infection, nasopharyngitis, burning, pyrexia, cough, nasal congestion, abdominal pain, sore throat, headache
Povidone-iodine (Betadine)	External antiseptic action	Apply as needed.	Rash, pruritus, local edema
Sertaconazole (Ertaczo)	Treatment of superficial dermatophytic and candidal infections	Apply 2 times/day.	Headache, drowsiness, pruritus, erythema
Silver sulfadiazine (Silvadene)	Prevention and treatment of infection in second- and third-degree burns; protection against conversion from partial- to full-thickness wounds	Apply 1-2 times/day.	Burning feeling at application site, rash, itching, increased skin sensitivity to sunlight
Tretinoin (Retin-A)	Treatment of acne vulgaris	Apply once daily at bedtime.	Transient pigmentation changes, photosensitivity, local inflammatory reactions (peeling, dry skin, stinging, pruritus)

Appendix E

Weights and Equivalents

METRIC SYSTEM

Weight

kilogram = kg = 1000 grams
gram = g = 1 gram
milligram = mg = 0.001 gram
microgram = μg = 0.001 milligram

Volume

liter = L = 1000 milliliters
milliliter = mL = 0.001 liter

HOUSEHOLD EQUIVALENTS–APPROXIMATE

Utensil	Volume
1 teaspoonful	5 ml
1 tablespoonful	15 ml
1 teacupful	120 ml
1 tumbler glass	240 ml
1 pint	480 ml

WEIGHT CONVERSION (KILOGRAMS TO POUNDS)

Kilograms (kg)	Pounds (lb)
1	2.2
10	22
15	33
20	44
40	88
60	132
80	176

Appendix F

Abbreviations

ā	before
aa	of each
ab	antibody
abd	abdomen
ABGs	arterial blood gases
ac	before meals *(ante cibum)*
ACE	angiotensin-converting enzyme
ACEI	angiotensin-converting enzyme inhibitor
Ach	acetylcholine
ACT	activated clotting time
ACTH	adrenocorticotropic hormone
ad lib	as desired
ADH	antidiuretic hormone
ADP	adenosine diphosphate
ADR	adverse drug reaction
AIDS	acquired immunodeficiency syndrome
aka	also known as
ALT	alanine aminotransferase, serum
ama	against medical advice
amb	ambulation
amp	ampule
ANA	antinuclear antibody
ant	anterior
ANUG	acute necrotizing ulcerative gingivitis
AP	anteroposterior
APAP	acetaminophen
APB	atrial premature beats
aPTT	activated partial thromboplastin time
ARC	AIDS-related complex
AROM	active range of motion
ASA	acetylsalicylic acid (aspirin)
asap	as soon as possible
ASHD	arteriosclerotic heart disease
AST	aspartate aminotransferase, serum
AV	atrioventricular
BAC	blood alcohol concentration
bid	twice a day *(bis in die)*

BM	bowel movement
BMR	basal metabolic rate
bol	bolus
BP	blood pressure
BPH	benign prostatic hypertrophy
bpm	beats per minute
BS	blood sugar
BUN	blood urea nitrogen
Bx	biopsy
c̄	with
C	Celsius (centigrade)
C section	Cesarean section
CA	cancer
Ca	calcium
CAD	coronary artery disease
cAMP	cyclic adenosine monophosphate
cap	capsule
cath	catheterization or catheterize
CBC	complete blood count
CCB	calcium channel blocker
CC	chief complaint
cc	cubic centimeter
cGMP	cyclic guanosine monophosphate
CHD	coronary heart disease
CHF	congestive heart failure
cm	centimeter
CML	chronic myeloid leukemia
CMV	cytomegalovirus I
CNS	central nervous system
CO_2	carbon dioxide
CoA	coenzyme A
c/o	complains of
CO	cardiac output
COMT	catechol-*O*-methyltransferase
con rel	controlled release
conc	concentration
COPD	chronic obstructive pulmonary disease
COX-2	cyclooxygenase-2
CPAP	continuous positive airway pressure
CPK	creatinine phosphokinase
CPR	cardiopulmonary resuscitation
CrCl	creatinine clearance
CRD	chronic respiratory disease
CRF	chronic renal failure
C&S	culture and sensitivity
CSF	cerebrospinal fluid

CTZ	chemoreceptor trigger zone
CV	cardiovascular
CVA	cerebrovascular accident
CVP	central venous pressure
$CysLT_1$	cysteinyl leukotriene receptor
D&C	dilation and curettage
del rel	delayed release
DIC	disseminated intravascular coagulation
DM	diabetes mellitus
DMARD	disease modifying antirheumatic drugs
DNA	deoxyribonucleic acid
DOB	date of birth
dr	dram
dsg	dressing
DVT	deep vein thrombosis
D_5W	5% glucose in distilled water
dx	diagnosis
EBV	Epstein-Barr virus
ECG	electrocardiogram (EKG)
EEG	electroencephalogram
EENT	ear, eye, nose, and throat
elix	elixir, hydroalcoholic solution containing active drug(s)
ENDO	endocrine systems
EPO	erythropoietin
EPS	extrapyramidal symptoms
ESR	erythrocyte sedimentation rate
ext rel	extended release
F	Fahrenheit
FBS	fasting blood sugar
FHT	fetal heart tones
FIo_2	inspired oxygen concentration
FSH	follicle-stimulating hormone
fx	fracture
g	gram
GABA	gamma-aminobutyric acid
gal	gallon
GERD	gastroesophageal reflux disease
GGTP	gamma-glutamyl transpeptidase
GHb	glycosylated hemoglobin
GI	gastrointestinal
G6PD	glucose-6-phosphate dehydrogenase
gr	grain
GR	glucocorticoid receptor
gtt	drop
GTT	glucose tolerance test
GU	genitourinary

Gyn	gynecology
HbA_{1c}	laboratory test for glycosylated hemoglobin
Hct	hematocrit
HCG	human chorionic gonadotropin
HDL	high-density lipoprotein
HEMA	hematologic system
Hgb	hemoglobin
HIV	human immunodeficiency virus
H&H	hematocrit and hemoglobin
H&P	history and physical examination
5-HIAA	5-hydroxyindoleacetic acid
HMG-CoA	3-hydroxy-3-methylglutaryl–coenzyme A reductase
5-HT	5-hydroxytryptamine (serotonin)
H_2O	water
HPA	hypothalamic-pituitary adrenocortical axis
HR	heart rate
HRT	hormone replacement therapy
hr	hour
hs	at bedtime *(hora somni)*
HSV	herpes simplex virus
HSV-2	herpes genitalis
hypo	hypodermically
Hx	history
IBS	irritable bowel syndrome
ICP	intracranial pressure
ICU	intensive care unit
IDDM	insulin-dependent diabetes mellitus
I&D	incision and drainage
IgG	immunoglobulin G
IL-2	interleukin-2
IM	intramuscular
immed rel	immediate release
inf	infusion
inh	inhalation
inj	injection
INR	international normalized ratio
INTEG	relating to integumentary structures
IOP	intraocular pressure
IPPB	intermittent positive pressure breathing
ITP	idiopathic thrombocytopenic purpura
IU	international units
IUD	intrauterine contraceptive device
IV	intravenous
IVP	intravenous piggy back
K	potassium
kg	kilogram

L or l	left
L	liter
lat	lateral
lb	pound
LDH	lactate dehydrogenase
LDL	low-density lipoprotein
LDL-C	low-density lipoprotein cholesterol
LE	lupus erythematosus
LFT	liver function tests
LH	luteinizing hormone
LHRH	luteinizing hormone-releasing hormone
liq	liquid
LLQ	left lower quadrant
LMP	last menstrual period
LOC	loss of consciousness
lot	lotion
loz	lozenge
LR	lactated Ringer's solution
LRI	lower respiratory infection
LVD	left ventricular dysfunction
m	meter
m^2	square meter
MAC	*Mycobacterium avium* complex
MAO	monoamine oxidase
max	maximum
META	metabolic
mEq	milliequivalent
mg	milligram
mcg (μg)	microgram
MI	myocardial infarction
min	minute
mixt	mixture
mL	milliliter
mm	millimeter
mo	month
MPA	mycophenolic acid
MS	musculoskeletal
MVA	motor vehicle accident
n	nanogram
Na	sodium
NC	nasal cannula
neg	negative
NIDDM	non–insulin-dependent diabetes mellitus
NKA	no known allergies
NMDA	*N*-methyl-D-aspartate
NMI	no middle initial

noc	nocturnal (night)
NPH	neutral protamine Hagedorn
NPO	nothing by mouth *(nil per os)*
NS	normal saline
NSAID	nonsteroidal antiinflammatory drug
NV	neurovascular
O_2	oxygen
OBS	organic brain syndrome
OC	oral contraceptive
OD	right eye *(oculus dexter)*
oint	ointment
OOB	out of bed
ophth	ophthalmic
OR	operating room
ORIF	open reduction, internal fixation
os	left eye *(ocular sinister)*
OTC	over the counter
ou	each eye *(oculus uterque)*
oz	ounce
p̄	after (post)
p	pulse
PABA	para-aminobenzoic acid
PAC	premature atrial contraction
pCO_2	arterial carbon dioxide tension (pressure tore)
pO_2	arterial oxygen tension (pressure)
PAT	paroxysmal atrial tachycardia
PBI	protein-bound iodine
PBP	penicillin-binding protein
pc	after meals *(post cibum)*
PCA	patient-controlled analgesia
PCN	penicillin
PE	physical examination
PG	prostaglandin
pH	hydrogen ion concentration
PMDD	premenstrual dysphoric disorder
PMS	premenstrual syndrome
PNS	peripheral nervous system
PO	by mouth *(per os)*
postop	postoperatively
PP	postprandial
ppm	parts per million
preop	preoperatively
prep	preparation
prn	as needed *(pro re nata)*
PSA	prostate-specific antigen
PT	prothrombin time

PTSD	posttraumatic stress disorder
PTT	partial thromboplastin time
PVC	premature ventricular contraction
PVD	peripheral vascular disease
q	every
qam	every morning
qd	every day
qh	every hour
qid	4 times a day
qod	every other day
qpm	every night
qt	quart
q2h	every 2 hours
q3h	every 3 hours
q4h	every 4 hours
q6h	every 6 hours
q12h	every 12 hours
qwk	every week
r	right
rap disintegr	rapidly disintegrating
RAR	retinoic acid receptor
RBC	red blood cell (count)
RDA	recommended dietary allowance
rec	rectal
REM	rapid eye movement
RESP	respiratory system
rhPDGF-BB	recombinant human platelet-derived growth factor
RNA	ribonucleic acid
R/O	rule out
ROAD	reversible obstructive airway disease
ROM	range of motion
RTI	respiratory tract infection
Rx	therapy, treatment, or prescription
$\bar{s}$	without
SA	sinoatrial
SAN	sinoatrial node
SC	subcutaneous
sec	second
SERM	elective estrogen receptor modulator
SGOT	serum glutamic-oxaloacetic transaminase (now AST)
SGPT	serum glutamic-pyruvic transaminase (now ALT)
SIADH	syndrome of inappropriate antidiuretic hormone
sig	patient dosing instructions on prescription label
SL	sublingual
SLE	systemic lupus erythematosus
slow rel	slow release

SMBG	self-monitored blood glucose
SMZ	sulfamethoxazole
SOB	short of breath
sol	solution
ss	one half
SSRI	serotonin selective reuptake inhibitor
stat	at once
STD	sexually transmitted disease
surg	surgical
sus rel	sustained release dose form
supp	suppository
Sx	symptoms
syr	syrup, a highly concentrated sucrose solution containing drug(s)
T	temperature
$T_{1/2}$	drug half-life
T_3	triiodothyronine
T_4	thyroxine
tab	tablet
TB	tuberculosis
TBG	thyroxine-binding globulin
tbsp	tablespoon
TCA	tricyclic antidepressant
TD	transdermal
temp	temperature
TG	total triglycerides
TIA	transient ischemic attack
tid	4 times daily *(ter in die)*
time rel	time release dose form
tinc	tincture, alcoholic solution of a drug
TMD	temporomandibular dysfunction
TMJ	temporomandibular joint
TMP	trimethoprim
TNF	tumor necrosis factor
top	topical
tPA	tissue plasminogen activator
TPN	total parenteral nutrition
TPR	temperature, pulse, respirations
TSH	thyroid-stimulating hormone
tsp	teaspoon
TT	thrombin time
Tx	treatment
U	unit
UA	urinalysis
ULDL	ultra-low-density lipoprotein
URI	upper respiratory infection

USP	*United States Pharmacopeia*
UTI	urinary tract infection
UV	ultraviolet
vag	vaginal
visc	viscous
VD	venereal disease
VHDL	very-high-density lipoprotein
VLDL	very-low-density lipoprotein
VO	verbal order
vol	volume
VPB	ventricular premature beats
VS	vital signs
WBC	white blood cell (count)
WHO	World Health Organization
wk	week
WNL	within normal limits
wt	weight
yr	year
>	greater than
<	less than
≠	not equal to
↑	increase
↓	decrease
2°	secondary

Appendix G

Dose Calculation by Weight

Manufacturer-recommended doses are based on extensive clinical trials and usually are intended for the average, healthy adult male of average weight and age. Thus age, sex, weight, and chronic diseases of the major organs of metabolism (liver) and excretion (kidney) may affect the usual safe and effective Food and Drug Administration–approved dose recommendations.

Creatine clearance, peak and trough blood levels, and symptomatic patient response often are used to titrate doses for a given therapeutic effect.

Doses for pediatric and geriatric patients require an adjustment downward from the usual dose.

Geriatric patients may be particularly susceptible to effects produced by central nervous system depressants or drugs that affect renal function.

No reliable general rule for dose calculations can supplant clinically derived doses, and many drug monographs now list doses for children based on a milligram per kilogram or milligram per pound basis. Children's doses also are based on a reduction of adult doses as determined by body surface area and weight.

Clark's rule has been used for many years as a general guide for calculating children's doses.

Clark's Rule:

$$\frac{\text{Child's weight (lb)}}{150} \times \text{Adult dose} + \text{Child's dose}$$

Weight Chart (kilograms to pounds) 1 kg = 2.2 lb

Kilograms (kg)	Pounds (lb)
10	22
20	44
25	55
30	66
35	77
40	88
45	99
50	110
55	121
60	132

Appendix H

Herbs and Other Natural Supplements

Aloe Vera

Aloe vera, Aloe barbadensis

Other Names: Burn plant, curaçao aloes

GENERAL INFORMATION

The term *aloe vera* conventionally refers to the gel within the aloe leaf. (The glands in the leaf surface contain a different and unsafe substance called "drug aloe" and are not present, save in trace amounts, in aloe gel products.) The major active ingredients of aloe vera gel are thought to be its polysaccharides, especially one called acemannan. Other potentially important constituents include sitosterols and lignins.

PROPOSED INDICATIONS AND USAGE

Aloe vera juice is credited widely with the ability to enhance skin regeneration after burns or wounds, but randomized clinical trials of aloe for speeding resolution of sunburn, skin damage caused by radiation therapy, and wounds generally have failed to find benefit. Based on the same putative tissue healing effect, aloe has been recommended for treatment of stomach ulcers and other gastrointestinal tract diseases, but there is no meaningful supporting evidence for these uses. Other claimed effects that lack supporting evidence from properly designed randomized clinical trials include immune stimulation and suppression of human immunodeficiency virus infection. (Acemannan, however, is a Food and Drug Administration–approved treatment for fibrosarcoma in cats and dogs.) Two randomized clinical trials indicate that oral aloe gel might have a hypoglycemic effect in type 2 diabetes, but it has been suggested that these benefits were due to trace contamination of the aloe gel with parts of the leaf glands, supplying some drug aloe.

Preliminary randomized clinical trials of moderate to low quality suggest that aloe vera cream may offer benefit for seborrhea, psoriasis, and genital herpes, reducing symptoms and speeding resolution. Other uses based on the claimed actions noted lack of randomized clinical trial support.

PRECAUTIONS

Drug aloe ("aloes"), a potent anthraquinone laxative produced from the aloe leaf rather than the gel, can cause hypokalemia and other effects in addition to diarrhea. Oral aloe gel does not present the same risks.

PATIENT INFORMATION

Aloe gel is a popular treatment for burns and wounds. However, no real evidence indicates that it works. In addition, aloe actually might make severe wounds heal more slowly.

Internal use of aloe gel has no proven benefits. However, some evidence indicates that oral aloe might reduce blood sugar levels in persons with diabetes. Advise patients that if they have diabetes, they should consult with their physician before taking this herb (or any other supplement). Keep in mind that if oral aloe does reduce blood sugar, a hypoglycemic reaction is possible.

DRUG INTERACTIONS

No drug interactions are known. However, the known immunomodulatory effects of acemannan conceivably could interfere with the action of immune-suppressant drugs. If aloe gel does indeed possess significant hypoglycemic effects, interactions with oral hypoglycemic agents or insulin might be a possibility.

PREGNANCY AND LACTATION

Maximum safe dosages for pregnant or lactating women, young children, or individuals with severe hepatic or renal disease are not known.

ADVERSE REACTIONS

Occasional hypersensitivity reactions

PROPOSED DOSAGE AND ADMINISTRATION

Topical aloe gel preparations typically are applied 3 to 4 times daily. Studies of aloe for diabetes treatment have used aloe vera gel at a dose of 1 tbs twice daily.

OCULAR CONSIDERATIONS

Ask why the product is being used. Treated conditions such as skin conditions, human immunodeficiency virus infection, and diabetes may have ocular manifestations or implications.

Bee Propolis

Other Names: Bee glue, bee putty, propolis

GENERAL INFORMATION

Bees coat the hive with propolis in much the same way human beings use paint and caulking on their homes. Propolis is a resinous compound made from tree sap and contains biologically active compounds called flavonoids. In vitro studies have found propolis to have activity against bacteria, viruses, and protozoans.

PROPOSED INDICATIONS AND USAGE

Evidence from preliminary controlled trials hints that topical propolis may be helpful for genital herpes, periodontal disease, and recovery from oral surgery. Other proposed uses include caries prevention, enhancing wound healing, and treatment of vaginal infections. Oral use of propolis has shown promise for acne rosacea and giardiasis.

PRECAUTIONS

Allergic reactions to topical propolis may occur and can involve painful redness, swelling, and oozing sores.

OCULAR CONSIDERATIONS

Propolis has been shown to have antiinflammatory effects in animal studies. The topical application of a water extract of propolis 1% drops has an inhibitory effect on corneal neovascularization on the rabbit cornea. The inhibitory effect was shown to be comparable to that of topical dexamethasone 0.1%. The effect of propolis partially may be due to its inhibitory effect on the activity of cyclooxygenase and lipooxygenase. (Hepsen IF, Er H, Cekic O: Topically applied water extract of propolis to suppress corneal neovascularization in rabbits, *Ophthalmic Res* 31[6]:426, 1999.)

In another study, a corneal alkali burn was induced on rabbit corneas. Topical 1% ethanolic extract of propolis and topical 1% dexamethasone were compared. Drugs were instilled 4 times a day for 7 days. Propolis had an antiinflammatory effect comparable to dexamethasone in this chemical corneal injury. (Ozturk F et al: The effect of propolis extract in experimental chemical corneal injury, *Ophthalmic Res* 32[1]:13, 2000.)

Methylprednisolone (5 mg/0.1 mL) and propolis (5 mg/0.16 mL) were compared for endotoxin-induced uveitis in rabbits. Drugs were delivered by anterior subtenon injection at the time of uveitis induction and at 4 and 8 hours after induction. The effects of methylprednisolone and propolis were similar. Propolis showed significant antiinflammatory effects on uveitis in rabbits. (Ozturk F et al: Effect of propolis on endotoxin-induced uveitis in rabbits, *Jpn J Ophthalmol* 43[4]:285, 1999.)

Bilberry Fruit

Vaccinium myrtillus

Other Names: Blueberry, huckleberry, hurtleberry, myrtilli fructus

GENERAL INFORMATION

Raw bilberry fruit contains 5% to 10% catechins, 30% invertose, and relatively small amounts of anthocyanosides and flavone glycosides. The pharmacokinetics of bilberry anthocyanosides are known only from animal studies. In male rats, plasma anthocyanosides achieve peak levels of 2 to 3 μg/mL at 15 minutes and decline rapidly within 2 hours, with an absolute bioavailability of only 1.2% of the administered dose. Anthocyanosides have received the most attention, and commercial bilberry products are standardized to anthocyanoside content. Some evidence suggests that anthocyanosides may increase cross-linkage of collagen fibers, normalize capillary permeability, inhibit collagen degradation, promote collagen biosynthesis, reduce inflammatory activity, and scavenge free radicals. Bilberry anthocyanosides have numerous effects in the retina, including enhancing recovery of rhodopsin and altering a variety of enzymatic reactions, although the clinical significance of these findings remains unclear. Like other flavonoids, at very high doses anthocyanosides inhibit platelet aggregation in vitro and in vivo. Bilberry leaves, as opposed to the much more commonly used fruit, have entirely different constituents and have been investigated for hypoglycemic and hypolipidemic effects.

PROPOSED INDICATIONS AND USAGE

Despite the absence of evidence showing efficacy, bilberry fruit is marketed widely for oral use in the prevention and treatment of eye disorders of all types, including poor night vision, macular degeneration, glaucoma, diabetic retinopathy, and cataracts. Bilberry also often is added to herb and supplement combinations intended for the treatment of chronic venous insufficiency/varicose veins. However, the evidence for other natural products such as horse chestnut, diosmin/hesperidin, oxerutins, and butcher's broom is considerably stronger.

PRECAUTIONS

Bilberry leaf may have hypoglycemic effects and should not be confused with bilberry fruit. Because bilberry anthocyanosides mildly inhibit platelet aggregation, bilberry possibly could have adverse effects in individuals with impaired hemostasis.

PATIENT INFORMATION

Extracts of bilberry fruit are marketed widely for improving night vision and helping the eyes in other ways. However, no real evidence exists that it works, and recent studies have found no effect. WARNING: Do not confuse bilberry leaf with bilberry fruit. The leaf can be toxic. The safety of bilberry fruit in pregnant or nursing women or young children has not been established. Individuals with severe liver or kidney disease should consult a physician before using this (or any other) supplement.

DRUG INTERACTIONS

Based on known antiplatelet effects, potentiation of anticoagulant and antiplatelet agents is possible.

PREGNANCY AND LACTATION

Safety in young children, pregnant or lactating women, or in individuals with severe hepatic or renal dysfunction has not been established. However, there are no known or suspected problems with such uses, and pregnant women have been given bilberry in clinical trials without apparent adverse effects.

ADVERSE REACTIONS

Bilberry fruit is a food and as such would appear to have a high safety threshold. Bilberry herbal extracts sold as medicinal products may contain artificially high levels of anthocyanosides. One drug-monitoring study of 2295 patients showed no serious side effects and only a 4% incidence of mild reactions such as gastrointestinal distress, skin rashes, and drowsiness. There are no known risks with overdosage of bilberry fruit; bilberry leaf, however, has been associated with toxicity.

PROPOSED DOSAGE AND ADMINISTRATION

The typical dose of bilberry is 160 mg twice a day of a fruit extract standardized to contain 25% bilberry anthocyanosides.

OCULAR CONSIDERATIONS

No reliable evidence indicates that bilberry has any medicinal effect in vision-related conditions. Two small, controlled studies of bilberry from the 1960s found short-term improvements in visual acuity in semidarkness and shortened time to dark adaptation and improved recovery from glare compared with placebo. Short-term benefits also were seen in a double-blind placebo-controlled study of 40 healthy subjects, which found that a single dose of bilberry extract improved pupillary photomotor response for 2 hours. However, more recent trials have failed to find improvements in night vision through the use of bilberry. For example, a 3-week double-blind crossover trial of 15 individuals found no immediate or delayed improvement in night vision attributable to bilberry extract (25% anthocyanosides) taken at a dose of 160 mg twice daily. Negative results were seen in a similar double-blind placebo-controlled crossover trial of 18 subjects and another of 16 subjects.

Weak evidence supports some potential benefits in other eye-related conditions. A pilot double-blind placebo-controlled trial of bilberry extract in 14 patients with diabetic and/or hypertensive retinopathy reported improvements as shown by ophthalmoscopic and angiographic examination. In a preliminary double-blind placebo-controlled trial of 50 individuals with mild cataracts (involving 62 eyes), a combination of vitamin E and bilberry slowed lens opacity progression. Animal studies suggest that bilberry can help prevent macular degeneration.

Black Cohosh

Cimicifuga racemosa, Cimicifugae racemosae rhizoma

Other Names: Black snakeroot, baneberry

BRAND NAMES

Remifemin (PhytoPharmica/Enzymatic Therapy) = Remifemin (Schaper and Brummer) in Europe

GENERAL INFORMATION

Black cohosh contains a variety of triterpene glycosides including actein, deoxyactein, cimigoside, cimicifugoside, and racemoside, as well as phytosterins, isoflavones, isoferulic acid, and miscellaneous volatile oils. Black cohosh extracts usually are standardized to deoxyactein content. Much of the apparent vasomotor and/or endocrine effect of black cohosh is believed to reside in the triterpene glycoside constituents, although the phytosterin and flavone derivatives also have been investigated. Black cohosh has been found in animal studies to inhibit pituitary luteinizing hormone production without affecting follicle-stimulating hormone or prolactin release. More recent human and animal studies have found no effect on luteinizing hormone or follicle-stimulating hormone and no estrogenic effects. Some preliminary evidence suggests that black cohosh may have selective action on estrogen receptors outside of the uterine area, making it a type of phyto-SERM.

PROPOSED INDICATIONS AND USAGE

Despite the paucity of evidence, black cohosh is marketed widely for the treatment of some menopausal symptoms and for other women's conditions such as premenstrual syndrome and dysmenorrhea.

PRECAUTIONS

The possibility of estrogenic effects outside the uterus suggests that black cohosh should be used with caution in conditions in which estrogen levels or activity are an issue. Safety in young children or in individuals with severe hepatic or renal dysfunction has not been established.

PATIENT INFORMATION

Black cohosh is marketed widely as a treatment for menopause. However, very little evidence indicates that it really works. Black cohosh often is described as a "natural estrogen"; however, recent studies indicate that black cohosh does not have any estrogen-like effects. In particular, there is no reliable indication that black cohosh can help prevent osteoporosis. Black cohosh should not be confused with the toxic herb blue cohosh. The safety of black cohosh in pregnant or nursing women or women with a history of breast cancer has not been established. Individuals with severe liver or kidney disease should consult a physician before using this (or any other) supplement.

DRUG INTERACTIONS

No drug interactions are known. However, formal drug interaction studies have not been performed, and interactions with estrogen and related hormones are possible. There are weak indications of potential interactions with antihypertensive medications.

PREGNANCY AND LACTATION

Traditional herbology contraindicates the use of black cohosh during pregnancy because of supposed increased risk of spontaneous abortion.

ADVERSE REACTIONS

Generally, black cohosh is well tolerated, producing only occasional mild gastrointestinal distress. Other occasionally reported side effects of unclear causal connection include headaches, weight gain, and breast tenderness.

PROPOSED DOSAGE AND ADMINISTRATION

The usual dosage of black cohosh is 1 or 2 tablets twice a day of a standardized extract such as Remifemin, which is manufactured to contain 1 mg of 27-deoxyactein per tablet. Commission E in Germany recommends the use of black cohosh for no more than 6 months because of the lack of long-term safety data in human beings.

OCULAR CONSIDERATIONS

Ask why the product is being used. Treated conditions such as menopause may have ocular manifestations or implications.

Butterbur

Petasites hybridus, P. albus, P. vulgaris

Other Names: Petasin, blatterdock, butterfly dock, capdockin, flapperdock, umbrella leaves

BRAND NAMES

Petadolex (Weber & Weber) = Petadolex (Weber & Weber) in Europe

GENERAL INFORMATION

The active ingredients of butterbur are thought to be angelic acid esters of sesquiterpine alcohols, including petasin, isopetasin, and furanopetasin. Petasin is unstable and spontaneously shifts into isopetasin. In vitro studies suggest that these substances may possess antiinflammatory, antispasmodic, antihistaminic, and antidopaminergic effects. Butterbur extracts appear to affect peptido-leukotrienes but not prostaglandins; the net effect may be gastric cytoprotection rather than gastric irritation. Furanopetasin extracts containing furanoeremophilanes have shown cytotoxic properties.

PROPOSED INDICATIONS AND USAGE

Two substantial double-blind studies indicate that butterbur extracts may be helpful for allergic rhinitis and related symptoms, including allergic conjunctivitis. In addition, two double-blind studies indicate that butterbur extracts may be helpful for migraine prophylaxis. Based on pharmacologic evidence suggesting that butterbur has spasmolytic and analgesic effects, butterbur also has been marketed for use in asthma, abdominal pain, tension headaches, back pain, bladder spasms, and gallbladder pain.

PRECAUTIONS

Unprocessed butterbur contains potentially hepatotoxic and carcinogenic pyrrolizidine alkaloids. These alkaloids must be removed during the manufacturing process to create a safe product. Raw butterbur may contain hepatotoxic and possibly carcinogenic pyrrolizidine alkaloids.

PATIENT INFORMATION

Some evidence suggests that butterbur extract may be helpful for the treatment of hayfever symptoms and to prevent migraine headaches. Butterbur extract also is marketed for other conditions such as asthma, tension headaches, and back pain, but there is no real evidence that it works for these conditions. Raw butterbur may contain hepatotoxic ingredients. These must be removed in a special manufacturing process to create a safe product.

DRUG INTERACTIONS

No drug interactions have been reported.

PREGNANCY AND LACTATION

Safety in pregnant or lactating women, young children, or individuals with severe hepatic or renal disease is not known.

ADVERSE REACTIONS

No significant side effects were reported in published clinical trials of standardized butterbur extracts.

PROPOSED DOSAGE AND ADMINISTRATION

The usual dosage of butterbur as a treatment for allergic rhinitis or as a migraine preventive is 50 mg 2 or 3 times daily of an extract that has been processed to remove pyrrolizidine alkaloids.

OCULAR CONSIDERATIONS

Butterbur may be helpful for the ocular (and other) symptoms of allergic rhinitis. (Schapowal A: Butterbur Ze339 for the treatment of intermittent allergic rhinitis: dose-dependent efficacy in a prospective, randomized, double-blind, placebo-controlled study, *Arch Otolaryngol Head Neck Surg* 130:1381, 2004.)

Carnitine

Alternate/Related Names:
L-Carnitine, L-acetyl-carnitine, propionyl-L-carnitine, acetyl-L-carnitine

GENERAL INFORMATION

Carnitine synthesis depends on the presence of vitamin B_6, vitamin C, niacin, and iron and is performed primarily in the liver, kidney, and brain. However, infants (especially preterm ones) cannot synthesize carnitine well and must rely on breast milk as an exogenous source. For this reason, formula should be fortified with carnitine. Orally administered L-carnitine reaches peak plasma concentrations in 3½ to 5 hours, with a half-life of 2 to 15 hours. Tracer studies in human beings suggest that exogenous carnitine is taken up rapidly and retained by the myocardium.

PROPOSED INDICATIONS AND USAGE

Promising but far from definitive evidence suggests that L-carnitine and propionyl-L-carnitine may be of use as adjunctive treatment for post–myocardial infarction cardioprotection, intermittent claudication, angina, and congestive heart failure. Acetyl-L-carnitine is marketed widely as a treatment for dementia, but overall the evidence is more negative than positive. Similarly, although L-carnitine is marketed widely as an ergogenic aid, studies have yielded contradictory results at best. Mixed evidence suggests that intravenously administered L-carnitine, in various forms, may offer cardioprotective effects in cardiac surgery and improve heart function in cardiogenic shock. Carnitines also have shown some promise for male infertility.

PRECAUTIONS

A single report suggests that patients undergoing hemodialysis might require reduced doses of carnitine. However, a more recent study suggests that hemodialysis causes a transient carnitine deficiency. In contrast to L-carnitine, D-carnitine is known to cause numerous problems by competitively inhibiting the L-form. DL-Carnitine has caused a myasthenia gravis–like syndrome in hemodialysis patients. Maximum safe dosage for young children, pregnant or lactating women, or persons with severe hepatic or renal disease has not been established.

PATIENT INFORMATION

Some evidence indicates that L-carnitine might be helpful in certain heart conditions, not as a replacement for standard medications but as a supplement to them. However, because of the serious nature of heart disease, it is not advisable for individuals with heart-related conditions to take carnitine (or any other supplement) except under the supervision of a physician. One form of carnitine, acetyl-L-carnitine, is marketed as a treatment for Alzheimer's disease and related conditions. However, on balance, the evidence suggests that it does not work. The maximum safe dosage of carnitine for pregnant or nursing women or young children has not been established. Individuals with severe liver or kidney disease should consult a physician before using this (or any other) supplement.

DRUG INTERACTIONS

No drug interactions are known. Formal drug interaction studies have not been performed.

ADVERSE REACTIONS

L-Carnitine in its three forms appears to be safe. In a 12-month drug-monitoring study involving more than 4000 patients with cardiovascular disease, the most common adverse effects were stomach discomfort (6%), nausea (4%), and diarrhea (2%).

PROPOSED DOSAGE AND ADMINISTRATION

Carnitine is used in its L-form, as L-carnitine, propionyl-L-carnitine, and acetyl-L-carnitine. The D- and DL-forms of carnitine should not be used. Generally, L-carnitine or propionyl-L-carnitine most often are recommended in heart-related conditions, whereas acetyl-L-carnitine is used in Alzheimer's and other central nervous system conditions. The daily dosage usually ranges from 1500 to 3000 mg for all forms, given in three divided doses.

OCULAR CONSIDERATIONS

Loss of carnitine may be related to the appearance of cataracts. A derivative of carnitine, acetylcarnitine, may prevent the formation of cataracts by a pharmacologic action, as has been shown for aspirin. (Pessotto P et al: In Experimental diabetes: the decrease in the eye of lens carnitine levels is an early important and selective event, *Exp Eye Res* 64(2):195, 1997.) Ask why the product is being used. Heart conditions may have ocular manifestations or implications.

Chasteberry

Vitex agnus castus

Alternate/Related Names:
Chaste tree

BRAND NAMES

Femaprin (Nature's Way) = Agnolyt (Madaus) in Europe

GENERAL INFORMATION

Chasteberry fruit contains 5% volatile oil and the iridoid glycosides agnoside and aucubin. Pharmacokinetic and pharmacodynamic data are lacking, as are meaningful studies on the species-specific constituents of chasteberry. In vitro, animal, and preliminary human trials in women suggest that chasteberry extracts inhibit prolactin release, apparently through dopaminergic stimulation of D_2-type receptor cells in the pituitary.

PROPOSED INDICATIONS AND USAGE

Preliminary evidence suggests that chasteberry may have use for cyclic mastalgia and general premenstrual syndrome symptoms.

Based on its antiprolactin effects, chasteberry also has been tried as a fertility drug. However, the two double-blind trials designed to evaluate this use were too small for the results to achieve statistical significance on primary endpoints. Chasteberry also has been tried as a treatment for secondary amenorrhea.

In addition, chasteberry is marketed as a treatment for menopause, but there is no supporting evidence for this use.

PRECAUTIONS

A clinical pharmacology study using high doses of chasteberry extract produced no more than mild nonspecific side effects, such as gastrointestinal disturbances. A fertility clinic has reported a single case of mild ovarian hyperstimulation in a woman who self-prescribed. Safety in young children and individuals with severe hepatic or renal disease has not been established.

PATIENT INFORMATION

Chasteberry is marketed as a treatment for a variety of conditions affecting women. Preliminary evidence suggests that it might offer benefit for cyclic breast discomfort and general premenstrual syndrome symptoms. However, there is no real evidence that it is helpful for any other conditions. NOTE: Instruct patients not to use chasteberry for amenorrhea (lack of menstruation) or irregular menstruation without first seeing a physician to rule out potentially dangerous causes of these conditions. Advise patients not to use chasteberry if they are taking other medications that affect their hormones.

DRUG INTERACTIONS

Based on its mechanism of action, chasteberry might interact with bromocriptine or other agents with endocrine or pituitary activity.

PREGNANCY AND LACTATION

Chasteberry definitely is not recommended for use in pregnancy and lactation because of its effects on prolactin.

ADVERSE REACTIONS

Widespread use of chasteberry in Germany has not led to any reports of significant adverse effects. In drug-monitoring studies enrolling more than 3000 participants, the rate of minor side effects was less than 2.5%, primarily nausea, headaches, and allergy.

PROPOSED DOSAGE AND ADMINISTRATION

Chasteberry dosages depend on the specific formulation. Follow label instructions.

OCULAR CONSIDERATIONS

Ask why the product is being used. Treated conditions such as menopause may have ocular manifestations or implications.

Chitosan

Alternate/Related Names:

Chitin

BRAND NAME

Liposan Ultra (Vanson, Inc.; U.S. product only)

GENERAL INFORMATION

Chitosan is a cationic polysaccharide containing polyglucosamine polymer chains with nonacetylated amines. Similarly to other forms of fiber, chitosan is thought to bind bile acids and dietary lipids. The solubility and activity of chitosan may be altered by the molecular weight of the particular product used.

PROPOSED INDICATIONS AND USAGE

Chitosan products are marketed widely as weight loss aids, although evidence from clinical trials is more negative than positive. Chitosan also frequently is included in supplement mixtures claimed to normalize cholesterol levels, again despite the lack of success in clinical trials.

PRECAUTIONS

Use of chitosan may further impair nutrition in malnourished individuals. Significant evidence indicates that long-term, high-dose chitosan supplementation can result in malabsorption of some crucial nutrients, including calcium, magnesium, selenium, and vitamins A, D, E, and K. In turn, this may create risk of osteoporosis in adults and growth retardation in children. For this reason, individuals using chitosan require general multinutrient supplementation. Chitosan may alter intestinal flora, potentially allowing overgrowth of pathogenic bacteria. Safety in individuals with severe hepatic or renal disease has not been established.

PATIENT INFORMATION

Chitosan is a form of fiber extracted from crustaceans. Chitosan is marketed widely as a weight loss aid. However, most studies have failed to find it effective. Chitosan also is said to reduce cholesterol levels, but it does not appear to be effective for this purpose. Other proposed uses of chitosan have no evidence at all behind them. Use of chitosan can cause digestive discomfort. In addition, chitosan can cause depletion of various nutrients. This may lead to a risk of osteoporosis in adults and growth retardation in children. Taking a multivitamin and mineral supplement might help prevent these side effects. Chitosan should not be used by pregnant or nursing women or young children. Individuals with severe liver or kidney disease should consult a physician before using this (or any other) supplement.

DRUG INTERACTIONS

No drug interactions are known.

PREGNANCY AND LACTATION

Because of its antinutrient effects, chitosan should not be used by pregnant or lactating women or young children.

ADVERSE REACTIONS

Gastrointestinal side effects such as discomfort, flatulence, increased stool bulkiness, bloating, and mild nausea may occur with use of chitosan. Increased water consumption may reduce these symptoms.

PROPOSED INDICATIONS AND USAGE

The usual dosage of chitosan is 3 to 6 g per day, taken in divided doses before meals.

OCULAR CONSIDERATIONS

Ask why the product is being used. Treated conditions such as hyperlipidemia may have ocular manifestations or implications.

Chromium Picolinate

Alternate/Related Names:

Chromium picolinate, chromium polynicotinate, chromium chloride, high-chromium

GENERAL INFORMATION

Evidence from animal trials and three reports of patients on total peripheral nutrition without chromium added has shown that chromium deficiency results in impaired glucose tolerance, elevated levels of serum insulin, weight loss, peripheral neuropathy, central nervous system disturbances, and elevated serum lipids. These signs and symptoms are refractory to insulin but reversible with chromium administration. For many years, it was said that chromium is found in foods in the form of a large molecular-weight substance called glucose tolerance factor. However, it now appears that the evidence indicating the existence of glucose tolerance factor was faulty, and the molecule does not in fact exist. Current evidence indicates that chromium acts by binding to a low-molecular-weight oligopeptide not found in foods; the chromium-bound oligopeptide facilitates the action of insulin receptor kinase. On this basis, chromium has been tried as a treatment for diabetes and prediabetic conditions.

PROPOSED DOSAGE AND ADMINISTRATION

The only meaningful evidence for benefit in diabetes was seen in a study that used a high dose of 1000 μg daily. Treatment at such supranutritional doses could cause symptoms of heavy metal toxicity in some patients (see Adverse Reactions). Chromium is marketed extensively as a weight loss aid, but the balance of the evidence is more negative than positive. Chromium has not been shown to be effective as an ergogenic aid.

PRECAUTIONS

Chromium supplementation above nutritional requirements is not recommended for individuals with renal or hepatic disease (see Adverse Reactions). Concerns also have been raised over the use of the picolinate form of chromium in individuals suffering from affective or psychotic disorders because picolinic acids can change levels of neurotransmitters. Maximum safe dosage for young children, pregnant or lactating women, or individuals with severe hepatic or renal disease has not been established.

PATIENT INFORMATION

Chromium is a mineral that is essential for good nutrition. Some evidence suggests that making sure to get enough chromium might improve blood sugar control and cholesterol levels. However, taking excessive doses of chromium could be dangerous. In addition, if the patient has diabetes, instruct the patient not to use chromium (or any other supplement) without consulting a physician. Chromium is marketed widely as a weight loss aid. However, most studies have found it ineffective for this purpose. No evidence exists that chromium improves sports performance. Pregnant or nursing women and individuals with liver or kidney disease should consult a physician before taking chromium.

DRUG INTERACTIONS

If chromium therapy proves successful, reduction in dosages of hypoglycemic agents may be necessary. Beta-blockers may reduce high-density lipoprotein cholesterol levels. According to a double-blind placebo-controlled trial of 72 men, chromium supplementation may correct this side effect, raising high-density lipoprotein levels in individuals. Simultaneous intake of calcium carbonate may impair chromium absorption.

PREGNANCY AND LACTATION

Because of the theoretical possibility of DNA damage, forms of chromium other than chromium picolinate may be preferable in pregnancy.

ADVERSE REACTIONS

Trivalent chromium, the form

taken in over-the-counter supplements, is generally well tolerated, and dosages within the nutritional recommendations given subsequently are believed to be safe. One case report has been published of anemia, thrombocytopenia, hemolysis, weight loss, and hepatic and renal toxicity in a woman taking 1200 to 2400 µg of chromium picolinate daily for 4 to 5 months. Another found acute interstitial nephritis in a woman taking only 600 µg of chromium daily for 6 weeks. There has been one report of acute generalized exanthematous pustulosis caused by chromium picolinate at a dose of 1000 µg daily. Several toxicologic studies have shown that hexavalent chromium can present health risks. Although this is not the form used nutritionally, there is some evidence that the nutritional trivalent form may be converted metabolically to hexavalent chromium when it is taken at high doses. Theoretical concerns also exist that chromium picolinate could cause adverse effects on DNA.

PROPOSED DOSAGE AND ADMINISTRATION

Estimated safe and adequate daily intakes of chromium are as follows: under 6 months, 10 to 40 µg; 6 months to 1 year, 20 to 60 µg; 1 to 3 years, 20 to 80 µg; 4 to 6 years, 30 to 120 µg; and over 7 years, 50 to 200 µg. For pregnant women, a dose of 4 µg/kg has been proposed. In studies of chromium for diabetes, a dose of 1000 µg daily has been used. However, case reports suggest the possibility of idiosyncratic toxic reactions at this dose (see Adverse Reactions).

OCULAR CONSIDERATIONS

Ask why the product is being used. Treated conditions such as diabetes may have ocular manifestations or implications.

Coenzyme Q_{10}

Alternate/Related Names:
CoQ_{10}

GENERAL INFORMATION

Coenzyme Q_{10} (CoQ_{10}) serves as a major redox component in the coupled mitochondrial mechanisms of electron transfer and oxidative phosphorylation. Certain illnesses such as congestive heart failure (CHF) have been associated with reduced tissue levels of CoQ_{10}. It has been suggested that mitochondrial dysfunction and consequent energy starvation caused by this relative deficiency and by other factors may be a primary physiologic disturbance in CHF and cardiomyopathies. Proponents of this view believe that CoQ_{10} supplementation may be a metabolically appropriate treatment for these conditions, improving myocardial aerobic energy production and hence cardiac function. In reperfusion after ischemia, CoQ_{10} may function by preventing oxidative damage to creatine kinase and other substances. Other authors have concluded that CoQ_{10} does not scavenge the free radicals produced in reperfusion but rather enhances the recovery of high-energy phosphates, thereby preventing Ca^{2+} overload. Bioavailability tests using low doses of oral CoQ_{10} (30 mg) show peak plasma levels of about 1 mg/L. Dietary CoQ_{10} appears to function like vitamin E in preventing lipid peroxidation and can exert a vitamin E–sparing effect.

PROPOSED INDICATIONS AND USAGE

CoQ_{10} may be useful adjunctive treatment in CHF, possibly improving functional capacity and decreasing the incidence of hospitalization. Other potential uses include cardioprotection during cardiac surgery and the treatment of cardiomyopathy and hypertension, but the evidence is weak at best. Coenzyme Q_{10} may be a useful repletion therapy in patients taking drugs that reduce endogenous CoQ_{10} levels, such as 3-hydroxy-3-methylglutaryl–coenzyme A reductase inhibitors, but this has not been proved. Similarly, CoQ_{10} might help prevent cardiac toxicity caused by doxorubicin, but more research is needed to establish this. Pilot trials suggest that CoQ_{10} might be useful in Duchenne's, Becker's, and the limb-girdle muscular dystrophies and in myotonic dystrophy, Charcot-Marie-Tooth disease, Kugelberg-Welander disease, Parkinson's disease, and migraine prophylaxis. Coenzyme Q_{10} is marketed widely for preventing heart disease and cancer, improving energy, aiding in weight loss, and enhancing sports performance, despite the lack of any meaningful evidence that it is effective for these purposes.

PRECAUTIONS

A study of hypertensive men unexpectedly found reduction of fasting glucose levels in the group treated with CoQ_{10}. However, another trial in diabetic patients found no effect on glycemic control. Nonetheless, serum glucose monitoring appears appropriate if diabetic patients begin using CoQ_{10} (to offset the potential CoQ_{10} depletion apparently caused by some oral hypoglycemic agents, for example). Avoid abrupt discontinuation of CoQ_{10} during treatment of CHF. Anecdotal reports indicate a CoQ_{10} withdrawal syndrome in CHF, leading to temporarily worsening failure.

PATIENT INFORMATION

Coenzyme Q_{10} is a substance that occurs naturally in the body. Coenzyme Q_{10} plays an important role in the process by which cells produce energy. Some evidence indicates that supplemental CoQ_{10} may be useful in CHF. However, because CHF is a dangerous illness, medical supervision is strongly advised before self-treatment with CoQ_{10} or any other supplement. Additionally, keep in mind that CoQ_{10} has been investigated only as an addition to standard treatment, not a substitute for it. Furthermore, discontinuation of CoQ_{10} by individuals with CHF may be dangerous. A wide variety of medications are believed to reduce CoQ_{10} levels or impair its action in the body. For this reason, supplemental CoQ_{10} has been advocated for persons taking these medications. However, no real evidence exists as yet that taking extra CoQ_{10} actually will provide any noticeable benefit. Coenzyme Q_{10} has been suggested for other heart-related conditions, such as high blood pressure, but there is little evidence that it is effective. Other proposed uses of CoQ_{10}, such as preventing heart disease and cancer, improving energy, aiding in weight loss, and enhancing sports performance, have no evidence behind them. The maximum safe dosage of CoQ_{10} for pregnant or nursing women or young children has not been established.

Individuals with severe liver or kidney disease should consult a physician before using this (or any other) supplement.

DRUG INTERACTIONS

One animal study suggests that CoQ_{10} can prolong the effects of antihypertensive drugs without increasing their maximum hypotensive effect. Coenzyme Q_{10} was found to reduce fasting glucose levels in a recent study of individuals with hypertension. This has led to the suggestion that a reduction in oral hypoglycemic dose may be necessary in individuals using CoQ_{10} for repletion therapy (or during concomitant use for any reason). However, another trial in diabetic patients found no effect on glycemic control.

PREGNANCY AND LACTATION

Maximum safe dosage in young children, pregnant or lactating women, or individuals with severe hepatic or renal disease has not been established.

ADVERSE REACTIONS

Coenzyme Q_{10} is generally well tolerated. In large double-blind and open studies lasting up to 1 year, no serious side effects or drug interactions were noted, and the incidence of minor side effects was generally less than 1.5%. A 6-year study of 143 patients showed no toxicity or intolerance.

PROPOSED DOSAGE AND ADMINISTRATION

The typical dose of CoQ_{10} ranges from 30 to 150 mg/day, given in two or three divided doses at the higher levels. This fat-soluble substance is better absorbed when taken in oil-based soft-gel form.

OCULAR CONSIDERATIONS

Ask why the product is being used. Treated conditions such as cardiovascular disease or congestive heart failure may have ocular manifestations or implications.

Coleus forskohlii

GENERAL INFORMATION

Coleus forskohlii could lower blood pressure and decrease muscle spasms. Forskolin appears to be responsible for much of this effect. Like certain drugs used for asthma, forskolin increases the levels of cyclic adenosine monophosphate. Cyclic adenosine monophosphate plays a major role in many cellular functions, and it can relax the muscles around the bronchial tubes.

PROPOSED INDICATIONS AND USAGE

Asthma, eczema, allergies; muscle contraction, menstrual cramps, irritable bowel syndrome (spastic colon); bladder pain; hypertension; glaucoma, psoriasis

PRECAUTIONS

Exercise caution when administering with blood pressure medications and blood thinners.

DRUG INTERACTIONS

Beta-blockers (such as clonidine or hydralazine) or blood-thinning drugs—such as warfarin (Coumadin), heparin, clopidogrel (Plavix), ticlopidine (Ticlid), or pentoxifylline (Trental)—should be used only under the supervision of a physician.

PROPOSED DOSAGE AND ADMINISTRATION

Common dosage is 50 mg 2 or 3 times a day (extract standardized to contain 18% forskolin). Because a 18% extract provides high levels, instruct patients to take *C. forskohlii* extracts only with a doctor's supervision.

OCULAR CONSIDERATIONS

Forskolin lowers the intraocular pressure of rabbits, monkeys, and human beings. Net aqueous humor inflow decreases, outflow facility remains unchanged, and ciliary blood flow increases in rabbits. Tolerance to the intraocular pressure lowering effect did not occur in rabbits after topical doses given every 6 hours for 15 days. (Caprioli J et al: Forskolin lowers intraocular pressure by reducing aqueous inflow, *Invest Ophthalmol Vis Sci* 25[3]:268, 1994.)

Creatine

Alternate/Related Names:
Creatine monohydrate

GENERAL INFORMATION

Creatine is a nitrogenous amine that is synthesized in the liver, kidneys, and pancreas from the amino acids glycine, arginine, and methionine. Endogenous and exogenous creatine are catabolized in the body to sarcosine and urea and thence to methylamine and glyoxylate. Excess creatine also is excreted in the urine. The normal requirement of about 2 g/day can be supplied by endogenous synthesis and by a diet that includes animal products. Vegetarians have lower levels of creatine in the serum and decreased output in the urine.

The phosphorylated form of creatine participates in energy generation via creatine kinase, contributing a phosphate group in the conversion of adenosine diphosphate to adenosine triphosphate. This reaction is rapid and reversible; however, stores of adenosine triphosphate and phosphocreatine can be exhausted within 10 seconds during high-intensity exercise. During periods of recovery, phosphocreatine is resynthesized. Creatine supplementation is thought to increase muscle reserves of phosphocreatine and aid resynthesis during rests between bouts of high-intensity exercise.

A single 20- to 30-g dose of creatine monohydrate has been found to raise plasma creatine concentrations to levels of 690 to 1000 µmol/L within 1 hour. The half-life of creatine in the plasma is 1 to $1\frac{1}{2}$ hours.

The potential mechanism of action of creatine in treatment of muscular disorders is not well elucidated. Diminished levels of creatine in muscle may be due to disturbances in ion homeostasis that result in decreased creatine transport into the cells. Diminished intramuscular creatine and phosphocreatine results in increased concentrations of lactic acid and hydrogen ions that may affect the contractile apparatus of the muscle directly. Acidosis also results in more rapid depletion of phosphocreatine and inhibits the enzymes of glycolysis.

PROPOSED INDICATIONS AND USAGE

Despite the lack of consistent evidence, creatine is marketed widely as a sports supplement. Based on highly preliminary evidence, creatine also has been tried for congestive heart failure; Duchenne's muscular dystrophy, McArdle's disease, and other neuromuscular disorders; congenital defects in creatine synthesis; mitochondrial disorders; progressive neurological disorders; and hyperlipidemia.

PRECAUTIONS

The preponderance of data documenting side effects is taken from short-term studies involving healthy and/or athletic subjects; large, systematic, long-term safety studies have not been performed. A long-term placebo-controlled study of 100 football players found no increase in injury or cramping during 1 year of creatine supplementation. Creatine does not appear to affect adversely the ability of the body to exercise under hot conditions.

Concerns have been expressed regarding creatine and renal function. Studies have not found any adverse effects on renal function among individuals with healthy kidneys. Nevertheless, there is one report of impaired renal functioning apparently attributable to creatine use in a healthy individual. Use of high-dose creatine is contraindicated in individuals with renal failure.

PATIENT INFORMATION

Creatine is marketed widely as a sports supplement. Some evidence indicates that it may be useful in high-intensity, repetitive burst exercise (such as repeated 10-second bursts of high-intensity exercise separated by 30-second rest periods); however, many studies have found no benefit. Creatine does not appear to be helpful for other forms of exercise. Creatine also sometimes is advocated for treatment of numerous conditions involving fatigue or muscle weakness, but no real evidence exists as yet that it is actually helpful. Individuals with kidney problems should not use creatine.

DRUG INTERACTIONS

No drug interactions with creatine have been reported, although most of the studies have prohibited concurrent use of other drugs, supplements, or steroids.

PREGNANCY AND LACTATION

Safety in pregnant or lactating women, young children, or individuals with severe hepatic disease has not been established.

ADVERSE REACTIONS

The most common side effect of creatine supplementation is weight gain from an increase in water content or in the diameter of fast-twitch (type II) glycolytic muscle fibers. Other side effects of creatine may include muscle cramping, dehydration, and gastrointestinal distress.

PROPOSED DOSAGE AND ADMINISTRATION

The most common proposed dosage schedule for creatine begins with a loading dose of 20 to 30 g creatine monohydrate (equivalent to 17.6 to 26.4 g creatine) for 5 to 7 days, usually ingested daily in four divided doses of 5 to 6 g. This is followed by doses of 2 g/day to maintain elevated creatine concentrations in the muscle. An alternative schedule avoids a loading dose and simply uses 3 g/day for 28 days. Combining carbohydrates with creatine may be helpful, perhaps because of insulin-augmented creatine accumulation or enhanced muscle glycogen supercompensation.

OCULAR CONSIDERATIONS

Ask why the product is being used. Treated conditions such as congestive heart failure or hyperlipidemia may have ocular manifestations or implications.

Dong Quai

Angelica sinensis

Alternate/Related Names: Dang quai, tang quai, dang kwai, dong kwai

GENERAL INFORMATION

Dong quai root contains numerous potentially active substances, including butylidene phthalide, ferulic acid, and beta-sitosterol. Nutritionally, dong quai root is a source of nicotinic acid, uracil, adenine, folinic acid, vitamin E, carotene, and a subnutritional amount of vitamin B_{12}. Dong quai does not appear to have estrogenic actions. In vitro and animal studies suggest that dong quai can cause uterine contractions and uterine relaxation, as well as suppress heart dysrhythmias, inhibit platelet aggregation, and lower blood pressure. However, the clinical relevance of these findings is not known.

PROPOSED INDICATIONS AND USAGE

Dong quai is sold widely as an ingredient in herbal mixtures said to be helpful for a variety of conditions, including menopausal syndrome, dysmenorrhea, amenorrhea, fibrocystic breast disease, and premenstrual syndrome. However, there is no evidence that dong quai is effective for any of these purposes and some evidence that it is ineffective for menopausal syndrome.

PRECAUTIONS

Chinese patent medicines containing dong quai are marketed widely; however, such products have been found in the past to contain unlisted, potentially dangerous pharmaceuticals and other contaminants. The furanocoumarin constituents of dong quai have been associated with photosensitivity.

PATIENT INFORMATION

Dong quai is a Chinese herb advocated as a treatment for various "women's conditions," such as menopause. However, there is no evidence that the herb is effective for any condition. Contrary to some reports, dong quai does not act as a "natural estrogen." Be cautious about using prepackaged dong quai formulas manufactured in Asia because there are reports of contamination with unlabeled prescription drugs, heavy metals, and other toxic substances.

DRUG INTERACTIONS

Dong quai may interact with warfarin. Because of its furanocoumarin content, dong quai might potentiate photosensitivity reactions if combined with photosensitizing drugs.

PREGNANCY AND LACTATION

Safety for young children, pregnant or lactating women, or individuals with severe hepatic or renal disease has not been established. One case report suggests that maternal dong quai usage caused hypertension in mother and child.

ADVERSE REACTIONS

Dong quai possesses a low order of toxicity. Reported side effects are rare and consist primarily of mild gastrointestinal distress and occasional allergic reactions. In addition, a man using a patent herb product containing dong quai developed gynecomastia, possibly because of adulteration of the product with a pharmaceutical estrogen.

PROPOSED DOSAGE AND ADMINISTRATION

Typical recommended dosages of dong quai vary widely.

OCULAR CONSIDERATIONS

Ask why the product is being used. Treated conditions such as menopause syndrome may have ocular manifestations or implications.

Eyebright

Euphrasia officinalis

GENERAL INFORMATION

Eyebright contains astringent substances and volatile oils may be slightly antibacterial. No evidence indicates that eyebright is effective for treating conjunctivitis or any other eye disease.

PROPOSED INDICATIONS AND USAGE

Conjunctivitis

PRECAUTIONS

Eyebright can cause tearing of the eyes, itching, redness, and many other symptoms, probably because of direct irritation.

PROPOSED DOSAGE AND ADMINISTRATION

Eyebright tea is made by boiling 1 tbs of the herb in a cup of water. The tea is used as an eye wash or is taken internally up to 3 times daily.

Fenugreek

Trigonella foenumgraecum

GENERAL INFORMATION

Although the mechanism of action of fenugreek is not fully understood, animal studies suggest that the seed fiber may impair glucose absorption in the intestines, among other potential mechanisms.

PROPOSED INDICATIONS AND USAGE

Scant preliminary evidence suggests that fenugreek seed may have hypoglycemic properties. Additional proposed uses parallel those of other high-fiber foods, such as preventing heart disease and cancer and aiding weight loss.

PRECAUTIONS

As a commonly eaten food, fenugreek seed generally is regarded as safe. The only common side effect is mild gastrointestinal distress when it is taken in high doses.

PATIENT INFORMATION

Fenugreek seed is a food spice that has been marketed as a treatment for diabetes. However, there has been little scientific study of this herb. Individuals with diabetes who use fenugreek should monitor blood sugar levels closely to avoid possible hypoglycemic reactions.

DRUG INTERACTIONS

Fenugreek seed conceivably could cause hypoglycemia in diabetic patients who use insulin or other hypoglycemic drugs.

PREGNANCY AND LACTATION

Extracts of fenugreek seed have been shown to stimulate uterine contractions in guinea pigs. For this reason, pregnant women should not take fenugreek in dosages higher than are used commonly as a spice (perhaps 5 g daily). Maximum safe dosages for young children, lactating women, and those with hepatic or renal disease have not been established.

ADVERSE REACTIONS

No adverse reactions have been reported other than mild, self-limited gastrointestinal distress.

PROPOSED DOSAGE AND ADMINISTRATION

The typical dosage is 5 to 33 g of defatted fenugreek seeds taken 3 times a day with meals. Because the seeds are somewhat bitter, they often are taken in capsule form or are added to foods.

OCULAR CONSIDERATIONS

Ask why the product is being used. Treated conditions such as diabetes may have ocular manifestations or implications.

Feverfew

Tanacetum parthenium

GENERAL INFORMATION

Feverfew contains many sesquiterpene lactones with an alpha-methylenebutyrolactone structure, of which the germacranolide parthenolide is the primary constituent. Feverfew also contains camphor, terpenes, and pyrethrin (used as an insecticide). The relative preponderance of these various constituents vary widely, depending on the variety of feverfew used and the conditions in which it was grown. In vitro studies suggest that feverfew extract can suppress prostaglandin production without an effect on cyclooxygenase. Furthermore, lactones (parthenolide and epoxyartemorin) isolated from feverfew have been found to have inhibitory effects, with inhibitory concentration (50%) values ranging from approximately 1 to 5 mcg/mL, irreversibly inhibiting eicosanoid generation. However, parthenolide-rich feverfew extracts have failed to show efficacy in clinical trials.

PROPOSED INDICATIONS AND USAGE

Feverfew is used widely in the United Kingdom for prophylaxis of chronic migraine headaches and has become popular in the United States as well. However, the evidence for its effectiveness is limited to a couple of dated preliminary trials using whole-leaf products; extracts standardized to parthenolide content have shown no benefit. Feverfew also is marketed as "herbal aspirin" for conditions such as fever and joint pain; however, feverfew, despite its name, does not appear to reduce fevers.

PRECAUTIONS

Chewing whole feverfew leaf can cause mouth sores. Safety definitely has not been established in pregnancy because feverfew has a folk history as an abortifacient. Safety for lactating women, young children, or individuals with severe hepatic or renal disease also has not been established.

PATIENT INFORMATION
Feverfew is an herb marketed for preventing migraine headaches. However, the evidence that it works is weak. Chewing whole feverfew can cause mouth sores. Individuals taking drugs that impair blood clotting should avoid feverfew. These drugs include warfarin (Coumadin), heparin, and aspirin. Safety for nursing women, young children, or individuals with severe liver or kidney disease has not been established.

DRUG INTERACTIONS
Because parthenolide affects platelet activity, use of caution is suggested with the concomitant use of feverfew and anticoagulants or antiplatelet agents.

PREGNANCY AND LACTATION
Pregnant women should not use feverfew.

ADVERSE REACTIONS
Feverfew is generally well tolerated. Animal studies have shown no adverse effects at 100 times the human daily dose; a median lethal dose has not been determined. In a 300-patient survey, 11.3% reported mouth ulcerations from chewing feverfew leaf, occasionally accompanied by general inflammation of tissues in the mouth, and 6.5% reported mild gastrointestinal distress. One report described a "postfeverfew syndrome" that consisted of withdrawal symptoms such as headache, insomnia, nervousness, and joint discomfort, but this pattern was not seen in another study.

PROPOSED DOSAGE AND ADMINISTRATION
In the past the daily dosage of feverfew used was 82 mg of dried leaf, containing 0.66% parthenolide. Subsequent dosage recommendations tended to concentrate on reproducing the same daily quantity of parthenolide. However, given the failures in clinical trials using parthenolide-rich extracts, it is no longer clear which forms of feverfew are effective or precisely at which dose they should be taken.

OCULAR CONSIDERATIONS
Ask why the product is being used. Treated conditions such as migraine headaches may have ocular manifestations or implications.

Gamma-Linolenic Acid

Alternate/Related Names:
Omega-6 oil(s), omega-6 fatty acids (Sources of gamma-linolenic acid include black currant seed oil, borage oil, evening primrose oil.)

BRAND NAMES
Efamol (Efamol Nutraceuticals) = Efamol (Efamol Ltd.) in Europe

GENERAL INFORMATION
The evening primrose has been bred artificially to produce plants with seeds that reliably yield 7% to 10% gamma-linolenic acid (GLA). Other evening primrose oil (EPO) constituents include saturated fats (10%), oleic acid (9%), and linoleic acid (72%). Because of the confounding effects of these other constituents, artificially purified GLA has been used in some studies. Borage and black currant oil also are used to supply GLA. Omega-6 fatty acids are essential nutrients for which the exact daily requirement is not known. The body pri-

marily uses dietary linoleic acid as a precursor, converting it to GLA in a rate-limiting step involving delta-6 desaturase. An elongase enzyme then creates dihomo-GLA, which can be converted to subscript 1-series prostaglandins and subscript 3-series leukotrienes. Additionally, delta-5 desaturase converts dihomo-GLA to arachidonic acid, with its subsequent possibly "unfavorable" prostaglandin and leukotriene metabolites.

PROPOSED INDICATIONS AND USAGE

Evening primrose oil has shown some promise for treatment of keratoconjunctivitis sicca. Evening primrose oil also is used widely in Europe to treat diabetic neuropathy, cyclic mastitis, and eczema, but it is not clear that it is effective for diabetic neuropathy, and substantial evidence exists that it is not effective for cyclic mastitis or eczema. Based on very weak evidence, GLA or EPO also have been advocated as treatments for obesity, chronic fatigue syndrome, rheumatoid arthritis, general premenstrual syndrome symptoms, Raynaud's phenomenon, Sjögren's disease, endometriosis, osteoporosis, and prostate disease.

PRECAUTIONS

It has been suggested that supplemental GLA might raise levels of arachidonic acid, with potential adverse consequences; however, none have been documented. Maximum safe dosage for young children, pregnant or lactating women, or individuals with severe renal or hepatic disease has not been established.

PATIENT INFORMATION

Evening primrose oil is a source of GLA, an essential fatty acid. Other sources of GLA include black currant oil and borage oil. Evening primrose oil and GLA are marketed widely for the treatment for eczema, diabetic neuropathy, cyclic breast pain, and many other conditions. However, most evidence suggests that they are not effective for cyclic mastitis and eczema.

The maximum safe dosage of GLA for pregnant or nursing women or young children has not been established. Individuals with severe liver or kidney disease should consult a physician before using this (or any other) supplement.

DRUG INTERACTIONS

No drug interactions are known.

ADVERSE REACTIONS

More than 4000 patients have participated in trials of GLA, primarily in the form of EPO. No adverse effects or significant differences in rate of side effects between the treated group and placebo group have been attributed to this treatment.

PROPOSED DOSAGE AND ADMINISTRATION

Because EPO is the most common form of GLA, dosages will be given in those terms.

For cyclic mastitis, the standard dosage of EPO is 3 g daily in two or three divided doses. Rheumatoid arthritis has been treated with 5 to 10 g daily, although one study used concentrated GLA equivalent to 30 g of EPO. Diabetic neuropathy typically is treated with 4 to 6 g daily. There may be value in combining lipoic acid with EPO when treating this condition. Children with eczema have been given 2 to 4 g daily. For all these conditions, the proposed minimum duration of treatment is several months.

OCULAR CONSIDERATIONS

Therapy with GLA and tear substitutes reduces ocular surface inflammation and improves dry eye symptoms. In one study the treated group received tablets containing GLA (15 mg) and linoleic acid (28.5 mg) twice daily for 45 days. Statistically significant improvements in symptoms, lissamine green staining, and ocular surface inflammation were seen in the treatment group compared with the placebo group. (Barabino S et al: Systemic linoleic and gamma-linolenic acid therapy in dry eye syndrome with an inflammatory component, *Cornea* 22[2]:97, 2003.)

Garlic

Allium sativum

Alternate/Related Names:

Allium spp.

BRAND NAMES

Kwai (Lichtwer Pharma) = Kwai (Lichtwer Pharma) in Europe

Kyolic (Wakanuga) = Kyolic (Wakanuga) in Europe

GENERAL INFORMATION

Fresh garlic contains 0.35% sulfur by weight, bound to cysteine and its derivatives. Some of the most investigated bioactive constituents or breakdown products include alliin, allicin, ajoene, allylpropyl sulfide, diallyl disulfide, diallyl trisulfide, s-allylcysteine, and vinyldithiins. Little to no allicin exists in an intact garlic bulb. However, when garlic is crushed or cut, the enzyme allinase is brought in contact with alliin, yielding allicin. At room temperature, the half-life of allicin is 3 hours, and 20 minutes of cooking suffices to degrade it entirely. Garlic oil and aged garlic possess neither alliin nor allicin and therefore are presumed to differ significantly in medical properties from fresh intact garlic and from garlic powder manufactured to contain alliin.

Pharmacokinetic studies in rats have found that alliin is absorbed well orally, reaching maximum serum concentrations within 10 minutes, and urinary measurements suggest a minimum absorption rate of 65% for allicin and 73% for vinyldithiins.

In vitro experiments on animal hepatocytes have found that allicin and (to a lesser extent) ajoene, s-allylcysteine, and related chemicals reduce cholesterol biosynthesis by inhibiting 3-hydroxy-3-methylglutaryl–coenzyme A reductase and 14-alpha-demethylase. However, current evidence suggests that garlic products have no meaningful effect on lipid profile in human beings.

Garlic extracts have been found to reduce blood pressure in dogs and rats. Fibrinolytic and antiplatelet activity also has been demonstrated in human, animal, and in vitro studies of various forms of garlic. Garlic powder and aged garlic have been found to produce antithrombotic effects, perhaps indicating a wide spectrum of active components.

Ajoene, alliin, allicin, vinyldithiins, and diallyl disulfide appear to inhibit platelet aggregation.

The apparent antihypertensive, fibrinolytic, and antiplatelet effects of garlic may be mediated through activation of nitric oxide synthetase. Garlic concentrates selenium in a readily absorbable form, which may explain partially its observed antioxidant and chemopreventive properties. In addition, the sulfuric components of garlic also may directly bind and inactivate reactive genotoxic metabolites.

PROPOSED INDICATIONS AND USAGE

Weak evidence suggests that garlic may possess antithrombotic, antihypertensive, and antioxidant actions, potentially leading to an overall antiatherosclerotic effect. Current evidence suggests it does not have meaningful hypolipemic actions.

PRECAUTIONS

Based on reports of increased bleeding following surgery, as well as other evidence of potential bleeding complications (see Patient Information, Drug Interactions, and Adverse Reactions sections), the European Scientific Cooperative on Phytotherapy recommends against using garlic before, during, or immediately after surgical procedures. For the same reason, it appears wise to caution against garlic use in the period before and after labor and delivery. Topical garlic can cause skin irritation, blistering, and even third-degree burns.

Based on theoretical reasons rather than case reports, garlic is not recommended for patients with brittle diabetes (possible hypoglycemic effect), pemphigus (activation by sulfur-containing compounds), organ transplants (possible activation of immune rejection), or acute rheumatoid arthritis (possible increase in autoimmunity).

Cooked garlic in dietary doses is presumed to be safe in pregnancy and lactation based on its extensive food use. However, there are few toxicity studies on the most commonly used garlic extracts and no studies on teratogenicity or embryotoxicity for any form of garlic. For this reason, avoid the use of standardized garlic extracts during pregnancy and in young children and individuals with severe hepatic or renal disease.

PATIENT INFORMATION

Garlic is marketed widely as an herb for lowering cholesterol and preventing cardiovascular disease. However, evidence suggests that garlic is only minimally effective, if at all, for high cholesterol. Garlic may help protect the heart in other ways, but the evidence is not strong. Garlic also is said to enhance the immune system and also act as a natural antibiotic. However, no scientific evidence exists for these claims. Garlic interferes with the ability of the blood to clot. For this reason, individuals taking anticoagulant drugs should not use garlic. These drugs include warfarin (Coumadin), aspirin, heparin, clopidogrel (Plavix), and pentoxifylline (Trental). Garlic also possibly could interact with other natural substances that interfere with blood clotting, such as ginkgo, policosanol, and high-dose vitamin E. Furthermore, garlic should be avoided in other circumstances where excessive bleeding is a risk, such as surgery and labor and delivery. Hemophiliacs also should avoid garlic. Individuals with human immunodeficiency virus infection should not use garlic because it might interfere with the actions of anti–human immunodeficiency virus medications or increase their side effects. The maximum safe dosage of garlic for pregnant or nursing women or young children has not been established. Individuals with severe liver or kidney disease should consult a physician before using this (or any other) herb.

DRUG INTERACTIONS

There are case reports of increased bleeding time in two patients combining warfarin and garlic supplements. Based on this, as well as evidence discussed previously, patients taking anticoagulants or antiplatelet agents should avoid using garlic extracts. Garlic conceivably could interact with other natural substances possessing anticoagulant or antithrombotic effects, such as ginkgo, policosanol, and high-dose vitamin E.

Garlic has been found to reduce plasma concentrations of saquinavir. In addition, two individuals with human immunodeficiency virus experienced severe gastrointestinal toxicity from ritonavir after taking garlic supplements.

PREGNANCY AND LACTATION

Garlic may possess significant antithrombotic and fibrinolytic actions, making its use risky in individuals with altered coagulation hemostasis, during pregnancy and labor and delivery, and within the perisurgical period.

ADVERSE REACTIONS

Based on its food use, garlic is on the Food and Drug Administration GRAS (generally recognized as safe) list. However, garlic in the diet usually is cooked. Typical standardized garlic products contain substances (such as alliin) not found in cooked garlic, making them more similar to raw garlic. There are few toxicity studies on these products. Only aged garlic has been well studied, and it lacks many active and potentially toxic components found in standardized garlic powder (and in raw garlic). One case report associated garlic supplement use with a spontaneous spinal epidural hematoma. However, in extensive clinical trials, standardized garlic extract and aged garlic powder have not been associated with serious side effects. The most common problem with garlic is the odor.

PROPOSED DOSAGE AND ADMINISTRATION

In most of the studies evaluating the proposed hypolipidemic effects of garlic, researchers used a dried form that supplies a daily dose of at least 10 mg of alliin, or a total allicin potential of 4 to 5 mg. However, not all manufacturers agree that allicin or alliin are at all relevant to the activity of garlic. The widely available deodorized form of garlic called Kyolic lacks allicin and many other constituents of garlic. Nonetheless, such products have provided positive results in studies and appear to have fewer gastric side effects. Garlic also sometimes is sold as an oil extract. Such products contain no allicin or alliin but high levels of ajoene, dithiins, and other breakdown products.

OCULAR CONSIDERATIONS

Ask why the product is being used. Treated conditions such as high cholesterol may have ocular manifestations or implications.

Ginkgo

Ginkgo biloba

GENERAL INFORMATION

Ginkgo is among the most widely prescribed herbs in Germany. German physicians consider it to be as effective as any drug treatment for Alzheimer's disease and other severe forms of memory and mental function decline.

PROPOSED INDICATIONS AND USAGE

Ginkgo appears to be effective for enhancing memory and mental function in Alzheimer's disease and milder forms of cognitive impairment. Weaker but still meaningful evidence supports benefit in intermittent claudication, premenstrual syndrome symptoms, and Raynaud's phenomenon. Very weak evidence hints at benefits for complications of diabetes, depression, glaucoma, macular degeneration, and vertigo. Despite early enthusiasm, ginkgo does not appear to be effective for tinnitus, altitude sickness, or reducing sexual side-effects of antidepressant drugs.

PRECAUTIONS

In clinical trials, use of ginkgo extract has been associated with few side effects. However, there have been several case reports of internal bleeding associated with use of ginkgo (spontaneous and following surgery). Therefore, those with bleeding disorders such as hemophilia should not use gingko, nor should anyone use it during the periods before or after surgery or labor and delivery.

Seizures also have been reported rarely with the use of ginkgo extract. Ginkgo seeds contain a toxic substance called 4-methoxypyridoxine and may cause seizures; although ginkgo products are made from the leafs and not the seeds, some ginkgo leaf products may be contaminated with ginkgo seeds. It also has been suggested that ginkgo, like tacrine, may have a direct proconvulsant effect, and for this reason those with epilepsy should avoid ginkgo.

In animal studies, ginkgo extract may cause the body to metabolize the drug nicardipine (a calcium channel blocker) more rapidly, thereby decreasing its effects.

Aminoglycoside antibiotics can cause hearing loss by damaging the nerve carrying hearing sensation from the ear. Ginkgo has been tried as a possible preventive for this side effect, but in one animal study, ginkgo increased the ototoxicity of amikacin. Individuals using aminoglycosides should avoid ginkgo.

Ginkgo might alter insulin release in persons with diabetes. Persons with diabetes should use ginkgo only under physician supervision.

DRUG INTERACTIONS

Antiplatelet drugs such as heparin, aspirin, clopidogrel (Plavix), ticlopidine (Ticlid), or pentoxifylline (Trental) might cause bleeding problems if combined with gingko. One study found no pharmacologic interaction between ginkgo and warfarin levels, but potentiation is still possible through combined effects on different aspects of the clotting system.

Combined use of ginkgo with natural substances with antiplatelet or anticoagulant thinning properties, such as garlic, phosphatidylserine, policosanol or high-dose vitamin E, also theoretically may cause bleeding problems.

Use of calcium channel blockers with ginkgo may reduce their effectiveness.

Use of aminoglycoside antibiotics with ginkgo may increase risk of hearing loss.

PROPOSED DOSAGE AND ADMINISTRATION

The standard dosage of ginkgo is 40 to 80 mg 3 times daily (50:1 extract standardized to contain 24% ginkgo-flavone glycosides).

OCULAR CONSIDERATIONS

Ginkgo extract at a dose of 120 mg daily for 8 weeks significantly improved the visual field in persons with glaucoma.

Use of ginkgo at a dose of 160 mg daily resulted in improved visual acuity for age-related maculopathy. Ginkgo at 240 mg per day compared with 60 mg daily showed improvement in vision for age-related maculopathy in both groups, but better results with the higher dose.

Use of *Ginkgo biloba* has been associated with spontaneous hyphema and retinal hemorrhages.

Ginseng

Panax ginseng

Alternate/Related Names: True ginseng, Asian ginseng, Chinese ginseng, Korean ginseng; American ginseng (P. quinquefolius)

BRAND NAMES

Ginsana (Pharmaton) = G115 (Pharmaton) in Europe

GENERAL INFORMATION

Panax ginseng contains 2% to 3% triterpenoid saponins named ginsenosides, of which 18 have been identified. Pharmacokinetic data on ginseng bioavailability are scarce. Aglycone metabolites of ginsenosides have been detected in the urine of human subjects taking ginseng orally, but only about 1.2% of the dose could be recovered over a 5-day period.

PROPOSED INDICATIONS AND USAGE

Ginseng is marketed widely in the United States as a stimulant, despite lack of any evidence that it exerts stimulant properties. In Europe, ginseng is considered an adaptogen, a substance that aids the response of the body to stress. However, little clinical evidence documents that ginseng actually possesses adaptogenic properties. Ginseng also is marketed for enhancing physical performance, prolonging life, and increasing sexual potency. However, the evidence base for these uses is weak to nonexistent. Ginseng sometimes is recommended for symptomatic relief in postmenopausal women, but a large trial found it ineffective.

Some evidence supports using ginseng as adjuvant therapy for diabetes and influenza vaccination.

PRECAUTIONS

Overstimulation and insomnia also have been reported with ginseng, and anecdotal evidence suggests that excessive doses may elevate blood pressure mildly. In addition, there has been one report of cerebral arteritis associated with ginseng use. However, because there have been numerous reports of adulteration of ginseng with other herbs, with germanium (a nephrotoxic substance), and with caffeine and other stimulants, it is not clear whether these reported side effects are actually due to ginseng itself. Reports in 1979 of a ginseng-abuse syndrome involving addiction, marked blood pressure elevation, agitation, severe sleeplessness, and hypersexuality have been discredited. Safety in pregnant or lactating women, young children, or individuals with severe hepatic or renal disease is not known.

PATIENT INFORMATION

Ginseng is an herb widely marketed as an energy booster. However, no evidence indicates that ginseng has any stimulant properties. Some proponents of ginseng claim that it helps the body adapt to stress (making it an adaptogen), but there is little evidence for this concept. Ginseng itself appears to be relatively safe. However, commercial ginseng products may at times be contaminated with unlisted stimulants or other hazardous substances. The safety of ginseng for pregnant or nursing women or young children has not been established. Individuals with severe liver or kidney disease should consult a physician before using this (or any other) supplement.

DRUG INTERACTIONS

One case report suggests that ginseng may inhibit CYP 3A4. According to another case report, *P. ginseng* may reduce the effectiveness of warfarin. However, a study in rats found no pharmacokinetic or pharmacodynamic interaction between warfarin and ginseng. There have been reports of apparent interaction between ginseng and phenelzine, resulting in headache, tremulousness, and maniclike symptoms. Whether this generalizes into a drug interaction with other monoamine oxidase inhibitors or drugs with monoamine oxidase inhibiting potential at high doses, such as selegiline, is not known. The ginseng involved in these case reports may have been contaminated with caffeine. One report indicates otherwise unexplained elevated digoxin levels in a patient taking digoxin and *Eleutherococcus*. (Because *Eleutherococcus* sometimes is substituted for *P. ginseng,* this finding is mentioned here.) However, this appears to have been a case of interference with a diagnostic test, rather than an actual elevation of digoxin. Based on results of clinical trials of ginseng for diabetes, concomitant use of ginseng possibly might require a reduction in insulin or oral hypoglycemic dose. Finally, if ginseng does have immunomodulatory actions as purported, interactions with immunosuppressive drugs are possible.

ADVERSE REACTIONS

Ginseng appears to present a low order of toxicity in short-term and long-term use, according to the results of studies in mice, rats, dogs, chickens, mink, deer, lambs, and dwarf pigs. Ginseng also does not appear to be teratogenic or carcinogenic. Studies of individual ginsenosides have shown little toxicity. Side effects from whole ginseng taken at appropriate doses are rare. Occasionally, women taking ginseng report menstrual abnormalities and breast tenderness. However, this side effect has not been documented formally, and large double-blind placebo-controlled trials have found no effects on sex hormones or gonadotropins.

PROPOSED DOSAGE AND ADMINISTRATION

The usual recommended daily dose of *P. ginseng* is 1 g crude herb or 200 g extract standardized to contain 4% to 7% ginsenosides, taken in two divided doses. In one study of American ginseng for diabetes, the dose used was 3 g.

OCULAR CONSIDERATIONS

Ask why the product is being used. Treated conditions such as menopause and diabetes may have ocular manifestations or implications.

Goldenseal

Hydrastis canadensis

GENERAL INFORMATION

Goldenseal contains berberine that inhibits or kills many microorganisms, including fungi, protozoa, and bacteria. Goldenseal often is used as a topical antibiotic for skin wounds and to treat viral mouth sores and superficial fungal infections, such as athlete's foot. No direct scientific evidence indicates that goldenseal is effective for any of these purposes. Goldenseal could be beneficial in treating sore throats and diseases of the digestive tract because it can contact the affected area directly.

PROPOSED INDICATIONS AND USAGE

Topical: Athlete's foot and other fungal infections, minor wounds, vaginal yeast infections

Oral: Congestive heart failure, dyspepsia, heart arrhythmias, high blood pressure, infectious diarrhea, irritable bowel syndrome, and urinary tract infections. No meaningful evidence exists to support any of these uses.

PRECAUTIONS

Topical use of goldenseal could cause photosensitivity. Individuals with elevated bilirubin levels (jaundice) also should avoid use of goldenseal.

PREGNANCY AND LACTATION

Pregnant women should not use goldenseal because goldenseal might cause uterine contractions. In addition, berberine might increase levels of bilirubin and also cause genetic damage.

PROPOSED DOSAGE AND ADMINISTRATION

For mouth sores and sore throats, goldenseal may be used as strong tea by boiling 0.5 to 1 g in a cup of water.

OCULAR CONSIDERATIONS

Topical treatment of trachoma with berberine has been studied in 32 microbiologically confirmed cases.

Berberine 0.2% was found to be superior compared with sulfacetamide 20% in the clinical course of trachoma and in achieving a fall in the serum antibody titers against *Chlamydia trachomatis* in the treated patients. (Khosla PK et al: Berberine, a potential drug for trachoma, *Rev Int Trach Pathol Ocul Trop Subtrop Sante Publique* 69:147, 1992). However, whole goldenseal products are not equivalent to these concentrated berberine formulations.

Guggul

Commiphora mukul

Alternate/Related Names:
Mukul myrrh, false myrrh, gum guggulu, gum guggul, gugulipid

GENERAL INFORMATION

Guggul contains a family of ketonic steroid compounds called guggulsterones. Most studies have used a standardized ethyl acetate extract of the resin, containing 4.09% total of two compounds known as Z- and E-guggulsterone. The mechanism of action of guggul is not known.

PROPOSED INDICATIONS AND USAGE

Studies performed in India have led to wide marketing of guggul as a hypolipidemic agent. However, the only U.S. trial found no benefit. Based on extremely weak evidence that guggul has thyroid-stimulating properties, guggul also has been marketed as a weight loss agent. However, no evidence indicates that guggul is effective, and one trial (the U.S. trial) found it ineffective. Very weak evidence has been used to justify marketing guggul for acne and diabetes.

PRECAUTIONS

Safety for pregnant or lactating women, young children, or individuals with hepatic or renal disease is not known.

PATIENT INFORMATION

Guggul is an extract of the mukul myrrh tree that is widely sold as a treatment for high cholesterol. However, the best study failed to find it effective. Guggul also is marketed as a weight loss treatment, but there is no evidence that it works, and one study found it ineffective. The safety of guggul for pregnant or nursing women or young children has not been established. Individuals with severe liver or kidney disease should consult a physician before using this (or any other) supplement.

DRUG INTERACTIONS

No drug interactions have been reported.

ADVERSE REACTIONS

In clinical trials of standardized guggul extract, no significant side effects other than occasional mild gastrointestinal distress have been seen. Laboratory tests conducted in the course of these trials did not reveal any alterations in hepatic or renal function, hematologic parameters, cardiac function, or blood chemistry. Animal studies reportedly found no evidence of toxicity.

PROPOSED DOSAGE AND ADMINISTRATION

Guggul is manufactured in a standardized form that provides a fixed amount of guggulsterones. The typical daily dose should provide 100 mg of guggulsterones.

OCULAR CONSIDERATIONS

Ask why the product is being used. Treated conditions such as hyperlipidemia may have ocular manifestations or implications.

Gymnema

Gymnema sylvestre

GENERAL INFORMATION

An ethanolic extract of gymnema leaves called GS4 is thought to contain the active constituents of the herb. In some low-quality human and animal studies, GS4 administration reportedly has resulted in reduced blood glucose levels. Histopathologic examination of pancreatic tissue in one quality study claimed to find evidence of an increase in the number of beta cells after GS4 supplementation. These findings have not been replicated in studies that are up to current scientific standards.

PROPOSED INDICATIONS AND USAGE

Poorly reported pilot studies provide weak evidence that gymnema may be an effective hypoglycemic agent.

PRECAUTIONS

Although gymnema has not been proved effective, if it were to reduce serum glucose, hypoglycemic reactions could occur. Monitoring of serum glucose therefore is recommended. Safety in pregnant or lactating women, young children, or individuals with severe hepatic or renal disease has not been established.

PATIENT INFORMATION

Gymnema is an herb sold as a treatment for diabetes. However, it has not been proved effective. NOTE: Do not substitute gymnema for standard diabetes therapy. In addition, keep in mind that if gymnema is added to standard therapy, it conceivably could cause a hypoglycemic reaction. The safety of gymnema for pregnant or nursing women or young children has not been established. Individuals with severe liver or kidney disease should consult a physician before using this (or any other) supplement.

DRUG INTERACTIONS

Gymnema theoretically could potentiate the action of insulin or other hypoglycemic medications.

ADVERSE REACTIONS

Gymnema appears to be well tolerated, although comprehensive safety testing has not been undertaken.

PROPOSED DOSAGE AND ADMINISTRATION

Gymnema extract usually is taken at a dosage of 400 to 600 mg daily. Some products are standardized to contain 24% gymnemic acid.

OCULAR CONSIDERATIONS

Ask why the product is being used. Treated conditions such as diabetes may have ocular manifestations or implications.

Hawthorn

Crataegus laevigata, C. monogyna, C. oxyacantha, C. pentagyna

BRAND NAMES

HeartCare (Nature's Way) = Crataegutt forte, WS 1442 (Schwabe) in Europe

GENERAL INFORMATION

The primary constituents of hawthorn include flavonoids (including quercetin and vitexin), oligomeric procyanidins (such as found in grape seed), catechins, purine derivatives, amines, triterpenoids, and aromatic carboxylic acids. Animal studies suggest that hawthorn extracts simultaneously increase the force, amplitude, and volume of cardiac contraction while lengthening the cardiac refractory period. This combination of effects may give hawthorn a particular safety factor when used in heart disease. Protection from myocardial reperfusion injury also has been seen in animal studies.

PROPOSED INDICATIONS AND USAGE

Considerable evidence indicates that hawthorn may be helpful in the treatment of New York Heart Association class I to III congestive heart failure. Hawthorn might offer safety advantages over digoxin in early congestive heart failure (CHF). However, although the long-term benefits of angiotensin-converting enzyme inhibitors have been established in numerous studies, no evidence indicates that hawthorn reduces the morbidity or mortality of CHF. Weaker evidence supports the use of hawthorn in angina. Based on animal trials, hawthorn also could be useful in the prevention of arrhythmias following myocardial infarction.

However, clinical trials in human beings are lacking. Hawthorn sometimes is recommended by herbalists as a treatment for minor, benign arrhythmias, but there is no scientific basis for this usage.

Hawthorn often is added to dietary products marketed for hypertension. However, no evidence indicates that hawthorn has any significant effect on blood pressure.

PRECAUTIONS

Commission E in Germany lists no known risks or contraindications with hawthorn. However, safety in young children, pregnant or lactating women, or individuals with severe renal or hepatic disease has not been established.

DRUG INTERACTIONS

Because hawthorn appears to possess cardioactive properties, the possibility of interaction with or potentiation of other cardiovascular drugs is likely.

ADVERSE REACTIONS

In clinical trials, hawthorn has been connected only with nonspecific side effects such as mild gastrointestinal distress and allergic reactions.

PROPOSED DOSAGE AND ADMINISTRATION

The standard dose of hawthorn is 100 to 300 mg 3 times daily of an extract standardized to contain about 2% to 3% flavonoids or 18% to 20% procyanidins. The effectiveness of hawthorn appears to require a 4- to 8-week course.

PATIENT INFORMATION

The herb hawthorn is marketed as a treatment for various heart conditions. Some evidence indicates that it may be helpful for CHF; however, CHF is a dangerous condition that should not be self-treated. Furthermore, although standard treatments have been shown to prevent serious complications of CHF, hawthorn has not been shown to provide the same benefit. Hawthorn has not been shown to reduce blood pressure or provide any other specific benefits for the heart. Instruct patients not to combine hawthorn with standard heart drugs except on the advice of a physician. The safety of hawthorn for pregnant or nursing women or young children has not been established. Individuals with severe liver or kidney disease should consult a physician before using this (or any other) supplement.

OCULAR CONSIDERATIONS

Ask why the product is being used. Treated conditions such as congestive heart failure may have ocular manifestations or implications.

Lipoic Acid

Alternate/Related Names:

Alpha-lipoic acid, thioctic acid

GENERAL INFORMATION

Alpha-lipoic acid is a vitamin-like substance that serves as a cofactor in the mitochondrial dehydrogenase reactions that lead to the formation of adenosine triphosphate. Certain illnesses may reduce levels of lipoic acid, such as diabetes, liver cirrhosis, and heart disease. Thus although lipoic acid is not ordinarily an essential nutrient, supplementation in such conditions may correct a relative deficiency.

PROPOSED INDICATIONS AND USAGE

Lipoic acid has been marketed extensively as a "super antioxidant" said to prevent heart disease and cancer. However, although lipoic acid is definitely an antioxidant, evidence for any therapeutic benefits remains weak. Weak evidence supports the use of oral lipoic acid in diabetic peripheral and autonomic neuropathy. Minimal evidence suggests that lipoic acid might retard the development of diabetic cataracts and provide benefits in heart disease and liver cirrhosis.

PRECAUTIONS

Maximum safe doses for young children, pregnant or lactating women, or persons with severe hepatic or renal disease have not been established.

PATIENT INFORMATION

Lipoic acid is a supplement that has been tried for diabetic neuropathy. However, little evidence indicates that lipoic acid is effective for this condition. Lipoic acid also is marketed as a super antioxidant for heart disease, cancer, and slowing down aging. However, these proposed uses have no real scientific foundation. The maximum safe dosage of lipoic acid for pregnant or nursing women or young children has not been established. Individuals with severe liver or kidney disease should consult a physician before using this (or any other) supplement.

DRUG INTERACTIONS

Formal drug interaction studies have not been performed. Based on pharmacologic studies, some concerns exist that lipoic acid might potentiate the effects of insulin or oral hypoglycemics, but this effect has not been seen in clinical trials.

ADVERSE REACTIONS

In a study of 509 type 2 diabetic patients, an oral lipoic acid dose of 1800 mg daily for 6 months was not associated with a greater incidence of side effects than placebo and did not affect glucose balance.

PROPOSED DOSAGE AND ADMINISTRATION

The typical dose of lipoic acid is 300 to 600 mg/day, taken in two to three divided doses. A dose of 800 mg/day has been used to treat cardiac autonomic neuropathy. The effects generally are seen within a few weeks.

OCULAR CONSIDERATIONS

Lipoic acid has shown some promise for treatment of glaucoma. Very weak evidence hints at possible activity for cataract prevention. Lipoic acid also may provide protection to the retina and ganglion cells from ischemia-reperfusion injuries. (Chidlow G et al: Alpha-lipoic acid protects the retina against ischemia-reperfusion, *Neuropharmacology* 43[6]:1015, 2002.)

Lutein

GENERAL INFORMATION

Lutein is a carotenoid that concentrates in the lens and retina. The yellow color of lutein may screen the retina and lens from damage caused by light of shorter wavelength. Lutein also may play a role in macular degeneration and cataract formation through its antioxidant effects.

PROPOSED INDICATIONS AND USAGE

Most proposed uses of lutein are ocular. See Ocular Considerations. Lutein also has been recommended, based on next to no evidence, for preventing atherosclerosis.

PROPOSED DOSAGE AND ADMINISTRATION

Dosing for lutein is not known, but estimates range from 5 to 30 mg daily. Maximum safe dosages for young children, pregnant or nursing women, or those with severe liver or kidney disease have not been established.

OCULAR CONSIDERATIONS

A small, 2-year double-blind placebo-controlled trial found some evidence that lutein may improve visual function in persons with cataracts. (Olmedilla B et al: Lutein, but not alpha-tocopherol, supplementation improves visual function in patients with age-related cataracts: a 2-year double-blind, placebo-controlled pilot study, *Nutrition* 19:21, 2003.) Another study found that lutein, or lutein plus antioxidants, can improve vision in persons with macular degeneration. (Richer S et al: Double-masked, placebo-controlled, randomized trial of lutein and antioxidant supplementation in the intervention of atrophic age-related macular degeneration: the Veterans LAST study [Lutein Antioxidant Supplementation Trial], *Optometry* 75:216, 2004.)

Lycopene

GENERAL INFORMATION

Lycopene is a carotenoid. Lycopene is present in human serum, liver, adrenal glands, lungs, prostate, colon, and skin at higher levels than other carotenoids. Lycopene has been shown to possess antioxidant and antiproliferative properties. Lycopene can be found in tomatoes and pink grapefruit.

PROPOSED INDICATIONS AND USAGE

Lycopene primarily has been advocated for the prevention or treatment of prostate cancer, but as yet the supporting evidence for this use is weak. Other proposed uses include treatment of exercise-induced asthma and male infertility and prevention of heart disease, intrauterine growth retardation, age-related maculopathy, cataracts, and preeclampsia.

PRECAUTIONS

Lycopene is believed to be a safe supplement, as evidenced by the fact that researchers felt comfortable giving it to pregnant women. However, maximum safe dosages are not known.

DRUG INTERACTIONS

Some drugs that lower cholesterol levels in the blood also may reduce levels of carotenoids such as lycopene. The fat substitute Olestra may decrease levels of lycopene in the blood.

PREGNANCY AND LACTATION

Some evidence indicates lycopene can help with prevention of complications during pregnancy. A preliminary double-blind trial hints that lycopene supplements may help prevent preeclampsia (a dangerous complication of pregnancy) and intrauterine growth retardation (inadequate growth of the fetus). Pregnant women should consult with a physician before taking any herbs or supplements.

PROPOSED DOSAGE AND ADMINISTRATION

The optimum dosage for lycopene has not been established. The amounts used in studies are in the range of 4 to 6.5 mg daily.

OCULAR CONSIDERATIONS

Lycopene has been shown to delay cataractogenesis in rats. (Gupta SK et al: Lycopene attenuates oxidative stress induced experimental cataract development: an in vitro and in vivo study, *Nutrition* 19[9]:794, 2003.)

Magnesium

Names: Magnesium chloride, magnesium citrate, magnesium fumarate, magnesium gluconate, magnesium malate, magnesium oxide, magnesium sulfate

GENERAL INFORMATION

Magnesium is the fourth most abundant mineral in the body and is essential to good health. Approximately 50% of total body magnesium is found in bone. The other half is found predominantly inside cells of body tissues and organs. Only 1% of magnesium is found in blood, but the body works hard to keep blood levels of magnesium constant.

Magnesium is needed for more than 300 biochemical reactions in the body. Dietary magnesium is absorbed in the small intestines. Magnesium is excreted through the kidneys.

PROPOSED INDICATIONS AND USAGE

There are numerous proposed uses of magnesium supplements.

Those uses with supporting evidence include preventing migraine headaches, enhancing glycemic control in diabetes, preventing noise-related hearing loss, and treating menstrual pain, pregnancy-induced leg cramps, premenstrual syndrome symptoms, and angina. Magnesium supplements also may have value as adjunctive treatment of congestive heart failure to combat furosemide-induced hypomagnesemia, which in turn may increase digoxin-related arrhythmias.

PRECAUTIONS

The most common complaint is loose stools. Persons with severe kidney or heart disease should not take magnesium (or any other supplement) except on the advice of a physician. One death was caused by excessive magnesium supplements in a developmentally and physically disabled child.

DRUG INTERACTIONS

Loop and thiazide diuretics, antineoplastic drugs, and antibiotics may increase the loss of magnesium in urine. Thus, taking these medications for long periods may contribute to magnesium depletion.

Magnesium binds tetracycline in the gut and decreases the absorption of tetracycline.

Many antacids and laxatives contain magnesium. When frequently taken in large doses, these drugs inadvertently can lead to excessive magnesium consumption and hypermagnesemia.

PROPOSED DOSAGE AND ADMINISTRATION

The official U.S. and Canadian recommendations for daily intake are as follows:

Infants: Birth to 6 months, 30 mg
7 to 12 months, 75 mg
Children: 1 to 3 years, 80 mg
4 to 8 years, 130 mg
Males: 9 to 13 years, 240 mg
14 to 18 years, 410 mg
19 to 30 years, 400 mg
31 years and older, 420 mg
Females: 9 to 13 years, 240 mg
14 to 18 years, 360 mg
19 to 30 years, 310 mg
31 years and older, 320 mg
Pregnant women 18 years and younger, 400 mg
19 to 30 years, 350 mg
31 to 50 years, 360 mg
Nursing women 18 years and younger, 360 mg
19 to 30 years, 310 mg
31 to 50 years, 320 mg

Supplemental dosages of magnesium ranges from the nutritional needs listed to as high as 600 mg daily.

The U.S. government has set the following upper limits:
Children 1 to 3 years, 65 mg
Children 4 to 8 years, 110 mg
Adults, 350 mg
Pregnant or nursing women, 350 mg

OCULAR CONSIDERATIONS

Ten patients with glaucoma (six with primary open-angle glaucoma, four with normal-tension glaucoma) with a digital cold-induced vasospasm were given magnesium (121.5 mg) twice a day for a month. After 4 weeks of treatment, the visual fields improved. Magnesium improved the peripheral circulation and had a beneficial effect on visual fields in glaucoma patients with vasospasm. (Gaspar AZ, Gasser P, Flammer J: The influence of magnesium on visual field and peripheral vasospasm in glaucoma, *Ophthalmologica* 209[1]:11, 1995.)

Melatonin

GENERAL INFORMATION

Melatonin is a natural hormone produced by the pineal gland. During daylight, the pineal gland in the brain produces serotonin. At night, the pineal gland stops producing serotonin and makes melatonin. Melatonin release helps trigger sleep.

PROPOSED INDICATIONS AND USAGE

Insomnia, jet lag, cancer, cluster headaches, epilepsy in children, fighting aging, immune support, preventing heart disease, reducing anxiety before surgery, and tardive dyskinesia

PRECAUTIONS

Melatonin has been shown to affect testosterone and estrogen metabolism in men and may impair sperm function. Melatonin can cause drowsiness, decreased mental attention for about 2 to 6 hours after use. Caution patients against driving or operating machinery for several hours after taking melatonin.

Some authorities recommend against using melatonin in persons with depression, schizophrenia, autoimmune diseases, and other serious illnesses. Melatonin might impair insulin action and glucose tolerance in menopausal women. Individuals with diabetes should seek physician supervision before using melatonin.

PROPOSED DOSAGE AND ADMINISTRATION

Melatonin is taken half an hour before bedtime. The optimum dose of melatonin is not clear.

OCULAR CONSIDERATIONS

Studies have shown agonists of melatonin receptors (5-MCA-NAT) have a strong ocular hypotensive effect in New Zealand white rabbits. (Pintor J et al: Ocular hypotensive effects of melatonin receptor agonists in the rabbit: further evidence for an MT3 receptor, *Br J Pharmacol* 138[5]:831, 2003.) Topical application of the melatonin receptor agonist reduces intraocular pressure in glaucomatous monkey eyes. (Serle JB et al: Effect of 5-MCA-NAT, a putative melatonin MT3 receptor agonist, on intraocular pressure in glaucomatous monkey eyes, *J Glaucoma* 13[5]:385, 2004.)

Oligomeric Proanthocyanidin Complexes

Alternate/Related Names:

Grape seed, PCOs (procyanidolic oligomers), maritime pine bark (Pinus pinaster), pycnogenol

BRAND NAMES

Grape Seed (PCO) Extract (PhytoPharmica/Enzymatic Therapy), Grapenol (Solaray), Grapeseed Extract (Thorne Research) = Endotelon (Sanofi/Labaz), LeucoSelect (Indena) in Europe

Pycnogenol (Horphag; U.S. product only)

GENERAL INFORMATION

The oligomeric proanthocyanidin complex (OPC) family includes a

APPENDIX H

variety of proanthocyanidins that are bound to each other in dimer, trimer, and larger molecules. In vitro studies suggest that OPCs increase collagen cross-linking, decrease capillary permeability, and block the effects of hyaluronidase, elastase, collagenase, and other enzymes that degrade connective tissue. In addition, they appear to chelate free iron molecules, prevent iron-potentiated lipid peroxidation, slow free radical production by reversibly inhibiting xanthine oxidase, and reduce the release and production of histamine and leukotrienes. The antioxidant effects of OPCs occur in polar and nonpolar media. However, the clinical relevance of these findings has yet to be established.

PROPOSED INDICATIONS AND USAGE

Preliminary evidence suggests that orally administered OPCs may be useful for chronic venous insufficiency and for speeding resolution of postsurgical or sports injury–related edema. Oligomeric proanthocyanidin complex products are advertised as "natural antihistamines," but an 8-week double-blind placebo-controlled trial of 49 individuals found no benefit with oral grape seed extract in the treatment of allergic rhinitis. In addition, OPCs have been recommended for diabetic retinopathy, impaired night vision, macular degeneration, capillary fragility, allergic rhinitis, and heart disease prevention, but there is little supporting evidence for these uses. Topical products containing OPCs are marketed widely with claims, largely unsubstantiated, that they can improve skin appearance and elasticity.

PRECAUTIONS

Maximum safe dosage in young children, pregnant or lactating women, and individuals with severe hepatic or renal disease has not been established.

PATIENT INFORMATION

Oligomeric proanthocyanidin complexes are an expensive supplement marketed for a great number of conditions. Weak evidence suggests that OPCs may be helpful for venous insufficiency (a condition related to varicose veins) and for swelling following surgery or sports injuries. Other uses of OPCs, such as preventing heart disease and treating eye conditions or improving skin tone, have no meaningful supporting evidence. One study found OPCs ineffective for allergies. The maximum safe dosage of OPCs for pregnant or nursing women or young children has not been established. Individuals with severe liver or kidney disease should consult a physician before using this (or any other) supplement.

DRUG INTERACTIONS

Based on the activity of other flavonoids, OPCs might potentiate the effects of anticoagulant and antiplatelet agents.

ADVERSE REACTIONS

In the double-blind studies of OPCs, no significant adverse reactions were seen, and the side-effect profile was similar to that of placebo.

PROPOSED DOSAGE AND ADMINISTRATION

Oligomeric proanthocyanidin complexes generally are taken in an oral dose of 150 to 600 mg daily. Topical creams are applied 1 to 2 times daily.

OCULAR CONSIDERATIONS

Visual performance after glare and adaptation to low luminances improved for a treated group of patients after 5 weeks. The treated group received four 50-mg tablets of OPCs a day in the study. (Corbe C, Boissin JP, Siou A: Light vision and chorioretinal circulation: study of the effect of procyanidolic oligomers [Endotelon], *J Fr Ophtalmol* 11[5]:453, 1988.)

In diabetic rats, OPCs enhanced the retinal antioxidant activities alone and in combination with beta-carotene. The rats received daily intraperitoneal doses (10 mg/kg). (Dene BA et al: Effects of antioxidant treatment on normal and diabetic rat retinal enzyme activities, *J Ocul Pharmacol Ther* 21[1]:28, 2005.)

Omega-3 Fatty Acids

Names: Fish oil, docosahexaenoic acid, eicosapentaenoic acid, omega-3 fatty acids, omega-3 oil

GENERAL INFORMATION

Fish oil contains omega-3 fatty acids, one of the two main classes of essential fatty acids. Omega-6 fatty acids are the other main type. Studies of the Inuit (Eskimo) people found that their diets contain an enormous amount of fat from fish, seals, and whales and that they seldom suffer heart attacks. Their sources of fat are high in omega-3 fatty acids. Omega-3 fatty acids found in fish oil can lower blood triglyceride levels, thin the blood, and decrease inflammation. Flaxseed oil also contains omega-3 fatty acids, although of a different kind. It has been suggested as a less smelly substitute for fish oil. However, flaxseed oil does not appear to be therapeutically equivalent to fish oil.

PROPOSED INDICATIONS AND USAGE

Dry eyes, retinitis pigmentosa, heart disease prevention, rheumatoid arthritis, allergies, asthma, attention deficit and hyperactivity disorder, bipolar disorder, borderline personality disorder, cancer treatment support, chronic fatigue syndrome, Crohn's disease, depression, diabetic neuropathy, dysmenorrhea, gout, human immunodeficiency virus support, hypertension, kidney stones, lupus, male infertility, migraine headaches, multiple sclerosis, osteoporosis, pregnancy support, prevention of premature birth, prostate cancer prevention, psoriasis, Raynaud's phenomenon, schizophrenia, sickle cell anemia, strokes (prevention), ulcerative colitis, and undesired weight loss caused by cancer.

PRECAUTIONS

The most common problem is fishy burps. Some fish oil products contain excessive levels of toxic substances such as organochlorines and PCBs (polychlorinated biphenyls). Fish oil has a mild blood-thinning effect and should not be combined with powerful blood-thinning medications such as warfarin (Coumadin) or heparin. Fish oil temporarily may raise the level of low-density lipoprotein cholesterol, but this effect may be short-lived.

DRUG INTERACTIONS

Instruct patients not to take fish oil if they are taking warfarin (Coumadin) or heparin, without the advice of a physician.

PROPOSED DOSAGE AND ADMINISTRATION

Dosages of fish oil are 3 to 9 g daily, but this is not the upper limit. In one study, patients have ingested 60 g daily.

OCULAR CONSIDERATIONS

Omega-3 fatty acids help to produce antiinflammatory factors and suppress proinflammatory cytokines. Suppression of cytokines can stimulate tear production. The clearing and thinning of meibomian gland oil has also been observed with omega-3 supplementation.

In one study, 208 patients with retinitis pigmentosa, aged 18 to 55 years, were assigned randomly to 1200 mg per day of docosahexaenoic acid plus vitamin A or control fatty acid plus vitamin A and were followed over 4 years. For patients with retinitis pigmentosa beginning vitamin A therapy, addition of docosahexaenoic acid slowed the course of disease for 2 years. Among patients on vitamin A for at least 2 years, a diet rich in omega-3 fatty acids slowed the decline in visual field sensitivity. (Berson EL et al: Further evaluation of docosahexaenoic acid in patients with retinitis pigmentosa receiving vitamin A treatment: subgroup analyses, *Arch Ophthalmol* 122[9]:1306, 2004).

Policosanol

Alternate/Related Names:
Octacosanol, 1-octacosanol, N-octacosanol, octacosyl alcohol, wheat germ oil

GENERAL INFORMATION

Policosanol contains several higher aliphatic primary alcohols. The main component is octacosanol, followed by triacontanol and hexacosanol. Policosanol appears to impair cholesterol synthesis between the acetate and mevalonate production steps. Policosanol also may increase receptor-dependent low-density lipoprotein processing, thereby reducing plasma low-density lipoprotein concentration. Policosanol reportedly exhibits dose-dependent antiplatelet actions comparable to 100 mg aspirin daily and may reduce lipid peroxidation.

PROPOSED INDICATIONS AND USAGE

Numerous double-blind trials conducted in Cuba by one research group indicate that policosanol is an effective treatment for hyperlipidemia. However, the lack of confirmation of these results by other independent researchers makes these results less than fully reliable; furthermore, the tested formulation of policosanol (sugarcane source) is not available in the United States, and the forms available in the United States (wheat germ and beeswax source) thus far have failed to prove effective. Policosanol also may be helpful for intermittent claudication. Policosanol also is marketed as sports supplements, but there is little evidence for any ergogenic effect.

Other proposed uses with minimal or no scientific support include for Parkinson's disease and amyotrophic lateral sclerosis.

PRECAUTIONS

The antiplatelet effects of policosanol suggest caution in individuals with bleeding disorders, as well as in the perioperative and around the labor and delivery period. The evidence from one human trial suggests that policosanol does not affect hepatic function. Nonetheless, safety in individuals with severe hepatic or renal disease has not been established.

PATIENT INFORMATION

Policosanol is a supplement marketed for reducing cholesterol. However, all supporting scientific studies were performed by a single research group in Cuba. These studies used policosanol made from sugarcane. The forms of policosanol available in the United States are made from wheat germ or beeswax instead and have not been shown to be effective. Policosanol interferes with the ability of the blood to clot. For this reason, individuals with bleeding disorders should not use policosanol, nor should those who use blood-thinning medications such as aspirin, warfarin (Coumadin), heparin, clopidogrel (Plavix), or pentoxifylline (Trental). In addition, policosanol might cause problems if it is combined with natural substances that thin the blood, such as garlic, ginkgo, white willow, and vitamin E.

DRUG INTERACTIONS

In studies, policosanol has not interacted with calcium channel antagonists, diuretics, or beta-blockers. However, policosanol does appear to potentiate the antiplatelet effects of aspirin. Therefore exercise caution when combining policosanol with any antiplatelet or anticoagulant agent. Policosanol possibly could potentiate the anticoagulant properties of supplements such as garlic, ginkgo, and high-dose vitamin E. According to one report, policosanol might impair the action of levodopa.

PREGNANCY AND LACTATION

Safety in pregnant or lactating women or in young children has not been established, although there are no known or suspected risks with policosanol in these populations. Individuals with severe liver or kidney disease should consult a physician before using this (or any other) supplement.

ADVERSE REACTIONS

Policosanol is generally well tolerated. In a drug-monitoring study that followed 27,879 patients for 2 to 4 years, adverse effects were reported in only 0.31% of participants and were primarily weight loss, excessive urination, and insomnia.

No signs of toxicity were observed in animals given very high doses of policosanol (as much as 620 times the maximum recommended dose).

PROPOSED DOSAGE AND ADMINISTRATION

Typical dosages of policosanol for lowering elevated cholesterol levels range from 5 to 10 mg twice daily. Results may require 2 months to develop.

OCULAR CONSIDERATIONS

Ask why the product is being used. Treated conditions such as hyperlipidemia may have ocular implications or ocular drug interactions.

Quercetin

Names: Quercetin chalcone

GENERAL INFORMATION

Quercetin is a bioflavonoid found in many foods, particularly apples, black tea, grapefruit, onions, and red wine.

PROPOSED INDICATIONS AND USAGE

Quercetin is marketed is a kind of natural cromolyn sodium, based on a few in vitro studies suggesting that it stabilizes mast cells and basophils. However, no clinical evidence supports any uses related to this proposed mechanism. Other proposed uses, including cancer and heart disease prevention, are largely theoretical.

PRECAUTIONS

Quercetin does not pass the Ames test, which is designed to identify chemicals that might be carcinogenic. However, most other evidence suggests that quercetin does not cause cancer but may help prevent cancer.

Use of quercetin in clinical trials has not been associated with any significant side effects beyond occasional allergic reactions and nonspecific digestive distress. However, despite in vitro evidence of chemoprevention, there are some indications that quercetin could have a carcinogenic effect under certain circumstances that are not well defined as yet.

PREGNANCY AND LACTATION

One study suggests that quercetin combined with other bioflavonoids in the diet of pregnant women might increase the risk of infant leukemia. Pregnant women probably should avoid quercetin supplements.

PROPOSED DOSAGE AND ADMINISTRATION

Dosage is 200 to 400 mg 3 times daily.

OCULAR CONSIDERATIONS

Dietary quercetin and metabolites are active in inhibiting oxidative damage in the lens and thus could play a role in prevention of cataract formation. (Cornish KM, Williamson G, Sanderson J: Quercetin metabolism in the lens: role in inhibition of hydrogen peroxide induced cataract, *Free Radic Biol Med* 33[1]:63, 2002.)

Quercetin protected the crystalline lens from calcium and sodium influx, which are early events leading to lens opacity. Quercetin helps to maintain lens transparency after an oxidative insult. (Sanderson J, McLauchlan WR, Williamson G: Quercetin inhibits hydrogen peroxide–induced oxidation of the rat lens, *Free Radic Biol Med* 26[5-6]:639, 1999.)

Red Clover

Trifolium pratense

Alternate/Related Names:
Wild clover, purple clover, trefoil

BRAND NAMES

Promensil (Novogen; clinically tested) = Promensil (Novogen) in Europe

GENERAL INFORMATION

Red clover contains numerous isoflavones, including most prominently biochanin A and formononetin, but also genistein and daidzein. Other constituents include coumarins, cyanogenic glycosides, and volatile oils.

Genistein and daidzein are found in soy and have been researched extensively for potential phytoestrogenic and chemopreventive properties. Biochanin A also appears to have phytoestrogenic action. Biochanin A also has been found in vitro to inhibit carcinogen activation; additionally, an in vitro study of human stomach cancer cell lines suggests that biochanin A inhibits cell growth through activation of a signal transduction pathway for apoptosis.

PROPOSED INDICATIONS AND USAGE

Despite extensive marketing as a treatment for menopausal symptoms, red clover isoflavones generally have failed to prove effective for this purpose in double-blind trials. Red clover isoflavones also generally have failed to prove effective for hyperlipidemia. Red clover in its whole form continues to be marketed for its archaic use as a "blood purifier."

PRECAUTIONS

Because red clover contains isoflavonoid constituents, its use in women with a history of hormone-sensitive cancer warrants caution. In addition, given its coumarin constituents, use of red clover in individuals with impaired hemostasis is questionable. Maximum safe dosages in individuals with severe hepatic or renal disease are not known. Because of its phytoestrogenic components, red clover is not recommended for use in pregnant or lactating women. Safety in young children has not been established.

PATIENT INFORMATION

Red clover extracts are marketed for the treatment of menopausal symptoms and reducing levels of cholesterol. However, in the largest and best studies, no benefits were seen. These extracts contain estrogen-like substances, which may present risks for pregnant or nursing women and for young children. These substances also might interact with blood-thinning medications. Whole red clover (as opposed to the extract) also sometimes is recommended for cancer treatment, but there is no evidence whatsoever that it is helpful for this purpose. Individuals with severe liver or kidney disease should consult a physician before using this (or any other) supplement.

DRUG INTERACTIONS

Based on the known actions of their isoflavone and coumarin constituents, red clover extracts potentially may interfere with hormone therapy and may potentiate the effect of anticoagulant pharmaceuticals.

ADVERSE REACTIONS

Red clover is on the Food and Drug Administration GRAS (generally recognized as safe) list and is included in many beverage teas. However, detailed safety studies have not been performed. Red clover isoflavones are a markedly different and much better researched product; no significant adverse effects have been reported in clinical trials, but there are theoretical concerns as described previously.

PROPOSED DOSAGE AND ADMINISTRATION

A typical dosage of red clover extract provides 40 to 160 mg isoflavones daily.

OCULAR CONSIDERATIONS

Ask why the product is being used. Treated conditions such as menopause and hyperlipidemia may have ocular implications or ocular drug interactions.

St. John's Wort

Hypericum perforatum, Hyperici herba

Other Names: Hypericum, kaimath weed, John's wort

GENERAL INFORMATION

St. John's wort is thought to raise levels of neurotransmitters in the brain (serotonin, norepinephrine, and dopamine). St. John's wort contains quinoids (hypericin, pseudohypericin), anthraquinones, flavonoids (hyperoside, quercitin, rutin), bioflavonoids, and a volatile oil. One of the pharmacologically active components is hypericin; another may be hyperfornin. The portions of the plant used are the aboveground parts harvested during the flowering season.

PROPOSED INDICATIONS AND USAGE

Considerable, if not entirely consistent, evidence indicates that St. John's wort is effective for major depression of mild to moderate severity. Other proposed uses—such as for anxiety, attention deficit disorder, insomnia, menopausal symptoms, premenstrual syndrome, seasonal affective disorder, human immunodeficiency virus infection, and diabetic neuropathy—lack and meaningful supporting evidence.

PRECAUTIONS

Side effects are generally minimal, but photosensitization, headache, nervousness, restlessness, hypomania, and constipation have been noted. Use St. John's wort with caution in severely depressed patients. The safety of St. John's wort during pregnancy and lactation is unknown. Avoid use of St. John's wort in patients with a history of seizure disorders or migraine.

DRUG INTERACTIONS

Use St. John's wort only with caution in patients taking other antidepressive medications, including monoamine oxidase inhibitors, tricyclic antidepressants, and selective serotonin reuptake inhibitors. It has been suggested that a risk of serotonin syndrome could occur with these antidepressants. Avoid indirect-acting sympathomimetics. Discontinue use 2 weeks before general anesthesia. Other drugs suggested to interact include metronidazole, caffeine, theophylline, digoxin, warfarin, cyclosporine, indinavir, possibly other human immunodeficiency virus drugs, oral contraceptives, losartan, and iron salts. St. John's wort possibly interacts with some cancer chemotherapy medications. Avoid drugs with a potential for photosensitivity.

PREGNANCY AND LACTATION

One animal study found no ill effects on the offspring of pregnant mice. However, these findings alone are not sufficient to establish St. John's wort as safe for use during pregnancy. Hypericin can accumulate in the nucleus of cells and directly bind to DNA. For this reason, pregnant or nursing women should avoid St. John's wort.

ADVERSE REACTIONS

The most common complaints were mild stomach discomfort (0.6%), allergic reactions (primarily rash; 0.5%), tiredness (0.4%), and restlessness (0.3%).

PROPOSED DOSAGE AND ADMINISTRATION

Typical dosing is 300 mg 3 times a day of an extract standardized to contain 0.3% hypericin; other products are standardized to hyperforin content. Some individuals report taking 500 mg twice a day or 600 mg in the morning and 300 mg in the evening. If the herb bothers the patient's stomach, instruct the patient to take it with food. Remind patients that the full effect takes 4 weeks to develop.

OCULAR CONSIDERATIONS

St. John's wort appears to have caused several cases of heart, kidney, and liver transplant rejection by interfering with the action of cyclosporine. Interaction with cyclosporine A in topical eye drop form is not known. Hypericin is a known photosensitizer. In one study, sun-sensitive persons who were given twice the normal dose of the herb showed a mild but measurable increase in reaction to ultraviolet radiation. These findings, along with other highly preliminary forms of evidence hint that regular use of St. John's wort might accelerate ultraviolet light damage of the eyes, potentially increasing the risk of cataracts and macular degeneration. However, these concerns remain largely theoretical.

Vitamin E

Names: Alpha tocopherol, D-tocopherol, DL-tocopherol, DL-alpha-tocopherol, tocopheryl succinate, tocopheryl acetate, D-alpha-tocopherol, D-delta-tocopherol, D-beta-tocopherol, D-gamma-tocopherol, mixed tocopherols

GENRAL INFORMATION

Vitamin E is involved in digestion and metabolism of polyunsaturated fats, decreases platelet aggregation, decreases blood clot formation, promotes normal growth and development of muscle tissue, and promotes prostaglandin synthesis.

Vitamin E is metabolized in the liver and is excreted in bile.

PROPOSED INDICATIONS AND USAGE

Incomplete evidence hints that vitamin E may be helpful for allergic rhinitis, preeclampsia, Alzheimer's disease, dysmennorhea, rheumatoid arthritis, restless legs syndrome, premenstrual syndrome, and diabetic cardiac autonomic neuropathy. Long-term use of vitamin E does not appear to help prevent cardiovascular disease or cancer (except, possibly, prostate cancer) and may increase risk of congestive heart failure.

PRECAUTIONS

Vitamin E use may impair hematologic response in patients with iron deficiency anemia.

Vitamin E has a blood-thinning effect that could lead to problems in certain situations. Vitamin E might enhance sensitivity to insulin and lead to a risk of blood sugar levels falling too low. Patients who are taking oral hypoglycemic medications should not take high-dose vitamin E without first consulting their physician. Strongly recommend to patients not to take any supplements while undergoing cancer chemotherapy, except on the advice of a physician.

DRUG INTERACTIONS

No drug interactions are known. However, vitamin E has antiplatelet actions and therefore could potentiate the effects of antiplatelet and anticoagulant drugs. Vitamin E also might potentiate oral hypoglycemic drugs.

PREGNANCY AND LACTATION

For pregnant women under 19 years of age, the upper limit is 800 mg.

PROPOSED DOSAGE AND ADMINISTRATION

The official U.S. recommendations for daily intake of vitamin E are as follows:

Infants: Birth to 6 months, 4 mg
7 to 12 months, 5 mg
Children: 1 to 3 years, 6 mg
4 to 8 years, 7 mg
9 to 13 years, 11 mg
Males and females 14 years and older, 15 mg
Pregnant women, 15 mg
Nursing women, 19 mg

Therapeutic dosage of vitamin E has not been established. Most studies have used 50 to 800 mg of synthetic vitamin E (DL-alpha-tocopherol) or 25 to 400 mg of natural vitamin E (D-alpha-tocopherol or mixed tocopherols). Safe upper limits are 1000 mg daily or 1500 IU of natural vitamin E and 1100 IU of synthetic vitamin E.

OCULAR CONSIDERATIONS

A 4-year double-blind placebo-controlled trial of almost 1200 patients with age-related maculopathy failed to find vitamin E alone helpful for preventing or treating age-related maculopathy. Vitamin E also has failed to prove effective for slowing the development of cataracts.

The use of vitamin E for uveitis has been demonstrated in animal studies. Intraocular inflammation was considerably smaller in the vitamin E supplemented group. (Pararajasegaram G, Sevanian A, Rao NA: Suppression of S antigen-induced uveitis by vitamin E supplementation, *Ophthalmic Res* 23[3]:121, 1991.)

Zinc

Names: Zinc sulfate, zinc gluconate, zinc citrate, zinc picolinate, chelated zinc

GENERAL INFORMATION

Zinc, an essential mineral, is found in almost every cell.

PROPOSED INDICATIONS AND USAGE

Oral use of zinc has been proposed for the treatment of numerous conditions. Those uses with some supporting evidence include for macular degeneration, acne, sickle cell anemia, and attention deficit disorder. However, for many of these conditions, potentially toxic doses of zinc must be used for benefit. Topical use of zinc as lozenge or nasal gel may have efficacy in respiratory infections.

PRECAUTIONS

Occasional stomach upset may occur when zinc is taken on an empty stomach. Zinc lozenges, designed for topical use, may have an unpleasant metallic taste. Prolonged oral zinc supplementation should be accompanied by supplementation of copper at 1 to 3 mg daily. Dosages of 100 mg zinc or more daily can cause a number of toxic effects: severe copper deficiency, impaired immunity, heart problems, and anemia.

DRUG INTERACTIONS

Zinc interferes with the absorption of antibiotics in the fluoroquinolone or tetracycline families if taken at the same time.

ADVERSE REACTIONS

Occasional stomach upset and metallic taste.

PROPOSED DOSAGE AND ADMINISTRATION

The official U.S. recommendations for daily intake of zinc are as follows:

Infants: Birth to 6 months, 2 mg
7 to 12 months, 3 mg
Children: 1 to 3 years, 3 mg
4 to 8 years, 5 mg
Males: 9 to 13 years, 8 mg
14 years and older, 11 mg
Females: 9 to 13 years, 8 mg
14 to 18 years, 9 mg
19 years and older, 8 mg
Pregnant women, 11 mg (13 mg if 18 years old or younger)
Nursing women, 12 mg (14 mg if 18 years old or younger)

Tolerable upper intake levels for zinc are as follows:

Infants: Birth to 6 months, 4 mg
7 to 12 months, 5 mg
Children: 1 to 3 years, 7 mg
4 to 8 years, 12 mg
9 to 13 years, 23 mg
Males and females: 14 to 18 years, 34 mg
19 years and older, 40 mg
Pregnant or nursing women, 40 mg (34 mg if 18 years old or younger)

OCULAR CONSIDERATIONS

A double-blind placebo-controlled trial looked at zinc with or without antioxidants on the progression of age-related maculopathy in 3640 patients. Participants were assigned to receive antioxidants (vitamin C, vitamin E, and beta-carotene), zinc (80 mg) and copper (2 mg), antioxidants plus zinc, or placebo. The results indicated that zinc alone or zinc plus antioxidants significantly slowed the progression of the disease.

Furthermore, in a double-blind study of 151 individuals, zinc supplements at a dose of 80 mg daily significantly spared vision loss in individuals with age-related macular degeneration. However, a double-blind study of 112 subjects found no prevention of macular degeneration in the second eye among individuals with exudative age-related macular degeneration in one eye.

Much weaker evidence hints the dietary requirement of zinc on a daily basis over many years might reduce the risk of developing macular degeneration later in life.

Appendix I

International Brand Names Index

International brand name (generic name)	Page no.

APPENDIX I

International brand name (generic name)	Page no.

International brand name (generic name)	Page no.

International brand name (generic name)	Page no.
Cotribase (sulfamethoxazole; trimethoprim)	514
Cotrim-Diolan (sulfamethoxazole; trimethoprim)	514
Cotrimel (sulfamethoxazole; trimethoprim)	514
Cotrix (sulfamethoxazole; trimethoprim)	514
Coumadan Sodico (warfarin sodium)	567
Coumadine (warfarin sodium)	567
Covospor (clotrimazole)	143
Covosulf (sulfacetamide)	511
Coxid (celecoxib)	106
Cozole (sulfamethoxazole; trimethoprim)	514
Cranoc (fluvastatin)	242
Cravit (levofloxacin)	324
Cravit Ophthalmic (levofloxacin)	324
Crecisan (minoxidil)	378
Cremosan (ketoconazole)	312
Cristapen (penicillin G potassium)	430
Crixan (clarithromycin)	133
Croanan Duo Dry Syrup (amoxicillin/clavulanate potassium)	37
Cromabak (cromolyn sodium)	149
Cromadoses (cromolyn sodium)	149
Cromal-5 Inhaler (cromolyn sodium)	149
Cromlex (cephalexin)	108
Cromo-Asma (cromolyn sodium)	149
Cromogen (cromolyn sodium)	149
Cromolyn (cromolyn sodium)	149
Crom-Ophtal (cromolyn sodium)	149
Cromoptic (cromolyn sodium)	149
Cronase (cromolyn sodium)	149
Cronitin (loratadine)	336
Cronopen (loratadine)	336
Cruor (bepridil)	67
Cryocriptina (bromocriptine mesylate)	80
Cryopril (captopril)	91
Cryosolona (methylprednisolone sodium succinate)	368
Cryptal (fluconazole)	229
Crysanal (naproxen)	395
Crystapen V (penicillin V potassium)	431
Cuivasil Spray (lidocaine)	330
Cumatil (phenytoin sodium)	441
Cuprofen (ibuprofen)	295
Curacne Ge (isotretinoin)	307
Curam (amoxicillin/clavulanate potassium)	37
Curatane (isotretinoin)	307
Curinflam (diclofenac)	177
Curyken (loratadine)	336
Cusicrom (cromolyn sodium)	149
Cusimolol (timolol maleate)	534
Cusimolol (travoprost)	548
Cusiviral (acyclovir)	17
Cutason (prednisone)	462
C-Vimin (ascorbic acid [vitamin C])	43
Cyben (cyclobenzaprine hydrochloride)	151
Cycin (ciprofloxacin hydrochloride)	128
Cyclabid (tetracycline hydrochloride)	528
Cyclidox (doxycycline)	199
Cyclimycin (minocycline hydrochloride)	376
Cyclivex (acyclovir)	17
Cyclo (acyclovir)	17
Cycloblastin (cyclophosphamide)	154
Cycloblastine (cyclophosphamide)	154
Cyclo-Cell (cyclophosphamide)	154
Cyclomed (acyclovir)	17
Cyclomidril (cyclopentolate hydrochloride; phenylephrine hydrochloride)	153
Cyclomydri (cyclopentolate hydrochloride)	152
Cyclopentol (cyclopentolate hydrochloride)	152
Cyclopentolat (cyclopentolate hydrochloride)	152
Cyclopentolat Thilo (cyclopentolate hydrochloride)	152
Cyclopentolate (cyclopentolate hydrochloride)	152
Cyclopentolate Eye Drops (cyclopentolate hydrochloride)	152
Cyclophar (cyclophosphamide)	154
Cyclor (cefaclor)	99
Cyclorax (acyclovir)	17
Cyclostad (acyclovir)	17
Cyclostin (cyclophosphamide)	154
Cyclostin N (cyclophosphamide)	154
Cyclovir (acyclovir)	17
Cygran (ranitidine hydrochloride/ranitidine bismuth citrate)	487
Cyheptine (cyproheptadine)	159
Cylat (cyproheptadine)	159
Cyllanvir (acyclovir)	17
Cymevan (ganciclovir sodium)	254
Cymeven (ganciclovir sodium)	254

International brand name (generic name)	Page no.
Fontex (fluoxetine hydrochloride)	237
Fonvicol (cefazolin sodium)	101
Forcan (fluconazole)	229
Forcanox (itraconazole)	310
Forken (amiodarone hydrochloride)	28
Formin (metformin hydrochloride)	353
Formyco (ketoconazole)	312
Fornidd (metformin hydrochloride)	353
Fortecortin (dexamethasone)	165
Fortfen SR (diclofenac)	177
Fosalan (alendronate sodium)	22
Foscovir (foscarnet sodium)	246
Fosinil (fosinopril)	248
Fosinorm (fosinopril)	248
Fosipres (fosinopril)	248
Fositen (fosinopril)	248
Fositens (fosinopril)	248
Fosmin (alendronate sodium)	22
Fovas (fosinopril)	248
Foxetin (fluoxetine hydrochloride)	237
Foxinon (norfloxacin)	410
Foxolin (amoxicillin)	33
Fozitec (fosinopril)	248
Fractal (fluvastatin)	242
Fractal LP (fluvastatin)	242
Franyl (furosemide)	250
Freejex (diclofenac)	177
Frekven (propranolol hydrochloride)	471
Frenal (cromolyn sodium)	149
Frina (propranolol hydrochloride)	471
Fristamin (loratadine)	336
Frixitas (alprazolam)	24
Froben (flurbiprofen)	239
Froben SR (flurbiprofen)	239
Frontal (alprazolam)	24
Frusedan (furosemide)	250
Frusema (furosemide)	250
Fudone (famotidine)	225
Fugacin (ofloxacin)	413
Fugen (ketoconazole)	312
Fugentin (amoxicillin/clavulanate potassium)	37
Fulgram (norfloxacin)	410
Fullcilina (amoxicillin)	33
Fuluson (fluorometholone acetate)	235
Fumay (fluconazole)	229
Fumelon (fluorometholone acetate)	235
Funazol (fluconazole)	229
Funazole Tabs (ketoconazole)	312
Funet (ketoconazole)	312
Fungarest (ketoconazole)	312
Fungata (fluconazole)	229
Fungaway (ketoconazole)	312
Fungazol Tabs (ketoconazole)	312
Fungicide (ketoconazole)	312
Fungicide Tabs (ketoconazole)	312
Fungicip (clotrimazole)	143
Fungicon (clotrimazole)	143
Fungiderm (clotrimazole)	143
Fungiderm-K (ketoconazole)	312
Funginoc (ketoconazole)	312
Funginox Tabs (ketoconazole)	312
Fungistin (clotrimazole)	143
Fungitrazol (itraconazole)	310
Fungizid (clotrimazole)	143
Fungoral (ketoconazole)	312
Furanthril (furosemide)	250
Furanturil (furosemide)	250
Furetic (furosemide)	250
Furix (furosemide)	250
Furmid (furosemide)	250
Furo-Basan (furosemide)	250
Furolnok (itraconazole)	310
Furomen (furosemide)	250
Furomex (furosemide)	250
Furo-Puren (furosemide)	250
Furorese (furosemide)	250
Furoscan (furosemide)	250
Furosix (furosemide)	250
Furovite (furosemide)	250
Fusid (furosemide)	250
Fuweidin (famotidine)	225
Fuxen (naproxen)	395
Gadoserin (diltiazem hydrochloride)	185
Galidrin (ranitidine hydrochloride/ ranitidine bismuth citrate)	487
Gantaprim (sulfamethoxazole; trimethoprim)	514
Gantin (gabapentin)	253
Gantrim (sulfamethoxazole; trimethoprim)	514
Garabiotic (gentamicin sulfate)	257
Garalone (gentamicin sulfate)	257
Garamicin (gentamicin sulfate)	257
Garamicina Cream (gentamicin sulfate)	257
Garamicina Crema (gentamicin sulfate)	257
Garamicina (gentamicin sulfate)	257
Garamicina Oftalmica (gentamicin sulfate)	257
Garbilocin (gentamicin sulfate)	257
Gardenal (phenobarbital)	436
Gardenale (phenobarbital)	436

International brand name (generic name)	Page no.

APPENDIX I

International brand name (generic name)	Page no.

Index

Entries can be identified as follows: Trade name (generic name).

Entries can be identified as follows: Trade name (generic name).

Entries can be identified as follows: Trade name (generic name).

D

Entries can be identified as follows: Trade name (generic name).

Entries can be identified as follows: Trade name (generic name).

Entries can be identified as follows: Trade name (generic name).

Entries can be identified as follows: Trade name (generic name).

M

N

Entries can be identified as follows: Trade name (generic name).

Entries can be identified as follows: Trade name (generic name).

Entries can be identified as follows: Trade name (generic name).

W

X

Y

Z

Entries can be identified as follows: Trade name (generic name).